CONTEMPORARY ASPECTS OF BIOMEDICAL RESEARCH:
DRUG DISCOVERY

CONTEMPORARY ASPECTS OF BIOMEDICAL RESEARCH:
DRUG DISCOVERY

Edited by

S. J. Enna
Department of Molecular & Integrative Physiology
University of Missouri-Kansas City
Kansas City, Kansas

Michael Williams
Department of Molecular Pharmacology and Biological Chemistry
Feinberg School of Medicine, Northwestern University
Chicago, Illinois

ADVANCES IN
PHARMACOLOGY

VOLUME 57

AMSTERDAM • BOSTON • HEIDELBERG • LONDON
NEW YORK • OXFORD • PARIS • SAN DIEGO
SAN FRANCISCO • SINGAPORE • SYDNEY • TOKYO
Academic Press is an imprint of Elsevier

Academic Press is an imprint of Elsevier
525 B Street, Suite 1900, San Diego, CA 92101-4495, USA
30 Corporate Drive, Suite 400, Burlington, MA 01803, USA
32 Jamestown Road, London NW1 7BY, UK
Radarweg 29, PO Box 211, 1000 AE Amsterdam, The Netherlands

First edition 2009

British Library Cataloguing in Publication Data
A catalogue record for this book is available from the British Library

Library of Congress Cataloging-in-Publication Data
A catalog record for this book is available from the Library of Congress

ISBN: 978-0-12-378642-5
ISSN: 1054-3589

For information on all Academic Press publications
visit our website at elsevierdirect.com

Printed and bound in USA
09 10 11 12   10 9 8 7 6 5 4 3 2 1

Working together to grow
libraries in developing countries

www.elsevier.com | www.bookaid.org | www.sabre.org

ELSEVIER   BOOK AID
             International   Sabre Foundation

Contents

Defining the Role of Pharmacology in the Emerging World of Translational Research

S. J. Enna and M. Williams

Anti-Inflammatory Agents as Cancer Therapeutics

Khosrow Kashfi

The Development and Pharmacology of Proteasome Inhibitors for the Management and Treatment of Cancer

Bruce Ruggeri, Sheila Miknyoczki, Bruce Dorsey, and Ai-Min Hui

Subtype-Selective GABA$_A$ Receptor Modulation Yields a Novel Pharmacological Profile: The Design and Development of TPA023

John R. Atack

Contributors

Numbers in parentheses indicate the pages on which the authors' contributions begin.

Abdel A. Abdel-Rahman (291) Department of Pharmacology and Toxicology, Brody School of Medicine at East Carolina University, Greenville, North Carolina 27834

John R. Atack (137) Department of Neuroscience, Johnson & Johnson Pharmaceutical Research and Development, Turnhoutseweg 30, Beerse, B-2340, Belgium

Vincent Castagné (381) Porsolt & Partners Pharmacology, 9 bis rue Henri Martin, 92100 Boulogne-Billancourt, France

Jerry R. Colca (237) Metabolic Solutions Development Company, 125 S. Kalamazoo Mall #202, Kalamazoo, Michigan 49007

Nicholas A. DeMartinis (187) Neuroscience Research Unit, Pfizer, Inc., Eastern Point Rd., Groton, Connecticut 06340 and Department of Psychiatry, University of Connecticut School of Medicine, Farmington, Connecticut 06030-6415

Bruce Dorsey (91) Discovery Research, Cephalon, Inc., West Chester, Pennsylvania 19380

S. J. Enna (1) Departments of Molecular and Integrative Physiology and of Pharmacology, Toxicology and Therapeutics, University of Kansas Medical Center, Kansas City, Kansas

Ai-Min Hui (91) Clinical Research, Cephalon, Inc., West Chester, Pennsylvania 19380

Jayesh Kamath (187) Department of Psychiatry, University of Connecticut School of Medicine, Farmington, Connecticut 06030-6415

Khosrow Kashfi (31) Department of Physiology and Pharmacology, Sophie Davis School of Biomedical Education, The City College of The City University of New York, New York, New York 10031

Jonathan L. Katz (253) Psychobiology Section, Medications Discovery Research Branch, Intramural Research Program, Department of Health and Human Services, National Institute on Drug Abuse, National Institutes of Health, Baltimore, Maryland 21224

Rolf F. Kletzien (237) Metabolic Solutions Development Company, 125 S. Kalamazoo Mall #202, Kalamazoo, Michigan 49007

Xia Li (247) Neuroscience Discovery Research, Lilly Research Laboratories, Eli Lilly and Company, Indianapolis, Indiana, 46285

Sheila Miknyoczki (91) Discovery Research, Cephalon, Inc., West Chester, Pennsylvania 19380

Paul C. Moser (381) Porsolt & Partners Pharmacology, 9 bis rue Henri Martin, 92100 Boulogne-Billancourt, France

Amy H. Newman (253) Medicinal Chemistry Section, Medications Discovery Research Branch, Intramural Research Program, Department of Health and Human Services, National Institute on Drug Abuse, National Institutes of Health, Baltimore, Maryland 21224

Roger D. Porsolt (381) Porsolt & Partners Pharmacology, 9 bis rue Henri Martin, 92100 Boulogne-Billancourt, France

Daniel U. Rabin (419) The France Foundation, Old Lyme, Connecticut 06371

Bruce Ruggeri (91) Discovery Research, Cephalon, Inc., West Chester, Pennsylvania 19380

Alexander Scriabine (419) Guilford, Connecticut 06437

Gianluigi Tanda (253) Psychobiology Section, Medications Discovery Research Branch, Intramural Research Program, Department of Health and Human Services, National Institute on Drug Abuse, National Institutes of Health, Baltimore, Maryland 21224

David A. Taylor (291) Department of Pharmacology and Toxicology, Brody School of Medicine at East Carolina University, Greenville, North Carolina 27834

Michael Williams (1) Department of Molecular Pharmacology and Biological Chemistry, Feinberg School of Medicine, Northwestern University, Chicago, Illinois 60611

Andrew Winokur (187) Department of Psychiatry, University of Connecticut School of Medicine, Farmington, Connecticut 06030-6415

Jeffrey M. Witkin (347) Neuroscience Discovery Research, Lilly Research Laboratories, Eli Lilly and Company, Indianapolis, Indiana, 46285

Preface

The decreased number of new drug approvals (NDAs) has been a topic of considerable debate over the past decade. While the research and development budgets in the pharmaceutical and biotechnology industries have increased approximately threefold in this time, the number of NDAs has remained constant with increasing attrition rates. In 2008, only 8% of the new chemical entities (NCEs) entering clinical trials were ultimately introduced to the market as compared to 14% in 1985. This has led to various initiatives, the most notable being the NIH Roadmap Initiative and the FDA's Critical Path and Phase 0 clinical trial initiatives, to enhance the biomedical science activities driving drug discovery.

All of these initiatives have focused on the need to train more scientists in the discipline of pharmacology to both enhance the characterization of NCEs preclinically to ensure that they are drug-like molecules and to provide the intellectual bridge between disease models and the human disease state. Pharmacology, as a unifying, hierarchically integrated, and technologically agnostic discipline is thus viewed as a key contributor to decreasing the attrition rates in new drug introductions.

It is appropriate therefore that in the present volume, leading pharmacologists from government, academia, and industry provide their perspective of current research activities, both basic and enabling, in drug discovery.

To start Volume 57, the Editors, Williams and Enna provide an overview addressing what is considered a major hurdle in bringing drugs to the clinic, that of translational research, which is described as the successful transition of drug-like NCEs with good efficacy and safety to clinical trials.

Next, Kashfi delivers an update on the role of inflammation in tumor initiation and growth and highlights new approaches to anti-inflammatory agents that have the potential to be used as novel anticancer drugs. In the same therapeutic area, Ruggeri, Miknyoczki, Dorsey, and Hui supply an update on the utility of proteasome inhibitors, namely bortezomib (Velacade®), the first agent of this drug class drug approved for the treatment of multiple myeloma, and compare early data on next-generation proteasome inhibitors with bortezomib.

Moving to drugs for CNS disease states, Atack gives an overview of a novel GABA$_A$ receptor modulator, TPA023 while DeMartinis, Kamath, and Winokur review therapeutic advances in the treatment of sleep disorders.

Colca and Kletzien discuss new approaches to the treatment of dyslipidemia and macrovascular disease, focusing on novel targets for next generation agents.

In the field of substance abuse, Tanda, Newman, and Katz review progress in the search for novel, atypical dopamine transport inhibitors that, based on animal data, may have the potential to treat cocaine dependence and possibly other types of addiction.

Taylor and Abdel-Rahman review hypertension, highlighting novel targets and new treatment regimens for existing antihypertensive medications.

Witkin and Li next offer a new perspective on approaches to treat depression, namely, compounds that interact with metabotropic glutamate receptors while Castagné, Moser, and Porsolt, in keeping with the theme of translational medicine, review the utility of preclinical models to assess efficacy and side effect liabilities of potential antipsychotic agents.

Finally, Scriabine and Rabin provide an update on new approaches for the treatment of fibrosis, an area of considerable unmet medical need.

With an explicit focus on the role of pharmacology in drug discovery in Volume 57, the Editors of *Advances in Pharmacology* seek to enhance the role and relevance of this serial publication to effectively document Contemporary Aspects of Biomedical Research.

The editors would like to sincerely thank the authors for their energy and enthusiasm in contributing to the present volume and Ms. Lynn LeCount for her guidance and skill sets, both administrative and people-related, in coordinating and collating the various submissions. Given the very tight timelines to have this volume published in 2009, Lynn's experience, consummate attention to detail, and good humor have made all the difference in maintaining the momentum and guiding this endeavor to a successful conclusion.

S. J. Enna
Kansas City, KS
Michael Williams
Chicago, IL

S. J. Enna[*] and M. Williams[†]

[*]Department of Molecular and Integrative Physiology, Department of Pharmacology,
Toxicology, and Therapeutics, University of Kansas Medical Center, Kansas City, Kansas
[†]Department of Molecular Pharmacology and Biological Chemistry, Feinberg School of
Medicine, Northwestern University, Chicago, Illinois 60611

Defining the Role of Pharmacology in the Emerging World of Translational Research

Abstract

Pharmacology is focused on studying the effects of endogenous agents and xenobiotics on tissue and organ function. Analysis of the concentration/response relationship is the foundation for these assessments as it provides quantifiable information on compound efficacy, potency, and, ultimately, side-effect liability and therapeutic index. Historically, pharmacology has been viewed as a unifying, hierarchically integrated, and technologically agnostic discipline. Besides being important in the development of new medications, pharmacological research has led to a better understanding

Advances in Pharmacology, Volume 57
1054-3589/08 $35.00
10.1016/S1054-3589(08)57001-3

of disease pathogenesis and progression. By defining the effects of compounds *in vitro* and *in vivo*, pharmacology has provided the means to validate, optimize, and advance new chemical entities (NCEs) to human testing. With the advent of molecular biology-based assay systems and a technology-driven (high-throughput screening, combinatorial chemistry, SNP mapping, systems biology) reductionistic focus, the integrated, hypothesis-driven pharmacological approach to drug discovery has been de-emphasized in recent years. This shift in research emphasis is now viewed by many as a major factor in the decline of new drug approvals and has led to various initiatives, the most notable being the Critical Path and Phase 0 clinical trial initiatives launched by the US Food and Drug Administration (FDA). These programs underscore the growing need for individuals trained in integrative pharmacology and having a background in molecular pharmacology to drive the drug discovery process and to fostering the translational research that is now considered vital for more rapidly identifying novel, more effective, and safer medications.

I. Introduction

Molecular pharmacology evolved in the mid-twentieth century as a result of advances in biochemistry. This approach to studying drug actions provided a potentially facile means for identifying sites that may be targeted for more precisely attacking the pathophysiology of disease processes. By adding to a systematic, heuristic framework for defining the mechanisms of disease causality, molecular pharmacology has become a critical component of the *in vitro/in vivo* hierarchy of assay systems used for evaluating hypotheses in the drug discovery process.

The importance of the contributions of molecular pharmacology to biomedical research is reflected in the number of Nobel Prizes in medicine awarded over the past 50 years for fundamental discoveries in disease causality and the manner in which drugs affect these processes. Thus, the prize has been given for discoveries relating to mechanisms for the storage, release, and inactivation of humoral transmitters; the action of hormones; signal transduction in the cardiovascular and nervous systems; peptide hormone production; regulation of cholesterol metabolism; and the establishment of modern mechanistic principles for drug treatment. With respect to the last topic, the Nobel Prize was awarded to Gertrude Elion, George Hichens, and Sir James Black for their discoveries relating to particular drug entities, namely azathioprine, acyclovir, and the H_2 receptor blocker cimetidine (http://nobelprize.org/nobel_prizes/medicine/laureates/index.html).

These successes solidified the molecular approach to drug discovery and this research orientation subsequently expanded to include gene cloning techniques, leading to an increased emphasis on transcriptional and translational processes as drug targets (Celis et al., 2000). However, the impact of the characterization of the human genome (International Human Genome Sequencing Consortium, 2004) has fallen far short of its predicted utility for, and impact on, drug discovery (Collins et al., 2003). While this is probably due, in part, to an oversimplification of the target validation process (Kopec, Bozyczko-Coyne, & Williams, 2005) and highly optimistic time lines, the human genome effort still has a far reaching influence in regard to the design of research programs aimed at defining drug mechanisms of action, efficacy, and side-effect profiles.

The late 1960s witnessed a resurgence of the receptor–ligand concept, at that time some 100 years old (Maehle, Prüll, & Halliwell, 2002). The delay in acceptance was due, in part, to the fact that it took time to convince a majority of biomedical scientists that drug receptors were cell surface entities through which medications exert their actions (Kenakin, 2009; Rang, 2006).

The notion that intracellular proteins might also function as drug targets was given little consideration, however. Thus, potential roles for small molecules interacting with DNA (Chenoweth & Dervan, 2009), ATP-binding proteins (e.g., protein kinases in cancer; Zhang, Yang, & Gray, 2009), NOD (nucleotide-binding and oligomerization domain)-like receptors (NLRs; Geddes, Magalhaes, & Girardin, 2009) of "omal" intracellular targets like the proteasome (Ruggeri, Miknyoczki, Dorsey, & Hui, 2009), the spliceosome (Rino & Carmo-Fonseca, 2009), and the inflammasome (Martinon & Tschopp, 2007) were not considered for many more years. Similarly proteostasis networks (Powers, Morimoto, Dillin, Kelly, & Balch, 2009), a fundamental role for mitochondrial dysfunction in disease etiology and drug treatment (Javadov, Karmazyn, & Escobales, 2009; Kita et al., 2004; Wu et al., 2009), and the use of antibodies (Brekke & Sandlie, 2003) and RNA interference (Dykxhoorn & Lieberman, 2005) were/are all novel concepts for therapeutics. Additionally, until recently, disease causality was rarely considered in terms other than as a binary event. Thus, in the mid- to late twentieth century, the prevailing view was that diseases were caused by tissue dysfunction with the progression spectrum reflecting the difference between the normal and diseased state. That disease states could reflect an imbalance or overexpression of a normal homeostatic defense process, such as parainflammation (Medzhitov, 2008), was a concept that evolved over time. Molecular pharmacology thus added a new dimension to the drug discovery paradigm with the provision of a molecular basis for tissue dysfunction (Enna, Fuerstein, Piette, & Williams, 2008).

The mapping of the human genome provided an additional certainty to the molecular equation such that it was believed that defects in a single gene would be found responsible for a particular disease. This led to an explosion in gene association studies with common conditions like Parkinson's disease, Type II diabetes, and hypertension being anticipated to be linked to a disease-specific gene variant that would be common to all those suffering from these conditions. However, once data were accumulated, unbridled optimism gave way to the realization that multiple factors, genetic and epigenetic, were usually causal for human disorders (Hardy & Singleton, 2009; Uher et al., 2009; Vogelstein, 2008; Wilgenbus et al., 2007; Williams, 2009).

Nonetheless, the molecular era of drug discovery, and the focus on developing targeted therapeutics, has yielded many important new drugs, including the statins for hypercholesterolemia (Mills et al., 2008), β-adreno-ceptor antagonists (Task Force, 2004), angiotensin-converting enzyme (ACE) inhibitors, calcium blockers (Neal et al., 2000), renin inhibitors (Villamil et al., 2007), and vasopressin V_2 antagonists (Miyazaki, Fujiki, Yamamura, Naka-mura, & Mori, 2007) for hypertension, the SSRI (selective 5-HT reuptake inhibitor) antidepressants (Wong, Perry, & Bymaster, 2005), and the anxio-lytic benzodiazepines (BZ) (Martin et al., 2007). While the selective cyclooxygenase (COX-2) inhibitors celecoxib, rofecoxib, and valdecoxib were withdrawn from the market because of an increased incidence of myocardial infarction and ischemic stroke associated with their use (Wong et al., 2005), these second-generation nonsteroidal anti-inflammatory drugs (NSAIDs) were highly effective as arthritis medications and had utility in the treatment of certain cancer types (Kashfi, 2009). Similarly, etanercept, infliximab, and adalimumab, biologics and antibodies that target the TNF-α receptor–ligand interaction, are important drugs for reducing the inflammatory consequences associated with rheumatoid, psoriatic and juvenile idiopathic arthritis, ankylosing spondylitis, and plaque psoriasis (Shealy & Visvanathans, 2008).

However, it is also noteworthy that many very useful medications, including clozapine for schizophrenia, pregabalin for neuropathic pain, modafinil for wake promotion, and valproic acid for epilepsy and biopolar disorder, have as yet no clearly defined molecular mechanism of action despite many years of research. Nonetheless, these compounds, through targets yet to be discovered or because of their non-selective interaction with multiple targets (Roth, Sheffler, & Kroeze, 2004), are effective medications. This reinforces the value of a more holistic, and perhaps a less target-oriented, approach to biomedical research like that traditionally embodied in the discipline of pharmacology.

II. Historical Perspective of Pharmacology

Throughout the past 150 years the intellectual underpinning of biomedical research has been the "lock and key" theory of hormone and drug action that led to the receptor concept (Kenakin, 2009; Rang, 2006).

Receptors thus represent the molecular targets through which chemical entities exert their effects (Changeux & Edelstein, 2005). The receptor concept originated from the seminal work of Ehrlich and Langley at the end of the nineteenth century (Parascandola, 1986) from their studies on the effects of compounds in bioassays and animal models. They hypothesized the presence of receptors, or receptive substances, on the basis of their findings, but in the absence of any direct, physical evidence for their existence. However, it was not until the mid-twentieth century that the *Torpedo* electroplax nicotinic cholinergic receptor was the first receptor to be isolated and characterized (Eldefrawi & Eldefrawi, 1972; Romine, Goodall, Peterson, & Bradley, 1974) and the 1980s before the first receptors, GPCRs, were cloned (Lefkowitz, 2004).

Receptor-based or biochemical pharmacology-driven drug discovery dominated biomedical research from the late 1950s through the early 1990s. This approach was greatly facilitated by the development of radioligand binding assays (Snyder, 2008) that made possible the rapid assessment of structure–activity relationships (SARs). The latter advance was ideal for drug discovery as it required the use of minimal amounts of compound, thereby lowering considerably the cost of screening. Thus, receptor binding assays provided a high-throughput means to iteratively evaluate and optimize NCEs for potency, efficacy, and target selectivity *in vitro* with incremental advances in throughput as new technologies were developed to automate the process (Comley, 2006). Whereas previously grams of NCE were required to assess initially its therapeutic potential, now 5–10 mg sufficed for this purpose allowing both targeted NCEs and synthetic chemical intermediates to be assessed for target interactions. After meeting criteria in a binding assay, NCEs could then be tested in more complex tissue and organ systems and/or intact animals to define their pharmacokinetic (PK) and phamacodynamic (PD) properties. While emphasis on biochemical pharmacology diminished somewhat in the mid-1990s with the ascendancy of molecular biology techniques (Williams, 2004), interest has now shifted back to a more biochemical and organ-based approach to drug discovery (Chiang, 2006; Schreiber, 2000). This is due to the realization that the biotechnology revolution failed to facilitate and, in fact, slowed small molecule drug discovery. Indeed, it can be argued, together with high-throughput screening technologies and combinatorial chemistry, that the tools of molecular biology fostered a biomedical research culture that was almost exclusively technology based, which was aptly described as "turn on the computer, turn off the brain" (Kubinyi, 2003). With the reemergence of biochemical pharmacology and an attendant focus on systems pharmacology (Jobe et al., 1994; Preusch, 2004; van der Greef & McBurney, 2005), NCEs are again being used to characterize, validate, and modulate putative drug targets while the targets, in turn, are being employed to characterize the efficacy and selectivity of NCEs *in vitro* before advancement to more costly and complex *in vivo* animal models (Millan, 2008).

Historically, evaluating NCE effects in organ systems or in whole animals has often led to ambiguous results. Many of the NCEs used in these complex systems were non-selective, having undergone limited, if any, molecular profiling, with responses more often than not reflecting the PK rather than the PD properties of the molecule. Thus, the testing of an NCE *in vitro* at a defined molecular target provided a more precise, albeit reductionistic, characterization of its ability to interact with the target, independent of its other properties. In fact, because receptor profiling studies (Roth et al., 2004) provided a broader understanding of the potency and selectivity of an NCE at receptors, enzymes, transporters, the Cyp_{450}, and kinome families, they are now an expected part of an Investigational New Drug (IND) submission package. However, the use of recombinant cell systems expressing a single drug target (Kenakin, 1996) has tended to make *in vitro* NCE SAR studies even more reductionistic. Rather than replacing the more holistic and empirical pharmacological approach, these customized *in vitro* systems have increased the need for scientists capable of placing the results of such work in the proper therapeutic context, the traditional role of the pharmacologist (Enna & Williams, 2009).

A recent example of an integrated pharmacological approach to drug discovery is that of the novel anxiolytic AC-5216 (Kita et al., 2004). This compound was synthesized as a potent (Ki = 0.3 nM), orally active agonist for the peripheral BZ receptor. Also known as the mitochondrial BZ receptor or translocator protein, this site is involved in the synthesis of endogenous neurosteroids that enhance GABAergic neurotransmission. Whole animal testing revealed that AC-5216 had anti-anxiety effects in mice in the Vogel-conflict test (0.1–3 mg/kg p.o.), the light/dark box (0.003–0.01 mg/kg p.o.), and social interaction tests (0.01–0.3 mg/kg p.o.). These actions were blocked by the peripheral BZ/mitochondrial BZ receptor antagonist, PK 11195 (3 mg/kg i.p.). Further behavioral tests revealed that AC-5216 was also active in the Porsolt forced swim test (3–30 mg/kg p.o.), a measure of antidepressant activity. Unlike the classical BZ, diazepam, AC-5216 did not produce muscle relaxation, nor did it affect memory or prolong hexobarbital sleep time at doses up to 1,000 mg/kg p.o. To the extent tested, AC-5216 represents the elusive non-BZ anxiolytic that has been the focus of active research since the discovery of the BZ receptor in 1977 (Briley & Nutt, 2000). Renamed XBD173, AC-5316 indirectly modulated GABAergic transmission in medial prefrontal cortex slices via a mechanism that was dependent on steroid biosynthesis (Rupprecht et al., 2009). XBD173 also was active in a CCK4-challenge model in panic-prone rats and in humans where it had fewer side effects than the BZ, alprazolam, thus validating the translocator protein (18 kD) as a novel target for anxiolytic drug discovery. XBD173 recently completed Phase II trials for generalized anxiety disorder although no details on the outcome have yet been provided (http://clinicaltrials.gov/ct2/show/NCT00108836?term=XBD173&rank=1).

III. Initiatives to Improve Drug Discovery Productivity _____

The fall in the number of new drug approvals has been extensively documented in both the scientific (Duyk, 2003; Edwards, Bountra, Kerr, & Willson, 2009; FDA, 2004; Kola, 2008; Kola & Landis, 2004; LoRusso, 2009; Milne, 2003) and lay (Shaywitz & Taleb, 2008) press. Despite major advances in preclinical research technologies, only 8% of NCEs that enter clinical trials are ultimately marketed, as compared to 14% in 1985. This decline has been attributed to a variety of causes. Included are the complexity, sophistication, or possible irrelevance of the technologies presently used in the drug discovery process; a lack of innovation due, in part, to centralized bureaucracies in large research organizations (Cuatrecasas, 2006; Duyk, 2003); the instability in the pharmaceutical industry driven by mergers and/or the subprime meltdown that have precluded any semblance of a strategic approach; investors who, by focusing on short-term returns, shortchange the lengthy process of drug discovery and have demoralized researchers (Dixon, Lawton, & Machin, 2009); scientists who no longer appear to be personally motivated in their scientific careers (Kubinyi, 2003); an overt disconnect between biomedical research and the realities of the human disease state (Horrobin, 2003); and a lack of training and consequent absence of pharmacologists (FDA, 2004; Williams, 2008).

To address this lack of productivity, the US National Institutes of Health (NIH) and the FDA launched the Roadmap (Zerhouni, 2003) and Critical Path Initiatives (FDA, 2004), respectively. In addition, the US Government Accounting Office (GAO) (2006) published a White Paper on factors that were deemed to be responsible for limiting new drug introductions. To quote from the GAO report, factors slowing drug development included "… limitations on the scientific understanding of how to translate chemical and biological discoveries into safe and effective drugs; business decisions by the pharmaceutical industry that influence the types of drugs developed; uncertainty regarding regulatory standards for determining whether a drug should be approved as safe and effective; and certain intellectual property protections that can discourage innovation." The GAO specifically recommended that a greater number of scientists must be trained in the techniques necessary to turn the discovery of chemical leads into effective medications. The GAO also advised there be a restructuring of the drug regulatory and review process to allow for conditional approvals based on the results of shorter clinical trials using a fewer number of patients. Conditional approvals would be used for moving agents forward that could be of benefit in conditions where treatments were currently lacking. It was also recommended that the length of patent coverage be extended to stimulate more innovation. Thus, these three separate government studies came to the same conclusions. Specifically, they all agreed that research based on the null hypothesis and a replenishment of the supply of scientists trained to move drug candidates from the chemistry laboratory, through animal testing and into the clinic, in short basic and clinical pharmacologists, were essential steps for increasing the number of novel and effective medications.

Similarly, despite optimistic beliefs that the present dearth of new compounds is but a transient phenomenon (LaMattina, 2009), pharmaceutical industry insiders have argued for the past 20 years that the drug discovery process must return to a more science-based approach if greater productivity is to be achieved (Cuatrecasas, 2006; Duyk, 2003; Milne, 2003; Shaywitz & Taleb, 2008; Weisbach & Moos, 1995; Williams, 2004). These arguments parallel and reinforce the recommendations of the FDA (2004) and GAO (2006) White Papers. Furthermore, Dixon et al. (2009) have debated as to whether "creating" (research) and "selling" (marketing) can continue to co-exist within a single vertical organization. Rather, they propose "vertical disintegration" as a new business model. With such a structure, drug discovery R&D would be an independent entity delivering compounds to separate commercial or philanthropic development organizations. This approach, therefore, encourages increased collaborations among scientists in academia, government, and industry (Brady, Winsky, Goodman, Oliveri, & Stover, 2009; Cuatrecasas, 2006; Conn & Roth, 2008), with industry bringing the strategic and tactical focus. In other words, because of its experience with regulatory issues, product manufacturing and clinical trials, the pharmaceutical industry is best at providing the translational component for drug discovery. This type of collaborative approach has already proven successful in the Gates TB Alliance and Medicines for Malaria Venture.

Francis Collins, the new head of the NIH, has enthusiastically endorsed these types of public–private partnerships. As the work performed in the academic and government laboratories can lower the product failure risk, pharmaceutical companies have an incentive to license drug candidates that are ready to enter clinical trials (Young, 2009). Thus, there is a growing consensus that the current model for drug discovery and development as practiced in large pharmaceutical firms is unsustainable (Dixon et al., 2009; FitzGerald, 2008, 2009) and that innovation must be sought elsewhere (Cuatrecasas, 2006).

A. The NIH Roadmap

The stated focus of the NIH Roadmap is to accelerate the rate of medical discovery. While some have criticized this effort for practical reasons (Marks, 2006), it is now well entrenched in the academic community.

As part of its strategy, the NIH established the Molecular Libraries Initiative (MLI) (Austin, Brady, Insel, & Collins, 2004) "to facilitate the use of HTS to identify small molecules ... to study cellular pathways ... in health and disease by rapidly and efficiently screening a large number of compounds that encompasses a broad range of novel targets and activities ... to increase the number of molecules available as potential drug candidates for further development by the public or private sector." To establish the MLI, the NIH has funded approximately 10 academic screening centers that, to date, have produced a number of publications and 62 NCEs. However, because no funding was provided for *in vivo* ADME or safety testing, these agents are, for the most part, tool compounds rather than drug leads (Kaiser, 2008).

In many respects, the core elements of the NIH Roadmap, especially the MLI, emulate the technology-based approaches utilized by the pharmaceutical industry over the past decade that are now being criticized as unproductive. This suggests that, like the current industry approach to drug discovery, the Roadmap initiative is probably due for a reassessment of its strategic and tactical objectives.

Success in federally funded drug discovery initiatives has had a checkered history. As one example, while the 1971 National Cancer Act gave the National Cancer Institute a charter to cure cancer, the incidence of this disease in the United States remains the highest in the world, with a death rate that has remained unchanged for over 50 years (193.9 per 100,000 in 1950 vs. 193.4 per 100,000 in 2002). This lack of progress is both surprising and disappointing given the billions of dollars spent over the past 40 years on improving treatment options, reducing cancer-related behaviors, such as smoking, and increasing efforts in early detection (Aggarwal, Danda, Shan Gupta, & Gehlot, 2009). Many are now coming to the realization that, as in other therapeutic areas, the greatest limitation for identifying new drugs for treating cancer are the deficiencies in the animal models used for testing NCEs (Aggarwal et al., 2009). Yet despite their many limitations (Hackam & Redelmeier, 2006), these animal models remain a key element of translational medicine (Cozzi, Fraichard, & Thiam, 2008; Mankoff, Brander, Ferrone, & Marincola, 2004). Given this, it has been argued that a greater emphasis be placed on improving animal models of human disease rather than to emphasize the screening of chemical libraries for leads that are then tested in animal systems known to have limited predictive validity with respect to human illness.

B. Translational Research

Translational research is generally viewed (Adams, 2008; Duyk, 2003; FitzGerald, 2005, 2007; LoRusso, 2009; Maienschein, Sunderland, Ankeny, & Robert, 2008; Wehling, 2008, 2009; Woolf, 2008b) as a "bench to bedside" discipline designed to direct the findings of basic research to the production of new medications (Woolf, 2008b). Translational research may also be viewed as important in fulfilling the desire of basic scientists to have their work used for the benefit of mankind (Wehling, 2008) and to ultimately reverse the decline in drug discovery productivity. Translational research has been further envisaged (i) a process for ensuring the bidirectional flow of information from the research laboratory to the clinic and vice versa (Sung et al., 2003) and (ii) as encompassing all elements of the drug development process from the initial screening for chemical leads to target identification to clinical proof of concept (FitzGerald, 2005). Many fear, however, that like the concept of target validation (Kopec et al., 2005), in its current form, the promise of translational medicine approach far exceeds the practicalities of what it can deliver in terms of facilitating the drug discovery process (Maienschein et al., 2008; Wehling, 2008). In FitzGerald's view, the centerpieces of the translational effort are the academic medical centers (AMCs) responsible for conducting clinical trials. To this end, the NIH has sponsored Clinical and Translation Science Awards (CTSAs) as part of the Roadmap initiative with some $500 million being earmarked through 2012 to fund 60 AMCs across the United States (FitzGerald, 2009; Woolf, 2008b). Similar efforts are underway in the United Kingdom under the auspices of the National Institute for Health Research (Adams, 2008) and in Europe as the European Advanced Translational Research Infrastructure in Medicine Network (EATRIS) (Wehling, 2009; Woolf, 2008b). All these programs focus on improving the outcomes from drug discovery R&D to enhance medical care. However, it has been noted (FitzGerald, 2009) that the existing AMCs are much less efficient than traditional contract research organizations (Moos & Mirsalis, 2009) that conduct the majority of clinical trials for the pharmaceutical industry. This has been ascribed to a perceived lack of necessary career incentives that may be viewed as conflicting with the ethos of biomedical research (Harris, 2005).

A major contributor to the confusion around translational research involves the definitions of "translational blocks." Termed T1 and T2 by the Institute of Medicine's Clinical Research Roundtable (Sung et al., 2003; Woolf, 2008b), T1 is generically considered as representing the translational component and is defined as "the transfer of new understandings of disease mechanisms gained in the laboratory into the development of new methods for diagnosis, therapy, and prevention and their first testing in humans." T2 involves translation in the context of the community and ambulatory care setting and is described as "the translation of results from clinical studies into everyday clinical practice and health decision making". Support of T2, which has been argued as being in need of a new name and emphasis (Woolf, 2008b), is essential for T1 to be successful and also for patients to derive maximal benefit from delivered health care. T2 involves studies in the community and ambulatory care setting.

A key element of any translational initiative is the development of cellular, tissue, and animal assays that can reliably predict human responses and facilitate the successful advancement of NCEs from the "bench" to the "bedside." This is a complex process involving the transition of potent, drug-like NCEs from cellular to animal assays and their subsequent transition to the clinic. As an initial step in developing a scientific basis for translational research and to reduce the concept to practice, Wehling (2009) has identified a number of key elements that form the basis of a scoring system (Table I) of determinants that must be considered when assessing the success or failure of a particular approach.

TABLE I   Translational Assessment

1. Target identification and validation
Animal evidence
  • *In vitro* evidence including animal genetics
  • *In vivo* evidence including animal genetics
  • Animal disease models
  • Animal safety models
  • Data from multiple species
Human evidence
  • Genetics
  • Model compounds and existing drugs
  • Clinical trials
2. Biomarkers for efficacy and safety prediction
  • Biomarker grading
  • Biomarker development
  • Biomarker validation
3. Proof-of-mechanism, proof-of-principle, and proof-of-concept testing
  • Biomarker strategy
  • Surrogate of clinical end-point strategy
4. Personalized medicine
  • Disease sub-classification and concentration of "responders"
  • Pharmacogenetics
5. Drug discovery
Chemical/pharmacological tractability
  • Lead identification
  • Lead optimization
  • Drugability
  • Potency, efficacy, selectivity, safety
Intellectual property
  • Patent strength
  • Freedom to operate
  • Patent expiration
Clinical dynamics
  • Unmet clinical need
  • Patient availability
  • Competitor (generics, proprietary, patent expiration)
  • Cost pressure via reimbursement or insurance mechanisms

Proposed scoring system for assessing the translatability of drug discovery projects to the clinic. Important feasibility parameters without direct translational implications are given in brackets (After Wehling, 2009).

C. Animal Models of Human Disease States

A major hurdle in the translational medicine undertaking is the fact that most preclinical animal models of disease generally lack predictive value with respect to the human condition under study. Indeed, the false positives that result from the present generation of animal assays are a major cause of NCE attrition in the clinic either because of lack of efficacy or the appearance of unacceptable side effects that were not detected preclinically. While there are notable, albeit retrospective, exceptions (Zambrowicz & Sands, 2003), this weakness in the conventional drug discovery process has not been resolved with the use of transgenic animals which themselves contribute additional confounds that further complicate data interpretation.

In therapeutic areas as diverse as pain (Rice et al., 2008), stroke (O'Collins et al., 2006), neurodegeneration (Lindner, McArthur, Deadwyler, Hampson, & Tariot, 2008), and substance abuse (Gardner, 2008), numerous agents that displayed substantial efficacy and safety in animal models, have failed in the clinic (Hackam & Redelmeier, 2006). Similarly, animal models used to interrogate the PK and PD effects of NCEs are in need of further refinement so they have predictive value with regard to human use. The poor translational record from animal models to humans has been attributed to poor preclinical methodologies (Green, 2008; Hackam, 2007; Perel et al., 2007), which include a lack of blinding and randomization, adequate powering/size, and an "optimization bias"; in that very often only positive results are reported.

An analysis of 76 peer reviewed animal studies (Hackam & Redelmeier, 2006) in a variety of therapeutic areas including obesity, cancer, irritable bowel disorder (IBD), stroke, diabetes, experimental autoimmune encephalomyelitis (EAE), multiple sclerosis (MS), hypertension, and sepsis led to the conclusion that "only about one-third (33%) of highly cited animal research translated at the level of human randomized trials." Of the 76 studies, 34 (45%) were "untested," for example, failed to reach Phase III (D.G. Hackam, personal communication), 28 (27%) were replicated, and 14 (18%) contraindicated. For those compounds whose effects were replicated, 8 were finally approved for human use. To place the studies analyzed in context, replication rates in human studies were slightly higher (44%; Ioannidis, 2005a) extending the question of rigor to the full spectrum of the biomedical research endeavor (Ioannidis, 2005b). Outcomes from the translational process have been further confounded by the underreporting of negative clinical trial outcomes (Ramsey & Scoggins, 2008; Turner, Matthews, Linardatos, Tell, & Rosenthal, 2008).

Other important reasons for the difficulty in translating laboratory animal data to the clinic are the inherent differences between rodent and human physiology and the likelihood that animal models are limited in their relationship to the actual human disease. This is certainly the case in areas where years of research have yet to yield improved treatments. In animal models of stroke, the species, experimental protocol, and timing of NCE administration have little resemblance to what occurs in humans and how the condition is treated (Hall, 2007; O'Collins et al., 2006).

In the field of psychiatry (Millan, 2008), many of the available models of human disease states, for example, schizophrenia and depression, actually evolved from the evaluation of the drugs discovered serendipitously to be of therapeutic benefit (Sneader, 2005). Accordingly, these are models of drug action rather than of the disease state (Millan, 2008). Similarly, models of Parkinson's (Meredith, Sonsalla, & Chesselet, 2008) and Alzheimer's diseases (Götz & Ittner, 2008) utilize chemical or surgical ablation techniques to mimic the human condition or employ transgenic animal models that overexpress certain gene products (Aβ or α-synuclein) that are thought to be associated with the disorder. These have a markedly different time course and severity than the human condition. For Alzheimer's disease, such assays are often paired with models of cognition impairment (Levin & Buccafusco, 2006; Lindner et al., 2008), even though the precise relationship of this impairment with the Alzheimer's phenotype is unclear. In the area of substance abuse (Volkow & Li, 2004) there are many sophisticated rodent models of drug dependence and relapse to cocaine, amphetamine, and alcohol (Gardner, 2008; Heidbreder, 2009). The most predictable, however, are those that involve human and non-human primates.

While animal models of acute and chronic pain are generally viewed as among the more robust preclinical tests, having been validated with the opioid analgesics and NSAIDs, there are serious issues with their face validity and relationship to the human disease state (Blackburn-Monro, 2004; Whiteside, Adedoyin, & Leventhal, 2008) as well as preclinical study design (Rice et al., 2008). Chief among the translational concerns is species differences in pain targets between rodents and human, the use of healthy animals as subjects, the time for pain onset and testing, and differences between spontaneous or natural pain and evoked pain (Blackburn-Monro, 2004), the latter being a hallmark of the majority of preclinical pain models (Rice et al., 2008). Despite significant progress in understanding the molecular pathophysiology of pain (Costigan, Scholz, & Woolf, 2009; Woolf, 2008a), these factors have no doubt contributed to the poor translatability of positive preclinical data.

The studies with NK1 receptor antagonists, typified by aprepitant (MK-869), are a prime example of this phenomenon. Thus despite robust preclinical results, several members of this compound class failed to display efficacy in the clinic, leading to a debate about the relationship between a role of NK1 in mediating pain in humans (Hill, 2000) and the drug-like properties of the first-in-class NCEs used that may have precluded them reaching their intended site of action (Laszlo & Fox, 2000). Subsequent studies (Bergstrom et al., 2004) using PET imaging demonstrated that aprepitant occupied NK1 receptors in the CNS, leading to the conclusion that NK1 was not associated with pain behaviors in humans (Whiteside et al., 2008), thus providing a rationale as to why the animal models in this instance had no predictive value with regard to this target approach. Other examples of a disconnect between animal data and human responses include α4β2 nicotinic agonists, like tebanicline (ABT-594) (Bannon et al., 1998). In this case, an NCE that was some 200 times more potent than morphine in various animal pain models had limited clinical efficacy due to side effects that were not detected in animal studies (Rueter, Honore, & Bitner, 2006). Moreover, clinical trials have indicated that the analgesic utility of TRPV1 antagonists, like SB-705498, are limited by effects on core temperature regulation (Caterina, 2008).

Collectively, such findings have led to renewed calls for creating animal models that are more indicative of clinical pain and that probably should be focused on supraspinal mechanisms (Whiteside et al., 2008). Operant models that integrate both the motor and motivational aspects of pain that may augment existing pain models, together with more consistent and transparent experimentation (Rice et al., 2008), will undoubtedly improve the predictive value of these assays.

D. The Yin and the Yang of Translational Outcomes

While there are ample reasons to conclude that preclinical (Yin) efficacy studies are flawed and result in the wrong target or wrong NCE being advanced to the clinical (Yang) trial arena, it is not always clear as to whether "failed" randomized clinical trials (RCTs) have themselves been conducted with sufficient rigor and transparency to yield scientifically valid results. Because of the costs associated with, and the competition for, patient recruitment, clinical trials are often undertaken with restrictions on the number of subjects and treatment arms making it difficult, if not impossible, to benchmark NCEs against standard of care. Analyses of failed Phase IIa (proof-of-concept) trials often reveal, with 20:20 hindsight, critical elements that should have been included in the initial study design. Added to this are delays in patient recruitment that slow the process and drive up costs, such as those that occur routinely at existing AMCs because of mandated ethical and scientific reviews and contractual challenges (FitzGerald, 2009). Kolata (2009) has reported that similar circumstances contribute to the lack of progress in cancer therapeutics (Aggarwal et al., 2009) noting that only 3% of adult patients participate in clinical trials in cancer focused on NCEs or new treatment regimens. Of the 6,500 trials registered on the website, clinicaltrials.gov, more than 1 in 5 of those sponsored by the NCI has failed to recruit a single patient while half do not recruit sufficient patients to adequately power the trials.

The FDA's exploratory IND guidance (FDA, 2006) is an additional initiative to expedite the clinical evaluation of NCEs and has led to the establishment of the Phase 0 clinical trial concept (Kinders et al., 2007; Kummar et al., 2008). This type of trial has no intended therapeutic or diagnostic intent being instead a continuation of preclinical discovery rather the initiation of development (LoRusso, 2009). The exploratory IND for a Phase 0 trial supports first-in-human NCE testing using subtherapeutic doses. Also known as microdoses, these are 1/100th of the NCE dose to a maximum of 100 μg that is required to yield a pharmacological effect in animals. An NCE is tested at this dose in a limited patient cohort (~10 individuals) for 7 days or less to measure drug–target effects for proof of concept and to assess PK/PD relationships in humans.

A useful Phase 0 trial requires that the mechanism of action of the NCE be precisely known as demonstration of a target interaction (PD) is a key outcome of a successful trial. In this context, LoRusso (2009) has noted that because the pan-kinase inhibitor, sorafenib, was originally developed as a selective inhibitor of B-Raf kinase and is now known to be several fold more active as an inhibitor of other kinases (Karaman et al., 2008), it would not have been a good candidate for Phase 0 trials as measuring B-Raf inhibition as a PD outcome would have failed to identify its antitumor activity. Another key aspect of the Phase 0 approach that defines the need for a more pharmacologically based approach is the need to identify and validate robust biomarkers that can be reliably used at multiple clinical sites. The potential impact of the Phase 0 program has been highlighted by the National Cancer Institute-sponsored Phase 0 trial with the Poly (ADP-ribose) polymerase (PARP) inhibitor, ABT-888. PK/PD data obtained in 5 months in a cohort of 13 patients allowed the initiation of combination studies earlier in the trials and at less expense than would have occurred using a conventional Phase I approach (Kummar et al., 2009).

E. Translation in Antidepressant Trials – Depressing?

The outcomes of clinical trials for drugs to treat depression (Blier, 2008; Kirsch, 2009; Kramer, 2005; Leventhal & Martell, 2005) have been a controversial topic with considerable focus on placebo responses. A meta-analysis (Kirsch, Moore, Scoboria, & Nicholls, 2002) of the efficacy data from 47 clinical trials covering the six most widely prescribed antidepressants approved between 1987 and 1999 – fluoxetine, paroxetine, sertraline, venlafaxine, nefazodone, and citalopram – determined that approximately 80% of the effect ascribed to drug was also seen in the placebo controls. This led to the oft-repeated claim that four out of six clinical trials for approved antidepressants routinely fail. In a follow-up analysis focusing on fluoxetine, paroxetine, venlafaxine, and nefazodone (Kirsch et al., 2008), it was further established that baseline severity was a critical component for drug-related responses, and that a *decreased* response to placebo rather than an *increased* drug response was frequently responsible for positive clinical results in this area. It was additionally determined that patients recruited into clinical trials were not representative of the average individual treated in practice (Wisniewski et al., 2009). The issue of antidepressant efficacy has been further clouded by the selective reporting of data in published findings (Turner & Rosenthal, 2008; Turner et al., 2008). Thus, publications covering 37 out of 74 FDA-registered trials indicated that 94% of these yielded positive results. However, an FDA analysis of the full cohort of 74 trials revealed that only 51% of the trials were positive, suggesting that antidepressants were less effective than the published data indicated. The issue of the placebo effect in clinical trials for psychiatric medications remains a highly controversial topic (Silberman, 2009).

Thus while considerable evidence exists as to why the translation of NCEs to the clinic based on non-clinical efficacy and safety data to the clinic may be flawed, it is equally possible that the actual data from clinical trials may also be flawed, reinforcing – to a major degree – the need for a bidirectional flow of information (Sung et al., 2003) on NCE efficacy as a planned part of the translational process through Phase IIa rather than a typical binary fault finding exercise across the translational divide.

IV. Pharmacology as an Enabling Science in Translational Research

A. Animals and Humans

The preclinical research that contributes to the selection of an IND candidate typically occurs in a relatively well-defined and controlled environment, with the tissue samples and subjects (animals) being studied being relatively uniform in their characteristics. Accordingly, the preclinical research process is relatively straightforward and economical, resulting in data that are generally highly reproducible. This contrasts markedly to the clinical situation where subjects are drawn from a diverse population and where there are many other variables not encountered in the laboratory setting, including differences in diagnostic criteria and stage of the disease. For instance, while schizophrenia can be viewed as a single disorder, there is in fact a major overlap in the symptoms of this condition with bipolar disorder (Marino, Knutsen, & Williams, 2008). Indeed, it has been suggested that schizophrenia may consist of 10 or more discrete disorders

(Marino et al., 2008). Similarly, there is a general view that because of considerable challenges with diagnosis, many of the NCEs evaluated as treatments for Alzheimer's disease are administered too late in the disease process, that has yet to be clearly understood (Hardy, 2009), to be of any real therapeutic benefit.

B. Compound Characterization

Drug discovery involves target selection for a given disease; the identification of compounds active at the target; the identification of NCEs that are potent, selective, and efficacious at the target; their optimization for drug-like properties; and their evaluation for safety and efficacy *in vitro* and *in vivo* (Table II; Ator, Mallamo, & Williams, 2007; Kenakin, 2009). In fact, NCE activity is most accurately described in terms of concentration parameters, for example, potency, functional efficacy, and affinity, for its target. Replicate efficacy determinations provide robust and critical information on the potential effectiveness of an NCE and can also be used to benchmark and prioritize its movement through the preclinical process to an IND.

C. From Cell to Animal

Prior to an NCE being evaluated in an animal model of human disease, it undergoes an intensive optimization cycle to enhance potency, efficacy, safety, and drug-like properties (Abdel-Rahman & Kauffman, 2004; Ator et al., 2007; Danhof et al., 2007; Duzic, Marino, & Williams, 2009; Kenakin, 2009). This process typically encompasses the iterative synthesis of some 300–1000 NCEs to generate a clinical candidate. In addition to the mandatory determination of concentration/dose dependence for biological activity and the derivation of a therapeutic index, the solubility, stability, and physical form of an NCE must also be assessed to ensure it has the appropriate drug-like characteristics. Other issues addressed as part of this process are whether an NCE can reach its site of action, produces a desired therapeutic effect, and is excreted before it is able to induce unwanted side effects (Hodgson, 2001).

The derivation of an SAR for the interaction of the NCE with its target provides critical information on its efficacy and the means to chemically differentiate positive attributes from those producing side effects. By defining in more detail the nature of the NCE interaction with its target (Kenakin, 2009), its kinetics, enthalpic and entropic binding energy (Freire, 2004), and residence time (Copeland, Pompliano, & Meek, 2007; Tummino & Copeland, 2008), it is possible to optimize pharmacological differences in members of a chemical series and between pharmacophores active at a target. For example, assessment of the efficacy of a series of HIV-1 protease

TABLE II   Drug Characteristics of an NCE

Synthesis and chemical properties
- Facile synthetic route from ready available starting materials; ≤8 steps with chiral and chemical purity >98%
- Good yields (>40%)
- Patentable
- Aqueous solubility at physiological pH >10–20 µg/ml
- Appropriate solid-state properties (stable crystal polymorph, optimal salt form)
- Suitable physical properties (e.g., pKa, cLogP [≤3], chemical stability)
- Rule of 5 guidelines

Potency
- Active and selective inhibition of human drug target
- Ki = 1–100 nM
- 20- to 100-fold selectivity versus other targets; ideally > 100-fold selective in panel of > 150+ targets (receptors/enzymes; Cerep/Millipore screens)
- Defined SAR for efficacy *and* safety
- Similarly active in both recombinant and native cell systems
- Active across species
- Active against molecular target in preclinical efficacy model

Efficacy
- Agonist or antagonist mechanism demonstrated in appropriate cellular systems (native and recombinant)
- Defined target kinetics profile
- Efficacy established in *ex vivo* system and accepted animal model(s) of disease state
- Plasma and target tissue levels in pharmacology experiments associated with efficacy and side effects (PK/PD model)

ADME properties
- Metabolically stable in liver S-9 preparation from multiple species, including human
- Caco-2 permeability; compound is permeable with little evidence for P-gp substrate activity
- Identification of primary metabolic pathways and routes of elimination
- Minimal potential for drug–drug interactions
- Absence of potent inhibition of CYP isozymes in human recombinant and microsomal systems
- Minimal induction of CYP3A4 in fresh human hepatocytes
- Minimal human P-gp interactions
- Protein binding (preclinical species and human); <98% bound, no marked species differences
- Single-dose rodent PK; appropriate extent and duration of exposure by intended route of administration, oral bioavailability >20%
- Rodent PK dose escalation and tolerability; dose-proportional increases in exposure
- Rodent PK fed/fasted
- Rodent repeat-dose PK/tolerability; no decrease in plasma levels after repeat dosing, compound is tolerated

Safety pharmacology
- Therapeutic index >30; optimally >100
- hERG inactive > 15–30 µM (if active, followed by patch clamp and telemeterized rat studies)
- ICH 7A profiling
    - o CV safety (blood pressure, heart rate, dP/dT, etc.)
    - o CNS safety (core battery studies, Category A, ICH7A)
    - o General behavioral observations
    - o Spontaneous motor activity

(Continued)

TABLE II (*Continued*)

---

o General anesthetic effects
o Potential synergism/antagonism with general anesthetics
o Convulsion effects (proconvulsant activity and synergy with convulsive agents)
o Effects on body temperature
o Effects on GI motility and renal function
o Repeat-dose PK/tolerability (nonrodent)
o Genetic toxicity (e.g., Ames, *in vitro* micronucleus, chromosomal aberrations), negative

---

After (Ator et al., 2007).

inhibitors revealed that NCEs with similar IC_{50} or Ki values had markedly different efficacy based on their residence time as determined by the dissociative half-life of their target–ligand complexes (Copeland et al., 2007).

While the ultimate goal of each drug discovery project is to find a patentable NCE in which each and every parameter (Table II) is optimized to maximize the therapeutic index, in actuality, as one parameter is optimized, another may be de-optimized. An NCE with excellent efficacy but poor bioavailability may lose biological activity as the pharmacophore is modified to improve its ADME properties. In many instances, a compromise needs to be reached where acceptable bioavailability is introduced with minimal to no loss of efficacy or target selectivity. In other instances, necessary modifications that improve bioavailability or toxicity can lead to an almost complete loss in NCE efficacy or the introduction of other, unwanted properties, such as hERG activity. In these cases it becomes necessary to initiate a search for a new pharmacophore for the target being interrogated.

D. From Animal to Human

In vitro assays used to define the characteristics of an NCE typically employ an isolated target, such as a human receptor recombinantly expressed in a cell line, under equilibrium conditions in a *closed system* (Tummino & Copeland, 2008). In these tests, the target and the signaling system are held constant, with the NCE concentration being the only variable. *In vivo*, however, the evaluation of an NCE is complicated by the presence of numerous uncontrolled variables in what is an *open system*. In this situation, the actions of an NCE at its target are confounded by the constantly changing concentrations of the NCE in the general circulation due to absorption, plasma protein binding, metabolism, and elimination.

For an orally active NCE to reach an intracellular receptor, it must be absorbed from the intestine into the systemic circulation, be transported to the target tissue with minimal first-pass metabolism, cross the cell membrane, and finally bind to its target. For a target within the brain, the blood–brain barrier must also be traversed. As interest in intracellular targets, such as the mitochondrion, increases, the task of delivering an NCE to its site of action can often be a greater challenge than optimizing its efficacy and safety. Additionally, in accessing an NCE target within a tissue or cell, large amounts of the NCE are present in the circulation, increasing the likelihood of NCE interactions with "collateral" proteins (Copeland et al., 2007) and the potential for side effects that would not necessarily be predicted from a target-binding profile. For these reasons, many highly potent and selective NCEs, as established by their favorable *in vitro* cellular and tissue activities, do not transition to the *in vivo* situation, making them unsuitable for development.

An additional consideration when studying the interaction of an NCE with its target is whether the target is actually disease specific. Chromosomal translocation, for example, t(2;5)(p23;q35) NPM in anaplastic lymphoma kinase (ALK), is a transforming event in the genesis of anaplastic large cell lymphoma (ALCL; Polgar et al., 2005). Because this is a demonstrably unique disease-associated event, therapeutic NCEs can be designed to target selectively the disease-associated kinase, thereby have the potential to improve the therapeutic index.

Demonstrating the dose-dependent efficacy of an NCE in an appropriate animal model can be used to inform the Phase I clinical trial design. When integrated with *in vitro* metabolic studies using transfected human CYP enzymes (Bu, Magis, Knuth, & Teitelbaum, 2000), CYP induction, species microsomal stability, and plasma protein binding, the dose-related duration of effect and time to onset can be used as a basis for transition an NCE from rodent to human (Caldwell, Masucci, Yan, & Hageman, 2004). For this, measuring the plasma or tissue concentration of an NCE is far more accurate and relevant than relying on the actual dose administered although this can be confounded if the NCE has long-lasting effects on gene transcription such that the biological half-life far exceeds that observed in the plasma.

Animal models are being extensively used to develop biomarkers to assess NCE efficacy in humans. Biomarkers are indicators of normal biological or disease-associated processes and can be used to assess pharmacological responses to NCEs. Examples of common biomarkers are body temperature for fever, blood pressure for stroke risk, serum cholesterol for cardiovascular risk, blood sugar for diabetes, and cognition for Alzheimer's and other neurodegenerative disorders (Day et al., 2008). In colorectal cancer, apoptosis signaling proteins are being developed as prognostic biomarkers (Hector & Prehen, 2009).

In the clinic, appropriately validated biomarkers can be used for diagnosing disease, for assessing disease severity, for guiding patient treatment, and assessing patient response to therapeutic intervention. Biomarkers can also be employed to determine the mechanism of action of an NCE, its biologically effective dose, and its therapeutic index, as well as to stratify patients in an attempt to identify those most likely to respond to treatment. Developing accurate and robust biomarkers for different diseases is a major challenge, with many false positives revealed when a biomarker fails to change as expected when there is improvement in the condition. Thus while disease association of a biomarker provides a retrospective assessment, it is the prospective use of a biomarker in disease progression and response that provides objective value. In systemic lupus erythematosus (SLE), double-stranded DNA (dsDNA) autoantibodies are a well-established biomarker of SLE and a component of the SLE Disease Activity Index (SLEDAI) used to diagnose and assess disease progression. However, in a Phase III SLE trial of abetimus, a synthetic double-stranded oligodeoxyribonucleotide that modulates B lymphocyte function, while anti-dsDNA antibody levels were reduced, there was no effect on prolonging time to renal flare, a key marker of SLE pathophysiology, in comparison to placebo (Cardiel et al., 2008), questioning the relevance of dsDNA as a biomarker of this aspect of SLE.

V. Conclusion

Translational research as a scientific discipline is very much in its infancy (Wehling, 2009), with numerous hurdles to overcome before it matures into an established approach for drug development. Clearly, much work remains to more effectively chart the path forward from a preclinical IND submission data set to a proof of concept in Phase IIa. Pharmacology has a key role to play in this process by providing the critical information required about the actions of an NCE *in vitro* and *in vivo*, as such data are vital in the design of Phase 0 and Phase I clinical trials. Importantly, there is a need to enhance communication between those conducting the clinical trials and preclinical scientists to ensure that the targets selected, the NCEs synthesized, and the animal models employed are relevant to the human disease state under investigation and that the data generated are used as part of a learning process to iteratively improve on next generation approaches either in terms of NCEs or next generation targets.

Since the late nineteenth century, the discipline of pharmacology has been synonymous with drug discovery, aiding in the understanding of disease pathophysiology, defining the mechanism of action of existing agents and identifying new therapeutics (Chast, 2008; Sneader, 2005). Thus, pharmacology is a key element of the FDA's Critical Path initiative (FDA, 2004), along with basic physiology and clinical pharmacology (FDA, 2006; Kinders et al., 2007; LoRusso, 2009).

For more than a generation, however, training in integrative pharmacology has been de-emphasized as graduates have been trained in molecular and genetic disciplines (Jobe et al., 1994; Williams, 2005). This has lead to a shortage of trained pharmacologists. Evidence for this is provided by the fact that the dose/concentration–response curve for drug studies has been increasingly replaced with gel scans or heat maps obtained following exposure to a single, often non-physiological, concentration of an NCE (Maddox, 1992). Moreover, very often such studies are conducted in the absence of a testable hypothesis (Firestein & Pisetsky, 2002), making it impossible to judge the significance of the findings in the broader context of drug discovery and development.

A major initiative to address this problem has been the NIH-sponsored Integrative and Organ Systems Pharmacology courses (Preusch, 2004). These workshops, conducted over a 2–3 week period at selected US universities, focus on increasing the understanding and appreciation for receptor theory as it pertains to drug discover and the use of animal models in biomedical research. Similar training programs exist in Europe (Collis, 2006). Together, these initiatives offer an antidote to biomedical research having "taken a wrong turn in [its] relationship to human disease" (Horrobin, 2003), in that they provide essential tools needed for transitioning translational research from "wishful thinking" (Wehling, 2008) to a *bona fide* science (Wehling, 2009).

Acknowledgments

The authors would like to thank Mark Ator, Jim Barrett, Emir Duzic, Gary Firestein, Garrett FitzGerald, Terry Kenakin, Dan Hackam, Jay Robert, Bruce Ruggeri, Peter Tummino, and Martin Wehling for their insights on the translational process in drug discovery.

Conflict Statement: S.J. Enna has no conflicts of interest with regard to the subject matter of this review. Michael Williams is a full-time employee of Cephalon, Inc., a biopharmaceutical company involved in the discovery, clinical evaluation, and marketing of drugs.

References

Abdel-Rahman, S. M., & Kauffman, R. E. (2004). The integration of pharmacokinetics and pharmacodynamics: Understanding dose-response. *Annual Review of Pharmacology and Toxicology, 44*, 111–136.

Adams, J. U. (2008). Building the bridge from bench to bedside. *Nature Reviews. Drug Discovery, 7*, 463–464.

Aggarwal, B. B., Danda, D., Shan Gupta, S., & Gehlot, P. (2009). Models for prevention and treatment of cancer: Problems vs. promises. *Biochemical Pharmacology, 78*, 1083–1094.

Ator, M. A., Mallamo, J. P., & Williams, M. (2007). Overview of drug discovery and development. In S. J. Enna, M. Williams, J. W. Ferkany, T. Kenakin, & R. D. Porsolt (Eds.), *Short protocols in pharmacology and drug discovery* (pp. 1-1–1-27). Hoboken, NJ: Wiley.

Austin, C. P., Brady, L. S., Insel, T. R., & Collins, F. S. (2004). NIH molecular libraries initiative. *Science, 306*, 1138–1139.

Bannon, A. W., Decker, M. W., Holladay, M. W., Curzon, P., Donnelly-Roberts, D., Putt-farcken, P. S., et al. (1998). Broad-spectrum, non-opioid analgesic activity by selective modulation of neuronal nicotinic acetylcholine receptors. *Science, 279,* 77–81.

Bergstrom, M., Hargreaves, R. J., Burns, H. D., Goldberg, M. R., Sciberras, D., Reines, S. A., et al. (2004). Human positron emission tomography studies of brain neurokinin 1 receptor occupancy by aprepitant. *Biological Psychiatry, 55,* 1007–1012.

Blackburn-Monro, G. (2004). Pain-like behaviors in animals – how human are they? *Trends in Pharmacological Sciences, 25,* 399–305.

Blier, P. (2008). Do antidepressants really work? *Journal of Psychiatry & Neuroscience, 33,* 89–90.

Brady, L. S., Winsky, L., Goodman, W., Oliveri, M. E., & Stover, E. (2009). NIMH initiatives to facilitate collaborations between industry, academia and government for the discovery and clinical testing of novel models and drugs for psychiatric disorders. *Neuropsychopharmacology, 34,* 229–243.

Brekke, O. H., & Sandlie, I. (2003). Therapeutic antibodies for human diseases at the dawn of the twenty-first century. *Nature Reviews. Drug Discovery, 2,* 52–62.

Briley, M., & Nutt, D. (2000). *Anxiolytics.* Berlin: Birkhauser.

Bu, H.-Z., Magis, L., Knuth, K., & Teitelbaum, P. (2000). High-throughput cytochrome P450 (CYP) inhibition screening via cassette probe-dosing strategy. I. Development of direct injection/on-line guard cartridge extraction tandem mass spectrometry for the simultaneous detection of CYP probe substrates and their metabolites. *Rapid Communications in Mass Spectrometry, 14,* 1619–1624.

Caldwell, G. W., Masucci, J. A., Yan, Z., & Hageman, W. (2004). Allometric scaling of pharmacokinetic parameters in drug discovery: Can human CL, V^{ss} and $t_{1/2}$ be predicted from *in vivo* rat data? *European Journal of Drug Metabolism and Pharmacokinetics, 29,* 122–143.

Cardiel, M. H., Tumlin, A., Furie, R. A., Wallace, D. J., Joh, T., Linnik, M. D., & the LJP 394-90-09 Investigator Consortium. (2008). Abetimus sodium for renal flare in systemic lupus erythematosus: Results of a randomized, controlled phase III trial. *Arthtitis and Rheumatism, 58,* 2470–2480.

Caterina, M. J. (2008). On the thermoregulatory perils of TRPV1 antagonism. *Pain, 136,* 3–4.

Celis, J. E., Kruhøffer, M., Gromova, I., Frederiksen, C., Ostergaard, M., Thykjaer, T., et al. (2000). Gene expression profiling: Monitoring transcription and translation products using DNA microarrays and proteomics. *FEBS Letters, 480,* 2–16.

Changeux, J.-P., & Edelstein, S. J. (2005). *Nicotinic acetylcholine receptors: From molecular biology to cognition* (pp. 1–21). New York: Odile Jacob.

Chast, F. (2008). A history of drug discovery. In C. G. Wermuth (Ed.), *The practice of medicinal chemistry* (3rd ed., pp. 3–62). Burlington, MA: Academic Press.

Chenoweth, D. M., & Dervan, P. B. (2009). Allosteric modulation of DNA by small molecules. *Proceedings of the National Academy of Sciences of the United States of America, 106,* 13175–13179.

Chiang, S. L. (2006). Chemical genetics: Use of high-throughput screening to identify small-molecule modulators of proteins involved in cellular pathways with the aim of uncovering protein function. In J. Huser (Ed.), *High throughput-screening in drug discovery* (pp. 1–13). Weinheim, Germany: Wiley-VCH.

Collins, F. S., Green, E. D., Guttmacher, A. E., Guyer, M. S., & the US National Human Genome Research Institute. (2003). A vision for the future of genomics research. *Nature, 422,* 835–847.

Collis, M. G. (2006). Integrative pharmacology and drug discovery – is the tide finally turning? *Nature Reviews. Drug Discovery, 5,* 377–380.

Comley, J. (2006). Tools and technologies that facilitate automated screening. In J. Huser (Ed.), *High throughput-screening in drug discovery* (pp. 37–73). Weinheim, Germany: Wiley-VCH.

Conn, P. J., & Roth, B. L. (2008). Opportunities and challenges of psychiatric drug discovery: Roles for scientists in academic, industry, and government settings. *Neuropsychopharmacology, 33*, 2048–2060.

Copeland, R. A., Pompliano, D. L., & Meek, T. D. (2007). Drug-target residence time and its implications for lead optimization. *Nature Reviews. Drug Discovery, 5*, 730–739.

Costigan, M., Scholz, J., & Woolf, C. J. (2009). Neuropathic pain: A maladaptive response of nervous system to damage. *Annual Review of Neuroscience, 32*, 1–32.

Cozzi, J., Fraichard, A., & Thiam, K. (2008). Use of genetically modified rat models for translational medicine. *Drug Discovery Today, 13*, 488–494.

Cuatrecasas, P. (2006). Drug discovery in jeopardy. *Journal of Clinical Investigation, 116*, 2837–2842.

Danhof, M., de Jongh, J., De Lange, E. C. M., Pasqua, O. D., Ploeger, B. A., & Voskuyl, R. A. (2007). Mechanism-based pharmacokinetic/pharmacodynamic modeling: Biophase distribution, receptor theory, and dynamical systems analysis. *Annual Review of Pharmacology and Toxicology, 47*, 357–400.

Day, M., Balci, F., Wan, H. I., Fox, G. B., Rutkowski, J. L., & Feuerstein, G. (2008). Cognitive endpoints as disease biomarkers: Optimizing the congruency of preclinical models to the clinic. *Current Opinion in Investigational Drugs, 9*, 696–707.

Dixon, J., Lawton, G., & Machin, P. (2009). Vertical disintegration: A strategy for pharmaceutical businesses in 2009? *Nature Reviews. Drug Discovery, 8*, 433.

Duyk, G. (2003). Attrition and translation. *Science, 302*, 603–605.

Duzic, E., Marino, M. J., & Williams, M. (2009). Receptor binding in drug discovery. In D. E. Abrahams & D. Rottella (Eds.), *Burger's medicinal chemistry and drug discovery* (7th ed.). Hoboken, NJ: Wiley, in press.

Dykxhoorn, D. M., & Lieberman, J. (2005). The silent revolution: RNA interference as basic biology, research tool, and therapeutic. *Annual Review of Medicine, 56*, 401–442.

Edwards, A. M., Bountra, C., Kerr, D. J., & Willson, T. M. (2009). Open access chemical and clinical probes to support drug discovery. *Nature Chemical Biology, 5*, 436–440.

Enna, S. J., Fuerstein, G., Piette, J., & Williams, M. (2008). Fifty years of biochemical pharmacology: The discipline and the journal. *Biochemical Pharmacology, 76*, 1–10.

Enna, S. J., & Williams, M. (2009). Challenges in the search for drugs to treat central nervous system disorders. *Journal of Pharmacology and Experimental Therapeutics, 329*, 404–411.

Eldefrawi, M. E., & Eldefrawi, A. T. (1972). Characterization and partial purification of the acetylcholine receptor from *Torpedo* electroplax. *Proceedings of the National Academy of Sciences of the United States of America, 69*, 1776–1780.

FDA. (2004). *Innovation/stagnation. Challenge and opportunity on the critical path to new medical products.* Bethesda, MD: Author. Retrieved from www.fda.gov/oc/initiatives/criticalpath/whitepaper.html

FDA. (2006). *Guidance for industry and reviewers. Exploratory IND Studies.* Retrieved from http://www.fda.gov/downloads/Drugs/GuidanceComplianceRegulatoryInformation/Guidances/ucm078933.pdf

Firestein, G. S., & Pisetsky, D. S. (2002). DNA microarrays: Boundless technology or bound by technology? Guidelines for studies using microarray technology. *Arthtitis and Rheumatism, 46*, 859–861.

FitzGerald, G. A. (2005). Anticipating change in drug development: The emerging era of translational medicine and therapeutics. *Nature Reviews. Drug Discovery, 4*, 815–818.

FitzGerald, G. A. (2007). Clinical pharmacology or translational medicine and therapeutics: Reinvent or rebrand and expand? *Clinical Pharmacology and Therapeutics, 81*, 17–18.

FitzGerald, G. A. (2008). Drugs, industry, and academia. *Science, 320*, 1539.

FitzGerald, G. A. (2009). Moving clinical research in academic medical centres up the value chain. *Nature Reviews. Drug Discovery, 8*, 597.

Freire, E. (2004). Isothermal titration calorimetry: Controlling binding forces in lead optimization. *Drug Discovery Today Technologies, 1,* 295–299.

GAO. (2006). *New drug development: Science, business, regulatory, and intellectual property issues cited as hampering drug development efforts.* Retrieved from http://www.gao.gov/htext/d0749.html

Gardner, E. L. (2008). Use of animal models to develop antiaddiction medications. *Current Psychiatry Reports, 10,* 377–338.

Geddes, K., Magalhaes, J. G., & Girardin, S. E. (2009). Unleashing the therapeutic potential of NOD-like receptors. *Nature Reviews. Drug Discovery, 8,* 465–479.

Götz, J., & Ittner, L. M. (2008). Animal models of Alzheimer's disease and frontotemporal dementia. *Nature Reviews. Neuroscience, 9,* 532–544.

Green, S. (2008). Animal research: Raise standards to protect patients. *Nature, 445,* 460.

Hackam, D. G. (2007). Translating animal research into clinical benefit. *British Medical Journal, 334,* 163–164.

Hackam, D. G., & Redelmeier, D. A. (2006). Translation of research evidence from animals to humans. *JAMA, 296,* 1731–1732.

Hall, E. D. (2007). Stroke. In *Comprehensive medicinal chemistry* II *(Vol. 6,* pp. 253–277). Oxford: Elsevier Ltd.

Hardy, J. (2009). The amyloid hypothesis of Alzheimer's disease: A critical reappraisal. *Journal of Neurochemistry, 110,* 1129–1134.

Hardy, J., & Singleton, A. (2009). Genomewide association studies and human disease. *New England Journal of Medicine, 360,* 1759–1768.

Harris, J. (2005). Scientific research is a moral duty. *Journal of Medical Ethics, 31,* 242–248.

Hector, S., & Prehen, J. H. M. (2009). Apoptosis signaling proteins as prognostic biomarkers in colorectal cancer: A review. *Biochimica et Biophysica ACTA(BBA) – Reviews on Cancer, 1795,* 117–129.

Heidbreder, C. (2009). Impulse and reward deficit disorders: Drug discovery and development. In R. A. McArthur & F. Borsini (Eds.), *Animal and translational models for CNS drug discovery (Vol. 3,* pp. 1–22). Burlington, MA: Academic Press.

Hill, R. G. (2000). NK1 (substance P) receptor antagonists – why are they not analgesic in humans? *Trends in Pharmacological Sciences, 21,* 244–246.

Hodgson, J. (2001). ADMET: Turning chemicals into drugs. *Nature Biotechnology, 19,* 722–726.

Horrobin, D. F. (2003). Modern biomedical research: An internally self-consistent universe with little contact with medical reality? *Nature Reviews. Drug Discovery, 2,* 151–154.

International Human Genome Sequencing Consortium. (2004). Finishing the euchromatic sequence of the human genome. *Nature, 431,* 931–945.

Ioannidis, J. P. A. (2005a). Contraindicated and initially stronger effects in highly cited clinical research. *JAMA, 294,* 218–228.

Ioannidis, J. P. A. (2005a). Why most published research findings are false. *PLoS Medicine, 2,* e124.

Javadov, S., Karmazyn, M., & Escobales, N. (2009). Mitochondrial permeability transition pore opening as a promising therapeutic target in cardiac diseases. *Journal of Pharmacology and Experimental Therapeutics, 330,* 670–678.

Jobe, P. C., Adams-Curtis, L. E., Burks, T. F., Fuller, R. W., Peck, C. C., Ruffolo, R. R., et al. (1994). The essential role of integrative biomedical sciences in protecting and contributing to the health and well being of our nation. *Physiologist, 37,* 79–84.

Kaiser, J. (2008). Industrial-style screening meets academic biology. *Science, 321,* 764–766.

Karaman, M. W., Herrgards, S., Treiber, D. K., Gallant, P., Atteridge, C. E., Campbell, B. T., et al. (2008). A quantitative analysis of kinase inhibitor selectivity. *Nature Biotechnology, 26,* 127–132.

Kashfi, K. (2009). Anti-inflammatory agents as cancer therapeutics. *Advances in Pharmacology, 57,* 31–89.

Kenakin, T. (1996). The classification of seven transmembrane receptors in recombinant expression systems. *Pharmacological Reviews, 48,* 413–463.

Kenakin, T. (2009). *A pharmacology primer. Theory, applications, and methods* (3rd ed.). Burlington, MA: Elsevier Academic Press.

Kita, A., Kohayakawa, H., Kinoshita, T., Ochi, Y., Nakamichi, K., Kurumiya, S., et al. (2004). Antianxiety and antidepressant-like effects of AC-5216, a novel mitochondrial benzodiazepine receptor ligand. *British Journal of Pharmacology, 142,* 1059–1072.

Kinders, R., Parchment, R. E., Ji, J., Kummar, S., Murgo, A. J., Gutierrez, M., et al. (2007). Phase 0 clinical trials in cancer drug development: From FDA guidance to clinical practice. *Molecular Interventions, 7,* 325–334.

Kirsch, I. (2009). *The emperor's new drugs: Exploding the antidepressant myth.* London: The Bodley Head.

Kirsch, I., Deacon, B. J., Huedo-Medina, T. B., Scoboria, A., Moore, T. J., & Johnson, B. T. (2008). Initial severity and antidepressant benefits: A meta-analysis of data submitted to the Food and Drug Administration. *PLoS Medicine, 5,* e45.

Kirsch, I., Moore, T. J., Scoboria, A., & Nicholls, S. S. (2002). The emperor's new drugs: An analysis of antidepressant medication data submitted to the U. S. Food and Drug Administration. *Prevention & Treatment,* article 23. Retrieved August 20, 2009, from http://alphachoices.com/repository/assets/pdf/EmperorsNewDrugs.pdf

Kola, I. (2008). The state of innovation in drug development. *Clinical Pharmacology and Therapeutics, 83,* 227–230.

Kola, I., & Landis, J. (2004). Can the pharmaceutical industry reduce attrition rates? *Nature Reviews. Drug Discovery, 3,* 711–716.

Kolata, G. (2009). Lack of study volunteers hobbles cancer fight. *New York Times,* August 3.

Kopec, K., Bozyczko-Coyne, D. B., & Williams, M. (2005). Target identification and validation in drug discovery: The role of proteomics. *Biochemical Pharmacology, 69,* 1133–1119.

Kramer, P. D. (2005). *Against depression.* New York: Viking.

Kubinyi, H. (2003). Drug research: Myths, hype and reality. *Nature Reviews. Drug Discovery, 2,* 665–668.

Kummar, S., Kinders, R., Gutierrez, M. E., Rubinstein, L., Parchment, R. E., Phillips, L. R., et al. (2009). Phase 0 clinical trial of the poly (ADP-ribose) polymerase inhibitor ABT-888 in patients with advanced malignancies. *Journal of Clinical Oncology, 27,* 2705–2711.

Kummar, S., Rubinstein, L., Kinders, R., Parchment, R. E., Gutierrez, M. E., Murgo, A. J., et al. (2008). Phase 0 clinical trials: Conceptions and misconceptions. *The Cancer Journal, 14,* 133–137.

LaMattina, J. L. (2009). *Drug truths. Dispelling the myths about pharma R & D.* Hoboken, NJ: Wiley.

Laszlo, A., & Fox, A. J. (2000). NK_1 receptor antagonists – are they really without effect in the pain clinic? *Trends in Pharmacological Sciences, 21,* 462–464.

Lefkowitz, R. J. (2004). Historical review: A brief history and personal retrospective of seven-transmembrane receptors. *Trends in Pharmacological Sciences, 8,* 413–422.

Leventhal, A. M., & Martell, C. R. (2005). *The myth of depression as disease: Limitations and alternatives to drug treatment.* Santa Barbara, CA: Praeger.

Levin, E. D., & Buccafusco, J. J. (2006). Animal models of cognitive impairment. Boca Raton, FL: CRC Press.

Lindner, M. D., McArthur, R. A., Deadwyler, S. A., Hampson, R. E., & Tariot, P. N. (2008). Development, optimization and use of preclinical behavioral models to maximize the productivity of drug discovery for Alzheimer's disease. In R. A. McArthur & F. Borsini (Eds.), *Animal and translational models for CNS drug discovery (Vol. 2,* pp. 93–157). Burlington, MA: Academic Press.

LoRusso, P. M. (2009). Phase 0 clinical trials: An answer to drug development stagnation? *Journal of Clinical Oncology, 27*, 2586–2588.

Maddox, J. (1992). Is molecular biology yet a science? *Nature, 335*, 201.

Maehle, A.-H., Prüll, C.-R., & Halliwell, R. F. (2002). The emergence of the drug receptor theory. *Nature Reviews. Drug Discovery, 1*, 637–641.

Maienschein, J., Sunderland, M., Ankeny, R. A., & Robert, J. S. (2008). The ethos and ethics of translational research. *American Journal of Bioethics, 8*, 43–51.

Mankoff, S. P., Brander, C., Ferrone, S., & Marincola, F. M. (2004). Lost in translation: Obstacles to translational medicine. *Journal of Translational Medicine, 2*, 14.

Marino, M. J., Knutsen, L. S. J., & Williams, M. (2008). Emerging opportunities for antipsychotic drug discovery in the postgenomic era. *Joruanl of Medicinal Chemistry, 51*, 1077–1107.

Marks, A. R. (2006). Rescuing the NIH before it is too late. *Journal of Clinical Investigation, 116*, 844.

Martin, J. L. R., Sainz-Pardo, M., Furukawa, T. A., Martin-Sanchez, E., Seoane, T., & Galan, C. (2007). Review: Benzodiazepines in generalized anxiety disorder: Heterogeneity of outcomes based on a systematic review and meta-analysis of clinical trials. *Journal of Psychopharmacology, 21*, 774–782.

Martinon, F., & Tschopp, J. (2007). Inflammatory caspases and inflammasomes: Master switches of inflammation. *Cell Death and Differentiation, 14*, 10–22.

Medzhitov, R. (2008). Origin and physiological roles of inflammation. *Nature, 454*, 428–435.

Meredith, G. E., Sonsalla, P. K., & Chesselet, M. F. (2008). Animal models of Parkinson's disease progression. *ACTA Neuropathologica, 115*, 385–389.

Millan, M. J. (2008). The discovery and development of pharmacotherapy for psychiatric disorders: A critical survey of animal and translational models and perspectives for their improvement. In R. A. McArthur & F. Borsini (Eds.), *Animal and translational models for CNS drug discovery (Vol. 1*, pp. 1–57). Burlington, MA: Academic Press.

Mills, E. J., Rachlis, B., Wu, P., Devereaux, P. J., Arora, P., & Perri, D. (2008). Primary prevention of cardiovascular mortality and events with statin treatments: A network meta-analysis involving more than 65,000 patients. *Journal of the American College of Cardiology, 52*, 1769–1781.

Milne, G. M., Jr. (2003). Pharmaceutical productivity – the imperative for new paradigms. *Annual Reports in Medicinal Chemistry, 38*, 383–396.

Miyazaki, T., Fujiki, H., Yamamura, Y., Nakamura, S., & Mori, T. (2007). Tolvaptan, an orally active vasopressin V2-receptor antagonist – pharmacology and clinical trials. *Cardiovascular Drug Reviews, 25*, 1–13.

Moos, W. H., & Mirsalis, J. C. (2009). Nonprofit organizations and pharmaceutical research and development. *Drug Development Research, 70*, in press.

Neal, B., MacMahon, S., Chapman, N., & Blood Pressure Lowering Treatment Trialists' Collaboration. (2000). Effects of ACE inhibitors, calcium antagonists, and other blood-pressure-lowering drugs: Results of prospectively designed overviews of randomised trials. Blood Pressure Lowering Treatment Trialists' Collaboration. *Lancet, 356*, 1955–1964.

O'Collins V. E., Macleod, M. R., Donnan, G. A., Horky, L. L., van der Worp, B. H., & Howells, D. W. (2006). 1,026 experimental treatments in acute stroke. *Annals of Neurology, 59*, 467–477.

Parascandola, J. (1986). The development of receptor theory. In M. J. Parnham & J. Bruinvels (Eds.), *Pharmacological methods, receptors & chemotherapy (Vol. 3*, pp. 129–158). Amsterdam: Elsevier/North Holland.

Perel, P., Roberts, E., Sena, E., Wheble, P., Briscoe, C., Sandercock, P., et al. (2007). Comparison of treatment effects between animal experiments and clinical trials: Systematic review. *British Medical Journal, 334*, 197–202.

Polgar, D., Leisser, C., Maier, S., Strasser, S., Ruger, B., Dettle, M., et al. (2005). Truncated ALK derived from chromosomal translocation t(2;5)(p23;q35) binds to the SH3 domain of p85-PI3K. *Mutatation Research, 570*, 9–15.

Powers, E. T., Morimoto, R. I., Dillin, A., Kelly, J. W., & Balch, W. E. (2009). Biological and chemical approaches to diseases of proteostasis deficiency. *Annual Review of Biochemistry, 78*, 959–991.

Preusch, P. C. (2004). Integrative and organ systems pharmacology: A new initiative from the National Institute of General Medical Sciences. *Molecular Interventions, 4*, 72–73.

Ramsey, S., & Scoggins, J. (2008). Commentary: Practicing on the tip of the information iceberg? Evidence of underpublication or registered clinical trials in oncology. *Oncologist, 13*, 925–929.

Rang, H. P. (2006). The receptor concept: Pharmacology's big idea. *British Journal of Pharmacology, 147*, S9–S16.

Rice, A. S. C., Cimino-Brown, D., Eisenach, J. C., Kontinen, V. K., Lacroix-Fralish, M., Machin, J. J., et al. (2008). Animal models and the prediction of efficacy in clinical trials of analgesic drugs: A critical appraisal and call for uniform reporting standards. *Pain, 139*, 243–247.

Rino, J., & Carmo-Fonseca, M. (2009). The spliceosome: A self-organized macromolecular amchine in the nucleus. *Trends in Cell Biology*. doi:10.1016/j.tcb.2009.05.004

Romine, W. O., Goodall, M. C., Peterson, J., & Bradley, R. J. (1974). The acetylcholine receptor. Isolation of a brain nicotinic receptor and its preliminary characterization in lipid bilayer membranes. *Biochimica et Biophysica ACTA, 367*, 316–325.

Roth, B. L., Sheffler, D. J., & Kroeze, W. K. (2004). Magic shotguns versus magic bullets: Selectively non-selective drugs for mood disorders and schizophrenia. *Nature Reviews. Drug Discovery, 3*, 353–359.

Rueter, L. F., Honore, P., & Bitner, R. S. (2006). The promise and limitation SOF broad sprectrum analgesics: Nicotinic acetylcholine receptors as potential candidates. In A. Lucas (Ed.), *Frontiers in pain research* (pp. 73–99). Hauppage, NY: Nova.

Ruggeri, B., Miknyoczki, S., Dorsey, B., & Hui, A.-M. (2009). The development and pharmacology of proteasome inhibitors for the management and treatment of cancer. *Advances in Pharmacology, 57*, 91–135.

Rupprecht, R., Rammes, G., Eser, D., Baghai, T. C., Schule, C., Nothdurfter, C., et al. (2009). Translocator protein (18 kD) as target for anxiolytics without benzodiazepine-like side effects. *Science, 325*, 490–493.

Schreiber, S. L. (2000). Target-oriented and diversity-oriented organic synthesis in drug discovery. *Science, 287*, 1964–1969.

Shaywitz, D., & Taleb, N. (2008, July, 29). Drug research needs serendipity. *Financial Times*. Retrieved November 8, 2008 from http://www.ft.com/cms/s/0/b735787c-5d9b-11dd-8129-000077b07658.html Accessed 8/11/08.

Shealy, D. J., & Visvanathans, S. (2008). Anti-TNF antibodies: Lessons from the past, roadmap for the future. *Handbook of Experimental Pharmacology, 181*, 101–129. Therapeutic Antibodies. Y. Chernajovsky & A. Nissim (Eds.).

Silberman, S. (2009). The placebo problem. *Wired*, September, 2009, 128/136.

Sneader, W. (2005). *Drug discovery: A history*. Chichester: Wiley.

Snyder, S. H. (2008). *Science and psychiatry. Groundbreaking discoveries in molecular neuroscience*, Washington, DC: American Psychiatric Press.

Sung, N. S., Crowley, W. F. Jr., Genel, M., Salber, P., Sandy, L., Sherwood, L. M., et al. (2003). Central challenges facing the national clinical research enterprise. *JAMA, 289*, 1278–1287.

Task Force on Beta-Blockers of the European Society of Cardiology. (2004). Expert consensus document on ß-adrenergic receptor blockers. *European Heart Journal, 25*, 1341–1362.

Tummino, P. J., & Copeland, R. A. (2008). Residence time of receptor-ligand complexes and its effect on biological function. *Biochemistry, 47*, 5481–5492.

Turner, E. H., Matthews, A. M., Linardatos, E., Tell, R. A., & Rosenthal, R. (2008). Selective publication of antidepressant trials and its influence on apparent efficacy. *New England Journal of Medicine, 358,* 252–260.

Turner, E. H., & Rosenthal, R. (2008). Efficacy of antidepressants. *BMJ, 336,* 516–517.

Uher, R., Huezo-Diaz, P., Perroud, N., Smith, R., Rietschel, M., Mors, O., et al. (2009). Genetic predictors of response to antidepressants in the GENDEP project. *Pharmacogenomics Journal, 9,* 225–233.

van der Greef, J., & McBurney, R. N. (2005). Rescuing drug discovery: *In vivo* systems pathology and systems pharmacology. *Nature Reviews. Drug Discovery, 4,* 961–967.

Villamil, A., Chrysant, S. G., Calhoun, D., Schober, B., Hsu, H., Matrisciano-Dimichino, L., et al. (2007). Renin inhibition with aliskiren provides additive antihypertensive efficacy when used in combination with hydrochlorothiazide. *Journal of Hypertension, 25,* 217–226.

Vogelstein, B., quoted in Hayden, E. C. (2008). Cancer complexity slows quest for cure. *Nature, 455,* 148.

Volkow, N. D., & Li, T. K. (2004). Drug addiction: The neurobiology of behavior gone awry. *Nature Reviews. Neuroscience, 5,* 963–970.

Wehling, M. (2008). Translational medicine: Science or wishful thinking? *Journal of Translational Medicine, 6,* 31. doi:10.1186/1479-5876-6-31.

Wehling, M. (2009). Assessing the translatability of drug projects: What needs to be scored to predict success? *Nature Reviews. Drug Discovery, 8,* 541–546.

Weisbach, J. A., & Moos, W. H. (1995). Diagnosing the decline of major pharmaceutical research laboratories: A prescription for drug companies. *Drug Development Research, 34,* 243–259.

Whiteside, G. T., Adedoyin, A., & Leventhal, L. (2008). Predictive validity of animal pain models? A comparison of the pharmacokinetic–pharmacodynamic relationship for pain drugs in rats and humans. *Neuropharmacology, 54,* 767–775.

Wilgenbus, K., Hill, R., Warrander, A., Kakkar, S., Steiness, E., & Wessel, R. (2007). What pharma wants. *Nature Biotechnology, 25,* 967–969.

Wisniewski, S. R., Rush, A. J., Nierenberg, A. A., Gaynes, B. N., Warden, D., Luther, J. L., et al. (2009). Can phase III trial results of antidepressant medications be generalized to clinical practice? A STAR*D report. *American Journal of Psychiatry, 166,* 599–607.

Williams, M. (2004). A return to the fundamentals of drug discovery? *Current Opinion in Investigational Drugs, 5,* 1–3.

Williams, M. (2005). Systems and integrative biology as alternative guises for pharmacology: Prime time for an iPharm concept? *Biochemical Pharmacology, 70,* 1707–1716.

Williams, M. (2008). Perseverance furthers? The role of the drug hunter in the postgenomic era. *Current Opinion in Investigational Drugs, 9,* 21–27.

Williams, M. (2009). Progress in Alzheimer's disease drug discovery: An update. *Current Opinion in Investigational Drugs, 10,* 23–34.

Wong, D. T., Perry, K. W., & Bymaster, F. P. (2005). The discovery of fluoxetine hydrochloride (prozac). *Nature Reviews. Drug Discovery, 4,* 764–774.

Woolf, C. J. (2008a). Novel analgesic development: From target to patient or patient to target? *Current Opinion in Investigational Drugs, 9,* 694–695.

Woolf, S. H. (2008b). The meaning of translational research and why it matters. *JAMA, 299,* 211–213.

Wu, J. J., Quijano, C., Chen, E., Liu, H., Cao, L., Fergusson, M. M., et al. (2009). Mitochondrial dysfunction and oxidative stress mediate the physiological impairment induced by the disruption of autophagy. *Aging, 1,* 425–437.

Young, D. (2009). Collins: End of stimulus funds could send NIH off cliff in '11. *BioWorld Today, 20*(158), 1/6.

Zambrowicz, B. P., & Sands, A. T. (2003). Knockouts model the 100 best-selling drugs – will they model the next 100? *Nature Reviews. Drug Discovery, 2*, 38–51.

Zerhouni, E. (2003). The NIH roadmap, *Science, 302*, 63–72.

Zhang, J., Yang, P. L., & Gray, N. S. (2009). Targeting cancer with small molecule kinase inhibitors. *Nature Reviews Cancer, 9*, 28–39.

Khosrow Kashfi

Department of Physiology and Pharmacology, Sophie Davis School of Biomedical
Education, The City College of The City University of New York, New York, 10031

Anti-Inflammatory Agents as Cancer Therapeutics

Abstract

Cancer prevention sometimes referred to as *tertiary prevention* or
chemoprevention makes use of specific xenobiotics or drugs to prevent,
delay, or retard the development of cancer. Over the last two decades or
so cancer prevention has made significant strides. For example, prevention
of lung cancer through smoking cessation; cervical cancer prevention
through regular Pap smear tests; colon cancer prevention through screening
colonoscopy; and prostate cancer reductions by prostate-specific antigen
measurements in conjunction with regular prostate examinations.
The seminal epidemiological observation that nonsteroidal anti-inflammatory drugs (NSAIDs) prevent colon and other cancers has provided the

Advances in Pharmacology, Volume 57
© 2009 Elsevier Inc. All rights reserved.

1054-3589/08 $35.00
10.1016/S1054-3589(08)57002-5

impetus to develop novel chemoprevention approaches against cancer. To that end, a number of "designer drugs" have been synthesized that are in different stages of development, evaluation, and deployment. Some include the cyclooxygenase-2-specific inhibitors (coxibs), nitric oxide-releasing NSAIDs (NO-NSAIDs and NONO-NSAIDs), hydrogen sulfide-releasing NSAIDs, modulators of the lipoxygenase pathway, prostanoid receptor blockers, and chemokine receptor antagonists. In addition to these novel agents, there are also a host of naturally occurring compounds/micronutrients that have chemopreventive properties. This chapter reviews these classes of compounds, their utility and mechanism(s) of action against the background of mediators that link inflammation and cancer.

I. Introduction

A. Inflammation and Its Connection to Neoplastic Progression

Inflammation as a fundamental response to injury has been recognized for many thousands of years. The Egyptians described abscesses and ulcers, and the Code of Hammurabi (2000 BC) detailed instructions on how to treat abscesses of the eye (Eisen, 1977). The Greek physician, Hippocrates may have been the first to regard inflammation as the beginning of a healing process, introducing words such as *edema* and *erysipelas* to describe its symptoms. The first comprehensive description of inflammatory symptoms can be found in *De Medicina*, written by Aulus Celsus (~25 BC–AD 38) who described the four symptoms of inflammation as *rubor, tumor, color*, and *dolor* (redness, swelling, heat, and pain; Ley, 2001). The fifth sign of inflammation, *functio laesa* (impaired function) was added by Galen of Pergamon some 100 years later (Ley, 2001). Figure 1 shows a cartoon depicting the five cardinal signs of inflammation (Lawrence, Willoughby, & Gilroy, 2002).

The functional relationship between inflammation and cancer was first proposed by Virchow in 1863, who noted the presence of leukocytes in neoplastic tissues (Balkwill & Mantovani, 2001). Since then, a considerable body of evidence has supported the concept that tumors can originate at the sites of infection or chronic inflammation (Mueller & Fusenig, 2004).

Acute inflammation is an adaptive host defense mechanism against infection or injury and is self-limiting; however, chronic inflammation may lead to various ailments including cancer (Schottenfeld & Beebe-Dimmer, 2006). For example, inflammatory diseases increase the risk of developing bladder, cervical, gastric, intestinal, esophageal, ovarian, prostate, and thyroid cancers (Mantovani, Allavena, Sica, & Balkwill, 2008). Key features of cancer-related inflammation include the infiltration of white blood cells, tumor-associated macrophages (TAMs), cytokines such as interleukin (IL)-1, IL-6, tumor necrosis factor-α (TNF-α), chemokines such as (C-C

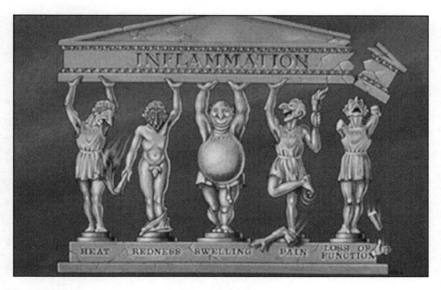

FIGURE 1   Cardinal signs of inflammation. This cartoon depicts five Greeks representing the cardinal signs of inflammation—heat, redness, swelling, pain, and loss of function. Reproduced with permission from *Nature Reviews Immunology, 2,* 787–795, copyright (2002) Macmillan Publishers Ltd.

motif) ligand 2 (CCL2) and CXCL8, acceleration of cell cycle progression and cell proliferation, evasion from apoptosis, and stimulation of tumor angiogenesis (Colotta, Allavena, Sica, Garlanda, & Mantovani, 2009; Kundu & Surh, 2008). Other evidence that links cancer and inflammation include the following: nonsteroidal anti-inflammatory drug (NSAID) use reducing the risk and mortality from certain cancers such as colon (Thun, Henley, & Patrono, 2002) and breast (Takkouche, Regueira-Mendez, & Etminan, 2008); inflammatory cells, chemokines and cytokines being present in the microenvironment of all tumors (Balkwill & Mantovani, 2001; Negus, Stamp, Hadley, & Balkwill, 1997); tumors further augmenting the inflammatory response by secreting cytokines and chemokines (Ariztia, Lee, Gogoi, & Fishman, 2006; Ben-Baruch, 2003), thus setting up a positive feed forward loop between inflammation and cancer (Ben-Baruch, 2003; Wyckoff et al., 2004); and finally, targeting inflammatory mediators such as IL-1 (Voronov et al., 2003) and TNF-α (Szlosarek & Balkwill, 2003) and transcription factors such as nuclear factor kappa-light-chain-enhancer of activated B cells (NF-κB) (Karin, 2006) and Signal transducer and activator of transcription 3 (STAT3) (Yu, Kortylewski, & Pardoll, 2007) decreases the incidence and spread of cancer (Mantovani et al., 2008).

Recently, two pathways (Fig. 2) have been proposed linking inflammation and cancer (Mantovani et al., 2008). An *extrinsic* pathway, driven by

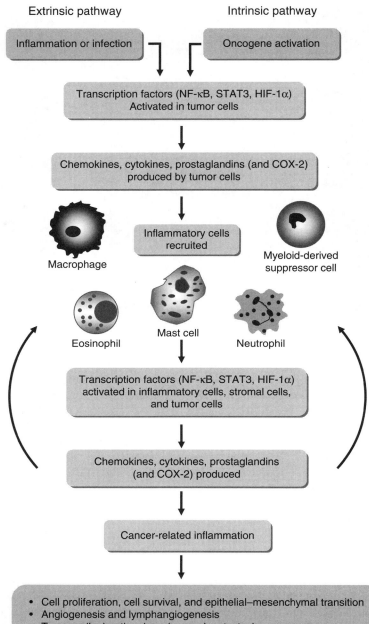

Extrinsic pathway   Intrinsic pathway

Inflammation or infection   Oncogene activation

Transcription factors (NF-κB, STAT3, HIF-1α)
Activated in tumor cells

Chemokines, cytokines, prostaglandins (and COX-2)
produced by tumor cells

Inflammatory cells
recruited

Macrophage

Myeloid-derived
suppressor cell

Eosinophil   Mast cell   Neutrophil

Transcription factors (NF-κB, STAT3, HIF-1α)
activated in inflammatory cells, stromal cells,
and tumor cells

Chemokines, cytokines, prostaglandins
(and COX-2) produced

Cancer-related inflammation

- Cell proliferation, cell survival, and epithelial–mesenchymal transition
- Angiogenesis and lymphangiogenesis
- Tumor cell migration, invasion, and metastasis
- Inhibition of adaptive immunity
- Altered response to hormones and chemotherapeutic agents

inflammatory conditions that increase cancer risk (e.g., inflammatory bowel disease); and an *intrinsic* pathway, driven by genetic alterations that cause inflammation and cancer (such as oncogenes). Proinflammatory cytokines (Balkwill, 2009) intersect these two pathways. Leukocytes are then recruited and activated. The cytokines activate the same key transcription factors in inflammatory cells, stromal cells, and tumor cells, resulting in more inflammatory mediators being produced and a cancer-related inflammatory microenvironment is then generated.

In both tumor and inflammatory cells, NF-κB is activated downstream of the toll-like receptor (TLR)-MyD88 pathway, and of the inflammatory cytokines TNF-α and IL-1. NF-κB induces the expression of inflammatory cytokines, adhesion molecules, cyclooxygenase-2 (COX-2), nitric oxide synthase (NOS), and angiogenic factors (Colotta et al., 2009). The role of NF-κB signaling in cancer development and progression has been reviewed elsewhere (Karin, 2006; Okamoto, Sanda, & Asamitsu, 2007). Needless to say, that an array of chemopreventive or chemotherapeutic agents target this transcription factor.

Akin to the two pathways discussed above, there are inducers and mediators of inflammation (Medzhitov, 2008). Inducers are the signals that initiate the inflammatory response, thus activating specialized sensors, which, in turn, promote production of specific mediators that alter the functional status of tissues and organs. Inducers may be (1) exogenous, either microbial (pathogen-associated molecular patterns, that function through dedicated receptors, and virulence factors) or nonmicrobial (allergens, irritants, toxic compounds) and (2) endogenous are signals produced by stressed or damaged tissues (Medzhitov, 2008). Inflammatory mediators can be classified into seven groups (Majno & Joris, 2004)

FIGURE 2   Pathways that connect inflammation and cancer. Cancer and inflammation are connected by two pathways: the intrinsic pathway and the extrinsic pathway. The intrinsic pathway is activated by genetic events that cause neoplasia. These events include the activation of various types of oncogene by mutation, chromosomal rearrangement or amplification, and the inactivation of tumor-suppressor genes. Cells that are transformed in this manner produce inflammatory mediators, thereby generating an inflammatory microenvironment in tumors for which there is no underlying inflammatory condition (e.g., breast tumors). By contrast, in the extrinsic pathway, inflammatory or infectious conditions augment the risk of developing cancer at certain anatomical sites (e.g., the colon, prostate, and pancreas). The two pathways converge and activate NF-κB, STAT3, and Hypoxia-inducible factor (HIF)-1α, in tumor cells. These, in turn, coordinate the production cytokines and chemokines, as well as the production of COX-2 derived PGE$_2$, which, in turn, recruit and activate various leukocytes. The cytokines activate the same key transcription factors in inflammatory cells, stromal cells, and tumor cells, resulting in more inflammatory mediators being produced and a cancer-related inflammatory microenvironment being generated. Reproduced with permission from *Nature, 454*, 436–444, copyright (2008) Macmillan Publishers Ltd.

according to their biochemical properties: vasoactive amines (histamine and serotonin), vasoactive peptides (substance P), fragments of complement components (anaphylatoxins, C3a, C4a, C5a), lipid mediators (eicosanoids, platelet-activating factors), inflammatory cytokines (TNF-α, IL-1, IL-6), chemokines, and proteolytic enzymes (elastin, cathepsins, matrix metallo-proteinases) (Medzhitov, 2008).

B. Chemokines and Cancer

Chemokines are a family of small (8–14 kDa) chemotactic cytokines comprising more than 46 members (Mackay, 2001). They are divided into four groups, C, CC, CXC, and CX3C, according to the number and spacing of the first two cysteine residues in the amino-terminal part of the protein. The CXC family can be further subdivided into two categories depending on the presence or absence of an "ELR motif" (glutamic acid–leucine–arginine) preceding the first cysteine residue in the protein (Strieter, Belperio, Phillips, & Keane, 2004). They function through G protein-coupled receptors (GPCRs) (Slettenaar & Wilson, 2006) that are one of the most important drug targets, with more than 30% of all US-marketed therapeutics directed toward them (Hopkins & Groom, 2002). To date, 19 chemokine receptors have been identified which are expressed on a variety of cells including immune cells, endothelial cells, and neurons; they are either constitutively activated or induced by cytokines (Horuk, 2001). Each receptor has a repertoire of chemokine ligands that can activate it. These range from CCR1, which has at least nine ligands, to specific receptors such as CCR8, which has only one (Murphy et al., 2000). Thus, it seems that there is a great degree of redundancy in the chemokine receptor system. This is accentuated further by the fact that some chemokines can bind with high affinity to more than one receptor; for example, CCL5 (or RANTES) can bind to CCR1, CCR3, and CCR5. By contrast, others such as CCL1 (or I-309) bind only a single receptor. In addition, chemokines that are agonists on one receptor can be antagonists for others (Ogilvie, Bardi, Clark-Lewis, Baggiolini, & Uguccioni, 2001).

Most cancers express an extensive network of chemokines and che-mokine receptors (Balkwill & Mantovani, 2001; Vicari & Caux, 2002). Selected chemokine receptors are often upregulated in a large number of common human cancers, including those of the breast, lung, prostate, colon, and melanoma (Tanaka et al., 2005; Vicari & Caux, 2002). Tumor-associated chemokines have at least five roles in the biology of primary and metastatic disease (Murphy, 2001): (1) control of leukocyte infiltration into the tumor, CCL2 is one of the most frequently detected CC chemokines in cancer (Mantovani et al., 2004), high levels of CCL5 are expressed stage II and III cancer (Luboshits et al., 1999; Yaal-Hahoshen et al., 2006); (2) manipulation of tumor immune response, regulatory

T cells express the chemokine receptor CCR4 and are attracted into ovarian cancer by tumor- and macrophage-derived CCL22 (Curiel et al., 2004); (3) regulation of angiogenesis, CXC chemokines regulate angiogenesis either positively or negatively depending on the presence or absence of the ELR motif (Strieter et al., 2004); (4) actions such as autocrine or paracrine growth and survival factors, CXCL1-3 are upregulated in melanoma and stimulate the growth of melanoma cells (Dhawan & Richmond, 2002), CXCL1 and CXCL8 stimulate proliferation of pancreatic cancer cells (Takamori, Oades, Hoch, Burger, & Schraufstatter, 2000); and (5) direct the movement of tumor cell themselves, stimulation of CXCR4-positive cancer cells with CXCL12 results in direct migration/invasion of cancer cells (Scotton, Wilson, Milliken, Stamp, & Balkwill, 2001). These have been reviewed in Slettenaar and Wilson (2006).

Examples of chemokines that are anti-carcinogenic are few. CCL2 has anticancer properties in pancreatic cancer, patients with high circulating CCL2 levels had higher survival rates than those with low levels, this effect was through macrophages (Monti et al., 2003).

II. Blocking Chemokines and or Chemokine Receptors as Approaches to Cancer Therapy

Targeting specific chemokines derived from tumors that may affect tumor angiogenesis are a promising area for the future. Antibodies to neutralize CXCL5 and CXCL8 reduced tumor growth, vascularity, and metastasis in experimental models of nonsmall-cell lung cancer (Arenberg et al., 1998, 1996). Neutralizing antibodies to CCL20 inhibited the growth of prostate cancer cells that overexpress CXCR4 in a tumor xenograft model (Beider et al., 2009).

Higher expression levels of selected chemokine receptors have been reported in many cancer cells compared to their normal counterparts. A partial list includes, for breast (CXCR3, CXCR4, CCR7, CXCR7, CCR5),ovarian (CXCR4), prostate (CXCR4, CXCR5, CCR9, CCR5, CX3CR1), pancreas (CXCR4, CXCR1/2, CCR6), bladder (CXCR4), colon (CXCR3, CXCR4, CCR6, CCR7, CXCR1/2), stomach (CCR7), and thyroid (CXCR4) (Wu, Lee, Chevalier, & Hwang, 2009). It appears that three receptors, CCR7, CXCR4, and CXCR7, are prominently expressed in cancer and more specifically in metastasis (Meijer, Ogink, & Roos, 2008; Zlotnik, 2006). Preclinical data suggest that inhibition of CXCR4 by neutralizing antibodies, siRNA against CXCR4, and antagonists such as AMD3100, MSX-122, or CTCE-9908, inhibit growth and reduce metastasis (Kim et al., 2008; Liang et al., 2004; Slettenaar & Wilson, 2006; Yoon et al., 2007). Another peptide-based CXCR4 receptor antagonist, TN14003, inhibited primary tumor growth and metastasis of head and neck cancer

TABLE I   Chemokine Receptor Antagonists Currently in Clinical Trials for Treatment
of Cancer

Target	Compound, company	Development status	Disease
CCR2	CNTO-888, Centocor	Phase I	Solid tumor
CCR4	KW-0761, Kyowa	Phase I	Haematological cancer
CCR9	CCX-282B, Chemocentrux	Phase II/III	IBD
	CCX-025, Chemocentrux	Phase I	IBD
CXCr4	AMD-3100, Gemzyme/Arnor Med	Phase II/III	Multiple myeloma, Non-Hodgkin's Lymphoma (NHL)
	CTCE-9908, Chemokine Therapeutics	Phase I	Ovarian/liver cancer
	MSX-122, Metastatix	Phase I (suspended)	Advanced solid tumor

This is a partial list as it pertains to cancer. There are a number of other clinical trials evaluating
potential agents and targets for, rheumatoid arthritis, multiple sclerosis, chronic obstructive
pulmonary disease, HIV, diabetes, asthma, and transplant rejection. Adapted from Wu and Lee
(2009).

cells in a mouse xenograft model (Yoon et al., 2007). Table I provides a
partial list of chemokine receptor antagonists currently in clinical trials
for treatment of cancer together with their status and the companies
involved.

Another possible use of chemokine receptor antagonists is to block angiogenesis. For example, neutralization of CXCR4 with blocking antibodies
resulted in a delay in tumor formation by CXCR4-expressing colon 38 tumor
cells, through inhibition of angiogenesis (Guleng et al., 2005).

III. Evidence that NSAIDs Protect Against Cancer

"An aspirin a day may keep cancer away." Cancer prevention entered a
new era with the observation that subjects using NSAIDs had lower incidence of colorectal cancer (Kune, Kune, & Watson, 1988). Over 30 epidemiological studies, collectively describing results on more than 1 million
subjects, have established NSAIDs as the prototypical chemopreventive
agents against many forms of cancer. In particular, three well-designed
randomized, double-blind trials of aspirin as a chemopreventive agent
against colorectal adenomas established its chemopreventive effect (Baron
et al., 2003; Benamouzig et al., 2003; Sandler et al., 2003). While this work
provided a much-needed proof of principle, it also made it clear that aspirin
may not be optimal for cancer prevention because of its shortcomings in

safety and efficacy. All studies to date strongly suggest that NSAIDs reduce the incidence of and mortality from colon cancer by about half (Wallace & Del Soldato, 2003). The use of NSAIDs is limited by their significant toxicity, which includes (1) gastrointestinal (GI) side effects, which range from dyspepsia to GI bleeding, obstruction, and perforation; (2) renal side effects; and (3) a large number of additional side effects, some of which are serious, ranging from hypersensitivity reactions to the distinct salicylate intoxication. Among patients using NSAIDs, up to 4% per year suffer serious GI complications and more than 8,000 deaths (Bjorkman, 1999). The gastric damage is caused through two mechanisms: (1) direct epithelial damage as a result of their acidic properties and (2) breakdown of mucosal defense mechanisms (leukocyte adherence, decreases in blood flow, and bicarbonate and mucus secretions) due to a reduction of mucosal prostaglandin (PG) synthesis (Wallace, 2008).

A. The COX Cascade

Cancer prevention by NSAIDs is, at least conceptually, largely based on effects on the eicosanoid pathways. In the presence of molecular oxygen, the COX (PGH2 synthase) pathway, through the COX component of PGH_2 synthase, produces the unstable intermediate PGG_2, which is rapidly converted to PGH_2 by the peroxidase activity of PGH_2 synthase. Specific isomerases convert PGH_2 to various PGs and thromboxane A_2 (TxA_2) (Kashfi & Rigas, 2005). Two isoforms of COX have been well characterized (Vane, Bakhle, & Botting, 1998). COX-1 is constitutively expressed in most tissues and is responsible for platelet aggregation, renal blood flow, and maintenance of the gastric mucosa. COX-1 is inhibited by traditional NSAIDs either reversibly or irreversibly, depending on the NSAID. COX-2, identified as an inducible isoform in inflamed and neoplastic tissues, is expressed constitutively in human kidney and brain.

The clinical usefulness of NSAIDs together with their serious side effects prompted the search for a "better NSAID." This led to the development of selective COX-2 inhibitors—the coxibs.

B. COX-2 Inhibition in Cancer Prevention

Since human colon cancers have elevated PGE_2 levels compared to uninvolved mucosa (Bennett, Civier, Hensby, Melhuish, & Stamford, 1987; Rigas, Goldman, & Levine, 1993) and COX-2 is overexpressed in 45% of colon adenomas and 85% of colon carcinomas (Eberhart et al., 1994), it was proposed that inhibition of COX-2, the isoform overexpressed in cancer, would arrest carcinogenesis. Extensive preclinical data supported this approach. Multiple cell culture studies indicated the potential efficacy of coxibs against cancer (Dannenberg & Subbaramaiah, 2003). In animal studies, deletion of COX-2 significantly decreased the number of intestinal tumors in Apc^{4716} mice (Oshima et al., 1996); interestingly, COX-1 deletion, also attenuated tumor formation in the same mice (Chulada et al., 2000). Animal studies using specific COX-2 inhibitors provided further support for the concept that COX-2 inhibition both prevents and regresses tumors arising from a variety of tissues, including colon, lung, breast, pancreas, and skin (Dannenberg & Subbaramaiah, 2003). This work, together with clinical trials (Steinbach et al., 2000), culminated in celecoxib receiving FDA approval for its use in patients with familial adenomatous polyposis.

The concept that COX-2 was central to carcinogenesis was challenged very early on when it was shown that both sulindac sulfide and piroxicam induced apoptosis in COX-2-expressing HT-29 and the COX-2-deficient HCT 15 human colon cancer cells (Hanif et al., 1996). Similar results were also reported with the COX-2-selective inhibitor, NS-398, in HT-29 and S/KS (COX-2-negative) human colon cancer cell lines (Elder, Halton, Hague, & Paraskeva, 1997). It is now well recognized that in addition to COX, traditional NSAIDs and coxibs can modulate many different signaling pathways such as NF-κB, phosphodiesterases, NSAID-activated gene (NAG-1), peroxisome proliferator-activated receptors (PPARs), the Wnt pathway, and cell kinetic effects (Kashfi & Rigas, 2005; Soh & Weinstein, 2003).

C. Cardiovascular Side Effects of NSAIDs

In patients with a low risk for GI damage, coxibs have been successful in limiting the upper GI ulceration associated with traditional NSAIDs (reviewed in 2008). However, in patients with comorbidities or other factors that increase the risk of GI ulceration, the benefits of coxibs over traditional NSAIDs is significantly reduced (Wallace, Viappiani, & Bolla, 2009).

Several large-scale clinical trials have shown that long-term use of coxibs and even traditional NSAIDs is associated with an increased risk of adverse myocardial events (2008; Antman et al., 2007). For example, the APPROVe (Adenomatous Polyp Prevention on Vioxx) study that was launched to evaluate the efficacy of rofecoxib in patients with previous history of colorectal adenomas showed that 3.5% of rofecoxib recipients and 1.9% of placebo recipients suffered myocardial infarctions or strokes during the trial. This prompted the termination of this and all related trials and voluntary withdrawal of rofecoxib. Inhibition of COX-2 in the vasculature leading to a reduction in prostacyclin (PGI_2) levels, thus reducing vasodilation with a consequence increase in thromboxane, was proposed as the underlying mechanism for this increased risk (FitzGerald & Patrono, 2001). However, other data strongly suggest that under certain conditions, traditional NSAIDs can also precipitate untoward cardiovascular events (Kearney et al., 2006). It has been suggested that COX-2 inhibition in the kidneys leading to decreases in PGI_2 could lead to increases in blood pressure and hence increases in myocardial infarctions and stroke (Singh et al., 2003).

IV. Inhibition of Prostanoid Receptors for Cancer Prevention

The physiological actions of the five primary prostanoids PGE_2, PGD_2, $PGF_{2\alpha}$, PGI_2, and TxA_2 are mediated, in part, via GPCRs. There are nine such receptors, eight of which (EP_{1-4}, DP, FP, IP, and TP) are classified according to the prostanoid ligand that each binds with greatest affinity (Breyer, Bagdassarian, Myers, & Breyer, 2001; Hata & Breyer, 2004). The ninth receptor, $CRTH_2$ or DP_2, is expressed on Th2 cells and binds PGD_2 (Hirai et al., 2001) (Fig. 3). The diverse effects of PGE_2 may result from its actions on four receptors, EP_{1-4}. The EP_2 and EP_4 (relaxant) receptors are G_s-type leading to cAMP accumulation; the EP_1 (constrictor) receptor increases intracellular calcium; and EP_3 (inhibitory) receptor is of the G_i-type. Activation of a given receptor may elicit varying responses in different cell types (Gardiner, 1986) and some may be quite important to cancer biology.

PGE_2 is believed to have an important role in colon cancer. Stimulation of EP_4 (but not EP_2) leads to phosphatidylinositol 3 (PI3)-kinase-dependent phosphorylation of extracellular signal-regulated kinase (ERK)1/2 (Fujino, Xu, & Regan, 2003); PI 3-kinase/EP_4 may also be involved in the wnt/β-catenin signaling pathway (Fujino, West, & Regan, 2002); EP_4 may modulate the PGE_2-stimulated proliferation of colon cancer cells (Pozzi et al., 2004).

PPAR-γ ligands inhibit human lung carcinoma cell growth by decreasing the expression of EP_2 receptors through ERK signaling and PPAR-γ-dependent and PPAR-γ-independent pathways (Han & Roman, 2004). IP, DP, and CRTH2 receptors are also coupled with the activation of G_s and linked to increases in cAMP; FP and TP signal by increasing intracellular calcium (Funk, 2001).

In a series of elegant experiments designed to determine the effects of prostanoid receptors on colon carcinogenesis, two approaches were used. The first, a genetic approach, examined the induction of aberrant crypt foci (ACFs) by the carcinogen azoxymethane (AOM) in knockout mice deficient in EP_{1-4}, DP, FP, IP, or TP (Mutoh et al., 2002; Watanabe et al., 1999). The results indicated that tumor reduction was only seen in EP_1 and EP_4 knockouts. The second approach made use of pharmacological antagonists of EP_1 and EP_4 receptors. Here using the AOM-induced ACF model and the *Min* mouse model, both EP_1 (ONO-8711 and ONO-8713) and EP_4 (ONO-AE2-227) receptor blockers reduced the number of ACFs and tumors formation, respectively (Mutoh et al., 2002; Niho et al., 2005; Watanabe et al., 1999). To ascertain the contribution of each of the two receptors to intestinal carcinogenesis, the combined effects of EP_1 and EP_4 antagonists were

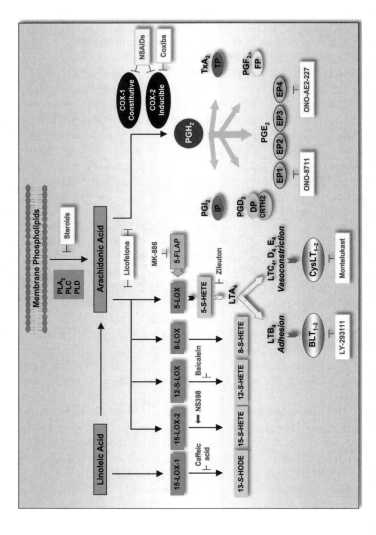

FIGURE 3 Overview of the eicosanoid pathway. Arachidonic acid, the substrate of the COX and LOX biosynthetic pathways, is derived from diet or synthesized from linoleic acid and is released from membrane phospholipids through a series of reactions requiring phospholipases. The COX pathway produces various prostaglandins and thromboxane; and the LOX pathways produce leukotrienes and hydroxyeicosatetraenoic acids. *Abbreviations:* phospholipases A₂, C, and D, PLA₂; PLC; PLD; prostaglandins (respective receptors), PGE₂ (EP₁₋₄); PGF₂α (FP); PGD₂ (DP, CRTH2); prostacyclin, PGI₂ (IP); thromboxane A₂, TxA₂ (TP). Leukotrienes, LTA₄, LTB₄, LTC₄, LTD₄, LTE₄; LTB₄ receptors, BLT₁₋₂; LTC₄, LTD₄, LTE₄ receptors, CysLT₁₋₂. 13-*S*-Hydroxyoctadecadienoic acid, 13-*S*-HODE; hydroxyeicosatetraenoic acid, HETE. T-shaped arrows: inhibition.

evaluated in APC1309 mice (Kitamura et al., 2003). The results showed additive effects of the two antagonists indicating independent mechanisms of action. Thus, combination treatment has potential for the chemoprevention of colon carcinogenesis.

Regarding other EP receptor types, the number of intestinal polyps in EP_2-deficient APC^{4716} mice was lower compared to the number of polyps in their APC^{4716} counterparts (Sonoshita et al., 2001). In contrast, enhancement of AOM-induced colon cancer development occurs in EP_3 knockout mice (Shoji et al., 2004). It should be noted that in most human colon cancer cell lines, EP_3 expression was not detectable and mRNA expression for EP_3 in human colon cancer was lower compared to normal mucosa (Shoji et al., 2004).

Aromatase, a product of the *CYP19* gene, catalyzes the synthesis of estrogens from androgens (Simpson et al., 1994). Aromatase-dependent estrogen biosynthesis has been linked to hormone-dependent breast carcinogenesis, and PGE_2 is a potent inducer of *CYP19* transcription via a cAMP-dependent mechanism *in vitro* (Cai, Kwintkiewicz, Young, & Stocco, 2007). Using agonists and antagonists of EP_2 and EP_4 receptors, together with mice that overexpressed COX-2 in the mammary gland and those in which the EP_2 receptor had been knocked out, it was determined that PGE_2 via EP_2 and EP_4 activates the cAMP $\rightarrow$ PKA $\rightarrow$ cAMP response element binding (CREB) pathway resulting in reciprocal changes in the interaction between breast cancer 1, early onset (BRCA1), p300, and the aromatase promoter I.3/II, which contributes, in turn, to enhanced *CYP19* transcription and increased aromatase activity (Subbaramaiah, Hudis, Chang, Hla, & Dannenberg, 2008). Thus, inhibitors of this pathway, including antagonists of EP_2 and EP_4, may be useful in reducing the risk of breast cancer.

V. LOX Cascades

Lipoxygenases (LOXs) are a family of nonheme iron-containing dioxygenases that are designated 5-, 8-, 12-, and 15-LOX, based on their regiospecificity of interaction with arachidonic acid (Funk, 2001) (Fig. 3). LOX metabolite levels are elevated in various cancers, including colon, breast, prostate, lung, skin, and esophageal (Kashfi & Rigas, 2005). Some LOX products are procarcinogenic, while others are anticarcinogenic (Shureiqi & Lippman, 2001).

The procarcinogenic LOXs and metabolites include 5-LOX and its products 5-(*S*)-hydroxyeicosatetraenoic acid (5-*S*-HETE) and LTB$_4$; 8-LOX and 8-*S*-HETE; and 12-*S*-LOX and 12-*S*-HETE. As shown in Fig. 3, 5-LOX, activated by the enzyme FLAP (5-LOX-activating protein, an 18-kDa membrane protein), converts arachidonic acid to 5-*S*-HETE, which, in turn, is converted to leukotrienes (LTs) LTA$_4$ and then to LTB$_4$ by a zinc metallohydrolase, LTA$_4$ hydrolase (Haeggstrom, 2000). LTs, potent inflammatory mediators, are synthesized in many cells and act through specific receptors. LTB_4 acts by stimulating members of BLT GPCRs (Poff & Balazy, 2004). LTD_4, LTE_4, and LTC_4 activate receptors belonging to the CysLT family (Capra, 2004) (Fig. 3). In several cancers (prostate, pancreatic, colon, testicular, and esophageal), 5-LOX is overexpressed and its manipulation may offer therapeutic or prevention opportunities (Kashfi & Rigas, 2005). Other procarcinogenic LOXs have been reviewed in Kashfi and Rigas (2005).

15-LOX-1 and 15-LOX-2 have anticarcinogenic effects. The preferred substrate for 15-LOX-1 is linoleic acid and for 15-LOX-2 is arachidonic acid (Brash, Boeglin, & Chang, 1997). 15-LOX-1 is the main enzyme for metabolizing linoleic acid into 13-S-HODE (Baer, Costello, & Green, 1991) and is the only 15-LOX isozyme found in the human colon epithelium (Ikawa, Kamitani, Calvo, Foley, & Eling, 1999). 13-S-HODE is linked to cellular differentiation and apoptosis, 15-LOX-1 expression levels are reduced in human colorectal cancers, NSAIDs induce its expression which is COX-2 independent (Shureiqi et al., 2000). Detailed review of anticarcinogenic LOXs has been given elsewhere (Kashfi & Rigas, 2005).

A. LOX Inhibitors

Modulation of the various LOX isozymes may be of therapeutic value. Such approaches to chemoprevention may include inhibition of 5-LOX, FLAP, and 12-S-LOX activities or the use of LT receptor antagonists. Some of these agents are briefly discussed below.

Early inhibitors of 5-LOX were nonselective antioxidants that had significant toxicity and lacked oral bioavailability (Kennedy, Chan, Ding, & Adrian, 2003). Zileuton, a specific 5-LOX inhibitor of N-hydroxyurea series (Carter et al., 1991), was the first orally active agent approved (1996) in the United States for treatment of bronchial asthma. It had antiproliferative properties in murine colon adenocarcinoma cell lines (Hussey & Tisdale, 1996). It prevented lung tumors and slowed the growth and progression of adenomas to carcinomas in mice treated with the carcinogen, vinyl carbamate (Gunning, Kramer, Lubet, Steele, & Pereira, 2000). In a xenograft model, using LoVo and HT-29 human colon cancer cells, zileuton inhibited tumor growth and reduced tumor mass (Melstrom et al., 2008). Zyflo, an extended release formulation of zileuton, in combination with celecoxib or alone reduced the incidence and size of pancreatic tumors in N-nitrosobis(2-oxopropyl)amine (BOP)-treated Syrian golden hamsters (Wenger et al., 2002). ABT-761 (Abbott Laboratories, IL, USA) is a second generation of hydroxyurea 5-LOX inhibitor which is much more potent than zileuton, a small placebo-controlled phase III clinical study in exercise-induced asthma demonstrated its clinical efficacy (Reid, 2001); however, in 2001 its development was discontinued (ThomsonPharma, 2009). There is considerable body of evidence linking LT signaling to the development of advanced atherosclerotic lesions (Back, 2009; Back &

Hansson, 2006; Funk, 2005). Hence, in 2005, ABT-761 was resurrected by VIA Pharmaceuticals (CA, USA) as VIA-2291 for the treatment of vascular inflammation in patients with atherosclerotic plaques. A phase II, randomized, double-blind, placebo-controlled study of VIA-2291 on atherosclerotic plaque and vascular inflammation in patients with carotid stenosis undergoing elective carotid endarterectomy was completed in 2008 (NCT00352417 at: http:// clinicaltrials.gov), the results of which are pending. In 2008, VIA initiated a phase II trial (NCT00552188; Fluorodeoxyglucose-positron emission tomography (FDG-PET) study) for vascular inflammation after an acute coronary syndrome event, this study is currently recruiting patients. There are no reports on the chemopreventive potentials of ABT-761/ VIA-2291.

AA-861 (Takeda) is a benzoquinone 5- and 12-LOX competitive inhibitor used for the treatment of bronchial asthma that has potent anti-inflammatory properties (Fujimura et al., 1986; Nakadate, Yamamoto, Aizu, & Kato, 1985). It has potent antiproliferative effects in leukemia (Tsukada, Nakashima, & Shirakawa, 1986), prostate (Ghosh & Myers, 1997), lung (Moody et al., 1998), esophageal (Hoque et al., 2005), bladder (Hayashi, Nishiyama, & Shirahama, 2006), colon (Ihara et al., 2007), breast (Hammamieh, Sumaida, Zhang, Das, & Jett, 2007), and neuroblastoma (Sveinbjornsson et al., 2008) cancer cell lines.

Two other LOX inhibitors, Nordihydroguaiaretic acid (NDGA) (GeroNova Research, NV, USA), a nonselective LOX inhibitor, and REV 5901 (Rhone-Poulenc Rorer Inc. merged with Hoechst Marion Roussel to form Aventis Pharma, PA, USA) a 5-LOX selective inhibitor, inhibited colon cancer cell proliferation in a time- and concentration-dependent manner (Melstrom et al., 2008).

B. FLAP Inhibitors

MK-886 (Merck, NJ, USA) is a potent inhibitor of FLAP that inhibits LT biosynthesis (Dixon et al., 1990; Miller et al., 1990). Its development for treatment of asthma was short lived when it was found that it inhibited a 50% of LT production in asthmatic patients (Friedman et al., 1993). MK-886 has chemopreventive properties in mice given the tobacco-specific carcinogen 4-(methylnitrosamino)-1-(3-pyridyl)-1-butanone (Rioux & Castonguay, 1998). In the vinyl carbamate model of lung cancer, MK-886 reduced lung tumor multiplicity by 37.8% and also decreased tumor size (Gunning, Kramer, Steele, & Pereira, 2002). MK-886 also inhibited intercellular adhesion molecule-1 (ICAM-1) in melanoma cells and may be useful for the treatment of melanoma metastasis (Wang et al., 2004). MK-886 inhibited isolated COX-1 activity and blocked the formation of the COX-1-derived products 12-HHT and TxB_2 in washed human platelets in response to collagen or exogenous arachidonic acid. Isolated COX-2 was less affected, and in A549 cells, MK-886 failed to suppress COX-2-dependent $PGF_{2\alpha}$ formation (Koeberle et al.,

2009). These observations indicate caution in interpreting data where MK-886 is used as a tool to determine the involvement of FLAP and/or 5-LOX pathways in respective experimental models.

Other FLAP inhibitors have also been developed for treatment of asthma, but have been abandoned due to poor clinical outcomes. For example, BAY-X1005 (Bayer, Leverkusen, Germany) was discontinued following disappointing phase III clinical trials (Steele et al., 1999).

C. LT Receptor Blockers

LTs exert their action through two GPCR classes, BLT receptors activated by LTB_4, and CysLT receptors activated by cysLTs (Brink et al., 2003). The BLT receptors are designated as BLT_1 and BLT_2, based on agonist affinity (Yokomizo, Izumi, & Shimizu, 2001). The receptors activated by cysLTs, $CysLT_1$ and $CysLT_2$, are characterized based on their sensitivity to antagonists developed for inhibition of LT-induced bronchoconstriction (Back, 2002).

Inhibition of LT receptors can also attenuate the actions of 5-LOX products. Pranlukast (Ono Pharmaceuticals, Tokyo, Japan) was the first LTD_4 receptor blocker to be introduced to the market acting at cysteinyl LT_1 receptor; however, it also blocks LTC_4 and LTE_4 (Keam, Lyseng-Williamson, & Goa, 2003). Montelukast (Merck) and zafirlukast (Merck) are other LTD_4 receptor antagonists used for the treatment of bronchial asthma. Studies evaluating the chemoprevention properties of these cysteinyl LT receptor blockers showed that pranlukast increased the sensitivity of human lung cancer cells to various chemotheraputic agents (Keam et al., 2003); zafirlukast reduced lung tumor multiplicity by 29.5% and decreased tumor size in a vinyl carbamate lung cancer model (Gunning et al., 2002).

The first LTB_4 receptor antagonist, SC-41930 (Searle, IL, USA), had anti-inflammatory activity in animal models of colitis (Fretland et al., 1990) and inhibited 5-LOX (Villani-Price et al., 1992), and LTB_4- and 12-R-HETE-stimulated proliferation of HT-29 and HCT-15 colon cancer cell lines (Bortuzzo et al., 1996). In pancreatic cancer and early pancreatic cancer lesions, 5-LOX and LTB_4 receptors are upregulated. LY293111 (Eli Lilly, IN, USA), another LTB_4 antagonist, inhibited growth of pancreatic cancer, and induced apoptosis both *in vitro* and *in vivo*, as well as enhancing the antipancreatic cancer effects of gemcitabine (Hennig et al., 2004). LY293111 exerts its anticancer effects through blockade of the LTB_4 receptor and PPAR-γ another potential target for prevention or treatment of cancer (Adrian, Hennig, Friess, & Ding, 2008). In a phase I trial, LY293111 was well tolerated by patients with no significant side effects (Ding, Talamonti, Bell, & Adrian, 2005). However, a randomized double-blind phase II clinical trial comparing gemcitabine plus LY293111 versus gemcitabine plus placebo in advanced adenocarcinoma of the pancreas, suggested that there was no benefit in adding LY293111 to gemcitabine (Saif et al., 2009). In anaplastic large-cell lymphoma, LY293111 dose dependently inhibited proliferation and induced complete G_1–S cell cycle arrest that was accompanied by upregulation of p27 and downregulation of cyclin E (Zhang et al., 2005). It also induced caspase-dependent apoptosis via activation of the intrinsic pathway (Tong, Ding, Talamonti, Bell, & Adrian, 2007; Zhang et al., 2005).

D. Dual COX/LOX Inhibitors

One potentially serious problem with inhibiting LOX or COX is the shuttling of substrate between pathways. For example, once 5-LOX has been inhibited, there may be more substrate available for the COX-2 or LOX pathways that are procarcinogenic. Conversely, inhibition of the COX pathway by NSAIDs could increase LTs (Gilroy, Tomlinson, & Willoughby, 1998). This subtle but potentially critical interplay between the various eicosanoid pathways could dictate the final result of therapeutic interventions directed at single enzymes. Hence, a novel approach is to develop agents that inhibit both 5-LOX and COX pathways (dual COX/LOX inhibitors).

Several chemically distinct dual inhibitors are in different stages of development and deployment. For example, the di-tert-butylphenol class has antioxidant and radical scavenging properties in addition to inhibiting both COX and LOX, *in vitro* and *in vivo*; examples of this class include darbufelone, tebufelone, and R-830 (Leval, Julemont, Delarge, Pirotte, & Dogne, 2002). Other classes include pyrazoles (FPL-62064, tepoxalin, ER-34122), thiophenes (RWJ-34122, L-652,343), and the pyrrolizines (licofelone or ML 3000) (Leval et al., 2002).

Licofelone is a substrate analog of arachidonic acid, which inhibits 5-LOX, COX-1, and COX-2 (Alvaro-Gracia, 2004). In a multicenter study comparing the efficacy of licofelone to that of naproxen in patients with osteoarthritis (OA), licofelone and naproxen were equieffective in reducing OA symptoms; however, licofelone significantly reduced cartilage volume loss over time, thus having a protective effect in patients with knee OA (Raynauld et al., 2009). Licofelone also prevents oral carcinogenesis at the postinitiation stage in a hamster model (Li, Sood, et al., 2005). Another dual COX/LOX inhibitor recently reported is NNU-hdpa [2-(4-hydroxyphenyl)-3-(3,5-dihydroxyphenyl) propenoic acid] which has anti-inflammatory activity, appears safe to the GI, and inhibits NF-κB activation (Xu et al., 2009).

Given the multitude of solid organ tumors in which the LOX pathway is upregulated, the development of LOX inhibitors may have far-reaching implications. Since LOX inhibitors appear to have limited side effects, they may constitute a useful chemopreventive class of compounds.

VI. Nitric Oxide-Releasing NSAIDs (NO-NSAIDS and NONO-NSAIDs)

A. Nitric Oxide Signaling

Nitric oxide (NO) is one of the ten smallest molecules found in nature. It is released intracellularly when L-arginine is oxidized by the enzyme nitric oxide synthase (NOS) of which there are three isoforms. Neuronal (nNOS, NOS1) and endothelial (eNOS, NOS3) are constitutive calcium-dependent forms of the enzyme that are regulated by negative feedback and release low fluxes of NO over a short period to regulate neural and vascular function, respectively (Stuehr, 1997). The third isoform (iNOS, NOS2), is calcium-independent, inducible, and produces supraphysiological concentrations of NO and is involved in immune surveillance. Most of NO signaling is through the second messenger, cGMP. For example, NO inhibits NF-κB activation thus controlling inflammation (Hattori, Kasai, & Gross, 2004; Katsuyama, Shichiri, Marumo, & Hirata, 1998). NO can also suppress expression of proinflammatory mediators in mast cells (Hogaboam, Befus, & Wallace, 1993), macrophages (Huang et al., 1998), and vascular smooth muscles (Naseem, 2005). NO regulates blood flow (Ignarro, Buga, Wood, Byrns, & Chaudhuri, 1987; Wallace & Miller, 2000), modulates platelet and leukocyte activation, adhesion, and aggregation (Wallace et al., 2009). NO in the vasculature is an important regulator of blood pressure since eNOS inhibition leads to an increase in systemic blood pressure (Sander, Chavoshan, & Victor, 1999). The role of NO in cancer has been quite perplexing, as both protective and cytotoxic responses have been observed (Ridnour et al., 2006; Wink et al., 1998; Xu, Liu, Loizidou, Ahmed, & Charles, 2002).

B. Rational for Developing NO-NSAIDs

The development of NO-NSAIDs (also known as COX-inhibiting nitric oxide donators, CINODs) (Wallace, Ignarro, & Fiorucci, 2002) represents a novel approach to reduce the side effects of NSAIDs alluded to above. Their development was based on the observation that NO has some of the same properties as PGs within the gastric mucosa. For example, NO increases blood flow, which reduces the effects of luminal irritants. NO also increases mucus and bicarbonate secretions thus modulating other components of the mucosal defense systems (Wallace & Miller, 2000). Therefore, coupling an NO-releasing moiety to an NSAID might deliver NO to the site of NSAID-induced damage, thereby decreasing gastric toxicity. This logic has proved to be quite successful. Animal studies have shown that many NO-NSAIDs are indeed safer to the GI mucosa than the parent NSAID (Davies et al., 1997; Elliott, McKnight, Cirino, & Wallace, 1995; Wallace et al., 1994a, 1994b). This has held true in human studies (Fiorucci, Santucci, Gresele, et al., 2003; Fiorucci, Santucci, Wallace, et al., 2003). It is also important to note that NO-NSAIDs inhibit the formation of COX-1- and COX-2-derived PGs *in vitro* and *in vivo* (Cirino, Wheeler-Jones, Wallace, Del Soldato, & Baydoun, 1996; Fiorucci et al., 1999; Wallace, McKnight, Del Soldato, Baydoun, & Cirino, 1995; Wallace et al., 1994b). For example, *meta*-NO-aspirin (*m*-NO-ASA, NCX 4016) inhibits platelet aggregation and TxB_2 formation in animals (Fiorucci et al., 1999) and completly inhibited TxB_2 generation in healthy human volunteers (Fiorucci, Santucci, Gresele, et al., 2003). In animals, NO-NSAIDs do not alter systemic arterial blood pressure since NO release appears to be a slow process; however, after NO-NSAID administration there is a significant increase in plasma nitrite/nitrate levels, consistent with a release of an NO in the systemic circulation (Burgaud, Riffaud, & Del Soldato, 2002).

C. Structural Features of NO-NSAIDs

NO-NSAIDs are traditional NSAIDs linked to a NO-releasing group via a chemical spacer. The three key structural components of any NO-NSAID are the traditional NSAID moiety; the spacer, which can be either aliphatic or aromatic; and the NO-releasing group, which is $-NO_3$ in all available nitrate esters (Fig. 4). In general, NO-NSAIDS are more potent in inhibiting the growth of various human cancer cell lines compared to their traditional parent NSAID (Kashfi et al., 2002). Aromatic spacers generate more potent NSAID derivatives than aliphatic ones (Kashfi, Nath, & Jacobs, 2007; Kashfi et al., 2005), and positional isomerism greatly influences all cell kinetic parameters that are important determinants of cellular mass. For example, the *ortho* and *para* positional isomers of NO-ASA were significantly more potent than the *meta* isomer in inhibiting the growth of HT-29 human colon cancer cells, inducing apoptosis, and inhibiting proliferation (Kashfi et al., 2005). Table II lists NO- and NONO-NSAIDs and their development status.

1. NO-Donor "Aspirin-Like" Compounds

As indicated above, positional isomers of NO-ASA were obtained by joining, through a simple ester bridge, the carboxylic acid group of aspirin with an NO-releasing ($-ONO_2$, nitrooxy) moiety, Fig. 4. A second generation of NO-releasing aspirins soon followed in which furoxan derivatives were the NO donors (Cena et al., 2003), (Fig. 5A). Unlike the first generation of NO-ASAs, which required enzymatic metabolism for NO release (Carini, Aldini, Orioli, & Maffei Facino, 2002; Gao, Kashfi, & Rigas, 2005; Grosser & Schroder, 2000), the furoxan–aspirin hybrids released NO in the presence of plasma, GSH, or albumin, that is through a mechanism requiring action of thiols (Turnbull et al., 2006). NO generation from furoxans could be enhanced by ascorbic acid (Turnbull et al., 2006). These agents significantly inhibited COX-1 activity (Turnbull et al., 2006), reduced TNF-α release from lipopolysaccharide (LPS)-treated macrophages, and inhibited

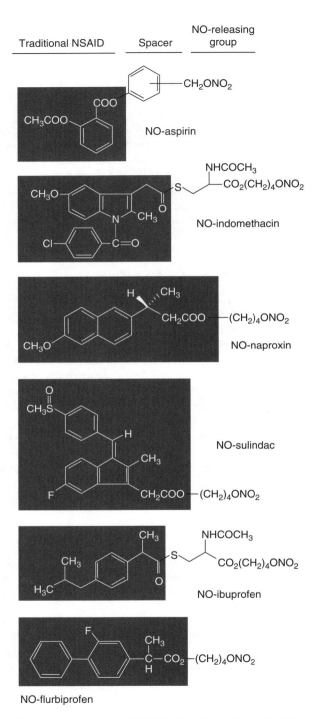

Traditional NSAID	Spacer	NO-releasing group

NO-aspirin

NO-indomethacin

NO-naproxin

NO-sulindac

NO-ibuprofen

NO-flurbiprofen

FIGURE 4 The chemical structures of NO-NSAIDs. The traditional NSAID is shown in the shaded box, the spacer molecule links the traditional NSAID to $-ONO_2$ which can release NO.

TABLE II   List of Different Classes of NO- and NONO-NSAIDs Underdevelopment, their Status, and the Companies Involved

Class	Drug	Status	Company
Nitrate esters	m-NO-ASA (NCX-4016)	Phase I trials (abandoned)	NicOx SA, France
	NO-flurbiprofen (HCT-1026)	Phase II trials	
	NO-naproxen (Napro-CINOD)	Phase III trials	
	NO-diclofenac (NCX-285)	Preclinical	
	NO-indomethacin (NCX-530)	Preclinical	
	NO-ketoprofen (HCT-2037)	Preclinical	
Dinitrate esters	NO-naproxen (NMI-1182)	Preclinical	Nitromed, USA
Nitrate ester coxibs	NO-rofecoxib	Phase II trials stopped (Vioxx^{TM} withdrawal)	Merck and Co., USA
	NO-valdecoxib (NMI-1093)	Preclinical	Nitromed, USA
Nitrosothiols	S-NO-diclofenac	Preclinical	
Furoxans	NO-ibuprofen	Preclinical	University of Turin, Italy
Diazenumdiolate	NONO-ASA	Preclinical	NCI, Frederick, USA
	NONO-ibuprofen	Preclinical	
	NONO-indomethacin	Preclinical	

NF-κB activation (Turnbull et al., 2008). Recently, a new class of NO-releasing "aspirin-like" compounds have been described in which the acetyl group on the aspirin has been replaced by acyl groups containing nitroxy NO-releasing moieties (Lazzarato et al., 2008) (Figs. 5B and C). These compounds have reduced gastrotoxicity compared to aspirin and have exhibited strong anti-inflammatory activity when evaluated in the carrageenan-induced paw edema in rats (Lazzarato et al., 2008).

D. NO-NSAIDs as Agents for Cancer Prevention

Preclinical studies have shown that NO-NSAIDs have chemopreventive properties. For example, NO-ASA, NO-sulindac, NO-ibuprofen, NO-indomethacin, NO-flurbiprofen, and NO-salicylic acid all have

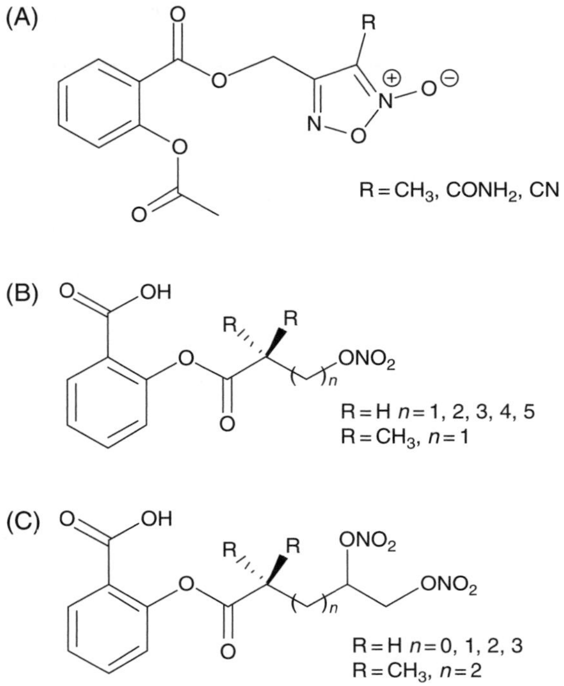

FIGURE 5 NO-donor "aspirin-like" compounds. A second generation of NO-releasing aspirin in which a furoxan derivative is the NO donor (A). In the "aspirin-like" compounds, the acetyl group on the aspirin has been replaced by acyl groups containing nitroxy NO-releasing moieties (B and C).

greater potency than their corresponding parent NSAID in inhibiting the growth of various cancer cells such as colon, prostate, lung, pancreas, skin, breast, and leukaemia (Huguenin et al., 2005; Kashfi et al., 2007, 2002; Nath, Labaze, Rigas, & Kashfi, 2005; Nath, Vassell, Chattopad-hyay, Kogan, & Kashfi, 2009; Tesei et al., 2005; Williams et al., 2001; Yeh et al., 2004). The studies evaluating the chemoprevention properties of NO-NSAIDs highlighted three key features: (1) NO enhanced the potency of NSAIDs in inhibiting cancer cell growth; (2) this enhanced potency was seen in cancers of various tissue origins; and (3) NO-ASA was consistently the most potent NO-NSAID in regard to these properties. What was also apparent was that the potency of an NSAID in inhibiting cell growth did not predict the potency of the corresponding NO-NSAID. For example, in comparing the growth inhibitory properties of ASA, sulindac, and indomethacin in a number of different cell lines (Kashfi et al., 2002), ASA was consistently the weakest of the three traditional NSAIDs; however, NO-ASA had the highest potency of all three NO derivatives, the magnitude of this reflected in the very large IC_{50} ratios of ASA/NO-ASA which exceeded those of the other NO-NSAIDS often by over 100-fold (Kashfi et al., 2002). The fact that nitration of different NSAIDs did not lead to the same cell growth inhibition, underscores the complexity of their effects on cell growth. The fact that the spacer molecule is not the same in all the NO-NSAIDs makes any efforts to define an underlying common mechanism difficult. The only shared structural feature amongst NO-NSAIDs is the $-ONO_2$ moiety, the NSAID component is a general pharmacological function and not a structural feature. This property, however, cannot account for the enhanced potency of the NO-NSAIDs.

The growth-inhibitory effects of NO-NSAIDs are due to enhanced cell death, reduced cell proliferation, and inhibition of cell cycle phase transitions. Of the NO-NSAIDs evaluated, NO-ASA was the only one that caused atypical cell death, for example, necrosis (Kashfi et al., 2002, 2005) and this may also occur *in vivo* (Ouyang, Williams, & Rigas, 2006).

I. NO-ASA Inhibits Carcinogenesis in Various Animal Models of Cancer

The first studies comparing the chemopreventive effects of ASA to that of *m*-NO-ASA (NCX 4016) were reported over a decade ago (Bak et al., 1998). In a rat model of colonic adenocarcinoma, the number of ACFs (an early preneoplastic lesion) were reduced after 4 weeks of treatment with aspirin by 64%, while *m*-NO-ASA produced an 85% reduction. The effect of *p*-NO-ASA (NCX 4040) was also evaluated in a *Min* (APC$^{Min/+}$) mouse model of intestinal cancer in which a truncating mutation in the Apc gene predisposed the mice to spontaneously develop intestinal tumors (Lipkin et al., 1999). In this study, tumor burden was used as an end point. Three weeks of treatment with *p*-NO-ASA had no effect on animal weight and there were no signs of overt toxicity including GI. *p*-NO-ASA reduced tumor growth by 55% but it did not affect cell proliferation in small intestinal mucosa (Williams et al., 2004). Given that tumors had already formed when NO-ASA was administered, it is evident that this compound not only had chemopreventive but also had chemotherapeutic properties. In another *Min* mice study, *p*-NO-ASA was more efficacious than *m*-NO-ASA in reducing the number of intestinal tumors (Kashfi et al., 2005), a finding consistent with the potency ranking of these two positional isomers based on their effects on cultured cells (Kashfi et al., 2002, 2005; Nath, Vassell, Chattopadhyay, Kogan, & Kashfi, 2009; Williams et al., 2001; Yeh et al., 2004). In F344 rats treated with the carcinogen, AOM to induce colon cancers, NO-indomethacin and *m*-NO-ASA suppressed both tumor incidence and multiplicity, with NO-indomethacin being more effective (Rao et al., 2006). In a series of *in vitro* studies using various human colon cancer cell lines, 5-flurouracil or oxaliplatin, both of which are used for the clinical management of colorectal cancer (Meyerhardt & Mayer, 2005), had additive effects when combined with *p*-NO-ASA (Leonetti et al., 2006). Using colon cancer xenografts, simultaneous treatment with p-NO-ASA and oxaliplatin or oxaliplatin followed by p-NO-ASA showed the same additive effects. However, treatment with p-NO-ASA followed by oxaliplatin showed synergistic interactions possibly by sensitization of the cancer cells to the cytotoxic effects of the antitumor agent (Leonetti et al., 2006). Finally, using Syrian golden hamsters and the carcinogen BOP to establish pancreatic cancer, compared to controls, m-NO-ASA reduced the incidence and multiplicity of pancreatic cancer by 88.9 and 94%, respectively, while ASA was without effect (Ouyang, Williams, Tsioulias, et al., 2006).

E. Molecular Targets of NO-ASA in Cancer

Apart from effects on cell kinetics, NO-ASA has multiple pleiotropic effects that involve NF-κB, Wnt, NOS, mitogen-activated protein kinase (MAPK), COX-2, PPAR, drug-metabolizing enzymes, reactive oxygen species, and pro- and anti-inflammatory cytokines.

1. Cell Kinetics

The effects of NO-ASA on cell renewal and cell death, two determinants of cell growth, have shown that NO-ASA inhibits cell proliferation (diminished expression of the proliferation marker PCNA) and enhances cell death by inducing apoptosis. It also blocks transitions of the cells through the cell cycle, mainly between G_1 and S (Kashfi et al., 2002, 2005; Williams et al., 2001).

2. NF-κB

p-NO-ASA profoundly affects the NF-κB–DNA interaction in cultured colon cancer cells decreasing it as early as 60 min after treatment, with similar results obtained with pancreatic cancer cell lines (Williams, Ji, Ouyang, Liu, and & Rigas, 2008; Williams et al., 2003). *In vivo*, compared to controls, p-NO-ASA decreased NF-κB activation in xenografts of estrogen receptor negative, ER(–), breast cancer cells (Kashfi & Nazarenko, 2006), and in intestinal epithelial cells of $APC^{min+/-}$ mice (Williams, Ji, Ouyang, Liu, & Rigas, 2008).

3. Wnt/β-Catenin Signaling

p-NO-ASA modulates the β-catenin signaling pathway in three different cancer cell lines of different origin (Gao, Liu, & Rigas, 2005; Nath, Kashfi, Chen, & Rigas, 2003; Nath, Labaze, Rigas, & Kashfi, 2005; Nath, Vassell, Chattopadhyay, Kogan, & Kashfi, 2009). One of the significant downstream genes dependent on β-catenin/T cell factor (TCF)-4 signaling is *cyclin D1*, which has been implicated in carcinogenesis (Moon, Kohn, De Ferrari, & Kaykas, 2004). Inhibition of this signaling pathway by low concentrations of p-NO-ASA was associated with reduced cyclin D1 expression suggesting that it may be an important disruptor of carcinogenesis. *In vivo*, NO-indomethacin and *m*-NO-ASA inhibited β-catenin expression in a standard AOM rat model of colorectal cancer (Rao et al., 2006).

4. Nitric Oxide Synthase

iNOS may have an important role in tumor development since increased expression occurs in breast (Thomsen et al., 1995), CNS (Cobbs, Brenman, Aldape, Bredt, & Israel, 1995), pancreas (Kasper, Wolf, Drebber, Wolf, & Kern, 2004), astrocytic gliomas (Hara & Okayasu, 2004), prostate (Aaltoma, Lipponen, & Kosma, 2001), acute myeloid leukaemia (Brandao, Soares, Salles, & Saad, 2001), and colon (Ambs et al., 1998) tumors. iNOS regulates COX-2 (Landino, Crews, Timmons, Morrow, & Marnett, 1996; Perez-Sala & Lamas, 2001) and its activity may be correlated with p53 mutations (Chiarugi, Magnelli, & Gallo, 1998), although this has not been replicated (Brandao et al., 2001). Importantly, iNOS inhibitors prevent colon cancer (Rao, Kawamori, Hamid, & Reddy, 1999; Takahashi et al., 2006). Various NO-NSAIDs inhibit the induction of iNOS in a macrophage cell line (Cirino et al., 1996). In HT-29 colon cancer cells, *p*-NO-ASA inhibits iNOS induction by cytokines (Williams et al., 2003) and also potently inhibits expression and enzymatic activity of iNOS (Spiegel et al., 2005). An NO chimera (GT-094), a nitrate containing an NSAID and disulfide pharmacophores, reduced iNOS levels in the AOM rat model of colorectal cancer (Hagos et al., 2007).

5. COX-2

The role of COX-2 and its inhibition in colon and other cancers has been the subject of considerable debate (Kashfi & Rigas, 2005; Soh & Weinstein, 2003). NO-NSAIDs, in general, and NO-ASA, in particular, were more potent than their corresponding traditional NSAIDs in inhibiting the growth of cultured HT-29 (expressing both COX-1 and COX-2) and HCT 15 (COX null) colon cancer cells (Williams et al., 2001; Yeh et al., 2004). Similar observations were made with the pancreatic cancer cell lines BxPC-3 (COX-1, COX-2 positive) and MIA PaCa-2 (COX null) (Kashfi et al., 2002). This raises an important and interesting question about the role of COX in cancer, since NO-ASA was equieffective and equipotent in both COX positive and COX negative cell lines. In HT-29 cells, *p*-NO-ASA at concentrations around its IC_{50} value for growth inhibition increased COX-2 expression by nearly ninefold. The induced enzyme was catalytically active (Williams et al., 2003). Similar findings were obtained with the DLD-1 colon cancer, BxPC-3 pancreatic cancer (Williams et al., 2003), and MCF-7 breast cancer cell lines (Nath, Vassell, Chattopadhyay, Kogan, & Kashfi, 2009). However, NO-indomethacin and *m*-NO-ASA also inhibited total COX including COX-2 activity and formation of PGE_2 in the AOM rat model of colon cancer (Rao et al., 2006). These results give caution in extrapolating cell culture data to *in vivo*. The mechanism(s) by which NO-ASA induces COX-2 is unclear, but may, in part, be Protein kinase C (PKC) dependent (Nath, Vassell, Chattopadhyay, Kogan, & Kashfi, 2009).

6. Peroxisome Proliferator-Activated Receptor δ

In matched normal and tumor samples from the colon, PPAR-δ mRNA was upregulated in colorectal carcinomas and endogenous PPAR-δ was transcriptionally responsive to PGI_2 (Gupta et al., 2000). Elevation of PPAR-δ expression in colorectal cancer cells was repressed by APC, an effect mediated by β-catenin/TCF-4-responsive elements in the PPAR-δ promotor (He, Chan, Vogelstein, & Kinzler, 1999). Sulindac blocked PPAR-δ from binding to its recognition sequences (He et al., 1999), and in SW480 colon cancer cells, sulindac sulfone decreased PPAR-δ expression more potently than the sulfide metabolite (Siezen et al., 2006). These data suggest that NSAIDs may, in part, inhibit tumorigenesis through inhibition of PPAR-δ. In *Min* mice, *m*- and *p*-NO-ASAs inhibited the expression of PPAR-δ in both histologically normal and tumor tissues. *m*-NO-ASA suppressed PPAR-δ expression in normal mucosa by 23% and in neoplastic tissue by 41%; *p*-NO-ASA suppressed PPAR-δ expression in normal mucosa by 27% and in neoplastic tissue by 55% (Ouyang et al., 2006).

7. Mitogen-Activated Protein Kinase

The MAPKs are a family of kinases that transduce signals from the cell membrane to the nucleus in response to a variety of stimuli modulating gene transcription and leading to biological response (Bode & Dong, 2004). MAPKs required for specialized cell functions, controlling cell proliferation, differentiation, and death are deregulated in several malignancies, including colon cancer, and may be involved in their pathogenesis. *p*-NO-aspirin treatment of colon cancer cells (HT-29 and SW480) activated c-Jun N-terminal kinase (JNK) and p38 along with their respective downstream transcription factors, cJun and ATF-2. NO-ASA stimulation of p38 was biphasic, with an initial increase in phosphorylation within the 60 min of treatment, and a second much stronger increase at 4 h (Hundley & Rigas, 2006).

8. Xenobiotic-Metabolizing Enzymes

Modulation of drug-metabolizing enzymes, leading to facilitated elimination of endogenous and environmental carcinogens, represents a successful strategy for cancer chemoprevention (Kwak, Wakabayashi, & Kensler, 2004) and is exemplified by dithiolethiones, that induce phase II metabolizing enzymes. These compounds inhibit tumorigenesis of environmental carcinogens in various animal models and in clinical trials, modulate the metabolism of the carcinogen, aflatoxin B1 (Kwak et al., 2004). In general, induction of phase II enzymes is an adequate strategy for protecting mammals against carcinogens and other forms of electrophile and oxidant toxicity. Chemopreventive agents induce the expression of phase II genes through their effects on the Keap1–Nrf2 complex (Lee & Surh, 2005). In the nucleus, the transcription factor Nrf2, a member of the NF-E2 family, dimerizes with Maf protein and binds to the antioxidant response element, a cis-acting regulatory element in the promoter region of phase II enzymes. A cytoplasmic actin-binding protein, Keap1, is an inhibitor of Nrf2 that sequesters it in the cytoplasm. Inducers dissociate this complex, allowing Nrf2 to translocate to the nucleus. Studies evaluating the effects of NO-ASA on xenobiotic-metabolizing enzymes have shown that m-NO-ASA induced the activity and expression of NAD(P)H:quinone oxireductase (NQO) and glutathione S-transferases (GSTs) in mouse hepatoma Hepa 1c1c7 and HT-29 human colon cancer cells (Gao, Kashfi, Liu, & Rigas, 2006). In *Min* mice, m-NO-ASA also induced the activities of NQO and GST in liver cytosolic and small intestine fractions but had no effect on the activity of these enzymes in the kidney, showing some degree of tissue of specificity (Gao et al., 2006). Expression of GST P1-1, GST A1-1, and NQO1 was induced in liver cytosols from *Min* mice; however, the expression of two phase I metabolizing enzymes, CypP450-1A1 and CypP450-2E1, were unaffected, suggesting that m-NO-ASA is a monofunctional inducer of phase II enzymes (Gao et al., 2006). m-NO-ASA also induced the translocation of Nrf2 into the nucleus, an effect that paralleled the induction of NQO1 and GST P1-1 (Gao et al., 2006).

9. Oxidative Stress

It has become evident that anticancer agents act, at least in part, by inducing reactive oxygen and nitrogen species (RONS). At low concentrations, RONS may protect the cell and at high concentrations can initiate biological damage, including cell death (Rigas & Sun, 2008). In evaluating the effects of p-NO-ASA in SW480 colon cancer cells, it was determined that the spacer in p-NO-ASA formed a conjugate with glutathione, depleting glutathione stores and thus induced a state of oxidative stress that led to apoptosis via activation of the intrinsic apoptosis pathway (Gao, Liu, et al., 2005). p-NO-ASA through induction of RONS also oxidized thioredoxin-1 (Sun & Rigas, 2008), an oxidoreductase that is involved in redox regulation of cell signaling (Arner & Holmgren, 2006; Maulik & Das, 2008).

10. Modulation of Proinflammatory Cytokines

m-NO-ASA inhibits cytokine production from endotoxin-stimulated human monocytes and macrophages (Fiorucci, Santucci, Cirino, et al., 2000) and when administered to mice, decreased IL-1β, IL-8, IL-12, IL-18, TNF-α, and INF-γ production and protected against concanavalin A-induced acute hepatitis (Fiorucci, Santucci, Antonelli, et al., 2000). The effect exerted by NO-ASA on cytokine production was COX-independent

(Santucci, Fiorucci, Di Matteo, & Morelli, 1995). Locally generated NO contributes to limit inflammation by inhibiting generation of proinflammatory cytokines and/or by enhancing the production of anti-inflammatory cytokines, IL-10 and TGFβ, resulting in downregulation of downstream mediators of inflammation including COX and NOS isoenzymes (Fiorucci, 2001; Fiorucci, Santucci, Antonelli, et al., 2000).

F. Biological Influence of the Spacer in NO-ASA

The defining entity in all NO-NSAIDs is NO. Structure–activity studies with NO-ASA indicated that NO was pivotal for its anticancer effects (Kashfi et al., 2005). However, careful reexamination regarding the contribution to the overall biological effect of each of the three structural components of NO-ASA in which the spacer joining the ASA to the NO-releasing moiety was aromatic, led to the surprising conclusion that the NO-releasing moiety was not required for the observed biological effects. Rather, the spacer was responsible for the biological actions of NO-ASA, with the NO-releasing moiety acting as a leaving group to facilitate the release and activation of the spacer to a quinone methide (QM) intermediate that acted as powerful electrophile such that the ASA component had little or no biological contribution (Dunlap et al., 2007; Hulsman et al., 2007; Kashfi & Rigas, 2007). On this basis, a series of o-, p-, and m-ester-protected hydroxy benzyl phosphates (EHBPs) were synthesized in which the – ONO_2 leaving group was replaced by a substituted phosphate and the ASA was replaced by an acetate. Electron-donating/withdrawing groups were also incorporated around the spacer to evaluate their effect on QM formation/stability and biological activity (Kodela, Chattopadhyay, et al., 2008). EHBPs inhibit the growth of various human cancer cell lines, indicating an effect independent of tissue type exercising pleotropic effects involving cell death as well as cell cycle phase transitions and that a QM if formed is influenced by the nature of the substitutes about the benzyl spacer (Kodela, Chattopadhyay, et al., 2008). Transient QMs and related electrophiles if formed during the metabolic activation of NO-ASA can lead to DNA alkylation and (reversible) adduct formation between the QM and deoxyadenosine, deoxyguanosine, deoxycytosine, or thymidine. Using deoxycytosine (dC), which has the potential to form only one (reversible) adduct, the relative reversibility of QM reaction versus bioactivity was determined using a series of EHBPs (Kodela, Rokita, Boring, Crowell, & Kashfi, 2008) that indeed showed a reversible dC adduct was formed, and that electron-donating/withdrawing groups significantly affected the rate of adduct formation/decomposition. As predicted, the m analog did not form a QM a finding consistent with the proposed mechanism of action of NO-ASA (Dunlap et al., 2007; Hulsman et al., 2007; Kashfi & Rigas, 2007).

G. NONO-NSAIDs

The production of NO from nitrate, released from the nitrate esters described above requires a three-electron reduction (Thatcher, Nicolescu, Bennett, & Toader, 2004). However, NONO-NSAIDs do not require redox activation before the release of NO (Velazquez, Praveen Rao, Citro, Keefer, & Knaus, 2007). These agents are based on linking a *N*-diazen-1-ium-1,2 diolate functional group to a classical NSAID (Fig. 6) yielding compounds

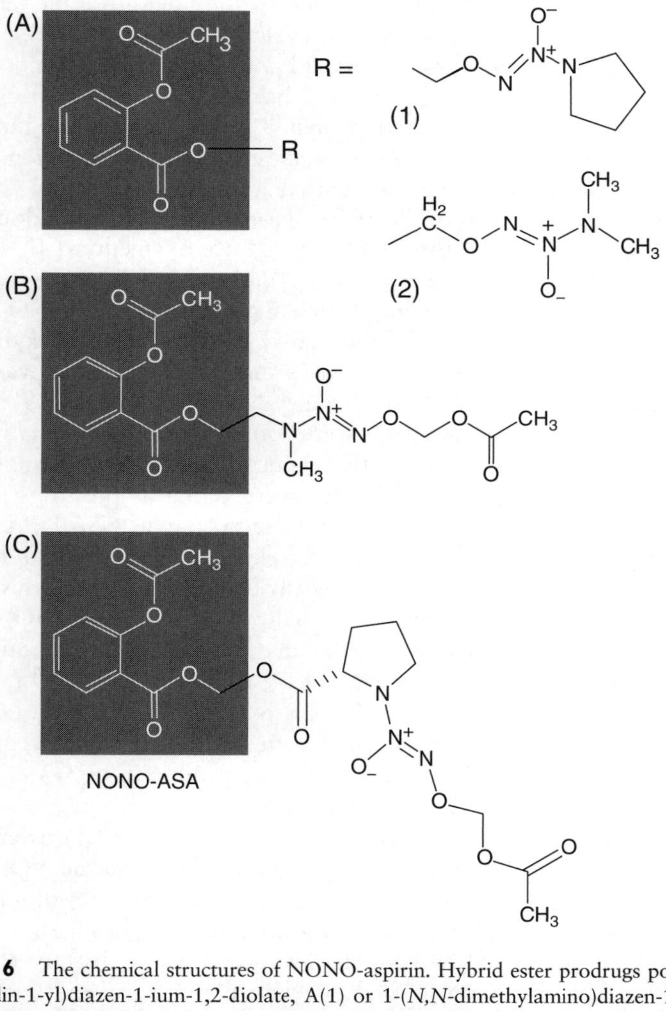

FIGURE 6 The chemical structures of NONO-aspirin. Hybrid ester prodrugs possessing a 1-(pyrrolidin-1-yl)diazen-1-ium-1,2-diolate, A(1) or 1-(*N,N*-dimethylamino)diazen-1-ium-1,2-diolate, A(2), moiety attached via a one-carbon methylene space to the carboxylic acid group of aspirin. In B, the NO-releasing moiety is O^2-acetoxymethyl 1-[*N*-(2-hydroxyethyl)-*N*-methylamino]diazen-1-ium-1,2-diolate. In C, the NO-releasing moiety is O^2-acetoxymethyl 1-[(2-hydroxymethyl) pyrrolidin-1-yl]diazen-1-ium-1,2-diolate.

that are not likely to lead to "nitrate tolerance" (Csont & Ferdinandy, 2005; Fung & Bauer, 1994; Hu Siu, et al., 2007) and also have the potential to generate two equivalents of NO (Velazquez et al., 2007). Another attractive attribute of these classes of NO-releasing compounds is their rich derivatization chemistry that facilitates the targeting of NO to specific target organ and/or tissue site (Keefer, 2003).

The first agent reported in this compound class had a NONOate (O^2-unsubstituted *N*-diazen-1-ium-1,2-diolate) attached via a one-carbon methylene spacer to the carboxylic acid group of a traditional NSAID (aspirin, ibuprofen, and indomethacin) (Velazquez, Praveen Rao, & Knaus, 2005) (Fig. 6A). *In vitro*, these agents did not inhibit the enzymatic catalytic activity of COX-1 or COX-2; however, they were equipotent to their traditional NSAID counterparts when evaluated in the carrageenan-induced rat paw anti-inflammatory model. Also, unlike their traditional parent NSAID, these agents had no significant gastric toxicity when given orally (Velazquez et al., 2005). A series NONO-NSAIDS (aspirin, ibuprofen, and indomethacin) was subsequently made that had an O^2-acetoxymethyl-1-[*N*-(2-hydroxyethyl)-*N*-methylamino]diazen-1-ium-1,2-diolate moiety as the NO donor (2-HEMA/NO) (Velazquez et al., 2007) (Fig. 6B). Here, the NO-donating moiety was attached via a two-carbon ethyl spacer to the carboxylic acid of the traditional NSAID, and because a secondary dialkyamine was used in their synthesis, the number of possible new NONO-NSAIDs was enormous. Like their predecessors, these agents were nonulcerogenic, and *in vitro* did not inhibit either COX-1 or COX-2 activity, but showed even better anti-inflammatory properties, suggesting that they were acting as prodrugs, requiring metabolic activation by an esterase to release the parent NSAID. A potential limitation was that hydrolysis would also release one equivalent of the corresponding nitrosoamines that are biologically toxic. To overcome this concern, a second generation of O^2-acetoxymethyl-protected (PROLI/NO)-releasing NONO-NSAIDs was developed where a diazeniumdiolate ion obtained from an amine like L-proline was used, the *N*-nitroso derivative of which is nontoxic (Velazquez, Chen, Citro, Keefer, & Knaus, 2008) (Fig. 6C). These agents were also nonulcerogenic, had better anti-inflammatory properties, and effective analgesic activity. They also produced up to 1.9 mol of NO/mol of compound (Velazquez et al., 2008).

NONO-NSAIDs are an attractive class of compounds; however, there are no data on their chemopreventive potential. Based on the NO-NSAIDs, one might expect these compounds to have potent chemoprevention properties. Recently, the antiulcerogenic, anti-inflammatory, analgesic, and antipyretic effects of an NONO-NSAID were compared directly to that of *m*-NO-ASA, together with effects on relevant biological markers such as gastric PGE_2 and lipid peroxidation levels, superoxide dismutase activity, and TNF-α, levels. In all aspects, the two classes of compounds were similar (K. Kashfi & C. A. Velazquez, unpublished data).

VII. Hydrogen Sulfide-Releasing NSAIDs _____

A. Hydrogen Sulfide Signaling

Hydrogen sulfide, H_2S, is a colorless gas with a strong odor that until recently was only considered to be a toxic environmental pollutant with little or no physiological significance. However, certain bacteria produce and utilize H_2S (Pace, 1997). Mammalian cells also produce H_2S, with rat serum having a concentration of $\sim46\,\mu M$ (Zhao, Zhang, Lu, & Wang, 2001). H_2S in low micromolar levels is also produced in other tissues, for example, brain (Abe & Kimura, 1996; Hosoki, Matsuki, & Kimura, 1997) and vascular tissue (Hosoki et al., 1997; Zhao et al., 2001). However, the highest levels of H_2S in the body (low millimolar levels) occur in the lumen of the colon (Magee, Richardson, Hughes, & Cummings, 2000) and are probably due to the nature of the luminal flora. Mitochondria of colonic epithelial cells can utilize H_2S as an inorganic substrate (Goubern, Andria-mihaja, Nubel, Blachier, & Bouillaud, 2007).

Most endogenous H_2S is produced from L-cysteine by two pyridoxal-5′-phosphate-dependent enzymes, cystathionine β-synthase (CBS) and cystathionine γ-lyase (CSE) (Bukovska, Kery, & Kraus, 1994; Erickson, Maxwell, Su, Baumann, & Glode, 1990). The activity of these enzymes is regulated by H_2S through negative feedback control. Expression of these enzymes is tissue specific, with some tissues requiring both CBS and CSE for H_2S generation, while in others only one of the enzymes is needed (Boehning & Snyder, 2003; Levonen, Lapatto, Saksela, & Raivio, 2000; Lu, O'Dowd, Orrego, & Israel, 1992; Meier, Janosik, Kery, Kraus, & Burkhard, 2001). H_2S can also be generated endogenously through none-nzymatic reduction of elemental sulfur (the concentration of which in blood is in the millimolar range (Westley & Westley, 1991)) using reducing equivalents supplied through the glycolytic pathway (Searcy & Lee, 1998). Signs and symptoms of H_2S toxicity are well known and are well above those produced endogenously. At concentrations of about 250 ppm, H_2S can cause pulmonary edema, and concentrations above 1,000 ppm are lethal. (Beauchamp, Bus, Popp, Boreiko, & Andjelkovich, 1984; Reiffenstein, Hulbert, & Roth, 1992.)

The functional role of H_2S at physiologically relevant concentrations in the brain appears to be mediated via activation of ATP-sensitive potassium channels (Wang, 2002). The same appears to be the case in the cardiovas-cular system since an i.v. bolus of H_2S transiently decreased blood pressure of rats, an effect that was mimicked by the K_{ATP} channel agonist, pinacidil; and blocked by application of glibenclamide, a K_{ATP} channel blocker (Zhao et al., 2001). It is noteworthy that both H_2S (Distrutti et al., 2006a) and NSAIDs (Ortiz et al., 2001) appear to exert their analgesic effects via K_{ATP} channels. H_2S is also a strong reducing agent and may function as an important redox controlling molecule (Kashiba, Kajimura, Goda, & Suematsu, 2002).

B. Anti-Inflammatory Effects of H$_2$S

The role of H$_2$S in inflammation and immunity is controversial, with some studies suggesting an anti-inflammatory effect, whereas others suggest a contribution to immune-mediated tissue injury. In the carrageenan-induced rat hindpaw model of inflammation, CSE and myeloperoxidase (MPO) activity were increased. Pretreatment with D,L-propargylglycine, a CSE inhibitor, reduced carrageenan-induced hindpaw edema in a dose-dependent manner (Bhatia, Sidhapuriwala, Moochhala, & Moore, 2005). Endotoxin administration to mice increased plasma, liver, and kidney H$_2$S levels that was accompanied by an increase in CSE gene expression in both liver and kidney. There was also histological evidence of lung, liver, and kidney tissue inflammatory damage. Administration of sodium hydrosulfide (an H$_2$S donor) resulted in histological signs of lung inflammation, increased lung and liver MPO activity, and increased plasma TNF-α levels (Li, Bhatia, et al., 2005). Elevated H$_2$S levels occur in the plasma of septic shock patients (Li, Bhatia, et al., 2005). Surprisingly, administration of NO-releasing flurbiprofen to LPS-treated rats resulted in a dose-dependent inhibition of liver H$_2$S synthesis and CSE mRNA levels (Anuar, Whiteman, Bhatia, & Moore, 2006; Anuar, Whiteman, Siau, et al., 2006). Together, these observations suggest a proinflammatory role for H$_2$S. H$_2$S may also act as a proinflammatory mediator in an animal model of pancreatitis (Bhatia, Wong, et al., 2005; Tamizhselvi, Moore, & Bhatia, 2007).

On the other hand, potent anti-inflammatory effects of H$_2$S have been reported. Administration of carrageenan into a rat air pouch resulted in infiltration of substantial numbers of leukocytes and neutrophils. Pretreatment with a number of different H$_2$S donors (NaHS, N-acetylcysteine, and Lawesson's reagent) reduced the number of leukocytes in a dose-dependent manner (Zanardo et al., 2006). This reduction was comparable to that seen by using diclofenac, the NOS inhibitor, L-NAME; or the steroid anti-inflammatory, dexamethasone. Pretreatment with β-cyanoalanine, a CSE inhibitor, reversed the inhibitory effects of N-acetylcysteine. Pretreatment with diclofenac, NaHS, or Na$_2$S similarly reduced carrageenan-induced rat paw edema while β-cyanoalanine showed a significant increase in paw swelling in response to carageenan (Zanardo et al., 2006). Through peroxynitrite scavenging, H$_2$S can inhibit tissue oxidative damage (Whiteman et al., 2004, 2005). H$_2$S has been shown to induce apoptosis in neutrophils (Mariggio et al., 1998), which could contribute to resolution of inflammation (Gilroy, Lawrence, Perretti, & Rossi, 2004). In LPS-stimulated microglia and astrocytes, H_2S donors inhibited TNF-α secretion, an anti-inflammatory effect, via inhibition of iNOS and p38 MAPK signaling pathways (Hu, Wong, Moore, & Bian, 2007). In the neuroblastoma cell line SH-SY5Y, H_2S inhibited rotenone (a toxin used *in vivo* and *in vitro* Parkinson's disease models)-induced cell apoptosis via regulation of p38- and JNK-MAPK pathway (Hu, Lu, Wu, Wong, & Bian, 2009). Thus, it appears that similar to NO, physiological concentrations of H_2S produce anti-inflammatory effects, whereas at higher concentrations, which can be produced endogenously in certain circumstances, the effects are proinflammatory (Li, Bhatia, & Moore, 2006; Wallace, 2007b).

C. H_2S Prevents Ulcer Formation Caused by NSAIDs and Promotes Ulcer Healing

Gastric mucosa can also produce H_2S that may contribute to its defense against luminal substances. Rats given various NSAIDs (aspirin, indomethacin, ketoprofen, or diclofenac), NaHS, or the combination of an NSAID plus NaHS were evaluated for gastric damage, effects on H_2S-synthesizing enzymes, gastric blood flow, and other parameters relevant to tissue injury (Fiorucci et al., 2005). NaHS significantly inhibited gastric mucosal injury, TNF-α, ICAM-1, and lymphocyte function-associated antigen-1 mRNA upregulation induced by aspirin. NaHS prevented the associated reduction of gastric mucosal blood flow and reduced ASA-induced leukocyte adherence in mesenteric venules. It did not however, alter suppression of PGE_2 synthesis by NSAIDs. Glibenclamide (K_{ATP} channel antagonist) and D,L-propargylglycine (CSE inhibitor) exacerbated, whereas pinacidil (K_{ATP} channel agonist) attenuated gastric injury caused by ASA. Exposure to NSAIDs reduced H_2S formation and mRNA and protein expression of CSE (Fiorucci et al., 2005). These results suggested that suppression of mucosal H_2S synthesis may represent another mechanism, in addition to inhibition of COX activity, through which NSAIDs produce GI damage (Wallace, 2007a).

To evaluate the ulcer healing properties of any GI-sparing agent, a chronic ulcer model is generally employed with acetic acid being used to produce gastric ulcers in rats, which highly resemble human ulcers in terms of pathological features and healing mechanisms (Okabe & Amagase, 2005). These ulcers respond well to antiulcer drugs such as the proton pump inhibitors and sucralfate (Okabe & Amagase, 2005). In this model, induction of gastric ulceration was associated with a increase in expression of CSE and CBS enzymes as well has H_2S levels, suggesting a defensive response (Wallace, Dicay, McKnight, & Martin, 2007). Ulcer healing was observed following administration of three chemically distinct (Lawesson's reagent, 4-hydroxyhiobenzamide, and H_2S-5-ASA) H_2S donors, and administration L-cysteine, a precursor of endogenous H_2S synthesis, also enhanced ulcer healing (Wallace, Dicay, et al., 2007). In evaluating the possible mechanisms through which H_2S accelerated ulcer healing, it was determined that the H_2S donors did not raise gastric pH or inhibit acid secretion; K_{ATP} channel agonists or antagonists had no affect on ulcer healing; ulcer healing was NO independent; and L-cysteine did not affect gastric levels of glutathione. Since H_2S is a vasodilator, it is possible that this may have contributed to healing process observed in this study (Wallace, Dicay, et al., 2007).

D. Hydrogen Sulfide-Releasing NSAIDs for Treatment of Inflammatory Diseases

Research in the field of hydrogen sulfide-releasing NSAIDs (HS-NSAIDs, Fig. 7) is in its infancy. To date, there have been no reports describing the effects of HS-NSAIDs in any *in vitro* studies of human cancer cell lines or in any *in vivo* animal models of cancer. There are some studies focusing on HS-diclofenac, HS-indomethacin, and HS-mesalamine for treatment and prevention of inflammatory bowl disease (IBD; Crohn's disease and ulcerative colitis), also their anti-inflammatory properties, and GI-sparing effects have been described.

IBD is a chronic disorder characterized by extensive ulceration and inflammation. The first-line therapy for mild-to-moderate IBD is up to 6 g/day of mesalamine (5-aminosalicylic acid), the mechanism of action of which is not well understood (Hanauer, 2006). The animal model used for evaluating various agents for treatment of IBD makes use of trinitrobenzene sulfonic acid (TNBS). This model is well characterized, and exhibits responsiveness to various therapies similar to those used for human IBD and shares many features with IBD in humans, particularly Crohn's colitis (Fiorucci et al., 2002; Morris et al., 1989). Using this model in mice, HS-mesalamine was more effective than mesalamine in reducing mucosal injury and disease activity (body weight loss, fecal blood, and diarrhea) and colonic granulocyte infiltration (Fiorucci et al., 2007). Treatment with mesalamine did not affect the expression of any of several proinflammatory cytokines/chemokines studied. TNBS colitis, like Crohn's colitis, is generally regarded as being driven by Th1 cytokines, including IL-1, IL-2 TNF-α, IFN-γ, and IL-12 (Sartor, 1997; Stallmach et al., 1999). The chemokine, RANTES, has also been implicated in the pathogenesis of colitis in this model (Ajuebor, Hogaboam, Kunkel, Proudfoot, & Wallace, 2001). Treatment with HS-mesalamine reduced the expression of mRNA for TNF-α, IFN-γ, IL-1, IL-2, IL-12 p40, and RANTES (Fiorucci et al., 2007). Using the same model in rats, HS-mesalamine modulated expression of colonic proinflammatory mediators, COX-2 and IL-1β (Distrutti et al., 2006b).

Traditional NSAID   H₂S-releasing moiety

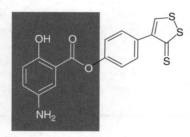

H₂S-diclofenac (ATB-337)

H₂S-indomethacin (ATB-343)

H₂S-mesalamine (ATB-429)

FIGURE 7   The chemical structures of HS-NSAIDs. The traditional NSAID is shown in the shaded box which is linked to the moiety that releases H₂S.

Importantly, HS-mesalamine also reduced visceral sensitivity and pain perception in conscious healthy and postcolitic, hypersensitive rats. These actions may involve K_{ATP} channels on afferent, sensitive spinal fibers (Distrutti et al., 2006b) and may have particular clinical significance since abdominal pain is one of the most debilitating symptoms of IBD.

HS-diclofenac had significant GI-sparing effects compared to diclofenac (Li et al., 2007; Wallace, Caliendo, Santagada, Cirino, & Fiorucci, 2007) and was equieffective in inhibiting both COX-1 and COX-2 enzymatic activity (Wallace, Caliendo, et al., 2007). It also reduced plasma IL-1β and TNF-α levels, while it elevated the anti-inflammatory, IL-10 (Li et al., 2007).

Similar GI-sparing effects have been observed with HS-indomethacin (Wallace, 2007b) and HS-mesalamine (Wallace, Dicay et al., 2007).

E. Is There an Interaction Between NO and H$_2$S?

This is a fascinating question the answer to which appears to be a resounding yes; however, the H$_2$S–NO interaction is quite complex. NO and H$_2$S share many similar actions, including modulation of leukocyte adherence to the vascular endothelium, both are "gasotransmitters," and both bind avidly to hemoglobin. The competition for the common hemoglobin sink can potentiate the biological activity of the other. NO can act as a ROS thus altering the reduced/oxidized glutathione balance; it can also inhibit enzymes and ion channels through S-nitrosylation (Wang, 2002). H$_2$S may also be involved in the reduction of thiols. Some examples of the metabolism and functions of NO and H$_2$S are given in Table III.

NO can increase CSE expression and activity in cultured vascular SMCs, as well as induce uptake of cystine by the cells. Endogenous H$_2$S production from rat aortic tissue can be increased by an NO donor (Zhao et al., 2001). Also, in the rat aortic tissue, NaHS enhanced the vasorelaxant effects of the NO donor, sodium nitroprusside (Hosoki et al., 1997). A putative hypothetical interaction between NO and H$_2$S in vascular tissue is depicted in Fig. 8.

TABLE III   Some Examples of the Metabolism and Function of Nitric Oxide and Hydrogen Sulfide

	NO	*H$_2$S*
Main substrates	L-arginine	L-cysteine
Generating enzymes	NO synthases	CBS, CSE
Inducer	Acetylcholin, endotoxin	NO
Inhibitor	L-NAME	D,L-propargylglycerine
Scavenger	Hemoglobin	Hemoglobin
Amino acid targets	Cysteine	?
Protein targets	cGMP, K$_{Ca}$ channel	K$_{ATP}$ channel, cAMP (?)
Half-life in solution	Seconds	Minutes
Production tissue source	EC > SMC	SMC, not in EC
Mucosal blood flow	Increased	Increased
Bicarbonate production	Increased	Unknown
Mucus secretion	Increased	Unknown
Cytoprotection	Yes	Yes
Epithelial cell proliferation	No	Yes

SMC, smooth muscle cell; EC, endothelial cell; L-NAME, N^G-nitro-L-arginine methyl ester. Partially adapted from Wang (2002) and Fiorucci (2009).

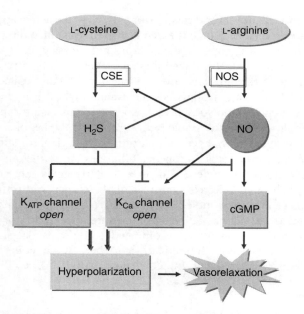

FIGURE 8   Putative interaction of H_2S and NO in vascular tissue. H_2S may decrease the expression level of NOS, while NO may increase the expression of CSE. H_2S may decrease the sensitivity of the cGMP pathways and also it may modify K_{Ca} channels to decrease their sensitivity to NO. Solid arrows indicate stimulatory, while T-shaped arrows indicate inhibitory inputs.

VIII. Natural Products for Cancer Prevention

We are what we eat. Hippocrates, ~480 BC, wrote "Positive health requires a knowledge of man's primary constitution and the powers of various foods, both those natural to them and those resulting from human skill." What Hippocrates called "man's primary constitution," today we call genetics and we may infer that foods "resulting from human skills" may be equated to diet (Pan, Lai, Dushenkov, & Ho, 2009). Worldwide, about 35% of all cancers are caused by poor diet (WHO, 2009), and this number is even higher in the case of colon cancer. Adding alcohol and cigarettes increases these numbers even more. Therefore, genetic predisposition accounts for a relatively small number of cancers.

A. Classification of Natural Bioactive Compounds

Many natural bioactive compounds interfere with the initiation, promotion, and progression of cancer by affecting intracellular signaling cascades involved in the inflammatory process (Pan & Ho, 2008). These compounds can be categorized into several classes (for each class the active ingredient and an example of a dietary source is given in parenthesis) including flavonoids, classified into seven groups, flavones (apigenin, parsley, celery), flavonols (quercetin, onion, broccoli), flavanones (naringenin, orange peel), flavanonols (silybin, milk thistle), flavanols (epicatechin (EC) and epigallocatechin-3-gallate, (EGCG), tea), isoflavones (genistein, soybean), and anthocyanidins (cyanidin, cherry and strawberry); isothiocyanates (sulforaphane, broccoli); terpenoids (all-*trans*-retinoic acid, grapes); polyphenolic compounds (resveratrol, grape, red wine; curcumin; tumeric; [6]-gingerol, ginger; carnosol, rosemary); carotenoids (lycopene, tomatoes, watermelon; β-carotene, carrots, leafy green vegetables); and omega-3-fatty acids (Eicosapentaenoic acid (EPA), fish oils). Selected examples of these agents affecting different types of cancer and their molecular targets are given in Table IV, a small number of which are discussed below. For more information of this general area, the following reviews are recommended (Buhr & Bales, 2009; Calviello, Serini, & Piccioni, 2007; Half & Arber, 2009; Pan et al., 2009; Reichrath, 2007; Yang, Wang, Lu, & Picinich, 2009).

I. Curcumin

Curcumin (diferuloylmethane), a polyphenol, is a major component of the spice, turmeric. It has anti-inflammatory properties and inhibits the

TABLE IV   Some Natural Anti-Inflammatory Compounds

Compound	Source	Cancer type	Molecular target
Curcumin	Tumeric	Colon, pancreas breast	COX, ROS, IL-8, MCP-1, TNF-α, angiogenesis
Resveratrol	Red grapes/wine, white helebore	Skin, colon	COX, ROS
β-carotene	Yellow/orange fruits vegetables	(Inflammation)	ROS
Quercetin	Cranberries and onions	Colon, lung, breast, skin	ROS, Ah-receptor
Ginseng	Panax plant root	Colon	TNF-α, NF-κB, angiogenesis
Vitamin D	Dairy, fish, various plants	Prostate, colon, breast	Cell cycle, Akt, ERK
Calcium	Dairy, nuts, Soy, seaweed	Prostate, colon, breast	Apoptosis
Omega-3 PUFAs	Fish, grains	Colon	Cell cycle, apoptosis, PPAR-γ

Abbreviations: COX, cyclooxygenase; ROS, reactive oxygen species; IL-8, interleukin-8; MCP-1, monocyte chemotactic protein-1; TNF-α, tumor necrosis factor-α; Ah-receptor, aryl hydrocarbon receptor; NF-κB, nuclear factor kappa-light-chain-enhancer of activated B cells; Erk, extracellular signal-regulated kinase; PPAR-γ, peroxisome proliferator-activated receptor-γ.

growth of a number of different human cancer cell lines. It is one of the most highly investigated natural products that affects many signaling pathways associated with inflammation and cancer. It inhibits iNOS (Brouet & Ohshima, 1995); induces the expression of phase II detoxifying enzymes such as GST (Appiah-Opong, Commandeur, Istyastono, Bogaards, & Vermeulen, 2009) and NADP(H):quinone oxidoreductase through modulation of the transcription factor Nrf2 (Ye, Hou, Zhong, & Zhang, 2007). Curcumin inhibits TNF-α-stimulated inflammatory cytokine production through modulating phosphorylation of p38, JNK, and activation of STAT3 and NF-κB in human endothelial cells (Kim et al., 2007). It also suppressed TPA-induced COX-2 expression by inhibiting NF-κB translocation and PKC activity (Garg, Ramchandani, & Maru, 2008). Recently, curcumin has been shown to suppress PGE_2 formation by reversibly blocking the expression of COX-2 and microsomal PGE_2 synthase-1 (Koeberle, Northoff, & Werz, 2009). It also inhibited proliferation of colon cancer by modulating Akt/mTOR signaling (Johnson et al., 2009). In a xenograft model, curcumin sensitized colorectal cancer cells to the antitumor and antimetastatic effects of capecitabine by suppressing the NF-κB cell signaling pathway (cyclin D1, c-myc, bcl-2, bcl-xL, cIAP-1, COX-2, ICAM-1, MMP-9, CXCR4, and VEGF) (Kunnumakkara et al., 2009).

The result of animal studies are promising, particularly with respect to colorectal cancer where oral administration of curcumin inhibited the development of intestinal adenomas in $APC^{Min/+}$ mice (Perkins et al., 2002) and have prompted several clinical trials to evaluate the effect of oral curcumin supplementation on IBD and precancerous colorectal lesions (National Institutes of Health, NCT00927485, NCT00779493, NCT00889161, available at: http://clinicaltrials.gov). One problem with curcumin is its low solubility; therefore, it is more likely to be effective as a preventative/therapeutic agent in cancers of the GI tract than other tissues.

2. Resveratrol

Resveratrol (3,4',5-trihydroxystilbene) belongs to a class of polyphenolic compounds called stilbenes (Aggarwal et al., 2004). The potential health benefits of resveratrol became of interest when its presence was reported in red wine, leading to speculation that resveratrol might help explain the "French Paradox" (Criqui & Ringel, 1994). Resveratrol inhibits the proliferation of a variety of human cancer cell lines, including those from breast, prostate, stomach, colon, pancreatic, and thyroid cancers. The underlying mechanism include, cell cycle arrest; upregulation of $p21^{Cip1/WAF1}$, p53, and Bax; downregulation of survivin, cyclin D1, cyclin E, Bcl-2, and Bcl-xL; and activation of caspases; suppression of activation of transcription factors, including NF-κB, AP-1, and Egr-1; inhibition of protein kinases including IκBα kinase, JNK, MAPK, Akt, PKC, PKD, and casein kinase II; and to downregulate products of genes like COX-2,

5-LOX, VEGF, IL-1, IL-6, and IL-8; reviewed in Aggarwal et al. (2004). Resveratrol suppressed IL-6-induced intracellular cell adhesion molecule-1 (ICAM-1) gene expression in endothelial cells (Wung, Hsu, Wu, & Hsieh, 2005), inhibited AOM-induced colon cancer in F344 rats (Tessitore, Davit, Sarotto, & Caderni, 2000); inhibited 7,12-dimethylbenz[a]anthracene (DMBA)-induced tumor incidence and tumor burden in a CD-1 mouse skin topical cancer model (Soleas, Grass, Josephy, Goldberg, & Diamandis, 2002); and suppressed DMBA-induced mammary carcinogenesis in rats (Banerjee, Bueso-Ramos, & Aggarwal, 2002). However, it moderately accelerated N-Nitroso-N-methylurea (MNU)-induced mammary carcinoma in rats (Sato et al., 2003).

3. Ginseng

Panax ginseng (Asian ginseng), *Panax pseudo-ginseng* (Japanese ginseng), and *Panax quinquefolius* (North American ginseng) represent primary sources of the herb commonly referred to as ginseng. Ginseng is composed of a mixture of glycosides, essential oils, and a variety of complex carbohydrates and phytosterols as well as amino acids and trace minerals (Duke, 1989). The principle active ingredient(s) of ginseng is a complex mixture of over 30 triterpenoid saponins commonly referred to as ginsenosides (Li, Mazza, Cottrell, & Gao, 1996) that are present in leaf, stem, and berries in addition to the traditionally harvested root. Ginseng has the potential to be used as chemopreventive agents in inflammation-mediated carcinogenesis.

Ginsan, a polysaccharide extracted from *P. ginseng*, inhibitied the p38 MAPK pathway (Jung et al., 2006); and genistein inhibited the activation of NF-κB and Akt signaling pathways (Banerjee, Li, Wang, & Sarkar, 2008), and inhibited NF-κB-dependent gene expression in TLR-4-stimulated dendritic cells (Dijsselbloem et al., 2007) blocking the production of TNF-α and IL-1β in phytohemagglutinin-treated macrophages (Kesherwani & Sodhi, 2007).

IX. Conclusion

In the same vein that during the past two decades cancer prevention has taken enormous strides, it may be argued that the next decade is going to be even more fruitful. A major need in chemoprevention is the development of effective and safe agents. NSAIDs in general including coxibs do not meet these criteria; hence, the development of NO- and HS-NSAIDs, and modulators of the COX/LOX pathway. While there are also limited data available on the safety of NO-NSAIDs, data on HS-NSAIDs have yet to be determined. Developing the appropriate pharmacological agents and identifying biomarkers that will aid in both monitoring response and selecting the best candidates for chemoprevention is key to the development of such agents.

When it comes to cancer treatment, there are no "magic bullets." This is a complex disease and as such requires a multipronged, mechanistically targeted approach. The elaboration of understanding of the various biochemical and signaling pathways involved in tumor cell growth has provided the tools to design agents that either augment or inhibit these potential targets. For example, the field of chemokine biology in tumor biology is essentially in its infancy. Preclinical studies indicate that reducing chemokine receptor function has the potential to reduce metastasis and reduce tumor growth, but the detailed mechanisms underlying these effects are only beginning to be understood. How these will translate into the development of effective therapies in the clinical setting has also to be addressed.

For many years, efforts to treat cancer concentrated on destruction of the tumor cell. Strategies to modulate the host microenvironment offer a new perspective with the targeting proinflammatory cytokines is a prime target. Naturally, many questions remain unanswered, for example, what is the best way to target cancer-related inflammation in patients with cancer?

Another example as to how understanding of the molecular events and agents that target them has helped developing strategies in treating cancer has been the identification of ROS as a mediator and critical proximal event for the actions of NO-ASA. Depletion of antioxidants, in particular GSH, may sensitize the tumor cells to chemotherapeutics. Therefore, developing other nontoxic GSH-depleting agents may be of considerable value in overcoming multidrug resistance.

No doubt, there are other mediators and pathways yet to be discovered that may help in identifying novel cancer therapeutics with "an ounce of prevention being better than a pound of cure."

Acknowledgments

I would like to thank Dr. Mitali Chattopadhyay for her critical comments and general help with the manuscript. This work was supported by National Institute of Health, NCI Division of Cancer Prevention, and PSC-CUNY.

Conflict of Interest: The author declares no potential conflict of interest.

References

Aaltoma, S. H., Lipponen, P. K., & Kosma, V. M. (2001). Inducible nitric oxide synthase (iNOS) expression and its prognostic value in prostate cancer. *Anticancer Research, 21*, 3101–3106.
Abe, K., & Kimura, H. (1996). The possible role of hydrogen sulfide as an endogenous neuromodulator. *Journal of Neuroscience, 16*, 1066–1071.

Adrian, T. E., Hennig, R., Friess, H., & Ding, X. (2008). The role of PPARgamma receptors and leukotriene B(4) receptors in mediating the effects of LY293111 in pancreatic cancer. *PPAR Research, 827096.*

Aggarwal, B. B., Bhardwaj, A., Aggarwal, R. S., Seeram, N. P., Shishodia, S., & Takada, Y. (2004). Role of resveratrol in prevention and therapy of cancer: Preclinical and clinical studies. *Anticancer Research, 24,* 2783–2840.

Ajuebor, M. N., Hogaboam, C. M., Kunkel, S. L., Proudfoot, A. E., & Wallace, J. L. (2001). The chemokine RANTES is a crucial mediator of the progression from acute to chronic colitis in the rat. *Journal of Immunology, 166,* 552–558.

Alvaro-Gracia, J. M. (2004). Licofelone—clinical update on a novel LOX/COX inhibitor for the treatment of osteoarthritis. *Rheumatology (Oxford), 43*(Suppl. 1), i21–i25.

Ambs, S., Merriam, W. G., Bennett, W. P., Felley-Bosco, E., Ogunfusika, M. O., Oser, S. M., et al. (1998). Frequent nitric oxide synthase-2 expression in human colon adenomas: Implication for tumor angiogenesis and colon cancer progression. *Cancer Research, 58,* 334–341.

Antman, E. M., Bennett, J. S., Daugherty, A., Furberg, C., Roberts, H., & Taubert, K. A. (2007). Use of nonsteroidal antiinflammatory drugs: An update for clinicians: A scientific statement from the American Heart Association. *Circulation, 115,* 1634–1642.

Anuar, F., Whiteman, M., Bhatia, M., & Moore, P. K. (2006). Flurbiprofen and its nitric oxide-releasing derivative protect against septic shock in rats. *Inflammation Research, 55,* 498–503.

Anuar, F., Whiteman, M., Siau, J. L., Kwong, S. E., Bhatia, M., & Moore, P. K. (2006). Nitric oxide-releasing flurbiprofen reduces formation of proinflammatory hydrogen sulfide in lipopolysaccharide-treated rat. *British Journal of Pharmacology, 147,* 966–974.

Appiah-Opong, R., Commandeur, J. N., Istyastono, E., Bogaards, J. J., & Vermeulen, N. P. (2009). Inhibition of human glutathione S-transferases by curcumin and analogues. *Xenobiotica, 39,* 302–311.

Arenberg, D. A., Keane, M. P., DiGiovine, B., Kunkel, S. L., Morris, S. B., Xue, Y. Y., et al. (1998). Epithelial-neutrophil activating peptide (ENA-78) is an important angiogenic factor in non-small cell lung cancer. *Journal of Clinical Investigation, 102,* 465–472.

Arenberg, D. A., Kunkel, S. L., Polverini, P. J., Glass, M., Burdick, M. D., & Strieter, R. M. (1996). Inhibition of interleukin-8 reduces tumorigenesis of human non-small cell lung cancer in SCID mice. *Journal of Clinical Investigation, 97,* 2792–2802.

Ariztia, E. V., Lee, C. J., Gogoi, R., & Fishman, D. A. (2006). The tumor microenvironment: Key to early detection. *Critical Reviews in Clinical Laboratory Sciences, 43,* 393–425.

Arner, E. S., & Holmgren, A. (2006). The thioredoxin system in cancer. *Seminars in Cancer Biology, 16,* 420–426.

Back, M. (2002). Functional characteristics of cysteinyl-leukotriene receptor subtypes. *Life Sciences, 71,* 611–622.

Back, M. (2009). Leukotriene signaling in atherosclerosis and ischemia. *Cardiocasular Drugs and Therapy, 23,* 41–48.

Back, M., & Hansson, G. K. (2006). Leukotriene receptors in atherosclerosis. *Annals of Medicine, 38,* 493–502.

Baer, A. N., Costello, P. B., & Green, F. A. (1991). In vivo activation of an omega-6 oxygenase in human skin. *Biochemical and Biophysical Research Communications, 180,* 98–104.

Bak, A. W., McKnight, W., Li, P., Del Soldato, P., Calignano, A., Cirino, G., et al. (1998). Cyclooxygenase-independent chemoprevention with an aspirin derivative in a rat model of colonic adenocarcinoma. *Life Sciences, 62,* 367–373.

Balkwill, F. (2009). Tumour necrosis factor and cancer. *Nature Reviews Cancer, 9,* 361–371.

Balkwill, F., & Mantovani, A. (2001). Inflammation and cancer: Back to Virchow? *Lancet, 357,* 539–545.

Banerjee, S., Bueso-Ramos, C., & Aggarwal, B. B. (2002). Suppression of 7,12-dimethylbenz(a) anthracene-induced mammary carcinogenesis in rats by resveratrol: Role of nuclear factor-kappaB, cyclooxygenase 2, and matrix metalloprotease 9. *Cancer Research, 62*, 4945–4954.

Banerjee, S., Li, Y., Wang, Z., & Sarkar, F. H. (2008). Multi-targeted therapy of cancer by genistein. *Cancer Letters, 269*, 226–242.

Baron, J. A., Cole, B. F., Sandler, R. S., Haile, R. W., Ahnen, D., Bresalier, R., et al. (2003). A randomized trial of aspirin to prevent colorectal adenomas. *New England Journal of Medicine, 348*, 891–899.

Beauchamp, R. O., Jr., Bus, J. S., Popp, J. A., Boreiko, C. J., & Andjelkovich, D. A. (1984). A critical review of the literature on hydrogen sulfide toxicity. *Critical Reviews in Toxicology, 13*, 25–97.

Beider, K., Abraham, M., Begin, M., Wald, H., Weiss, I. D., Wald, O., et al. (2009). Interaction between CXCR4 and CCL20 pathways regulates tumor growth. *PLoS One, 4*, e5125.

Benamouzig, R., Deyra, J., Martin, A., Girard, B., Jullian, E., Piednoir, B., et al. (2003). Daily soluble aspirin and prevention of colorectal adenoma recurrence: One-year results of the APACC trial. *Gastroenterology, 125*, 328–336.

Ben-Baruch, A. (2003). Host microenvironment in breast cancer development: Inflammatory cells, cytokines and chemokines in breast cancer progression: Reciprocal tumor-micro-environment interactions. *Breast Cancer Research, 5*, 31–36.

Bennett, A., Civier, A., Hensby, C. N., Melhuish, P. B., & Stamford, I. F. (1987). Measurement of arachidonate and its metabolites extracted from human normal and malignant gastrointestinal tissues. *Gut, 28*, 315–318.

Bhatia, M., Sidhapuriwala, J., Moochhala, S. M., & Moore, P. K. (2005). Hydrogen sulphide is a mediator of carrageenan-induced hindpaw oedema in the rat. *British Journal of Pharmacology, 145*, 141–144.

Bhatia, M., Wong, F. L., Fu, D., Lau, H. Y., Moochhala, S. M., & Moore, P. K. (2005). Role of hydrogen sulfide in acute pancreatitis and associated lung injury. *The FASEB Journal, 19*, 623–625.

Bjorkman, D. J. (1999). Current status of nonsteroidal anti-inflammatory drug (NSAID) use in the United States: Risk factors and frequency of complications. *American Journal of Medicine, 107*, 3S–8S; discussion 8S–10S.

Bode, A. M., & Dong, Z. (2004). Targeting signal transduction pathways by chemopreventive agents. *Mutation Research, 555*, 33–51.

Boehning, D., & Snyder, S. H. (2003). Novel neural modulators. *Annual Review of Neuroscience, 26*, 105–131.

Bortuzzo, C., Hanif, R., Kashfi, K., Staiano-Coico, L., Shiff, S. J., & Rigas, B. (1996). The effect of leukotrienes B and selected HETEs on the proliferation of colon cancer cells. *Biochimica et Biophysica Acta, 1300*, 240–246.

Brandao, M. M., Soares, E., Salles, T. S., & Saad, S. T. (2001). Expression of inducible nitric oxide synthase is increased in acute myeloid leukaemia. *Acta Haematologica, 106*, 95–99.

Brash, A. R., Boeglin, W. E., & Chang, M. S. (1997). Discovery of a second 15S-lipoxygenase in humans. *Proceedings of the National Academy of Sciences, USA, 94*, 6148–6152.

Breyer, R. M., Bagdassarian, C. K., Myers, S. A., & Breyer, M. D. (2001). Prostanoid receptors: Subtypes and signaling. *Annual Review of Pharmacology and Toxicology, 41*, 661–690.

Brink, C., Dahlen, S. E., Drazen, J., Evans, J. F., Hay, D. W., Nicosia, S., et al. (2003). International Union of Pharmacology XXXVII. Nomenclature for leukotriene and lipoxin receptors. *Pharmacological Reviews, 55*, 195–227.

Brouet, I., & Ohshima, H. (1995). Curcumin, an anti-tumour promoter and anti-inflammatory agent, inhibits induction of nitric oxide synthase in activated macrophages. *Biochemical and Biophysical Research Communications, 206*, 533–540.

Buhr, G., & Bales, C. W. (2009). Nutritional supplements for older adults: Review and recommendations-part I. *Journal of Nutrition for the Elderly, 28,* 5–29.

Bukovska, G., Kery, V., & Kraus, J. P. (1994). Expression of human cystathionine beta-synthase in Escherichia coli: Purification and characterization. *Protein Expression and Purification, 5,* 442–448.

Burgaud, J. L., Riffaud, J. P., & Del Soldato, P. (2002). Nitric-oxide releasing molecules: A new class of drugs with several major indications. *Current Pharmaceutical Design, 8,* 201–213.

Cai, Z., Kwintkiewicz, J., Young, M. E., & Stocco, C. (2007). Prostaglandin E2 increases cyp19 expression in rat granulosa cells: Implication of GATA-4. *Molecular and Cellular Endocrinology, 263,* 181–189.

Calviello, G., Serini, S., & Piccioni, E. (2007). n-3 polyunsaturated fatty acids and the prevention of colorectal cancer: Molecular mechanisms involved. *Current Medicinal Chemistry, 14,* 3059–3069.

Capra, V. (2004). Molecular and functional aspects of human cysteinyl leukotriene receptors. *Pharmacological Research, 50,* 1–11.

Carini, M., Aldini, G., Orioli, M., & Maffei Facino, R. (2002). In vitro metabolism of a nitroderivative of acetylsalicylic acid (NCX4016) by rat liver: LC and LC-MS studies. *Journal of Pharmaceutical and Biomedical Analysis, 29,* 1061–1071.

Carter, G. W., Young, P. R., Albert, D. H., Bouska, J., Dyer, R., Bell, R. L., et al. (1991). 5-lipoxygenase inhibitory activity of zileuton. *Journal of Pharmacology and Experimental Therapeutics, 256,* 929–937.

Cena, C., Lolli, M. L., Lazzarato, L., Guaita, E., Morini, G., Coruzzi, G., et al. (2003). Antiinflammatory, gastrosparing, and antiplatelet properties of new NO-donor esters of aspirin. *Journal of Medicinal Chemistry, 46,* 747–754.

Chiarugi, V., Magnelli, L., & Gallo, O. (1998). Cox-2, iNOS and p53 as play-makers of tumor angiogenesis (review). *International Journal of Molecular Medicine, 2,* 715–719.

Chulada, P. C., Thompson, M. B., Mahler, J. F., Doyle, C. M., Gaul, B. W., Lee, C., et al. (2000). Genetic disruption of Ptgs-1, as well as Ptgs-2, reduces intestinal tumorigenesis in Min mice. *Cancer Research, 60,* 4705–4708.

Cirino, G., Wheeler-Jones, C. P., Wallace, J. L., Del Soldato, P., & Baydoun, A. R. (1996). Inhibition of inducible nitric oxide synthase expression by novel nonsteroidal anti-inflammatory derivatives with gastrointestinal-sparing properties. *British Journal of Pharmacology, 117,* 1421–1426.

Cobbs, C. S., Brenman, J. E., Aldape, K. D., Bredt, D. S., & Israel, M. A. (1995). Expression of nitric oxide synthase in human central nervous system tumors. *Cancer Research, 55,* 727–730.

Colotta, F., Allavena, P., Sica, A., Garlanda, C., & Mantovani, A. (2009). Cancer-related inflammation, the seventh hallmark of cancer: Links to genetic instability. *Carcinogenesis, 30,* 1073–1081.

Criqui, M. H., & Ringel, B. L. (1994). Does diet or alcohol explain the French paradox? *Lancet, 344,* 1719–1723.

Csont, T., & Ferdinandy, P. (2005). Cardioprotective effects of glyceryl trinitrate: Beyond vascular nitrate tolerance. *Pharmacology and Therapeutics, 105,* 57–68.

Curiel, T. J., Coukos, G., Zou, L., Alvarez, X., Cheng, P., Mottram, P., et al. (2004). Specific recruitment of regulatory T cells in ovarian carcinoma fosters immune privilege and predicts reduced survival. *Nature Medicine, 10,* 942–949.

Dannenberg, A. J., & Subbaramaiah, K. (2003). Targeting cyclooxygenase-2 in human neoplasia: Rationale and promise. *Cancer Cell, 4,* 431–436.

Davies, N. M., Roseth, A. G., Appleyard, C. B., McKnight, W., Del Soldato, P., Calignano, A., et al. (1997). NO-naproxen vs. naproxen: Ulcerogenic, analgesic and anti-inflammatory effects. *Alimentary Pharmacology and Therapeutics, 11,* 69–79.

Desai S. P., Solomon, D. H., Abramson, S. B., Buckley, L., Crofford, L. J., Cush, J. C., Lovell, D, J., Saag, K. G. (2008). Recommendations for use of selective and nonselective nonsteroidal antiinflammatory drugs: An American College of Rheumatology white paper. *Arthtitis and Rheumatism*, *59*, 1058–1073.

Dhawan, P., & Richmond, A. (2002). Role of CXCL1 in tumorigenesis of melanoma. *Journal of Leukocyte Biology*, *72*, 9–18.

Dijsselbloem, N., Goriely, S., Albarani, V., Gerlo, S., Francoz, S., Marine, J. C., et al. (2007). A critical role for p53 in the control of NF-kappaB-dependent gene expression in TLR4-stimulated dendritic cells exposed to Genistein. *Journal of Immunology*, *178*, 5048–5057.

Ding, X. Z., Talamonti, M. S., Bell, R. H., Jr., & Adrian, T. E. (2005). A novel anti-pancreatic cancer agent, LY293111. *Anticancer Drugs*, *16*, 467–473.

Distrutti, E., Sediari, L., Mencarelli, A., Renga, B., Orlandi, S., Antonelli, E., et al. (2006a). Evidence that hydrogen sulfide exerts antinociceptive effects in the gastrointestinal tract by activating KATP channels. *Journal of Pharmacology and Experimental Therapeutics*, *316*, 325–335.

Distrutti, E., Sediari, L., Mencarelli, A., Renga, B., Orlandi, S., Russo, G., et al. (2006b). 5-Amino-2-hydroxybenzoic acid 4-(5-thioxo-5H-[1,2]dithiol-3yl)-phenyl ester (ATB-429), a hydrogen sulfide-releasing derivative of mesalamine, exerts antinociceptive effects in a model of postinflammatory hypersensitivity. *Journal of Pharmacology and Experimental Therapeutics*, *319*, 447–458.

Dixon, R. A., Diehl, R. E., Opas, E., Rands, E., Vickers, P. J., Evans, J. F., et al. (1990). Requirement of a 5-lipoxygenase-activating protein for leukotriene synthesis. *Nature*, *343*, 282–284.

Duke, J. A. (1989). *Ginseng: A concise hand book*. Algonac, MI: Reference Publication Inc.

Dunlap, T., Chandrasena, R. E., Wang, Z., Sinha, V., Wang, Z., & Thatcher, G. R. (2007). Quinone formation as a chemoprevention strategy for hybrid drugs: Balancing cytotoxicity and cytoprotection. *Chemical Research in Toxicology*, *20*, 1903–1912.

Eberhart, C. E., Coffey, R. J., Radhika, A., Giardiello, F. M., Ferrenbach, S., & Dubois, R. N. (1994). Up-regulation of cyclooxygenase 2 gene expression in human colorectal adenomas and carcinomas. *Gastroenterology*, *107*, 1183–1188.

Eisen, V. (1977). Past and present views of inflammation. *Agents and Actions. Supplements*, *3*, 9–16.

Elder, D. J. E., Halton, D. E., Hague, A., & Paraskeva, C. (1997). Induction of apoptotic cell death in human colorectal carcinoma cell lines by a cyclooxygenase-2 (COX-2)-selective nonsteroidal anti-inflammatory drug—independence from COX-2 protein expression. *Clinical Cancer Research*, *3*, 1679–1683.

Elliott, S. N., McKnight, W., Cirino, G., & Wallace, J. L. (1995). A nitric oxide-releasing nonsteroidal anti-inflammatory drug accelerates gastric ulcer healing in rats. *Gastroenterology*, *109*, 524–530.

Erickson, P. F., Maxwell, I. H., Su, L. J., Baumann, M., & Glode, L. M. (1990). Sequence of cDNA for rat cystathionine gamma-lyase and comparison of deduced amino acid sequence with related Escherichia coli enzymes. *Biochemical Journal*, *269*, 335–340.

Fiorucci, S. (2001). NO-releasing NSAIDs are caspase inhibitors. *Trends in Immunology*, *22*, 232–235.

Fiorucci, S., Antonelli, E., Distrutti, E., Del Soldato, P., Flower, R. J., Clark, M. J., et al. (2002). NCX-1015, a nitric-oxide derivative of prednisolone, enhances regulatory T cells in the lamina propria and protects against 2,4,6-trinitrobenzene sulfonic acid-induced colitis in mice. *Proceedings of the National Academy of Sciences, USA*, *99*, 15770–15775.

Fiorucci, S., Antonelli, E., Distrutti, E., Rizzo, G., Mencarelli, A., Orlandi, S., et al. (2005). Inhibition of hydrogen sulfide generation contributes to gastric injury caused by anti-inflammatory nonsteroidal drugs. *Gastroenterology*, *129*, 1210–1224.

Fiorucci, S., Antonelli, E., Santucci, L., Morelli, O., Miglietti, M., Federici, B., et al. (1999). Gastrointestinal safety of nitric oxide-derived aspirin is related to inhibition of ICE-like cysteine proteases in rats. *Gastroenterology, 116*, 1089–1106.

Fiorucci, S., Orlandi, S., Mencarelli, A., Caliendo, G., Santagada, V., Distrutti, E., et al. (2007). Enhanced activity of a hydrogen sulphide-releasing derivative of mesalamine (ATB-429) in a mouse model of colitis. *British Journal of Pharmacology, 150*, 996–1002.

Fiorucci, S., Santucci, L., Antonelli, E., Distrutti, E., Del Sero, G., Morelli, O., et al. (2000). NO-aspirin protects from T cell-mediated liver injury by inhibiting caspase-dependent processing of Th1-like cytokines. *Gastroenterology, 118*, 404–421.

Fiorucci, S., Santucci, L., Cirino, G., Mencarelli, A., Familiari, L., Soldato, P. D., et al. (2000). IL-1 beta converting enzyme is a target for nitric oxide-releasing aspirin: New insights in the antiinflammatory mechanism of nitric oxide-releasing nonsteroidal antiinflammatory drugs. *Journal of Immunology, 165*, 5245–5254.

Fiorucci, S., Santucci, L., Gresele, P., Faccino, R. M., Del Soldato, P., & Morelli, A. (2003). Gastrointestinal safety of NO-aspirin (NCX-4016) in healthy human volunteers: A proof of concept endoscopic study. *Gastroenterology, 124*, 600–607.

Fiorucci, S., Santucci, L., Wallace, J. L., Sardina, M., Romano, M., del Soldato, P., et al. (2003). Interaction of a selective cyclooxygenase-2 inhibitor with aspirin and NO-releasing aspirin in the human gastric mucosa. *Proceedings of the National Academy of Sciences, USA, 100*, 10937–10941.

FitzGerald, G. A., & Patrono, C. (2001). The coxibs, selective inhibitors of cyclooxygenase-2. *New England Journal of Medicine, 345*, 433–442.

Fretland, D. J., Widomski, D., Tsai, B. S., Zemaitis, J. M., Levin, S., Djuric, S. W., et al. (1990). Effect of the leukotriene B4 receptor antagonist SC-41930 on colonic inflammation in rat, guinea pig and rabbit. *Journal of Pharmacology and Experimental Therapeutics, 255*, 572–576.

Friedman, B. S., Bel, E. H., Buntinx, A., Tanaka, W., Han, Y. H., Shingo, S., et al. (1993). Oral leukotriene inhibitor (MK-886) blocks allergen-induced airway responses. *American Review of Respiratory Disease, 147*, 839–844.

Fujimura, M., Sasaki, F., Nakatsumi, Y., Takahashi, Y., Hifumi, S., Taga, K., et al. (1986). Effects of a thromboxane synthetase inhibitor (OKY-046) and a lipoxygenase inhibitor (AA-861) on bronchial responsiveness to acetylcholine in asthmatic subjects. *Thorax, 41*, 955–959.

Fujino, H., West, K. A., & Regan, J. W. (2002). Phosphorylation of glycogen synthase kinase-3 and stimulation of T-cell factor signaling following activation of EP2 and EP4 prostanoid receptors by prostaglandin E2. *Journal of Biological Chemistry, 277*, 2614–2619.

Fujino, H., Xu, W., & Regan, J. W. (2003). Prostaglandin E2 induced functional expression of early growth response factor-1 by EP4, but not EP2, prostanoid receptors via the phosphatidylinositol 3-kinase and extracellular signal-regulated kinases. *Journal of Biological Chemistry, 278*, 12151–12156.

Fung, H. L., & Bauer, J. A. (1994). Mechanisms of nitrate tolerance. *Cardiovascular Drugs and Therapy, 8*, 489–499.

Funk, C. D. (2001). Prostaglandins and leukotrienes: Advances in eicosanoid biology. *Science, 294*(5548), 1871–1875.

Funk, C. D. (2005). Leukotriene modifiers as potential therapeutics for cardiovascular disease. *Nature Reviews Drug Discovery, 4*, 664–672.

Gao, J., Kashfi, K., Liu, X., & Rigas, B. (2006). NO-donating aspirin induces phase II enzymes in vitro and in vivo. *Carcinogenesis, 27*, 803–810.

Gao, J., Kashfi, K., & Rigas, B. (2005). In vitro metabolism of nitric oxide-donating aspirin: The effect of positional isomerism. *Journal of Pharmacology and Experimental Therapeutics, 312*, 989–997.

Gao, J., Liu, X., & Rigas, B. (2005). Nitric oxide-donating aspirin induces apoptosis in human colon cancer cells through induction of oxidative stress. *Proceedings of the National Academy of Sciences, USA, 102*, 17207–17212.

Gardiner, P. J. (1986). Characterization of prostanoid relaxant/inhibitory receptors (psi) using a highly selective agonist, TR4979. *British Journal of Pharmacology, 87*, 45–56.

Garg, R., Ramchandani, A. G., & Maru, G. B. (2008). Curcumin decreases 12-O-tetradeca-noylphorbol-13-acetate-induced protein kinase C translocation to modulate downstream targets in mouse skin. *Carcinogenesis, 29*, 1249–1257.

Ghosh, J., & Myers, C. E. (1997). Arachidonic acid stimulates prostate cancer cell growth: Critical role of 5-lipoxygenase. *Biochemical and Biophysical Research Communications, 235*, 418–423.

Gilroy, D. W., Lawrence, T., Perretti, M., & Rossi, A. G. (2004). Inflammatory resolution: New opportunities for drug discovery. *Nature Reviews Drug Discovery, 3*, 401–416.

Gilroy, D. W., Tomlinson, A., & Willoughby, D. A. (1998). Differential effects of inhibitors of cyclooxygenase (cyclooxygenase 1 and cyclooxygenase 2) in acute inflammation. *European Journal of Pharmacology, 355*, 211–217.

Goubern, M., Andriamihaja, M., Nubel, T., Blachier, F., & Bouillaud, F. (2007). Sulfide, the first inorganic substrate for human cells. *The FASEB Journal, 21*, 1699–1706.

Grosser, N., & Schroder, H. (2000). A common pathway for nitric oxide release from NO-aspirin and glyceryl trinitrate. *Biochemical and Biophysical Research Communications, 274*, 255–258.

Guleng, B., Tateishi, K., Ohta, M., Kanai, F., Jazag, A., Ijichi, H., et al. (2005). Blockade of the stromal cell-derived factor-1/CXCR4 axis attenuates in vivo tumor growth by inhibiting angiogenesis in a vascular endothelial growth factor-independent manner. *Cancer Research, 65*, 5864–5871.

Gunning, W. T., Kramer, P. M., Lubet, R. A., Steele, V. E., & Pereira, M. A. (2000). Chemoprevention of vinyl carbamate-induced lung tumors in strain A mice. *Experimental Lung Research, 26*, 757–772.

Gunning, W. T., Kramer, P. M., Steele, V. E., & Pereira, M. A. (2002). Chemoprevention by lipoxygenase and leukotriene pathway inhibitors of vinyl carbamate-induced lung tumors in mice. *Cancer Research, 62*, 4199–4201.

Gupta, R. A., Tan, J., Krause, W. F., Geraci, M. W., Willson, T. M., Dey, S. K., et al. (2000). Prostacyclin-mediated activation of peroxisome proliferator-activated receptor delta in colorectal cancer. *Proceedings of the National Academy of Sciences, USA, 97*, 13275–13280.

Haeggstrom, J. Z. (2000). Structure, function, and regulation of leukotriene A4 hydrolase. *American Journal of Respiratory and Critical Care Medicine, 161*, S25–S31.

Hagos, G. K., Carroll, R. E., Kouznetsova, T., Li, Q., Toader, V., Fernandez, P. A., et al. (2007). Colon cancer chemoprevention by a novel NO chimera that shows anti-inflammatory and antiproli-ferative activity in vitro and in vivo. *Molecular Cancer Therapeutics, 6*, 2230–2239.

Half, E., & Arber, N. (2009). Colon cancer: Preventive agents and the present status of chemoprevention. *Expert Opinion on Pharmacotherapy, 10*, 211–219.

Hammamieh, R., Sumaida, D., Zhang, X., Das, R., & Jett, M. (2007). Control of the growth of human breast cancer cells in culture by manipulation of arachidonate metabolism. *BMC Cancer, 7*, 138.

Han, S., & Roman, J. (2004). Suppression of prostaglandin E2 receptor subtype EP2 by PPARgamma ligands inhibits human lung carcinoma cell growth. *Biochemical and Biophysical Research Communications, 314*, 1093–1099.

Hanauer, S. B. (2006). New lessons: Classic treatments, expanding options in ulcerative colitis. *Colorectal Disease, 8*(Suppl. 1), 20–24.

Hanif, R., Pittas, A., Feng, Y., Koutsos, M. I., Qiao, L., Staiano-Coico, L., et al. (1996). Effects of nonsteroidal anti-inflammatory drugs on proliferation and on induction of apoptosis in colon cancer cells by a prostaglandin-independent pathway. *Biochemical Pharmacology, 52*, 237–245.

Hara, A., & Okayasu, I. (2004). Cyclooxygenase-2 and inducible nitric oxide synthase expression in human astrocytic gliomas: Correlation with angiogenesis and prognostic significance. *Acta Neuropathologica, 108*, 43–48.

Hata, A. N., & Breyer, R. M. (2004). Pharmacology and signaling of prostaglandin receptors: Multiple roles in inflammation and immune modulation. *Pharmacology and Therapeutics, 103*, 147–166.

Hattori, Y., Kasai, K., & Gross, S. S. (2004). NO suppresses while peroxynitrite sustains NF-kappaB: A paradigm to rationalize cytoprotective and cytotoxic actions attributed to NO. *Cardiovascular Research, 63*, 31–40.

Hayashi, T., Nishiyama, K., & Shirahama, T. (2006). Inhibition of 5-lipoxygenase pathway suppresses the growth of bladder cancer cells. *International Journal of Urology, 13*, 1086–1091.

He, T. C., Chan, T. A., Vogelstein, B., & Kinzler, K. W. (1999). PPARdelta is an APC-regulated target of nonsteroidal anti-inflammatory drugs. *Cell, 99*, 335–345.

Hennig, R., Ding, X. Z., Tong, W. G., Witt, R. C., Jovanovic, B. D., & Adrian, T. E. (2004). Effect of LY293111 in combination with gemcitabine in colonic cancer. *Cancer Letters, 210*, 41–46.

Hirai, H., Tanaka, K., Yoshie, O., Ogawa, K., Kenmotsu, K., Takamori, Y., et al. (2001). Prostaglandin D2 selectively induces chemotaxis in T helper type 2 cells, eosinophils, and basophils via seven-transmembrane receptor CRTH2. *Journal of Experimental Medicine, 193*, 255–261.

Hogaboam, C. M., Befus, A. D., & Wallace, J. L. (1993). Modulation of rat mast cell reactivity by IL-1 beta. Divergent effects on nitric oxide and platelet-activating factor release. *Journal of Immunology, 151*, 3767–3774.

Hopkins, A. L., & Groom, C. R. (2002). The druggable genome. *Nature Reviews Drug Discovery, 1*, 727–730.

Hoque, A., Lippman, S. M., Wu, T. T., Xu, Y., Liang, Z. D., Swisher, S., et al. (2005). Increased 5-lipoxygenase expression and induction of apoptosis by its inhibitors in esophageal cancer: A potential target for prevention. *Carcinogenesis, 26*, 785–791.

Horuk, R. (2001). Chemokine receptors. *Cytokine and Growth Factor Reviews, 12*, 313–335.

Hosoki, R., Matsuki, N., & Kimura, H. (1997). The possible role of hydrogen sulfide as an endogenous smooth muscle relaxant in synergy with nitric oxide. *Biochemical and Biophysical Research Communications, 237*, 527–531.

Hu, L. F., Lu, M., Wu, Z. Y., Wong, P. T., & Bian, J. S. (2009). Hydrogen sulfide inhibits rotenone-induced apoptosis via preservation of mitochondrial function. *Molecular Pharmacology, 75*, 27–34.

Hu, L. F., Wong, P. T., Moore, P. K., & Bian, J. S. (2007). Hydrogen sulfide attenuates lipopolysaccharide-induced inflammation by inhibition of p38 mitogen-activated protein kinase in microglia. *Journal of Neurochemistry, 100*, 1121–1128.

Hu, R., Siu, C. W., Lau, E. O., Wang, W. Q., Lau, C. P., & Tse, H. F. (2007). Impaired nitrate-mediated dilatation could reflect nitrate tolerance in patients with coronary artery disease. *International Journal of Cardiology, 120*, 351–356.

Huang, F. P., Niedbala, W., Wei, X. Q., Xu, D., Feng, G. J., Robinson, J. H., et al. (1998). Nitric oxide regulates Th1 cell development through the inhibition of IL-12 synthesis by macrophages. *European Journal of Immunology, 28*, 4062–4070.

Huguenin, S., Vacherot, F., Fleury-Feith, J., Riffaud, J. P., Chopin, D. K., Bolla, M., et al. (2005). Evaluation of the antitumoral potential of different nitric oxide-donating nonsteroidal anti-inflammatory drugs (NO-NSAIDs) on human urological tumor cell lines. *Cancer Letters, 218*, 163–170.

Hulsman, N., Medema, J. P., Bos, C., Jongejan, A., Leurs, R., Smit, M. J., et al. (2007). Chemical insights in the concept of hybrid drugs: The antitumor effect of nitric oxide-donating aspirin involves a quinone methide but not nitric oxide nor aspirin. *Journal of Medicinal Chemistry, 50*, 2424–2431.

Hundley, T. R., & Rigas, B. (2006). Nitric oxide-donating aspirin inhibits colon cancer cell growth via mitogen-activated protein kinase activation. *Journal of Pharmacology and Experimental Therapeutics, 316*, 25–34.

Hussey, H. J., & Tisdale, M. J. (1996). Inhibition of tumour growth by lipoxygenase inhibitors. *British Journal of Cancer, 74*, 683–687.

Ignarro, L. J., Buga, G. M., Wood, K. S., Byrns, R. E., & Chaudhuri, G. (1987). Endothelium-derived relaxing factor produced and released from artery and vein is nitric oxide. *Proceedings of the National Academy of Sciences, USA, 84*, 9265–9269.

Ihara, A., Wada, K., Yoneda, M., Fujisawa, N., Takahashi, H., & Nakajima, A. (2007). Blockade of leukotriene B4 signaling pathway induces apoptosis and suppresses cell proliferation in colon cancer. *Journal of Pharmacological Sciences, 103*, 24–32.

Ikawa, H., Kamitani, H., Calvo, B. F., Foley, J. F., & Eling, T. E. (1999). Expression of 15-lipoxygenase-1 in human colorectal cancer. *Cancer Research, 59*, 360–366.

Johnson, S. M., Gulhati, P., Arrieta, I., Wang, X., Uchida, T., Gao, T., et al. (2009). Curcumin inhibits proliferation of colorectal carcinoma by modulating Akt/mTOR signaling. *Anticancer Research, 29*, 3185–3190.

Jung, S. H., Woo, M. S., Kim, S. Y., Kim, W. K., Hyun, J. W., Kim, E. J., et al. (2006). Ginseng saponin metabolite suppresses phorbol ester-induced matrix metalloproteinase-9 expression through inhibition of activator protein-1 and mitogen-activated protein kinase signaling pathways in human astroglioma cells. *International Journal of Cancer, 118*, 490–497.

Karin, M. (2006). Nuclear factor-kappaB in cancer development and progression. *Nature, 441*, 431–436.

Kashfi, K., Borgo, S., Williams, J. L., Chen, J., Gao, J., Glekas, A., et al. (2005). Positional isomerism markedly affects the growth inhibition of colon cancer cells by nitric oxide-donating aspirin in vitro and in vivo. *Journal of Pharmacology and Experimental Therapeutics, 312*, 978–988.

Kashfi, K., Nath, N., & Jacobs, L. (2007). *Flurbiprofen benzyl nitrate (FBN) modulates ß-catenin expression and inhibits growth of human epidermoid carcinoma A-431 cells.* 10th International Conference on "Eicosanoids & Other Bioactive Lipids in Cancer, Inflammation & Related Diseases", September 16–19, Montreal, Canada.

Kashfi, K., & Nazarenko, A. (2006). Nitric oxide-releasing aspirin suppresses NF-κB signaling in estrogen receptor negative breast cancer cells in vitro and in vivo: An effect through reactive oxygen species. *AACR: Fifth Annual International Conference on Frontiers in Cancer Prevention Research*, Boston, MA.

Kashfi, K., & Rigas, B. (2005). Non-COX-2 targets and cancer: Expanding the molecular target repertoire of chemoprevention. *Biochemical Pharmacology, 70*, 969–986.

Kashfi, K., & Rigas, B. (2007). The mechanism of action of nitric oxide-donating aspirin. *Biochemical and Biophysical Research Communications, 358*, 1096–1101.

Kashfi, K., Ryan, Y., Qiao, L. L., Williams, J. L., Chen, J., Del Soldato, P., et al. (2002). Nitric oxide-donating nonsteroidal anti-inflammatory drugs inhibit the growth of various cultured human cancer cells: Evidence of a tissue type-independent effect. *Journal of Pharmacology and Experimental Therapeutics, 303*, 1273–1282.

Kashiba, M., Kajimura, M., Goda, N., & Suematsu, M. (2002). From O_2 to H_2S: A landscape view of gas biology. *Keio Journal of Medicine, 51*, 1–10.

Kasper, H. U., Wolf, H., Drebber, U., Wolf, H. K., & Kern, M. A. (2004). Expression of inducible nitric oxide synthase and cyclooxygenase-2 in pancreatic adenocarcinoma: Correlation with microvessel density. *World Journal of Gastroenterology, 10*, 1918–1922.

Katsuyama, K., Shichiri, M., Marumo, F., & Hirata, Y. (1998). NO inhibits cytokine-induced iNOS expression and NF-kappaB activation by interfering with phosphorylation and

degradation of IkappaB-alpha. *Arteriosclerosis, Thrombosis, and Vascular Biology, 18*
(11), 1796–1802.

Keam, S. J., Lyseng-Williamson, K. A., & Goa, K. L. (2003). Pranlukast: A review of its use in
the management of asthma. *Drugs, 63*(10), 991–1019.

Kearney, P. M., Baigent, C., Godwin, J., Halls, H., Emberson, J. R., & Patrono, C. (2006). Do
selective cyclo-oxygenase-2 inhibitors and traditional non-steroidal anti-inflammatory
drugs increase the risk of atherothrombosis? Meta-analysis of randomised trials. *BMJ,
332*, 1302–1308.

Keefer, L. K. (2003). Progress toward clinical application of the nitric oxide-releasing
diazeniumdiolates. *Annual Review of Pharmacology and Toxicology, 43*, 585–607.

Kennedy, T. J., Chan, C. Y., Ding, X. Z., & Adrian, T. E. (2003). Lipoxygenase inhibitors for
the treatment of pancreatic cancer. *Expert Review of Anticancer Therapy, 3*, 525–536.

Kesherwani, V., & Sodhi, A. (2007). Involvement of tyrosine kinases and MAP kinases in the
production of TNF-alpha and IL-1beta by macrophages in vitro on treatment with
phytohemagglutinin. *Journal of Interferon and Cytokine Research, 27*, 497–505.

Kim, S. Y., Lee, C. H., Midura, B. V., Yeung, C., Mendoza, A., Hong, S. H., et al. (2008).
Inhibition of the CXCR4/CXCL12 chemokine pathway reduces the development of
murine pulmonary metastases. *Clinical and Experimental Metastasis, 25*, 201–211.

Kim, Y. S., Ahn, Y., Hong, M. H., Joo, S. Y., Kim, K. H., Sohn, I. S., et al. (2007). Curcumin
attenuates inflammatory responses of TNF-alpha-stimulated human endothelial cells.
Journal of Cardiovascular Pharmacology, 50, 41–49.

Kitamura, T., Itoh, M., Noda, T., Tani, K., Kobayashi, M., Maruyama, T., et al. (2003).
Combined effects of prostaglandin E receptor subtype EP1 and subtype EP4 antagonists
on intestinal tumorigenesis in adenomatous polyposis coli gene knockout mice. *Cancer
Science, 94*, 618–621.

Kodela, R., Chattopadhyay, M., Nath, N., Cieciura, L. Z., Pospishil, L., Boring, D., et al.
(2008). *Ester-protected hydroxybenzyl phosphates (EHBP) inhibit the growth of various
cultured human cancer cells: Evidence of a tissue type-independent effect.* In AACR:
Seventh Annual International Conference on Frontiers in Cancer Prevention Research,
Washington, DC.

Kodela, R., Rokita, S. E., Boring, D., Crowell, J. A., & Kashfi, K. (2008). *Bioactivated
chemotherapeutic agents based on ester-protected hydroxybenzyl phosphates (EHBP)
for reversible addition to cellular nucleophiles.* In AACR: Seventh Annual International
Conference on Frontiers in Cancer Prevention Research, Washington, DC.

Koeberle, A., Northoff, H., & Werz, O. (2009). Curcumin blocks prostaglandin E2 biosynthesis
through direct inhibition of the microsomal prostaglandin E2 synthase-1. *Molecular
Cancer Therapeutics, 8*, 2348–2355.

Koeberle, A., Siemoneit, U., Northoff, H., Hofmann, B., Schneider, G., & Werz, O. (2009). MK-
886, an inhibitor of the 5-lipoxygenase-activating protein, inhibits cyclooxygenase-1 activity
and suppresses platelet aggregation. *European Journal of Pharmacology, 608*, 84–90.

Kundu, J. K., & Surh, Y. J. (2008). Inflammation: Gearing the journey to cancer. *Mutation
Research, 659*, 15–30.

Kune, G., Kune, S., & Watson, L. (1988). Colorectal cancer risk, chronic illnesses, operations,
and medications: Case-control results from the Melbourne Colorectal Cancer Study.
Cancer Research, 48, 4399–4404.

Kunnumakkara, A. B., Diagaradjane, P., Anand, P., Kuzhuvelil, H. B., Deorukhkar, A.,
Gelovani, J., et al. (2009). Curcumin sensitizes human colorectal cancer to capecitabine
by modulation of cyclin D1, COX-2, MMP-9, VEGF and CXCR4 expression in an
orthotopic mouse model. *International Journal of Cancer, 125*, 2187–2197.

Kwak, M. K., Wakabayashi, N., & Kensler, T. W. (2004). Chemoprevention through the
Keap1-Nrf2 signaling pathway by phase 2 enzyme inducers. *Mutation Research, 555*,
133–148.

Landino, L. M., Crews, B. C., Timmons, M. D., Morrow, J. D., & Marnett, L. J. (1996). Peroxynitrite, the coupling product of nitric oxide and superoxide, activates prostaglandin biosynthesis. *Proceedings of the National Academy of Sciences, USA, 93*, 15069–15074.

Lawrence, T., Willoughby, D. A., & Gilroy, D. W. (2002). Anti-inflammatory lipid mediators and insights into the resolution of inflammation. *Nature Reviews Immunology, 2*, 787–795.

Lazzarato, L., Donnola, M., Rolando, B., Marini, E., Cena, C., Coruzzi, G., Guaita, E., Morini, G., Fruttero, R., Gasco, A., et al. (2008). Searching for new NO-donor aspirin-like molecules: A new class of nitrooxy-acyl derivatives of salicylic acid. *Journal of Medicinal Chemistry, 51*, 1894–1903.

Lee, J. S., & Surh, Y. J. (2005). Nrf2 as a novel molecular target for chemoprevention. *Cancer Letters, 224*, 171–184.

Leonetti, C., Scarsella, M., Zupi, G., Zoli, W., Amadori, D., Medri, L., et al. (2006). Efficacy of a nitric oxide-releasing nonsteroidal anti-inflammatory drug and cytotoxic drugs in human colon cancer cell lines in vitro and xenografts. *Molecular Cancer Therapeutics, 5*, 919–926.

Leval, X., Julemont, F., Delarge, J., Pirotte, B., & Dogne, J. M. (2002). New trends in dual 5-LOX/COX inhibition. *Current Medicinal Chemistry, 9*, 941–962.

Levonen, A. L., Lapatto, R., Saksela, M., & Raivio, K. O. (2000). Human cystathionine gamma-lyase: Developmental and in vitro expression of two isoforms. *Biochemical Journal, 347*, 291–295.

Ley, K. (2001). *Physiology of inflammation.* Oxford: Oxford University Press.

Li, L., Bhatia, M., & Moore, P. K. (2006). Hydrogen sulphide—a novel mediator of inflammation? *Current Opinion in Pharmacology, 6*, 125–129.

Li, L., Bhatia, M., Zhu, Y. Z., Zhu, Y. C., Ramnath, R. D., Wang, Z. J., et al. (2005). Hydrogen sulfide is a novel mediator of lipopolysaccharide-induced inflammation in the mouse. *The FASEB Journal, 19*, 1196–1198.

Li, L., Rossoni, G., Sparatore, A., Lee, L. C., Del Soldato, P., & Moore, P. K. (2007). Anti-inflammatory and gastrointestinal effects of a novel diclofenac derivative. *Free Radical Biology and Medicine, 42*, 706–719.

Li, N., Sood, S., Wang, S., Fang, M., Wang, P., Sun, Z., et al. (2005). Overexpression of 5-lipoxygenase and cyclooxygenase 2 in hamster and human oral cancer and chemopreventive effects of zileuton and celecoxib. *Clinical Cancer Research, 11*, 2089–2096.

Li, T. S. C., Mazza, G., Cottrell, A. C., & Gao, L. (1996). Ginsenosides in roots and leaves of American ginseng. *Journal of Agricultural and Food Chemistry, 44*, 717–720.

Liang, Z., Wu, T., Lou, H., Yu, X., Taichman, R. S., Lau, S. K., et al. (2004). Inhibition of breast cancer metastasis by selective synthetic polypeptide against CXCR4. *Cancer Research, 64*, 4302–4308.

Lipkin, M., Yang, K., Edelmann, W., Xue, L., Fan, K., Risio, M., et al. (1999). Preclinical mouse models for cancer chemoprevention studies. *Annals of the New York Academy of Sciences, 889*, 14–19.

Lu, Y., O'Dowd, B. F., Orrego, H., & Israel, Y. (1992). Cloning and nucleotide sequence of human liver cDNA encoding for cystathionine gamma-lyase. *Biochemical and Biophysical Research Communications, 189*, 749–758.

Luboshits, G., Shina, S., Kaplan, O., Engelberg, S., Nass, D., Lifshitz-Mercer, B., et al. (1999). Elevated expression of the CC chemokine regulated on activation, normal T cell expressed and secreted (RANTES) in advanced breast carcinoma. *Cancer Research, 59*, 4681–4687.

Mackay, C. R. (2001). Chemokines: Immunology's high impact factors. *Nature Immunology, 2*, 95–101.

Magee, E. A., Richardson, C. J., Hughes, R., & Cummings, J. H. (2000). Contribution of dietary protein to sulfide production in the large intestine: An in vitro and a controlled feeding study in humans. *American Journal of Clinical Nutrition, 72*, 1488–1494.

Majno, G., & Joris, I. (2004). *Cells, tissues, and disease: Principals of general pathology.* Oxford: Oxford University Press.

Mantovani, A., Allavena, P., Sica, A., & Balkwill, F. (2008). Cancer-related inflammation. *Nature, 454,* 436–444.

Mantovani, A., Allavena, P., Sozzani, S., Vecchi, A., Locati, M., & Sica, A. (2004). Chemokines in the recruitment and shaping of the leukocyte infiltrate of tumors. *Seminars in Cancer Biology, 14,* 155–160.

Mariggio, M. A., Minunno, V., Riccardi, S., Santacroce, R., De Rinaldis, P., & Fumarulo, R. (1998). Sulfide enhancement of PMN apoptosis. *Immunopharmacology and Immunotoxicology, 20,* 399–408.

Maulik, N., & Das, D. K. (2008). Emerging potential of thioredoxin and thioredoxin interacting proteins in various disease conditions. *Biochimica et Biophysica Acta, 1780,* 1368–1382.

Medzhitov, R. (2008). Origin and physiological roles of inflammation. *Nature, 454,* 428–435.

Meier, M., Janosik, M., Kery, V., Kraus, J. P., & Burkhard, P. (2001). Structure of human cystathionine beta-synthase: A unique pyridoxal 5′-phosphate-dependent heme protein. *Embo Journal, 20,* 3910–3916.

Meijer, J., Ogink, J., & Roos, E. (2008). Effect of the chemokine receptor CXCR7 on proliferation of carcinoma cells in vitro and in vivo. *British Journal of Cancer, 99,* 1493–1501.

Melstrom, L. G., Bentrem, D. J., Salabat, M. R., Kennedy, T. J., Ding, X. Z., Strouch, M., et al. (2008). Overexpression of 5-lipoxygenase in colon polyps and cancer and the effect of 5-LOX inhibitors in vitro and in a murine model. *Clinical Cancer Research, 14,* 6525–6530.

Meyerhardt, J. A., & Mayer, R. J. (2005). Systemic therapy for colorectal cancer. *New England Journal of Medicine, 352,* 476–487.

Miller, D. K., Gillard, J. W., Vickers, P. J., Sadowski, S., Leveille, C., Mancini, J. A., et al. (1990). Identification and isolation of a membrane protein necessary for leukotriene production. *Nature, 343,* 278–281.

Monti, P., Leone, B. E., Marchesi, F., Balzano, G., Zerbi, A., Scaltrini, F., et al. (2003). The CC chemokine MCP-1/CCL2 in pancreatic cancer progression: Regulation of expression and potential mechanisms of antimalignant activity. *Cancer Research, 63,* 7451–7461.

Moody, T. W., Leyton, J., Martinez, A., Hong, S., Malkinson, A., & Mulshine, J. L. (1998). Lipoxygenase inhibitors prevent lung carcinogenesis and inhibit non-small cell lung cancer growth. *Experimental Lung Research, 24,* 617–628.

Moon, R. T., Kohn, A. D., De Ferrari, G. V., & Kaykas, A. (2004). WNT and beta-catenin signalling: Diseases and therapies. *Nature Reviews Genetics, 5,* 691–701.

Morris, G. P., Beck, P. L., Herridge, M. S., Depew, W. T., Szewczuk, M. R., & Wallace, J. L. (1989). Hapten-induced model of chronic inflammation and ulceration in the rat colon. *Gastroenterology, 96,* 795–803.

Mueller, M. M., & Fusenig, N. E. (2004). Friends or foes—bipolar effects of the tumour stroma in cancer. *Nature Reviews Cancer, 4,* 839–849.

Murphy, P. M. (2001). Chemokines and the molecular basis of cancer metastasis. *New England Journal of Medicine, 345,* 833–835.

Murphy, P. M., Baggiolini, M., Charo, I. F., Hebert, C. A., Horuk, R., Matsushima, K., et al. (2000). International union of pharmacology. XXII. Nomenclature for chemokine receptors. *Pharmacological Reviews, 52,* 145–176.

Mutoh, M., Watanabe, K., Kitamura, T., Shoji, Y., Takahashi, M., Kawamori, T., et al. (2002). Involvement of prostaglandin E receptor subtype EP(4) in colon carcinogenesis. *Cancer Research, 62,* 28–32.

Nakadate, T., Yamamoto, S., Aizu, E., & Kato, R. (1985). Inhibition of mouse epidermal 12-lipoxygenase by 2,3,4-trimethyl-6-(12-hydroxy-5,10-dodecadiynyl)-1,4-benzoquinon e (AA861). *Journal of Pharmacy and Pharmacology, 37,* 71–73.

Naseem, K. M. (2005). The role of nitric oxide in cardiovascular diseases. *Molecular Aspects of Medicine, 26,* 33–65.

Nath, N., Kashfi, K., Chen, J., & Rigas, B. (2003). Nitric oxide-donating aspirin inhibits beta-catenin/T cell factor (TCF) signaling in SW480 colon cancer cells by disrupting the nuclear beta-catenin-TCF association. *Proceedings of the National Academy of Sciences, USA, 100,* 12584–12589.

Nath, N., Labaze, G., Rigas, B., & Kashfi, K. (2005). NO-donating aspirin inhibits the growth of leukemic Jurkat cells and modulates beta-catenin expression. *Biochemical and Biophysical Research Communications, 326,* 93–99.

Nath, N., Vassell, R., Chattopadhyay, M., Kogan, M., & Kashfi, K. (2009). Nitro-aspirin inhibits MCF-7 breast cancer cell growth: Effects on COX-2 Expression and Wnt/beta-catenin/TCF-4 signaling. *Biochemical Pharmacology, 15,* 1298–1304.

Negus, R. P., Stamp, G. W., Hadley, J., & Balkwill, F. R. (1997). Quantitative assessment of the leukocyte infiltrate in ovarian cancer and its relationship to the expression of C-C chemokines. *American Journal of Pathology, 150,* 1723–1734.

Niho, N., Mutoh, M., Kitamura, T., Takahashi, M., Sato, H., Yamamoto, H., et al. (2005). Suppression of azoxymethane-induced colon cancer development in rats by a prostaglandin E receptor EP1-selective antagonist. *Cancer Science, 96,* 260–264.

Ogilvie, P., Bardi, G., Clark-Lewis, I., Baggiolini, M., & Uguccioni, M. (2001). Eotaxin is a natural antagonist for CCR2 and an agonist for CCR5. *Blood, 97,* 1920–1924.

Okabe, S., & Amagase, K. (2005). An overview of acetic acid ulcer models—the history and state of the art of peptic ulcer research. *Biological and Pharmaceutical Bulletin, 28,* 1321–1341.

Okamoto, T., Sanda, T., & Asamitsu, K. (2007). NF-kappa B signaling and carcinogenesis. *Current Pharmaceutical Design, 13,* 447–462.

Ortiz, M. I., Castaneda-Hernandez, G., Rosas, R., Vidal-Cantu, G. C., & Granados-Soto, V. (2001). Evidence for a new mechanism of action of diclofenac: Activation of K+ channels. *Proceedings of the Western Pharmacology Society, 44,* 19–21.

Oshima, M., Dinchuk, J. E., Kargman, S. L., Oshima, H., Hancock, B., Kwong, E., et al. (1996). Suppression of intestinal polyposis in $Apc^{\Delta716}$ knockout mice by inhibition of cyclooxygenase 2 (COX-2). *Cell, 87,* 803–809.

Ouyang, N., Williams, J. L., & Rigas, B. (2006). NO-donating aspirin isomers downregulate peroxisome proliferator-activated receptor (PPAR)δ expression in APCmin/+ mice proportionally to their tumor inhibitory effect: Implications for the role of PPARδ in carcinogenesis. *Carcinogenesis, 27,* 232–239.

Ouyang, N., Williams, J. L., Tsioulias, G. J., Gao, J., Iatropoulos, M. J., Kopelovich, L., et al. (2006). Nitric oxide-donating aspirin prevents pancreatic cancer in a hamster tumor model. *Cancer Research, 66,* 4503–4511.

Pace, N. R. (1997). A molecular view of microbial diversity and the biosphere. *Science, 276,* 734–740.

Pan, M. H., & Ho, C. T. (2008). Chemopreventive effects of natural dietary compounds on cancer development. *Chemical Society Reviews, 37,* 2558–2574.

Pan, M. H., Lai, C. S., Dushenkov, S., & Ho, C. T. (2009). Modulation of inflammatory genes by natural dietary bioactive compounds. *Journal of Agricultural and Food Chemistry, 57,* 4467–4477.

Perez-Sala, D., & Lamas, S. (2001). Regulation of cyclooxygenase-2 expression by nitric oxide in cells. *Antioxidants & Redox Signaling, 3,* 231–248.

Perkins, S., Verschoyle, R. D., Hill, K., Parveen, I., Threadgill, M. D., Sharma, R. A., et al. (2002). Chemopreventive efficacy and pharmacokinetics of curcumin in the min/+ mouse, a model of familial adenomatous polyposis. *Cancer Epidemiology, Biomarkers & Prevention, 11,* 535–540.

Poff, C. D., & Balazy, M. (2004). Drugs that target lipoxygenases and leukotrienes as emerging therapies for asthma and cancer. *Current Drug Targets—Inflammation & Allergy, 3*, 19–33.

Pozzi, A., Yan, X., Macias-Perez, I., Wei, S., Hata, A. N., Breyer, R. M., et al. (2004). Colon carcinoma cell growth is associated with prostaglandin E2/EP4 receptor-evoked ERK activation. *Journal of Biological Chemistry, 279*, 29797–29804.

Rao, C. V., Kawamori, T., Hamid, R., & Reddy, B. S. (1999). Chemoprevention of colonic aberrant crypt foci by an inducible nitric oxide synthase-selective inhibitor. *Carcinogenesis, 20*, 641–644.

Rao, C. V., Reddy, B. S., Steele, V. E., Wang, C. X., Liu, X., Ouyang, N., et al. (2006). Nitric oxide-releasing aspirin and indomethacin are potent inhibitors against colon cancer in azoxymethane-treated rats: Effects on molecular targets. *Molecular Cancer Therapeutics, 5*, 1530–1538.

Raynauld, J. P., Martel-Pelletier, J., Bias, P., Laufer, S., Haraoui, B., Choquette, D., et al. (2009). Protective effects of licofelone, a 5-lipoxygenase and cyclo-oxygenase inhibitor, versus naproxen on cartilage loss in knee osteoarthritis: A first multicentre clinical trial using quantitative MRI. *Annals of the Rheumatic Diseases, 68*, 938–947.

Reichrath, J. (2007). Vitamin D and the skin: An ancient friend, revisited. *Experimental Dermatology, 16*, 618–625.

Reid, J. J. (2001). ABT-761 (Abbott). *Current Opinion in Investigational Drugs, 2*, 68–71.

Reiffenstein, R. J., Hulbert, W. C., & Roth, S. H. (1992). Toxicology of hydrogen sulfide. *Annual Review of Pharmacology and Toxicology, 32*, 109–134.

Ridnour, L. A., Thomas, D. D., Donzelli, S., Espey, M. G., Roberts, D. D., Wink, D. A., et al. (2006). The biphasic nature of nitric oxide responses in tumor biology. *Antioxidants & Redox Signaling, 8*, 1329–1337

Rigas, B., Goldman, I. S., & Levine, L. (1993). Altered eicosanoid levels in human colon cancer. *Journal of Laboratory and Clinical Medicine, 122*, 518–523.

Rigas, B., & Sun, Y. (2008). Induction of oxidative stress as a mechanism of action of chemopreventive agents against cancer. *British Journal of Cancer, 98*, 1157–1160.

Rioux, N., & Castonguay, A. (1998). Inhibitors of lipoxygenase: A new class of cancer chemopreventive agents. *Carcinogenesis, 19*, 1393–1400.

Saif, M. W., Oettle, H., Vervenne, W. L., Thomas, J. P., Spitzer, G., Visseren-Grul, C., et al. (2009). Randomized double-blind phase II trial comparing gemcitabine plus LY293111 versus gemcitabine plus placebo in advanced adenocarcinoma of the pancreas. *Cancer Journal, 15*, 339–343.

Sander, M., Chavoshan, B., & Victor, R. G. (1999). A large blood pressure-raising effect of nitric oxide synthase inhibition in humans. *Hypertension, 33*, 937–942.

Sandler, R. S., Halabi, S., Baron, J. A., Budinger, S., Paskett, E., Keresztes, R., et al. (2003). A randomized trial of aspirin to prevent colorectal adenomas in patients with previous colorectal cancer. *New England Journal of Medicine, 348*, 883–890.

Santucci, L., Fiorucci, S., Di Matteo, F. M., & Morelli, A. (1995). Role of tumor necrosis factor alpha release and leukocyte margination in indomethacin-induced gastric injury in rats. *Gastroenterology, 108*, 393–401.

Sartor, R. B. (1997). Pathogenesis and immune mechanisms of chronic inflammatory bowel diseases. *American Journal of Gastroenterology, 92*, 5S–11S.

Sato, M., Pei, R. J., Yuri, T., Danbara, N., Nakane, Y., & Tsubura, A. (2003). Prepubertal resveratrol exposure accelerates N-methyl-N-nitrosourea-induced mammary carcinoma in female Sprague–Dawley rats. *Cancer Letters, 202*, 137–145.

Schottenfeld, D., & Beebe-Dimmer, J. (2006). Chronic inflammation: A common and important factor in the pathogenesis of neoplasia. *CA: A Cancer Journal for Clinicians, 56*, 69–83.

Scotton, C. J., Wilson, J. L., Milliken, D., Stamp, G., & Balkwill, F. R. (2001). Epithelial cancer cell migration: A role for chemokine receptors? *Cancer Research, 61*, 4961–4965.

Searcy, D. G., & Lee, S. H. (1998). Sulfur reduction by human erythrocytes. *Journal of Experimental Zoology, 282*, 310–322.

Shoji, Y., Takahashi, M., Kitamura, T., Watanabe, K., Kawamori, T., Maruyama, T., et al. (2004). Downregulation of prostaglandin E receptor subtype EP3 during colon cancer development. *Gut, 53*, 1151–1158.

Shureiqi, I., Chen, D., Lotan, R., Yang, P., Newman, R. A., Fischer, S. M., et al. (2000). 15-Lipoxygenase-1 mediates nonsteroidal anti-inflammatory drug-induced apoptosis independently of cyclooxygenase-2 in colon cancer cells. *Cancer Research, 60,* 6846–6850.

Shureiqi, I., & Lippman, S. M. (2001). Lipoxygenase modulation to reverse carcinogenesis. *Cancer Research, 61,* 6307–6312.

Siezen, C. L., Tijhuis, M. J., Kram, N. R., van Soest, E. M., de Jong, D. J., Fodde, R., et al. (2006). Protective effect of nonsteroidal anti-inflammatory drugs on colorectal adenomas is modified by a polymorphism in peroxisome proliferator-activated receptor delta. *Pharmacogenetics and Genomics, 16,* 43–50.

Simpson, E. R., Mahendroo, M. S., Means, G. D., Kilgore, M. W., Hinshelwood, M. M., Graham-Lorence, S., et al. (1994). Aromatase cytochrome P450, the enzyme responsible for estrogen biosynthesis. *Endocrine Reviews, 15,* 342–355.

Singh, G., Miller, J. D., Huse, D. M., Pettitt, D., D'Agostino, R. B., & Russell, M. W. (2003). Consequences of increased systolic blood pressure in patients with osteoarthritis and rheumatoid arthritis. *Journal of Rheumatology, 30,* 714–719.

Slettenaar, V. I., & Wilson, J. L. (2006). The chemokine network: A target in cancer biology? *Advanced Drug Delivery Reviews, 58,* 962–974.

Soh, J. W., & Weinstein, I. B. (2003). Role of COX-independent targets of NSAIDs and related compounds in cancer prevention and treatment. *Progress in Experimental Tumor Research, 37,* 261–285.

Soleas, G. J., Grass, L., Josephy, P. D., Goldberg, D. M., & Diamandis, E. P. (2002). A comparison of the anticarcinogenic properties of four red wine polyphenols. *Clinical Biochemistry, 35,* 119–124.

Sonoshita, M., Takaku, K., Sasaki, N., Sugimoto, Y., Ushikubi, F., Narumiya, S., et al. (2001). Acceleration of intestinal polyposis through prostaglandin receptor EP2 in Apc(Delta 716) knockout mice. *Nature Medicine, 7,* 1048–1051.

Spiegel, A., Hundley, T. R., Chen, J., Gao, J., Ouyang, N., Liu, X., et al. (2005). NO-donating aspirin inhibits both the expression and catalytic activity of inducible nitric oxide synthase in HT-29 human colon cancer cells. *Biochemical Pharmacology, 70,* 993–1000.

Stallmach, A., Wittig, B., Giese, T., Pfister, K., Hoffmann, J. C., Bulfone-Paus, S., et al. (1999). Protection of trinitrobenzene sulfonic acid-induced colitis by an interleukin 2-IgG2b fusion protein in mice. *Gastroenterology, 117,* 866–876.

Steele, V. E., Holmes, C. A., Hawk, E. T., Kopelovich, L., Lubet, R. A., Crowell, J. A., et al. (1999). Lipoxygenase inhibitors as potential cancer chemopreventives. *Cancer Epidemiology, Biomarkers & Prevention, 8,* 467–483.

Steinbach, G., Lynch, P. M., Phillips, R. K., Wallace, M. H., Hawk, E., Gordon, G. B., et al. (2000). The effect of celecoxib, a cyclooxygenase-2 inhibitor, in familial adenomatous polyposis. *New England Journal of Medicine, 342,* 1946–1952.

Strieter, R. M., Belperio, J. A., Phillips, R. J., & Keane, M. P. (2004). CXC chemokines in angiogenesis of cancer. *Seminars in Cancer Biology, 14,* 195–200.

Stuehr, D. J. (1997). Structure-function aspects in the nitric oxide synthases. *Annual Review of Pharmacology and Toxicology, 37,* 339–359.

Subbaramaiah, K., Hudis, C., Chang, S. H., Hla, T., & Dannenberg, A. J. (2008). EP2 and EP4 receptors regulate aromatase expression in human adipocytes and breast cancer cells. Evidence of a BRCA1 and p300 exchange. *Journal of Biological Chemistry, 283,* 3433–3444.

Sun, Y., & Rigas, B. (2008). The thioredoxin system mediates redox-induced cell death in human colon cancer cells: Implications for the mechanism of action of anticancer agents. *Cancer Research, 68*, 8269–8277.

Sveinbjornsson, B., Rasmuson, A., Baryawno, N., Wan, M., Pettersen, I., Ponthan, F., et al. (2008). Expression of enzymes and receptors of the leukotriene pathway in human neuroblastoma promotes tumor survival and provides a target for therapy. *The FASEB Journal, 22*, 3525–3536.

Szlosarek, P. W., & Balkwill, F. R. (2003). Tumour necrosis factor alpha: A potential target for the therapy of solid tumours. *The Lancet Oncology, 4*, 565–573.

Takahashi, M., Mutoh, M., Shoji, Y., Sato, H., Kamanaka, Y., Naka, M., et al. (2006). Suppressive effect of an inducible nitric oxide inhibitor, ONO-1714, on AOM-induced rat colon carcinogenesis. *Nitric Oxide, 14*, 130–136.

Takamori, H., Oades, Z. G., Hoch, O. C., Burger, M., & Schraufstatter, I. U. (2000). Autocrine growth effect of IL-8 and GROalpha on a human pancreatic cancer cell line, Capan-1. *Pancreas, 21*, 52–56.

Takkouche, B., Regueira-Mendez, C., & Etminan, M. (2008). Breast cancer and use of non-steroidal anti-inflammatory drugs: A meta-analysis. *Journal of the National Cancer Institute., 100*, 1439–1447.

Tamizhselvi, R., Moore, P. K., & Bhatia, M. (2007). Hydrogen sulfide acts as a mediator of inflammation in acute pancreatitis: In vitro studies using isolated mouse pancreatic acinar cells. *Journal of Cellular and Molecular Medicine, 11*, 315–326.

Tanaka, T., Bai, Z., Srinoulprasert, Y., Yang, B. G., Hayasaka, H., & Miyasaka, M. (2005). Chemokines in tumor progression and metastasis. *Cancer Science, 96*, 317–322.

Tesei, A., Ulivi, P., Fabbri, F., Rosetti, M., Leonetti, C., Scarsella, M., et al. (2005). In vitro and in vivo evaluation of NCX 4040 cytotoxic activity in human colon cancer cell lines. *Journal of Translational Medicine, 3*, 7.

Tessitore, L., Davit, A., Sarotto, I., & Caderni, G. (2000). Resveratrol depresses the growth of colorectal aberrant crypt foci by affecting bax and p21(CIP) expression. *Carcinogenesis, 21*, 1619–1622.

Thatcher, G. R., Nicolescu, A. C., Bennett, B. M., & Toader, V. (2004). Nitrates and NO release: Contemporary aspects in biological and medicinal chemistry. *Free Radical Biology and Medicine, 37*, 1122–1143.

Thomsen, L. L., Miles, D. W., Happerfield, L., Bobrow, L. G., Knowles, R. G., & Moncada, S. (1995). Nitric oxide synthase activity in human breast cancer. *British Journal of Cancer, 72*, 41–44.

ThomsonPharma. (2009). Retrieved from http://www.thomsonscientific.com/thomsonpharma/modules/clinical/

Thun, M. J., Henley, S. J., & Patrono, C. (2002). Nonsteroidal anti-inflammatory drugs as anticancer agents: Mechanistic, pharmacologic, and clinical issues. *Journal of the National Cancer Institute, 94*, 252–266.

Tong, W. G., Ding, X. Z., Talamonti, M. S., Bell, R. H., & Adrian, T. E. (2007). Leukotriene B4 receptor antagonist LY293111 induces S-phase cell cycle arrest and apoptosis in human pancreatic cancer cells. *Anticancer Drugs, 18*, 535–541.

Tsukada, T., Nakashima, K., & Shirakawa, S. (1986). Arachidonate 5-lipoxygenase inhibitors show potent antiproliferative effects on human leukemia cell lines. *Biochemical and Biophysical Research Communications, 140*, 832–836.

Turnbull, C. M., Cena, C., Fruttero, R., Gasco, A., Rossi, A. G., & Megson, I. L. (2006). Mechanism of action of novel NO-releasing furoxan derivatives of aspirin in human platelets. *British Journal of Pharmacology, 148*, 517–526.

Turnbull, C. M., Marcarino, P., Sheldrake, T. A., Lazzarato, L., Cena, C., Fruttero, R., et al. (2008). A novel hybrid aspirin-NO-releasing compound inhibits TNFalpha release from LPS-activated human monocytes and macrophages. *Journal of Inflammation (London), 5*, 12.

Vane, J. R., Bakhle, Y. S., & Botting, R. M. (1998). Cyclooxygenases 1 and 2. *Annual Review of Pharmacology and Toxicology, 38*, 97–120.

Velazquez, C., Praveen Rao, P. N., & Knaus, E. E. (2005). Novel nonsteroidal antiinflammatory drugs possessing a nitric oxide donor diazen-1-ium-1,2-diolate moiety: Design, synthesis, biological evaluation, and nitric oxide release studies. *Journal of Medicinal Chemistry, 48*, 4061–4067.

Velazquez, C. A., Chen, Q. H., Citro, M. L., Keefer, L. K., & Knaus, E. E. (2008). Second-generation aspirin and indomethacin prodrugs possessing an O(2)-(acetoxymethyl)-1-(2-carboxypyrrolidin-1-yl)diazenium-1,2-diolate nitric oxide donor moiety: Design, synthesis, biological evaluation, and nitric oxide release studies. *Journal of Medicinal Chemistry, 51*, 1954–1961.

Velazquez, C. A., Praveen Rao, P. N., Citro, M. L., Keefer, L. K., & Knaus, E. E. (2007). O2-acetoxymethyl-protected diazeniumdiolate-based NSAIDs (NONO-NSAIDs): Synthesis, nitric oxide release, and biological evaluation studies. *Bioorganic and Medicinal Chemistry, 15*, 4767–4774.

Vicari, A. P., & Caux, C. (2002). Chemokines in cancer. *Cytokine and Growth Factor Reviews, 13*, 143–154.

Villani-Price, D., Yang, D. C., Walsh, R. E., Fretland, D. J., Keith, R. H., Kocan, G., et al. (1992). Multiple actions of the leukotriene B4 receptor antagonist SC-41930. *Journal of Pharmacology and Experimental Therapeutics, 260*, 187–191.

Voronov, E., Shouval, D. S., Krelin, Y., Cagnano, E., Benharroch, D., Iwakura, Y., et al. (2003). IL-1 is required for tumor invasiveness and angiogenesis. *Proceedings of the National Academy of Sciences, USA, 100*, 2645–2650.

Wallace, J. L. (2007a). Building a better aspirin: Gaseous solutions to a century-old problem. *British Journal of Pharmacology, 152*, 421–428.

Wallace, J. L. (2007b). Hydrogen sulfide-releasing anti-inflammatory drugs. *Trends In Pharmacological Sciences, 28*, 501–505.

Wallace, J. L. (2008). Prostaglandins, NSAIDs, and gastric mucosal protection: Why doesn't the stomach digest itself? *Physiological Reviews, 88*, 1547–1565.

Wallace, J. L., Caliendo, G., Santagada, V., Cirino, G., & Fiorucci, S. (2007). Gastrointestinal safety and anti-inflammatory effects of a hydrogen sulfide-releasing diclofenac derivative in the rat. *Gastroenterology, 132*, 261–271.

Wallace, J. L., & Del Soldato, P. (2003). The therapeutic potential of NO-NSAIDs. *Fundamental and Clinical Pharmacology, 17*, 11–20.

Wallace, J. L., Dicay, M., McKnight, W., & Martin, G. R. (2007). Hydrogen sulfide enhances ulcer healing in rats. *The FASEB Journal, 21*, 4070–4076.

Wallace, J. L., Ignarro, L. J., & Fiorucci, S. (2002). Potential cardioprotective actions of no-releasing aspirin. *Nature Reviews Drug Discovery, 1*, 375–382.

Wallace, J. L., McKnight, W., Del Soldato, P., Baydoun, A. R., & Cirino, G. (1995). Antithrombotic effects of a nitric oxide-releasing, gastric-sparing aspirin derivative. *Journal of Clinical Investigation, 96*, 2711–2718.

Wallace, J. L., & Miller, M. J. (2000). Nitric oxide in mucosal defense: A little goes a long way. *Gastroenterology, 119*, 512–520.

Wallace, J. L., Reuter, B., Cicala, C., McKnight, W., Grisham, M. B., & Cirino, G. (1994). A diclofenac derivative without ulcerogenic properties. *European Journal of Pharmacology, 257*, 249–255.

Wallace, J. L., Reuter, B., Cicala, C., McKnight, W., Grisham, M. B., & Cirino, G. (1994). Novel nonsteroidal anti-inflammatory drug derivatives with markedly reduced ulcerogenic properties in the rat. *Gastroenterology, 107*, 173–179.

Wallace, J. L., Viappiani, S., & Bolla, M. (2009). Cyclooxygenase-inhibiting nitric oxide donators for osteoarthritis. *Trends in Pharmacological Sciences, 30*, 112–117.

Wang, R. (2002). Two's company, three's a crowd: Can H2S be the third endogenous gaseous transmitter? *The FASEB Journal, 16*, 1792–1798.

Wang, Y., Zhou, B., Li, J., Cao, Y. B., Chen, X. S., Cheng, M. H., et al. (2004). Inhibitors of 5-lipoxygenase inhibit expression of intercellular adhesion molecule-1 in human melanoma cells. *Acta Pharmacologica Sinica, 25*, 672–677.

Watanabe, K., Kawamori, T., Nakatsugi, S., Ohta, T., Ohuchida, S., Yamamoto, H., et al. (1999). Role of the prostaglandin E receptor subtype EP1 in colon carcinogenesis. *Cancer Research, 59*, 5093–5096.

Wenger, F. A., Kilian, M., Achucarro, P., Heinicken, D., Schimke, I., Guski, H., et al. (2002). Effects of Celebrex and Zyflo on BOP-induced pancreatic cancer in Syrian hamsters. *Pancreatology, 2*, 54–60.

Westley, A. M., & Westley, J. (1991). Biological sulfane sulfur. *Analytical Biochemistry, 195*, 63–67.

Whiteman, M., Armstrong, J. S., Chu, S. H., Jia-Ling, S., Wong, B. S., Cheung, N. S., et al. (2004). The novel neuromodulator hydrogen sulfide: An endogenous peroxynitrite "scavenger"? *Journal of Neurochemistry, 90*, 765–768.

Whiteman, M., Cheung, N. S., Zhu, Y. Z., Chu, S. H., Siau, J. L., Wong, B. S., et al. (2005). Hydrogen sulphide: A novel inhibitor of hypochlorous acid-mediated oxidative damage in the brain? *Biochemical and Biophysical Research Communications, 326*, 794–798.

WHO. (2009). *Global strategy on diet, physical activity and health*. Retrieved from http://www. who.int/dietphysicalactivity/publications/facts/cancer/en/

Williams, J. L., Borgo, S., Hasan, I., Castillo, E., Traganos, F., & Rigas, B. (2001). Nitric oxide-releasing nonsteroidal anti-inflammatory drugs (NSAIDs) alter the kinetics of human colon cancer cell lines more effectively than traditional NSAIDs: Implications for colon cancer chemoprevention. *Cancer Research, 61*, 3285–3289.

Williams, J. L., Ji, P., Ouyang, N., Liu, X., & Rigas, B. (2008). NO-donating aspirin inhibits the activation of NF-kappaB in human cancer cell lines and Min mice. *Carcinogenesis, 29*, 390–397.

Williams, J. L., Kashfi, K., Ouyang, N., del Soldato, P., Kopelovich, L., & Rigas, B. (2004). NO-donating aspirin inhibits intestinal carcinogenesis in Min (APC(Min/+)) mice. *Biochemical and Biophysical Research Communications, 313*, 784–788.

Williams, J. L., Nath, N., Chen, J., Hundley, T. R., Gao, J., Kopelovich, L., et al. (2003). Growth inhibition of human colon cancer cells by nitric oxide (NO)-donating aspirin is associated with cyclooxygenase-2 induction and beta-catenin/T-cell factor signaling, nuclear factor-kappaB, and NO synthase 2 inhibition: Implications for chemoprevention. *Cancer Research, 63*, 7613–7618.

Wink, D. A., Vodovotz, Y., Laval, J., Laval, F., Dewhirst, M. W., & Mitchell, J. B. (1998). The multifaceted roles of nitric oxide in cancer. *Carcinogenesis, 19*, 711–721.

Wu, X., Lee, V. C., Chevalier, E., & Hwang, S. T. (2009). Chemokine receptors as targets for cancer therapy. *Current Pharmaceutical Design, 15*, 742–757.

Wung, B. S., Hsu, M. C., Wu, C. C., & Hsieh, C. W. (2005). Resveratrol suppresses IL-6-induced ICAM-1 gene expression in endothelial cells: Effects on the inhibition of STAT3 phosphorylation. *Life Sciences, 78*, 389–397.

Wyckoff, J., Wang, W., Lin, E. Y., Wang, Y., Pixley, F., Stanley, E. R., et al. (2004). A paracrine loop between tumor cells and macrophages is required for tumor cell migration in mammary tumors. *Cancer Research, 64*, 7022–7029.

Xu, G. L., Liu, F., Ao, G. Z., He, S. Y., Ju, M., Zhao, Y., et al. (2009). Anti-inflammatory effects and gastrointestinal safety of NNU-hdpa, a novel dual COX/5-LOX inhibitor. *European Journal of Pharmacology, 611*, 100–106.

Xu, W., Liu, L. Z., Loizidou, M., Ahmed, M., & Charles, I. G. (2002). The role of nitric oxide in cancer. *Cell Research, 12*, 311–320.

Yaal-Hahoshen, N., Shina, S., Leider-Trejo, L., Barnea, I., Shabtai, E. L., Azenshtein, E., et al. (2006). The chemokine CCL5 as a potential prognostic factor predicting disease progression in stage II breast cancer patients. *Clinical Cancer Research, 12,* 4474–4480.

Yang, C. S., Wang, X., Lu, G., & Picinich, S. C. (2009). Cancer prevention by tea: Animal studies, molecular mechanisms and human relevance. *Nature Reviews Cancer, 9,* 429–439.

Ye, S. F., Hou, Z. Q., Zhong, L. M., & Zhang, Q. Q. (2007). Effect of curcumin on the induction of glutathione S-transferases and NADP(H):quinone oxidoreductase and its possible mechanism of action. *Yao Xue Xue Bao, 42,* 376–380.

Yeh, R. K., Chen, J., Williams, J. L., Baluch, M., Hundley, T. R., Rosenbaum, R. E., et al. (2004). NO-donating nonsteroidal antiinflammatory drugs (NSAIDs) inhibit colon cancer cell growth more potently than traditional NSAIDs: A general pharmacological property? *Biochemical Pharmacology, 67,* 2197–2205.

Yokomizo, T., Izumi, T., & Shimizu, T. (2001). Leukotriene B4: Metabolism and signal transduction. *Archives of Biochemistry and Biophysics, 385,* 231–241.

Yoon, Y., Liang, Z., Zhang, X., Choe, M., Zhu, A., Cho, H. T., et al. (2007). CXC chemokine receptor-4 antagonist blocks both growth of primary tumor and metastasis of head and neck cancer in xenograft mouse models. *Cancer Research, 67,* 7518–7524.

Yu, H., Kortylewski, M., & Pardoll, D. (2007). Crosstalk between cancer and immune cells: Role of STAT3 in the tumour microenvironment. *Nature Reviews Immunology, 7,* 41–51.

Zanardo, R. C., Brancaleone, V., Distrutti, E., Fiorucci, S., Cirino, G., & Wallace, J. L. (2006). Hydrogen sulfide is an endogenous modulator of leukocyte-mediated inflammation. *The FASEB Journal, 20,* 2118–2120.

Zhang, W., McQueen, T., Schober, W., Rassidakis, G., Andreeff, M., & Konopleva, M. (2005). Leukotriene B4 receptor inhibitor LY293111 induces cell cycle arrest and apoptosis in human anaplastic large-cell lymphoma cells via JNK phosphorylation. *Leukemia, 19,* 1977–1984.

Zhao, W., Zhang, J., Lu, Y., & Wang, R. (2001). The vasorelaxant effect of H(2)S as a novel endogenous gaseous K(ATP) channel opener. *EMBO Journal, 20,* 6008–6016.

Zlotnik, A. (2006). Chemokines and cancer. *International Journal of Cancer, 119,* 2026–2029.

Bruce Ruggeri*, Sheila Miknyoczki*, Bruce Dorsey*, and Ai-Min Hui†

*Discovery Research, Cephalon, Inc., West Chester, Pennsylvania 19380
†Clinical Research, Cephalon, Inc., West Chester, Pennsylvania 19380

The Development and Pharmacology of Proteasome Inhibitors for the Management and Treatment of Cancer

Abstract

The ubiquitin–proteasome complex is an important molecular target for the design of novel chemotherapeutics. This complex plays a critical role in signal transduction pathways important for tumor cell growth and survival, cell-cycle control, transcriptional regulation, and the modulation of cellular stress responses to endogenous and exogenous stimuli. The sensitivity of transformed cells to proteasome inhibitors

Advances in Pharmacology, Volume 57
1054-3589/08 $35.00
10.1016/S1054-3589(08)57003-7

and the successful design of treatment protocols with tolerable, albeit narrow, therapeutic indices have made proteasome inhibition a viable strategy for cancer treatment. Clinical validation of the proteasome as a molecular target was achieved with the approval of bortezomib, a boronic acid proteasome inhibitor, for the treatment of multiple myeloma and mantle cell lymphoma. Several "next-generation" proteasome inhibitors (carfilzomib and PR-047, NPI-0052, and CEP-18770) representing distinct structural classes (peptidyl epoxyketones, β-lactones, and peptidyl boronic acids, respectively), mechanisms of action, pharmacological and pharmacodynamic activity profiles, and therapeutic indices have now entered clinical development. These agents may expand the clinical utility of proteasome inhibitors for the treatment of solid tumors and for specific non-oncological, i.e., inflammatory disease, indications as well. This chapter addresses the biology of the proteasome, the medicinal chemistry and mechanisms of action of proteasome inhibitors currently in clinical development, the preclinical and clinical pharmacological and safety profiles of bortezomib and the newer compounds against hematological and solid tumors. Future directions for research and other applications for this novel class of therapeutics agents are considered in this chapter.

I. Introduction

Because of the higher sensitivity of cancer cells to the cytotoxic effect of proteasome inhibition, blockade of the uniquitin–proteasome system could be of value in the treatment of a large number of human malignancies. Given this potential, the discovery and development of anti-proteasome drugs with a favorable pharmaceutical profile and enhanced tolerability is an area of active investigation (Adams, 2003; Adams et al., 1999; Bennett & Kirk, 2008; Chauhan et al., 2005; Piva et al., 2008; Williamson et al., 2006; Yang, Zonder, & Dou, 2009). The 26S proteasome is a multisubunit complex comprised of a 20S core and two 19S regulatory subunits. The proteasome plays a critical role in cytoplasmic protein processing and ATP-dependent degradation of polyubiquitinated proteins in maintaining cellular homeostasis. The proteasome complex catalyzes at least five distinct proteolytic functions, including chymotryptic, tryptic, and peptidylglutamyl-like activities. Because the chymotrypsin-like activity appears to be responsible for the most important biological functions, it is the major focus of proteasome inhibitor drug discovery programs (Adams, 2003; Ludwig, Khayat, Giaccone, & Facon, 2005; Piva et al., 2008; Sterz et al., 2008; Yang et al., 2009). Nonetheless, the therapeutic benefit of inhibiting a broader spectrum of proteolytic activities mediated by the proteasome is the focus of several next-generation proteasome inhibitors (Bennett & Kirk, 2008; Chauhan et al., 2005; Feling et al., 2003). The clinical success of bortezomib as an anticancer agent increased the interest in developing a next generation of proteasome inhibitors (Bennett & Kirk, 2008; Hoeller & Dikic, 2009). Currently, there are four proteasome inhibitors representing three different structural classes (peptide boronic acids, β-lactones, and peptide epoxyketones) in clinical development. Bortezomib (Millenium Pharmaceuticals, Inc.) and CEP-18770 (Cephalon, Inc.) are representatives of the boronic acid class, with NPI-0052 (salinosporamide A; Nereus Pharmaceuticals, Inc.) representing the β-lactone class, and carfilzomb (PR-171) and the related PR-047 (Proteolix, Inc.) being members of the peptidyl epoxyketone class of agents (Bennett & Kirk, 2008; Orlowski & Kuhn, 2008; Sterz et al., 2008). Although beyond the scope of this chapter, there are several natural products, including green tea polyphenols, isoflavones, and dithiocarbamates that display non-selective, micromolar potency as inhibitors of the mammalian proteasome *in vitro* and *in vivo* (Yang et al., 2009). Although clinical studies are underway to assess the efficacy of these naturally occurring agents as treatments for solid tumors (colon, pancreatic, lung, breast, prostate, glioma, and melanoma), to date the evidence suggests that they are primarily chemo-preventive rather than chemotherapeutic (Yang et al., 2009). Presented below is an overview of proteasome biology and of the medicinal chemistry and mechanisms of action of proteasome inhibitors currently in clinical development. The preclinical and clinical pharmacological and safety profiles of these compounds in hematological and solid tumors are also presented, with consideration given to future directions in this area of research, and the potential uses of this novel class of inhibitors as therapeutic agents in oncology.

II. Molecular and Biological Roles of the Proteasome Complex in Cellular Homeostasis and Disease

The ubiquitin–proteasome complex is integral to the regulation of multiple processes critical in cellular homeostasis. These include cell-cycle control, transcriptional regulation, cellular stress responses, antigen presentation and immune surveillance, and the regulation of signal transduction pathways essential for growth, angiogenesis, and cell survival (Adams, 2003; Adams et al., 1999; Bennett & Kirk, 2008; Ciechanover, 1994; Daniel, Kuhn, Kazi, & Dou, 2005; Ludwig et al., 2005; Fig. 1). The 26S form of the proteasome is comprised of 19S regulatory units flanking the 20S proteasome catalytic core. The 19S units are essential for the recognition and conformational unfolding of ubiquitin-tagged proteins for proteolytic degradation by the 20S complex. The 20S proteasome

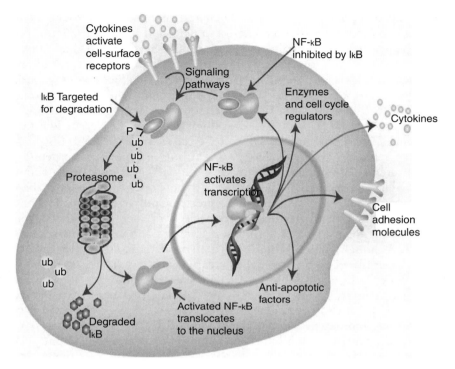

FIGURE I   Critical role of ubiquitin–proteasome signaling pathway in cellular homeostasis and survival.

complex consists of a hollow, multimeric, barrel-shaped structure consisting of two outer ring and two inner ring substructures. Seven outer ring α1–α7 subunits covalently associated with seven inner ring β1–β7 subunits comprise the 20S core and provide both catalytic and conformational flexibility to the proteasome complex. At least five distinct proteolytic functions are catalyzed by the proteasome complex which displays chymotryptic, tryptic, and petidylglutamyl-like activities. In lymphoid tissues, or after induction with interferon γ, these proteasome subunits are replaced by their immunoproteasomal counterparts, termed β1i, β2i, and β5i, to form the immunoproteasome. Because the chymotrypsin-like activity appears to be responsible for the more important biological functions relating to tumor growth and progression, historically it has received the greatest interest in designing and developing proteasome inhibitors as chemotherapeutic agents (Adams, 2003; Bennett & Kirk, 2008; Chauhan, Singh et al., 2008; Demo et al., 2007; Dorsey et al., 2008; Kuhn et al., 2007; Ludwig et al., 2005; Piva et al., 2008). As discussed below, several next-generation proteasome inhibitors have a broader proteolytic inhibitory profile than targeting the chymotrypsin-like activity alone (Bennett & Kirk, 2008; Chauhan et al., 2008; Demo et al., 2007; Kuhn et al., 2007). It remains to be established clinically whether this broader activity profile conveys an improved therapeutic benefit and tolerability profile relative to that achieved by bortezomib's inhibition of primarily the chymotrypsin-like activity of the proteasome (see Section VII).

The ubiquitin–proteasome pathway (UPP) is the major nonlysosomal route for the degradation of proteins that are misfolded, oxidized, or otherwise damaged. Consequently, inhibition of the proteasome prevents this targeted proteolysis, affecting multiple signaling cascades within the cell, disrupting the normal homeostatic mechanisms which ultimately results in tumor cell death. The activation of the transcription factor NF-κB, a key regulator of the acute inflammatory response and the immediate early response to pathogens, is also regulated by the UPP (Adams, 2003; Bennett & Kirk, 2008; Daniel et al., 2005; Rajkumar, Richardson, Hideshima, & Anderson, 2005; Sterz et al., 2008). In addition, NF-kB activates cell survival pathways in response to stress stimuli that normally trigger apoptosis. The active form of NF-κB is comprised of two subunits, p50 and p65, which are maintained as inactive, cytosolic species by complexing with an inhibitor, IκBα. Following stimulus-dependent phosphorylation and ubiquitination of IκBα, the proteasome catalyzes degradation of the regulatory molecule. Activated NF-κB translocates to the nucleus where it promotes the expression of a variety of genes essential for cell survival, proliferation, angiogenesis, and cellular invasiveness and metastasis. Among those genes regulated by NF-κB are pro-inflammatory cytokines and angiogenic factors such as IL-6, IL-8, and VEGF; several cellular adhesion molecules important for tumor adhesion and angiogenesis; and critical anti-apoptotic modulators such as Bcl2 and Bcl-xL. Thus, the suppression of NF-κB activation through proteasome inhibition and IκB stabilization lowers the apoptotic threshold and renders tumor cells more susceptible to pro-apoptotic signals (Adams, 2003; Chauhan et al., 2008; Demo et al., 2007; Mitsiades et al., 2002a,b, 2003; Piva et al., 2008; Rajkumar et al., 2005). Indeed, certain malignancies, such as multiple myeloma (MM) and mantle cell lymphoma, known to be most responsive to proteasome inhibition have elevated levels of NF-κB (Bogner, Peschel, & Decker, 2006; Sterz et al., 2008). This fact provides additional compelling evidence for the role of NF-κB modulation in those malignancies that respond to proteasome inhibitors.

Preclinical studies demonstrate that malignant and highly proliferative cells are more susceptible to proteasome inhibition than normal cells due, in large measure, to the coordinated regulation in the latter of both the cell-cycle and apoptotic pathways in response to endogenous and exogenous stressors (Adams, 2003; Delic et al., 1998; Drexler, 1997; Orlowski & Kuhn, 2008; Rajkumar et al., 2005; Sterz et al., 2008). This characteristic provides a measure of tumor selectivity to proteasome modulation. A substantial body of preclinical data (Adams, 2003; Cavo, 2006; Chauhan et al., 2003, 2008; Demo et al., 2007; Joazeiro et al., 2006; Ludwig et al., 2005; Piva et al., 2008; Rajkumar et al., 2005) generated in both solid and hematologic tumors provide additional mechanistic information as to why proteasome modulation is an effective approach for the treatment of certain malignancies. Importantly, the precise mechanism(s) for the proteasome inhibition anti-tumor activity appear to be tumor-type or tumor model specific (Bennett & Kirk, 2008). In addition, the profile of anti-tumor efficacy in a given tumor type is dictated by the binding kinetics and reversibility of specific proteasome subunit inhibition, the magnitude and duration of the tumor inhibition, and the optimal treatment schedules and therapeutic indices observed within a particular cancer patient population. While a comprehensive assessment of the multiple mechanisms of anti-tumor activity for each of the individual proteasome inhibitors in clinical development is beyond the scope of this chapter, the profile of bortezomib, the first and only FDA-approved member of this class (Adams, 2003; Bross et al., 2004; Richardson, Mitsiades et al., 2006), is presented to enable a comparison with the newer agents undergoing clinical development (Table I). When taken together, the data indicate that the mechanism of action of proteasome inhibitors includes one or more of the following (Adams, 2003; Cavo, 2006; Joazeiro et al., 2006; Orlowski & Kuhn, 2008; Piva et al., 2008; Sterz et al., 2008) (Fig. 2):

- Elevation of the levels of I-κB, resulting in inhibition of NF-κB-mediated regulation of angiogenic cytokines and adhesion molecules (ICAM-1, VCAM-1, and E-selectin), thereby affecting tumor cell–stromal cell interactions important for tumor cell survival and tumor angiogenesis.
- Induction of apoptosis of tumor cells and restored sensitivity of chemo- and radio-resistant tumor cells to cytotoxic therapies through elevation of I-κB and the resultant suppression of NF-κB-mediated cell survival pathways.
- Induction of the degradation of proteins involved in cell-cycle regulation, including cyclins of the A, B, C, and D classes, and the stabilization of the p53 protein, resulting in cellular apoptosis.
- Increased levels of cell-cycle inhibitors, including p21, p27, and members of the p15 p19 INK family of cyclin D-CDK4/6, resulting in G_1-S cell-cycle arrest and apoptosis.
- Activation of JNK-signaling pathways which in turn promote activation of caspase-3- and caspase-8-dependent cell death pathways.

TABLE I Summary of *In vitro* and *In vivo* Preclinical Profiles of Proteasome Inhibitors Currently in Clinical Development[a]

Compound	Mechanism of action	Enzyme IC_{50} (nM)	Cell viability IC_{50} (nM)	Active in vivo dose (mg/kg)	Tumor type	Response
Bortezomib	CT-L reversible	7 ± 2.0	3.9^b	0.5–1.6 i.v., 2q7d	Hematological and solid	PR; CR; prolonged survival
CEP-18770	CT-L reversible	3.8 ± 1.0	5–22	1.5–4 i.v. or 7.8–13 mg/kg p.o., 2q7d	Hematological and solid	PR; CR; prolonged survival
Carfilzomib	CT-L irreversible	6 ± 2.0	2–20	5 i.v., qd×2	Hematological and solid	TGI
NPI-0052	CT-L; T-L Irreversible	3.5 ± 0.3	<10	0.15–0.50 p.o., 2q7d	Hematological	CR; prolonged survival
PR-047	CT-L irreversible	82	<1–180	30 qd×2	Hematological and solid	TGI

[a] Abbreviations: CT-L, chymotrypsin-like; T-L, trypsin-like; PR, partial regression; CR, complete regression; TGI, tumor growth inhibition.
[b] Average over NCI 60 panel.

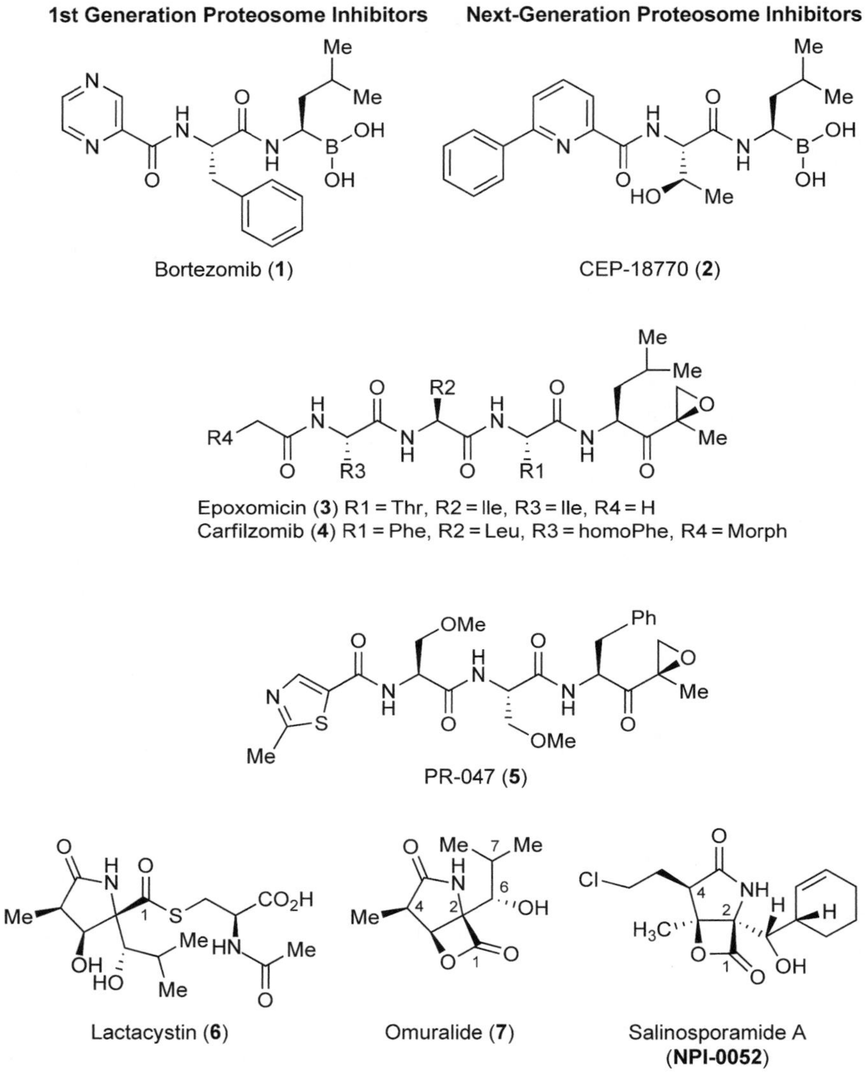

FIGURE 2   Structures of the first-generation proteasome inhibitors, bortezomib, epoxomicin, carfilzomib, lactacystin, and omuralide, and structures of the next-generation CEP-18770, PR-047, and salinosporamide A.

III. Historical Perspective of Proteasome Inhibitors in Development: Chemistry and Primary Mechanisms of Action

A. Dipeptidyl Boronic Acids: Bortezomib and CEP-18770

The first reported proteasome inhibitors were found to be slow-binding, reversible inhibitors of the peptide aldehyde and peptide α-keto ester class (Vinitsky, Michaud, Powers, & Orlowski, 1992). However, these agents lacked specificity for the proteasome because the aldehyde functionality reacts with a wide range of serine and cysteine proteases. To identify more selective proteasome inhibitors, the aldehyde functionality was systematically replaced with other chemical groups known to interact with serine, threonine, and cysteine proteases. This effort led to the synthesis of a highly potent and selective dipeptidyl boronic ester inhibitor of proteasome chymotrypsin-like activity (Iqbal et al., 1996). Subsequently, scientists at ProScript, Inc., reported a series of boronic acid peptides, including MG 341 or PS-341, which was later renamed bortezomib (Fig. 2). This compound displays a high degree of selectivity and affinity ($K_i = 0.6$ nM) for the 26S proteasome (Adams & Stein, 1996; Adams et al., 1999). The selectivity of bortezomib is over 500-fold greater for the proteasome complex than for thrombin, elastase, cathepsin G, and chymotrypsin. The boronic acid moiety of this chemical class is a critical determinate for their selectivity because of its tendency to interact with strong nucleophiles, such as oxygen, and extremely weaker nucleophiles, such as cysteine. The next generation of orally active dipeptidyl boronic acids, which was disclosed recently, is best exemplified by CEP-18770 (Fig. 2; Dorsey et al., 2008; Piva et al., 2008).

As demonstrated with bortezomib and CEP-18770, dipeptidyl boronic acids preferentially target the β5 subunit of the 26S proteasome. Although the X-ray crystal structure of bortezomib complexed with the yeast proteasome shows each catalytic subunit occupied by the inhibitor, this is an artifact of the inhibitor concentration used during crystal soaking (Groll, Berkers, Ploegh, & Ovaa, 2006). Analysis of bortezomib bound to the β5 chymotrypsin-like site reveals that the tetrahedral boron atom is covalently bound to the nucleophilic oxygen atom of Thr1Oγ (Fig. 3A). An acidic hydroxyl group of the boron acid is stabilized within the oxyanion hole and hydrogen bonded to Gly47N, while the second hydroxyl group is attached through intra-molecular hydrogen binding to Thr1 N-terminal atom. As this type of hydrogen bonding interaction is unique to the N-terminal threonine proteasome, it helps to explain the additional affinity and selectivity that is a characteristic of the boronic acid class of proteasome inhibitors as compared to other mammalian serine proteases.

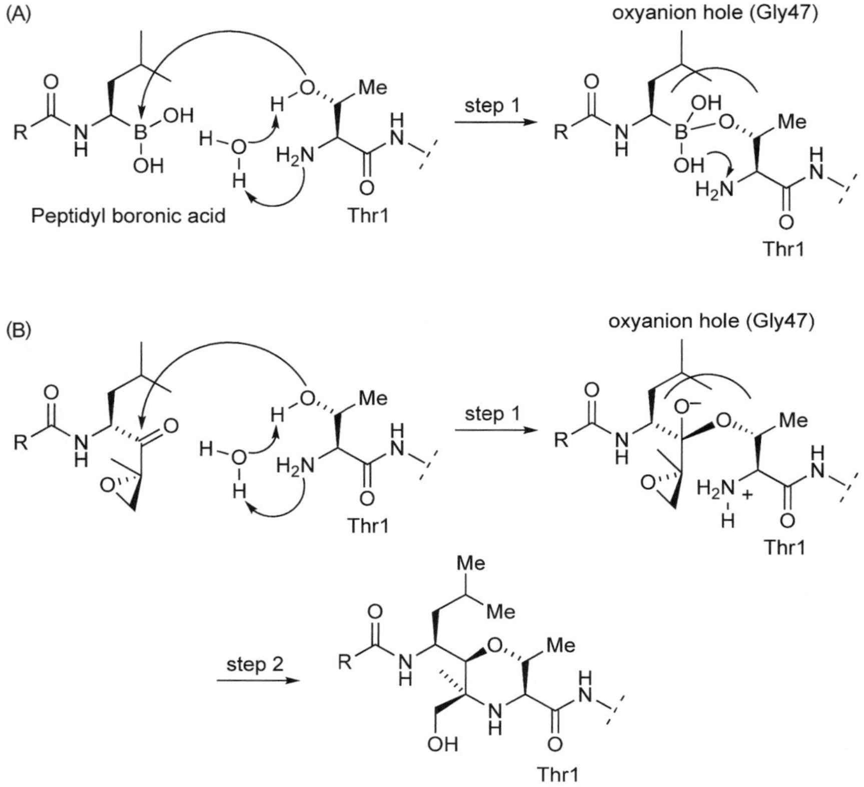

(A)

oxyanion hole (Gly47)

step 1

Peptidyl boronic acid   Thr1

Thr1

(B)

oxyanion hole (Gly47)

step 1

Thr1

Thr1

step 2

Thr1

FIGURE 3 (A) Schematic representation of a peptidyl boronic acid proteasome inhibitor bound to the chymotrypsin-like active site illustrating the tetrahedral boron, the boronic hydroxyl group filling an oxyanion hole and intra-molecule hydrogen bonding of the boronic hydroxyl and ThrN1. (B) Schematic representation of the proposed formation of a morpholino adduct with a representative ketoexpoxide.

B. Peptidyl Epoxyketones: Carflizomib and PR-047

Epoxomicin (Fig. 2), a naturally occurring peptidyl epoxyketone, was first isolated from the *Actinomycetes* strain Q996-17 (Hanada et al., 1992). Biotinylated epoxomicin binding studies revealed covalent attachment to the proteasome, primarily affecting the chymotryptic-like activity (Sin et al., 1999). As represented in Fig. 3B, the crystal structure of yeast 20S proteasome complexed with epoxomicin reveals the formation of an unusual six-membered morpholino ring (Groll, Kim, Kairies, Huber, & Crews, 2000). Activation of $Thr1O\gamma$ by water and nucleophilic attack of the Thr1 oxygen on the carbonyl atom of the epoxyketone (Fig. 3B, step 1) generate a hemiacetal. Similar to the complex with dipeptidyl boronic acids, the negative charge on the hemiacetal oxygen is stabilized by Gly47 in the oxyanion hole. In step 2, an intra-molecular cyclization starts with the nucleophilic attack by ThrN1 on the C2 position of the epoxide. Following Baldwin's rules of ring closure, this favorable 5 Exo-Tet ring closure generates the six-membered morpholino ring (Baldwin, 1976). The ability of ketoepoxide-class inhibitors to covalently bind to the proteasome in this bidentate fashion provides a structural explanation for the proteasome selectivity observed with this pharmacophore.

A tetrapeptidyl ketoepoxide such as epoxomicin has poor drug-like properties. To improve its physiochemical properties, the amino-acid substitutions were optimized and a morphilino ring was introduced on the N-terminal acetyl. This modification resulted in carfilzomib (CFZ) (Demo et al., 2007), a compound that inhibits proteasome chymotrypsin-like activity similar to epoxomicin. Like bortezomib, CFZ is administered intravenously for over 6 months on a biweekly or more frequent dosing schedule. An orally active CFZ analog was subsequently designed. Truncation of the tetrapeptidyl core to a tripeptide results in minor loss of potency and, following a systematic amino-acid optimization process, PR-047 was identified as an orally active, potent, and chymotrypsin-like selective proteasome inhibitor with favorable pharmacological properties (Zhou et al., 2009). As discussed below, CFZ and PR-047 are irreversible proteasome inhibitors that presumably bind in a manner similar to that described for epoxomicin (Fig. 3B).

C. Natural Product Inhibitors: Lactacystin, Omuralide, and NPI-0052

The natural product lactacystin (Fig. 2), an antibiotic *Streptomyces* spp. metabolite, was first identified on the basis of cell growth inhibition and its ability to induce neurite outgrowth (Omura et al., 1991). Subsequently, lactacystin was found to specifically inhibit the trypsin-like, chymotrypsin-like, and peptidylglutamyl-peptide hydrolyzing activity of the 20S proteasome (Fenteany et al., 1995). The putative mechanism of action of either lactacystin or omuralide is the covalent modification of the N-terminal threonine residue of subunit β5 of the mammalian 20S proteasome through a C-4 reactive carbonyl. As illustrated in Fig. 4A, cyclization of the lactacystin, with concomitant loss of the leaving group N-acetylcysteine (not shown), generates the reactive β-lactone (omuralide), found similarly in NPI-0052 (Fig. 4B). Nucleophilic addition of the threonine hydroxyl moiety opens the strained β-lactone ring forming a covalent complex with catalytic subunits of the proteasome. Subsequent X-ray crystallographic studies of complexes of the 20S proteasome with omuralide and salinosporamide A confirmed this hypothesis (Groll, Huber, & Potts, 2006; Groll et al., 1997).

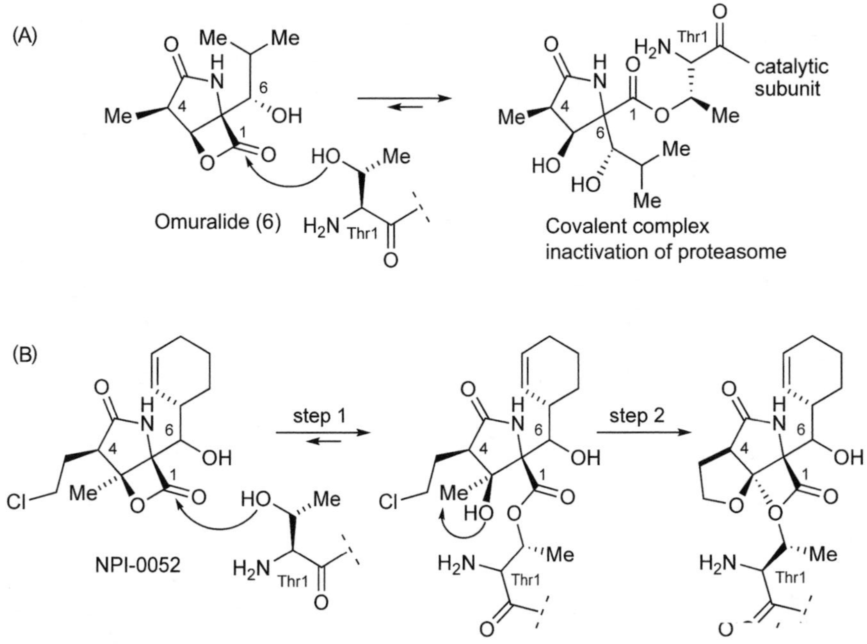

FIGURE 4 Inhibition of proteasome active sites by β-lactones. (A) Addition of Thr1Oγ to the C1 carbonyl of omuralide to generate a covalent complex. (B) Schematic representation of ThrOγ addition to NPI-0052, followed by step 2 in which the newly generated tertiary hydroxyl group at C3 displaces the chlorine atom to form at cyclic ether moiety.

Salinosporamide A, also known as NPI-0052, irreversibly inhibits all three catalytic activities of the 20S proteasome and is a secondary metabolite of the marine actinomycete, *Salinispora tropica* (Feling et al., 2003). Structurally, NPI-0052 shares the β-lactone-γ-lactam bicyclic ring core with omuralide but is more lipophilic because of the cyclohexene ring in place of the isopropyl group at C-7 and the chloroethyl group in place of the methyl moiety at C-4. These differences may account for the superior potency of NPI-0052 over omuralide. However, an alternative hypothesis on the relative potencies takes into account the role of the electrophilic chloride atom (Macherla et al., 2005). As illustrated in Fig. 4B, the first step of proteasome inhibition by NPI-0052 includes opening of the β-lactone with the N-terminal threonine hydroxyl of 20S proteasome. Although energetically unfavorable, this first step is potentially reversible since the newly formed tertiary hydroxyl moiety can revert back to the ester functionality and regenerate NPI-0052. However, a second reaction option is available for NPI-0052. In this case, the tertiary hydroxyl group reacts with the terminal chloroethyl group to form a cyclic ether (Fig. 4B, step 2). This is followed by the loss of HCl, which precludes the regeneration of β-lactone and helps drive the formation of an irreversible complex with the proteasome. Cyclic ether formation with NPI-0052 has been demonstrated in hydrolysis experiments and confirmed by X-ray crystallography. Additional insights obtained from the structural analyses of NPI-0052 include the role played by the cyclic ether to block access of water required to cleave the newly formed threonine ester, the role of the ether oxygen to stabilize the fully protonated threonine amine, and the importance of the additional lipophilicity in the hydrophobic binding pocket occupied by the cyclohexenyl ring (Groll, Huber, & Potts 2006).

IV.   Preclinical *In Vitro* and *In Vivo* Pharmacology of Proteasome Inhibitors in Hematological and Non-hematological Cancers

A.   Studies with Bortezomib

Bortezomib was the first reversible inhibitor of the chymotrypsin-like activity of the 26S mammalian proteasome to be extensively studied (Adams, 2003; Bross et al., 2004; Orlowski & Kuhn, 2008; Rajkumar et al., 2005). In human MM cell lines and freshly isolated primary MM cells, bortezomib directly inhibits cell proliferation by cell-cycle arrest at G2/M, inhibits NF-κB activation by stabilizing IκBα, and induces apoptosis at low nanomolar concentrations (Adams, 2003; Bross et al., 2004; Ling et al., 2003; Rajkumar et al., 2005). In addition, bortezomib confers on resistant MM cells a renewed sensitivity to chemotherapeutic agents such as doxorubicin, melphalan, and dexamethasone (Adams, 2003; Hideshima et al., 2001). When screened against the National Cancer Institute panel of 60 tumor cell lines (NCI-60), the average IC_{50} value for bortezomib was 3.9 nM, indicating that it is cytotoxic for a variety of non-hematological cancers (Adams, 2003; Hideshima et al., 2001; Mitsiades et al., 2002a; Mitsiades et al., 2002b). Bortezomib induces apoptosis in various tumor cells through multiple mechanisms, including the modulation of a number of pro-apoptotic proteins. The mechanism of action of bortezomib includes the stabilization of pro-apoptotic Bax and downregulation of Bcl-2, enhancement of the levels of the cyclin-dependent kinase inhibitors p21 and p27, and the stabilization of activated p53/PUMA complexes. Bortezomib induces cell-cycle arrest at the G1/S and G2/M interfaces (Adams, 2003; Adams et al., 1999; Hideshima et al., 2001; Rajkumar et al., 2005; Williams & McConkey, 2003). In addition, bortezomib-mediated inhibition of NF-κ B-mediated transcription through stabilization of its inhibitor IκB results in the inhibition of transcription of multiple cytokines and angiogenic factors. This group includes tumor necrosis factor, IL-1, IL-6, VEGF, several key stress response enzymes such as COX-2 and NO, and the cellular adhesion molecules ICAM, VCAM, and E-selectin. These cellular adhesion molecules inhibit MM cell attachment to the bone marrow stromal cells, thereby contributing to the effects of bortezomib on tumor cell growth, apoptosis, angiogenesis, and malignant progression (Adams et al., 1999; Concannon et al., 2007; Cusack et al., 2001; Hideshima et al., 2001, 2003; Richardson et al., 2006). More recent studies have demonstrated that bortezomib-mediated proteasome inhibition results in the accumulation and aggregation of misfolded proteins in the endoplasmic reticulum resulting in the activation of the unfolded protein response (UPR) pathway. The UPR triggers multiple signaling cascades, resulting in activation of both adaptive anti-apoptotic and pro-apoptotic responses when tumor cells are exposed to severe endogenous and exogenous stress, such as hypoxia, glucose deprivation, or reactive oxygen species (Nawrocki et al., 2005; Ron & Walter, 2007; Saito et al., 2009). Several studies have demonstrated that bortezomib administration sensitizes solid tumors, such as pancreatic, cervical, breast, and squamous cell carcinomas, to UPR-mediated apoptosis under stress conditions (Fribley, Zeng, & Wang, 2004; Nawrocki et al., 2005). Other studies have shown that the induction of the UPR pathway and autophagy induced by bortezomib and hypoxia (Fels et al., 2008) or bortezomib and reactive oxygen species (Szokalska et al., 2009) results in a massive tumor necrotic response. These findings suggest that the precise mechanism(s) and conditions within the tumor microenvironment influencing bortezomib-mediated UPR apoptosis are likely to be tumor type dependent.

In vivo, the administration of bortezomib (0.5–1.0 mg/kg i.v., 2q7d) to immune-deficient mice bearing human MM xenografts results in significant inhibition of tumor growth and induction of apoptosis, complete regressions, prolonged survival, and marked tumor anti-angiogenic efficacy (Adams et al., 1999; Hideshima et al., 2001; LeBlanc et al., 2002). As suggested by the tumor cytotoxicity profile in the NCI-60 panel of tumor lines, bortezomib demonstrates dose-related anti-tumor efficacy against several non-hematological xenografts, including melanoma (1.25 mg/kg peritumorally 2q7d), lung and squamous cell carcinomas (1–2 mg/kg i.p., 3q7d), pancreatic ductal adenocarcinomas (1 mg/kg i.v., 2q7d), and prostate carcinomas (1 mg/kg i.v., 3q7d) (Adams et al., 1999; Hideshima et al., 2001; Ludwig et al., 2005; Nawrocki et al., 2002; Sunwoo et al., 2001; Williams et al., 2003). Evaluation of bortezomib in combination with standard-of-care chemotherapeutics such as doxorubicin, etoposide, and irinotecan, or radiation revealed significant chemo- and/or radio-sensitization in human and murine xenograft models of melanoma, lung, pancreatic, breast and colon carcinoma (Adams, 2003; Amiri, Horton, LaFleur, Sosman, & Richmond, 2004; Bold, Virudachalam, & Mcconkey, 2001; Cusack et al., 2001; Ludwig et al., 2005; Russo et al., 2001; Teicher, Ara, Herbst, Palombella, & Adams, 1999). This data suggests that, in addition to its direct multimechanism pro-apoptotic effects, bortezomib enhances tumor chemo- and radio-sensitivity and can overcome tumor drug resistance. Significant enhancement of *in vivo* anti-tumor efficacy, with up to a 60–100% complete response, was demonstrated with bortezomib and photodynamic therapy in a variety of solid tumor xenograft models (Szokalska et al., 2009). Moreover, numerous preclinical studies demonstrate that bortezomib potentiates the anti-tumor activity of novel therapies for MM, including lenalidomide, arsenic trioxide, and inhibitors of histone deacetylase or protein kinase C, and when used in combination therapies with next-generation proteasome inhibitors such as NPI-0052 (Campbell et al., 2007; Chauhan et al., 2008; Deleu et al., 2009; Pei, Dai, & Grant, 2004; Podar et al., 2007). Taken together these data demonstrate that bortezomib inhibits growth, induces apoptosis or necrosis, and overcomes resistance to standard chemotherapeutic agents. Such findings contributed significantly to its advancement to clinical trials as a treatment for MM and variety of hematologic and solid tumors.

The marked ability of bortezomib to inhibit growth and induce apoptosis in primary human MM isolates, human MM cell lines, and s.c. human MM xenografts, and the correlation between magnitude and duration of proteasome inhibition with anti-tumor efficacy *in vitro* and *in vivo* (Orlowski & Kuhn, 2008; Richardson et al., 2006) provided a compelling rationale for its initial clinical assessment in this aggressive malignancy. The ability of bortezomib to synergize with dexamethasone and sensitize both primary human MM isolates and chemo-resistant MM cell lines to melphalan and doxorubicin (Hideshima et al., 2001, 2003) provided additional support for clinical studies in MM patients. Moreover, a series of preclinical and clinical studies in MM tumor xenograft models and patients demonstrated that bortezomib therapy, both alone and in combination with HDAC inhibitors (Deleu et al., 2009), has a significant benefit in reducing MM tumor burden and modulates bone homeostasis, inhibiting osteoclastogenesis, and stimulating osteoblast differentiation to reduce the debilitating osteolytic manifestations of MM (Terpos, Sezer, Croucher, & Dimopoulos, 2007; von Metzler et al., 2007). In retrospect, these preclinical and subsequent clinical studies demonstrated the beneficial efficacy of bortezomib both directly against MM cells and on the MM microenvironment of the host in having a positive impact on the clinical manifestations of this disease.

In advance of initial clinical trials with bortezomib in MM patients, preclinical toxicological studies were performed in rodents and monkeys. These studies identified hematological (lymphoid depletion, anemia, myelosuppression), cardiovascular (elevated heart rate, hypotension, and bradycardia), gastrointestinal, nephrotoxic, and neurological effects manifested by a steep dose–toxicity response relationship at i.v. doses greater than or equal to $0.9 \, mg/m^2$ and greater than or equal $0.6 \, mg/m^2$ for neurotoxicity (Adams, 2003; Adams et al., 1999; Bross et al., 2004; Richardson et al., 2006). Ex vivo pharmacodynamic (PD) studies in rats and primates revealed dose-related inhibition of 20S proteasome chymotrypsin-like activity reaching approximately 90% at its maximum-tolerated dose of bortezomib in these species and returning to baseline within 72 h following administration (Adams, 2003; Adams et al., 1999; Bross et al., 2004). These PD and corresponding pharmacokinetic and tissue distribution profiles in rodents and primates were critical for establishing a target range for human proteasome inhibition of 60–80% to achieve optimal efficacy while minimizing toxicity (Adams, 2003; Bross et al., 2004; Lightcap et al., 2000). The relatively narrow therapeutic index, rapid systemic clearance, and extended elimination half-life of bortezomib supported the application of ex vivo PD assays for monitoring the extent of proteasome inhibition in subsequent clinical studies with bortezomib and next-generation proteasome inhibitors.

B. Studies with CEP-18770

As noted above, CEP-18770 is an orally active and reversible boronic acid inhibitor of predominantly the chymotrypsin-like activity of the mammalian proteasome. Its preclinical profile has been described in detail (Dorsey et al., 2008; Piva et al., 2008). The proteasome inhibitory activity of CEP-18770 in an isolated human erythrocyte proteasome fluorimetric kinetic assay of chymotrypsin-like proteasome activity shows comparable potency to that of bortezomib, with IC_{50} values for both of approximately 3.0 nM. Analysis of CEP-18770 and bortezomib in the MOLT-4 cellular system shows comparable chymotrypsin-like inhibitory activity with IC_{50} values of 14 and 21 nM for CEP-18770 and bortezomib, respectively.

CEP-18770 displays a similar spectrum of tumor cytotoxicity (EC_{50} values less than 50 nM) to that of bortezomib against a panel of solid and hematological tumor cell lines. An analysis of CEP-18770 and bortezomib against 10 human MM cell lines, including RPMI-8226 and U266 cells, reveals comparable dose-related low nanomolar cytotoxic activity, as well as comparable profiles for inhibition of constitutive activation of NF-kB signaling, the degradation of the proteasome-regulated proteins, IkBα and XIAP, and reduced NF-kb-mediated expression of cellular adhesion molecules, cytokines, and angiogenic factors by human MM cells (Piva et al., 2008). Cell viability and apoptosis assays of primary CD138-positive explants from 13 MM patients indicate that CEP-18770 and bortezomib exposures cause a comparable concentration-related pro-apoptotic activity *ex vivo*, with complete MM cell death at 20 nM and IC_{50} values of approximately 4 nM for both inhibitors. In direct comparative studies, CEP-18770 inhibits human M-CSF-RANKL-mediated osteoclastogenesis *in vitro* to a greater extent than bortezomib and is significantly less cytotoxic than bortezomib against normal human bone marrow progenitor cells, human bone marrow stromal cells, and human intestinal epithelial cells *in vitro* suggesting a potential tumor-selective activity profile.

The pharmacokinetic profiles of CEP-18770 are similar to those observed for bortezomib in rats and mice (Adams, 2003; Adams et al., 1999; Bross et al., 2004; Richardson et al., 2006). They are characterized by linear increases in plasma exposure upon i.v. administration, prolonged permanence in the systemic circulation with a long terminal elimination half-life, low systemic clearance reflecting limited first-pass metabolism, and a large distribution volume. In contrast to bortezomib, CEP-18770 is well absorbed and displays an oral bioavailability of 39 and 54% in mice and rats, respectively (Dorsey et al., 2008). The pharmacokinetic and chymotrypsin-like proteasome inhibition profile of CEP-18770 reveals a sustained (72–80 h) dose-related inhibition of tumor proteasome activity within the 60–80% therapeutic window across a range of i.v. and oral doses (Piva et al., 2008). The PD profile of CEP-18770 in normal peripheral murine tissues declines below this threshold by 8–10 h after i.v. administration. Despite similarities in the binding kinetics and potencies of CEP-18770 and bortezomib against normal cell and tumor cell line lysates, in human MM xenograft models CEP-18770 inhibits the tumor versus normal tissue β1 and β5 chymotrypsin-like proteasome subunit activity to a significantly greater extent than bortezomib. Collectively these findings suggest that CEP-18770 has a more distinctive tumor PD and tumor β1 and β5 proteasome subunit inhibition profile than that observed with equi-active doses of bortezomib (Berkers et al., submitted). In accord with these tumor PD data, CEP-18770 (1.5–4.0 mg/kg i.v., q2d7) displays dose-related inhibition of human RPMI 8266 MM xenograft growth, induces complete tumor regressions, and results in a sustained incidence of tumor-free mice at its maximum-tolerated dose, surpassing the efficacy of bortezomib in this model (Piva et al., 2008). Oral administration of CEP-18770 (10–13 mg/kg, q2d7) results in a similar incidence of complete tumor regressions as that observed with i.v. administration, with anti-tumor efficacy consistent with its tumor PD and apoptosis induction profiles in this human MM model. Subsequent studies (Sanchez et al., 2008) demonstrated that the combination of CEP-18770 with standard regimens of melphalan or bortezomib induces synergistic inhibition of MM cell line viability *in vitro*. In bortezomib and melphalan-sensitive (LAGκ1A) and -resistant (LAGκ1B) primary human MM xenograft models, administration of CEP-18770 (1–3 mg/kg i.v., 2qd7, or 10 mg/kg p.o., 2qd7) completely prevents the growth of both melphalan-sensitive and melphalan-resistant MM tumors. The combination of CEP-18770 and bortezomib on standard 2qd7 administration regimens induces complete regression of bortezomib-sensitive tumors and markedly delays the progression of bortezomib-resistant tumors compared to treatment with either agent alone (Sanchez et al., 2008). CEP-18770 administration (3–4 mg/kg i.v., q2d7) also demonstrated significant efficacy in systemic murine and human non-Hodgkin's lymphoma models, and cisplatin-resistant ovarian tumor xenografts compared to controls and bortezomib-treated mice (Piva et al., 2008). The efficacy of CEP-18770 against aggressive human solid tumor orthotopic xenografts is particularly noteworthy. Administration of CEP-18770 (3 mg/kg i.v., q2d7 × 8 weeks) in an orthotopic human pancreatic ductal carcinoma model reduced primary tumor burden and hepatic metastatic tumor burden as well as the severity of progressive cancer cachexia characteristic of this malignancy. Similarly, marked reductions in primary tumor burden and localized tumor dissemination in the thoracic cavity are observed with chronic CEP-18770 administration (3 mg/kg i.v., q2d7 × 8 weeks) in an orthotopic non-small-cell lung adenocarcinoma model in mice (Ruggeri et al., unpublished data). This data demonstrate both the efficacy and the favorable therapeutic index of this inhibitor in metastatic models of highly aggressive human solid tumors.

In summary, CEP-18770 is similar to bortezomib in terms of its biochemical and *in vitro* anti-tumor pharmacological profiles. This is particularly true in MM and other hematological malignancies. However, the two differ with respect to tumor proteasome β5 and β1 subunit binding and their tumor versus normal tissue PD inhibition profiles. Also, CEP-18770 differs from bortezomib in its marked anti-osteoclastogenic activity, in its superior anti-tumor efficacy in several models of human MM and solid orthotopic solid tumors, and in its more favorable cytotoxicity profile against normal human epithelial cells, bone marrow progenitors, and bone marrow-derived stromal cells (Dorsey et al., 2008; Piva et al., 2008; Sanchez et al., 2008). Nonclinical safety pharmacology studies with CEP-18770 suggest favorable cardiovascular, arrhythmogenic, and hemodynamic profiles in rats and monkeys and provide evidence for diminished peripheral neuropathy during treatment, and improved recovery in nerve conduction velocity in rodents upon cessation of CEP-18770 administration as compared to equi-active i.v. doses of bortezomib (Ruggeri et al., unpublished data). Together these studies provided the support for the advancement of CEP-18770 into clinical development.

C. Studies with CFZ and PR-047

Carfilzomib (PR-171) is an epoxyketone-based, irreversible, selective inhibitor of the chymotrypsin-like proteasome activity that specifically targets the $\beta5$ and $\beta5i$ subunits of the proteasome and immunoproteasome, respectively. Carfilzomib has a high degree of proteasome selectivity with little or no off-target activity against a panel of 12 proteases, making it superior to bortezomib in this regard (Arastu-Kapur, Shenk, Parlati, & Bennett, 2008). In addition, its cellular (Molt-4) chymotrypsin-like inhibitory activity is essentially equivalent to its enzymatic activity, with IC_{50} values of 3–6 nM (Bennett & Kirk, 2008; Demo et al., 2007). Concentrations of CFZ that inhibit proteasome chymotrypsin-like activity greater than 80% also inhibit tumor cell proliferation in a concentration-dependent manner (IC_{50} values of less than 10 nM) in both hematologic and non-hematologic carcinoma cell lines. The hematological tumors cell lines are more sensitive than solid tumor cell lines (Demo et al., 2007; Stapnes et al., 2007). Of note is the observation that CFZ is more potent than bortezomib in its anti-proliferative and pro-apoptotic effects against chemo-naive primary MM samples and cell lines with brief treatments that mimic *in vivo* exposure (Demo et al., 2007; Kuhn et al., 2007). This preclinical profile of CFZ mirrors that observed in phase II clinical studies of CFZ in bortezomib-resistant relapsed and refractory MM patients who failed first-line therapies. In a panel of bortezomib-sensitive and bortezomib-resistant human MM cell lines, and bortezomib-resistant cell lines derived from primary CD138-positive MM patient samples, CFZ inhibits cell proliferation, induces apoptosis, and overcomes cellular resistance at low nanomolar concentrations. In this regard, the preclinical activity of CFZ against bortezomib-resistant MM *in vitro* is similar to the profiles observed for the boronic acid proteaseome inhibitor, CEP-18770. Moreover, as with bortezomib, CFZ exposure overcomes tumor resistance to melphalan, dexamethasone, and doxorubicin and acts synergistically with dexamethasone to enhance JNK activation and induce apoptosis through activation of both intrinsic and extrinsic apoptotic pathways (Kuhn et al., 2007). Similar to the efficacy seen in MM cell lines and samples, CFZ monotherapy produces anti-proliferative and pro-apoptotic responses superior to bortezomib against primary samples from patients with acute lymphoblastic leukemia, chronic lymphocytic leukemia, and acute myelogenous leukemia (Kuhn et al., 2007). It also demonstrates synergistic anti-tumor activity when administered *in vitro* in combination with idarubicin, cytarabine, and valproic acid (Stapnes et al., 2007). The ability of CFZ to overcome bortezomib resistance in preclinical tests, as well as its synergistic tumor cytotoxic profile with several standard-of-care therapeutic agents, suggests that this agent may provide an alternative for MM patients that have relapsed or progressed through bortezomib treatment (Bennett & Kirk, 2008).

Pharmacodynamic studies with single-dose administration of CFZ (4 mg/kg i.v.) to rats and monkeys result in greater than 80% inhibition of chymotrypsin-like activity in normal tissues. The half-life of CFZ is approximately 24 h, with 5-day consecutive dosing of CFZ (2 mg/kg i.v.) being well tolerated in rats and resulting in a sustained (greater than 80%) inhibition of chymotrypsin-like proteasome activity *in vivo* (Demo et al., 2007). Consecutive day dosing of CFZ (5 mg/kg i.v., qd × 2) in anti-tumor efficacy studies with B cell and Burkitt's lymphoma and colorectal xenografts was more efficacious than bortezomib delivered on the standard clinical schedule of 1 mg/kg i.v., 2q7d. Responses are, however, limited to tumor growth inhibition, with no sustained tumor stasis or tumor regressions reported in these models (Demo et al., 2007; Kuhn et al., 2007). The anti-tumor efficacy of CFZ compared to bortezomib is attributed to the high degree of chymotrypsin-like target selectivity and the irreversible nature of proteasome inhibition, the latter necessitating proteasome complex turnover and resynthesis to achieve full recovery of biological activity (Bennett & Kirk, 2008; Demo et al., 2007). This hypothesis challenges the conventional wisdom that inhibition of the chymotrypsin-like activity of the proteasome in a reversible and recoverable fashion as with bortezomib and CEP-18770 is the optimal approach for targeting the proteasome as an anti-cancer therapy. Carfilzomib is currently in phase II clinical development as a treatment for MM and non-Hodgkin's lymphoma (Bennett & Kirk, 2008; Demo et al., 2007).

The convenience of an orally active proteasome inhibitor with the efficacy and tolerability profile of CFZ led to the development of PR-047, a tripeptide epoxyketone analog of CFZ (Zhou et al., 2009). PR-047 displays an IC_{50} of 82 nM against the chymotrypsin-like activity of the proteasome and cellular IC_{50} values of 43–71 nM (Muchamuel et al., 2008; Peese, 2009; Zhou et al., 2009). Thus, PR-047 is approximately 6- to 12-fold less potent in its enzyme and cellular inhibitory activity than CFZ (Demo et al., 2007; Kuhn et al., 2007). Nonetheless, the *in vitro* cytotoxicity profile of PR-047 against a range of solid and hematological tumor cell lines is comparable to CFZ, with cell viability IC_{50} values of 1–176 nM (Muchamuel et al., 2008; Zhou et al., 2009).

PR-047 is orally active in mouse (17%), rat (21%), and dog (39%) and causes greater than 80% inhibition of proteasome chymotrypsin-like activity in rats and dogs. It is comparable to i.v. CFZ in the onset and duration of its PD activity, with a minimum oral dose for 80% inhibition of chymo-trypsin-like activity of 10 mg/kg compared to the 2 mg/kg i.v. dose for CFZ (Muchamuel et al., 2008; Zhou et al., 2009). Similarly, the oral anti-tumor efficacy reported for PR-047 in human non-Hodgkin's lymphoma, MM, colon, and non-small-cell lung carcinoma xenografts at 30 mg/kg qd × 2 was generally comparable to CFZ (5 mg/kg i.v.) in magnitude, with favorable tolerability and significant tumor growth inhibition, but in the absence of tumor stasis or regressions (Muchamuel et al., 2008; Peese, 2009).

The preclinical and clinical toxicity profiles observed following multiple administrations of other proteasome inhibitors necessitated schedules that allow for recovery of proteasome activity between doses. Despite similarities in the overall cardiovascular, gastrointestinal, and hematological toxicities of CFZ and PR-047 to those of bortezomib, the magnitude and severity of peripheral neuropathy and neurohistopathology observed in rodents were substantially less compared to bortezomib in rodents and primates (Kirk et al., 2008). These observations mirror those observed in phase II clinical studies with CFZ as discussed below. Consequently, the favorable tolerabil-ity profiles in rodents and primates observed with intensive sequential-day administration of PR-047 and CFZ are a distinguishing feature of the overall profile of these epoxyketone-class proteasome inhibitors compared to other inhibitors such as bortezomib. The explanation for this apparent difference in tolerability with sequential-day administration remains to be determined, although it may be related to their highly selective chymotrypsin-like inhibi-tory activity and minimal off-target protease activity (Arastu-Kapur et al., 2008; Bennett & Kirk, 2008). Based upon these findings, PR-047 was recom-mended in 2008 for clinical development as a treatment for hematological and solid tumors (Muchamuel et al., 2008; Peese, 2009).

D. Studies with NPI-0052

An orally active, lactacystin-based fermentation product derived from *Salinospora* spp., NPI-0052, irreversibly inhibits all three proteolytic activ-ities of the proteasome, with preference for inhibition of the chymotrypsin-like and trypsin-like activities (Chauhan et al., 2005; Williamson et al., 2006). *In vitro*, NPI-0052 has an IC_{50} of less than 10 nM against the NCI-60 panel of tumor cell lines and induces apoptosis in both hematolo-gical and solid tumor cell lines. Likewise, it induces apoptosis in primary CD138-positive MM explants from patients resistant to conventional thera-pies and to bortezomib, but displays reduced cytotoxicity against normal human bone marrow stromal cells and lymphocytes (Chauhan et al., 2005, 2008; Cusack et al., 2006; Feling et al., 2003; Miller et al., 2007; Ruiz et al., 2006). Further, at concentrations less than 100 nM, NPI-0052 suppresses RANKL-induced osteoclastogenesis and TNFα-induced tumor cell invasion and angiogenesis through inhibition of the NF-κB pathway. Moreover,

NPI-0052 induces synergistic growth inhibition, JNK and Hsp70 activation, and induction of UPR signaling, culminating in the induction of apoptosis of both chemo-naive and bortezomib-resistant MM cell lines *in vitro*. It has a similar effect on primary CD138-positive MM patient samples *ex vivo* when administered in combination with bortezomib, dexamethasone, and doxorubicin (Ahn et al., 2007; Chauhan et al., 2008). Transduction pathway studies in MM cells revealed additional evidence that NPI-0052 inhibits the NF-κB pathway two- to six-fold more potently than bortezomib. Unlike bortezomib, CEP-18770, CFZ, and PR-047, NPI-0052-induces apoptosis predominately through the FADD–caspase-8-mediated death pathway, while both intrinsic (caspase-9-mediated) and extrinsic (caspase-8-mediated) pathways are required for induction of apoptosis by the other classes of proteasome inhibitors now in clinical development (Bennett & Kirk, 2008; Chauhan et al., 2005, 2008; Piva et al., 2008).

Repeated administration of NPI-0052 (0.25 or 0.5 mg/kg p.o.) results in higher and more sustained inhibition (73–85%) of proteasome chymotrypsin-like activity as compared to 1 mg/kg i.v. bortezomib. Moreover, NPI-0052 penetrates the blood–brain barrier and inhibits chymotrypsin-like proteasome activity by more than 90% when administered at 0.4–1 mg/kg i.v. (Cusack et al., 2006; Williamson et al., 2006). While this compound is the only proteasome inhibitor currently in clinical development that crosses the blood–brain barrier, its effectiveness against brain malignancies has yet to be explored (Bennett & Kirk, 2008). Anti-tumor efficacy studies demonstrate that administration of NPI-0052 at 0.25–0.50 mg/kg, p.o. 2q7d inhibits human MM xenograft growth, prolongs overall survival of tumor-bearing mice, and reduces tumor recurrence in 57% of tumor-bearing mice. These oral doses were well tolerated. Chronic administration of NPI-0052 for up to 12 weeks did not result in peripheral neurotoxicity, suggesting a favorable and distinct tolerability profile (Chauhan et al., 2005, 2008). In combination studies, administration of NPI-0052 (0.025–0.075 mg/kg i.v.) and bortezomib (0.5 mg/kg i.v.) induces synergistic apoptosis and anti-tumor efficacy against MM and plasmacytoma xenografts (Chauhan et al., 2005, 2008). Moreover, administration of NPI-0052 (0.25 mg/kg p.o., 2q7d) in combination with oxaliplatin, irinotecan, avastin, and 5-fluorouracil significantly improves the tumoricidal response of these agents in models of chronic lymphocytic leukemia and colon carcinoma without increasing toxicity (Chauhan *et al.*, 2005, 2008; Cusack *et al.*, 2006; Ruiz *et al.*, 2006). These data demonstrate the anti-tumor activity of NPI-052 alone and its synergistic effects when used in combination with conventional chemotherapeutic agents or bortezomib in MM and other cancers as well. These findings, together with its broad proteasome subunit inhibition profile, and its oral bioavailability and tolerability, provided the rationale for advancing NPI-0052 to clinical trials in 2006 as a potential treatment for solid tumors and lymphoma. Most recently, the role for NPI-0052 in modulating the epithelial-mesenchymal transition

(EMT) critically important in tumor metastasis has been demonstrated (Baritaki et al, 2009). Exposure of DU-145 human prostate carcinoma cells to NPI-0052 inhibited the expression of the NFkB-regulated zinc-finger transcription factor, Snail, de-repressing the induction of the metastasis tumor suppressor, Raf kinase inhibitor protein (RKIP). Phenotypically, the exposure of prostatic carcinoma tumor cells to NPI-0052 suppressed the expression of mesenchymal gene products and morphology, and inhibited the chemotactic and invasive properties of tumor cells, consistent with a modulatory role of NPI-0052 in the EMT process (Baritaki et al, 2009). Additional studies are warranted to verify and extend these observations to other tumor types.

V. Clinical Studies with Proteasome Inhibitors _____

A. Bortezomib in MM and MCL: Clinical PDs, Efficacy, and Safety as Monotherapy

Several phase I trials of bortezomib monotherapy were completed in 123 patients with a variety of advanced solid tumor and hematological cancers. These studies established a maximum-tolerated dose of $1.3 \, mg/m^2$ when administered i.v. on days 1, 4, 8, and 11 of a 21-day cycle, with dose-limiting toxicities of sensory neurotoxicity, hypotension, and tachycardia. Bortezomib administration results in a rapid and dose-related inhibition of 20S proteasome chymotrypsin-like activity in peripheral white blood cells, with inhibition plateauing at 65–70% relative to baseline (Bross et al., 2004; Orlowski et al., 2002). This indicates an optimally efficacious dose of 1.0 to $1.3 \, mg/m^2$ in this patient population. Although initial indications of clinical activity were observed in a limited number of specific solid tumors, including hormone-refractory prostate cancer and non-small-cell lung cancer, complete remissions and partial remissions were observed only in MM patients. These clinical responses were accompanied by corresponding reductions in systemic immunoglobulin levels in MM patients (Aghajanian et al., 2002; Orlowski et al., 2002). These clinical findings were unprecedented in the management of MM and served as the basis for pivotal phase II trials of bortezomib in relapsed and refractory MM. The CREST study demonstrated significant partial and complete response rates with bortezomib alone in 30% of patients in the $1.0 \, mg/m^2$ group and 38% of patients in the $1.3 \, mg/m^2$ group. The subjects were heavily pretreated advanced MM patients who demonstrated manageable toxicities and overall response rates of 44 and 62% when bortezomib was combined with dexamethasone in the 1.0 and $1.3 \, mg/m^2$ bortezomib treatment groups, respectively (Jagannath et al., 2004; Richardson et al., 2003). The SUMMIT trial confirmed these observations, demonstrating an overall response rate of 35% with 10% complete remissions and 18% partial remissions, and a 1-year median duration of response in heavily pretreated, refractory MM patients receiving the standard twice weekly bortezomib regimen of $1.3 \, \text{mg/m}^2$ (Richardson et al., 2003). Bortezomib was subsequently granted accelerated FDA approval in 2003 for the treatment of MM in patients who had relapsed after two or more treatment regimens and were resistant to their last treatment regimen. More recently, follow-up survival analyses of the CREST trial data reveal a 5-year overall survival of 45 and 32% for MM patients in the 1.0 and $1.3 \, \text{mg/m}^2$ bortezomib treatment groups, respectively (Jagannath et al., 2008; Yang et al., 2009). In these initial phase II trials (Jagannath et al., 2004; Ludwig et al., 2005; Richardson et al., 2003), 50% of MM patients experienced serious adverse events on the standard regimen of bortezomib ($1.3 \, \text{mg/m}^2$/dose twice weekly × 2 weeks followed by a 10-day rest period for a maximum of 8 cycles), and in subsequent trials (Dispenzieri, 2005; Richardson et al., 2005), 75% of patients experienced grade 3–4 adverse events, with approximately one-third of patients discontinuing treatment as a result of adverse events. Among the most significant toxicities noted in these phase II studies with bortezomib were peripheral neuropathy, orthostatic hypotension, thrombocytopenia, neutropenia, anemia, pyrexia, gastrointestinal toxicity and diarrhea, nausea, vomiting, and asthenia. These toxicities were nonetheless deemed predictable and clinically manageable facilitating the development and subsequent widespread use of bortezomib for the treatment of MM (Bennett & Kirk, 2008; Dispenzieri, 2005; Richardson et al., 2005; Sterz et al., 2008).

The superiority of bortezomib ($1.3 \, \text{mg/m}^2$ regimen) in the management of relapsed and refractory MM relative to the standard of care, which consisted of dexamethasone, 40 mg orally on days 1–4, 9–12, and 17–20 in four 5-week cycles, was confirmed in an international, open-label phase III APEX study involving 669 patients. The overall response rates in this study were 38 and 18%, with median duration of response of 8 and 5.6 months achieved for bortezomib and dexamethasone, respectively (Richardson et al., 2005). These pivotal data confirmed the clinical efficacy and survival benefit of bortezomib monotherapy in relapsed MM patients, resulting in its full FDA approval in 2005 (Kane, Farrell, Sridhara, & Pazdur, 2006). The results also provided further support for initiating additional combination studies of bortezomib with traditional standard-of-care chemotherapy in the management of MM. In addition, these clinical findings provided the impetus for additional clinical trials examining the efficacy of bortezomib in a variety of additional hematological and solid tumors. More recently, extended follow-up analyses of the APEX patient population data confirmed that bortezomib monotherapy is superior to dexamethasone in relapsed and refractory MM patients, with higher response rates, longer duration of response, and improved overall 1-year survival rates. With bortezomib treatment, MM patients achieved significantly higher partial responses (38% versus 18%; $p < 0.001$) and complete responses (6% versus

<1%; p< 0.001) as compared to dexamethasone treatment. The median time to disease progression was also longer in the bortezomib arm than in patients treated with dexamethasone (6.2 versus 3.5 months; p < 0.001) (Richardson et al., 2007).

The efficacy and safety of bortezomib monotherapy in newly diagnosed, chemo-naive MM patients were investigated recently (Richardson et al., 2009). Sixty-four patients received 1.3 mg/m^2 bortezomib on days 1, 4, 8, and 11, for up to eight 21-day cycles. Bortezomib treatment achieved an overall response in 41% of patients including 9% with either complete remission or near-complete remission, and 32% incidence of partial remission, with a median duration of response of 8.4 months. The median time to disease progression was 17 months, and the estimated 1-year survival was 92% in this patient population. Pretreatment sensory neuropathy was observed in 20% of patients, with new or worsening neuropathy observed in 63% of those participating. Although this incidence of neuropathy is higher than in earlier reports with MM patients, most neuropathies were reversible upon discontinuation of bortezomib treatment (Richardson et al., 2009).

Subsequent to full FDA approval for the treatment of MM, bortezomib received approval for the treatment of relapsed patients with mantle cell lymphoma (Kane et al., 2007). This was based on the results of two pivotal phase II multicenter prospective studies (PINNACLE) conducted in relapsed mantle cell lymphoma patients. These studies demonstrated significant 33–46% overall response rates, 8% complete response rates, and 9.2–10 month median duration of response (Belch et al., 2007; Fisher et al., 2006). The safety profile observed in these studies was comparable to that observed in MM patients, with peripheral neuropathy (13%), fatigue (12%), and thrombocytopenia (11%) being the major adverse events (Fisher et al., 2006; Sterz et al., 2008).

Goy et al. (2009) reported the results from an extended follow-up analysis of the phase II PINNACLE study. This analysis confirmed the substantial single-agent efficacy of bortezomib in patients with relapsed and refractory mantle cell lymphoma (Goy et al., 2009). After a median follow-up of 26 months, the median overall survival was 23.5 months, with a median time to disease progression of 6.7 months. The median duration of response was 9.2 months overall, with a 1-year survival of 91% in responders (Goy et al., 2009). Similarly, O'Connor et al. (2009) reported results from a multicenter phase II study of bortezomib in 40 patients with heavily pretreated mantle cell lymphoma. Responses were observed in 19 patients (47%), including 5 complete remissions and 14 partial remissions. The overall response rate was similar with relapsed and refractory patients (50% versus 43%). There was no significant difference in progression-free survival between the relapsed (5.6 months) and refractory (3.9 months) patients (O'Connor et al., 2009). These data suggest that single-agent bortezomib is an effective therapy for the treatment of refractory and heavily pretreated mantle cell lymphoma patients.

B. Combination Therapies with Bortezomib in MM

Early clinical trials examining the safety and efficacy of bortezomib in combination with dexamethasone, doxorubicin, melphalan, prednisone, and thalidomide in newly diagnosed MM patients showed promising results (Ludwig et al., 2005; Rajkumar et al., 2005). During the past 5 years, bortezomib has been investigated extensively in combination with cytotoxic agents, immunomodulatory drugs, and glucocorticoids in the treatment of newly diagnosed and relapsed/refractory MM patients.

I. Combinations of Bortezomib with Melphalan

Based on the results of a phase III VISTA trial, bortezomib in combination with melphalan and prednisone was approved as first-line treatment for patients with newly diagnosed MM who are ineligible for high-dose therapy. The trial was conducted in 682 patients with untreated MM to compare melphalan–prednisone with bortezomib–melphalan–prednisone combination therapy (San Miguel et al., 2008). Patients were randomized to receive a 6-week cycle melphalan ($9\,mg/m^2$) and prednisone ($60\,mg/m^2$) on days 1–4, either alone or with bortezomib ($1.3\,mg/m^2$), on days 1, 4, 8, 11, 22, 25, 29, and 32 during cycles 1–4, and on days 1, 8, 22, and 29 during cycles 5–9. The bortezomib–melphalan regimens displayed superiority over melphalan alone in terms of time to progression (24 versus 17 months, $P < 0.001$), response rate (71% versus 35%, $P<0.001$), complete remissions (30% versus 4%, $P < 0.001$), median duration of response (20 versus 13 months), and overall survival. Thus, 13% in the bortezomib group and 22% of the control group died after a median follow-up of 16 months ($P = 0.008$). While patients in the bortezomib–melphalan group had more treatment-related adverse events, there were no significant differences in grade 4 events or treatment-related deaths between the groups (San Miguel et al., 2008). This trial was terminated early when it became clear that bortezomib–melphalan combination therapy was superior to melphalan alone as first-line treatment for newly diagnosed MM patients who are ineligible for high-dose therapy.

Berenson et al. (2009) have reported initial results from a single-arm, multicenter phase II study to assess combined therapy with bortezomib, ascorbic acid, and melphalan in patients with untreated MM (Berenson et al., 2009). Subjects received up to eight 28-day cycles of bortezomib ($1.0\,mg/m^2$) on days 1, 4, 8 and 11, and ascorbic acid (1 g) and melphalan ($0.1\,mg/kg$) on days 1–4, followed by maintenance bortezomib $1.3\,mg/m^2$ twice weekly until disease progression. Responses were achieved in 23 of 31 (74%) evaluable patients, including five (16%) complete, nine (29%) partial, and nine (29%) minimal responses. Disease control was achieved in 29 (94%) patients, including 6 (19%) with stable disease. While this steroid-free, bortezomib-containing regimen demonstrates efficacy and tolerability, the durability of the responses remains to be determined.

2. Combinations of Bortezomib with Pegylated Liposomal Doxorubicin

In 2007, based on a phase III study, the FDA approved the combination therapy of bortezomib and pegylated liposomal doxorubicin (PLD) for the treatment of bortezomib-naive patients who had progressed after at least one prior line of therapy (Orlowski et al., 2007). The efficacy of doxorubicin in MM treatment was established initially with the combination of vincristine–doxorubicin–dexamethasone therapy in the 1980s (Alexanian, Barlogie, & Tucker, 1990; Barlogie, Smith, & Alexanian, 1984). One of the mechanisms of doxorubicin resistance is activation of NF-κB (Wang, Mayo, & Baldwin, 1996). Since bortezomib inhibits NF-κB activity, it was hypothesized that the combination of bortezomib and doxorubicin might prevent chemo-resistance to doxorubicin (Ma et al., 2003). Based on this rationale, a combination of bortezomib and PLD was first evaluated in a phase I study with 42 patients with hematological cancers, including 24 with MM (Orlowski et al., 2005). In these studies, bortezomib ($1.3\,\text{mg/m}^2$) administered on days 1, 4, 8, and 11 in combination with PLD ($30\,\text{mg/m}^2$) on day 4 of a 21-day cycle was identified as the optimal treatment regimen. Among 22 evaluable MM patients, 72% achieved responses, including 36% complete or near-complete responses, and 36% partial responses. With extended follow-up, median overall survival was 38.3 months with the median time to progression of 9.3 months (Biehn et al., 2007). These results led to a multicenter, randomized phase III study of patients with relapsed/refractory MM to compare bortezomib monotherapy with the bortezomib and PLD in combination (Orlowski et al., 2007). The 646 patients in this study were randomized to receive either bortezomib alone ($1.3\,\text{mg/m}^2$) or bortezomib in combination with PLD ($30\,\text{mg/m}^2$). Although the response rates were not higher with the combination regimen versus bortezomib alone (44% versus 41%), the time to progression (9.3 versus 6.5 months, $p = 0.000004$) and duration of response (10.2 versus 7.0 months, $p = 0.0008$) were significantly better with the combination therapy. The 15-month survival was 76% with the combination regimen and 65% with bortezomib alone ($p = 0.03$). Grade 3 and 4 events were more frequent, however, in the combination group (80%) compared with bortezomib alone (64%), with increased incidences of grade 3–4 neutropenia, thrombocytopenia, asthenia, fatigue, diarrhea, and hand–foot syndrome (Orlowski et al., 2007). Additional studies suggest a potential clinical benefit for the combination of bortezomib and PLD administration as salvage therapy in MM patients (Braccalenti et al., 2007), in relapsed MM patients who failed thalidomide and lenilidomide treatment (Sonneveld et al., 2008) and in high-risk MM patients who relapsed within 1 year of stem cell transplantation therapy (Kumar et al., 2007). These findings await confirmation from additional clinical studies.

3. Combinations of Bortezomib with Cyclophosphamide and Glucocorticoids

Preliminary clinical data have suggested that a regimen of bortezomib in combination with cyclophosphamide and glucocorticoids is an effective treatment for newly diagnosed or relapsed MM. A phase I/II trial of the combination of weekly versus twice weekly bortezomib–cyclophosphamide–prednisone in patients with relapsed/refractory MM was reported (Reece et al., 2008). It was found that the bortezomib regimens tested (1.3 mg/m^2 on days 1, 4, 8, and 11, and 1.5 mg/m^2 on days 1, 8, and 15, each on a 28-day cycle) could be safely administered with cyclophosphamide (300 mg/m^2 per week) and prednisone. With the 1.5 mg/m^2 bortezomib dose administered weekly, the overall response rate, including complete and partial remissions and minor responses, was 95%, with a complete responses reported for more than 50% of patients. The weekly bortezomib regimen resulted in fewer instances of grade 3 thrombocytopenia and grade 1–2 peripheral neuropathies.

The anti-myeloma efficacy of the combination of cyclophosphamide, bortezomib, and dexamethasone in untreated MM was recently assessed in a phase II trial (Reeder et al., 2009). Thirty-two newly diagnosed patients received bortezomib (1.3 mg/m^2) on days 1, 4, 8, and 11, cyclophosphamide (300 mg/m^2) on days 1, 8, 15, and 22, and dexamethasone (40 mg) on days 1–4, 9–12, and 17–20 on a 28-day cycle for four cycles. Of this group, 88% experienced a partial remission or better, with 61% of patients exhibiting very good partial responses or better, and 39% complete or near-complete responses (Reeder et al., 2009).

A phase I/II trial of bortezomib with cyclophosphamide and dexamethasone as induction therapy prior to stem cell transplantation was conducted in younger patients with newly diagnosed MM (Kropff et al., 2009). After establishing the maximum-tolerated dose, patients were treated with bortezomib (1.3 mg/m^2) on days 1, 4, 8, and 11, dexamethasone (40 mg) on the day of and the day after bortezomib administration, and cyclophosphamide (900 mg/m^2) on day 1. The overall response rate at the maximum-tolerated dose was partial responses or better in 92% of the subjects. These preliminary data suggested that the bortezomib–cyclophosphamide–dexamethasone combination regimen is an effective induction therapy in younger MM patients eligible for stem cell transplantation.

4. Combinations of Bortezomib with Immunomodulatory Agents

Thalidomide was the first immunomodulatory agent approved for the treatment of MM. In relapsed MM, the response rate to thalidomide monotherapy is 32% (Singhal et al., 1999), with the addition of dexamethasone to thalidomide improving this response to 40–50% (von Lilienfeld-Toal et al., 2008). The combination regimen of bortezomib–thalidomide–dexamethasone improved the response rate further to 53–65% in patients with relapsed/

refractory MM based upon the findings of two small phase II studies (Ciolli, Leoni, Gigli, Rigacci, & Bosi, 2006; Pineda-Roman et al., 2008).

Lenalidomide, a structural analog of thalidomide, has a similar mechanism of action but more potent biologic activity. When combined with dexamethasone, lenalidomide induced response rates of 55–60% in relapsed/refractory MM (Dimopoulos et al., 2007; Weber et al., 2007). The combination of bortezomib–lenalidomide–dexamethasone was more effective in those with relapsed/refractory disease than lenalidomide–dexamethasone, achieving partial remission in 68% and complete or near-complete remission in 21% of the subjects (Richardson, Lonial, et al., 2008). The overall response rate to bortezomib–lenalidomide–dexamethasone combination therapy in newly diagnosed MM patients is reported to be almost 100% (Richardson, Jagannath, et al., 2008). The final results of these studies are yet to be reported.

Wolf et al. (2008) reported a retrospective study aimed at evaluating the utility of bortezomib re-treatment in patients with relapsed/refractory MM (Wolf et al., 2008). A total of 22 patients who participated in the phase II (SUMMIT or CREST) or phase III (APEX) registration studies were subsequently re-treated off protocol with bortezomib-based therapy. These individuals received either bortezomib alone or a bortezomib-containing regimen following at least a 60-day hiatus from the first bortezomib treatment. The overall response rate for bortezomib re-treatment was 50%, including 9% complete responses. Therapy was discontinued due to unmanageable toxicities in two patients during re-treatment. Bortezomib re-treatment may, nonetheless, represent a viable option for relapsed or refractory MM patients who have been previously exposed to this agent.

As discussed above, preclinical bortezomib administration in combination with HDAC inhibitors (Deleu et al., 2009; Terpos et al., 2007) has a synergistic benefit in reducing MM tumor burden *in vitro* and *in vivo*. Histone deacetylase inhibitors inhibit HDAC6 function and disrupt the aggresomal pathway of protein degradation, an alternative protein disposal pathway whose activation has been associated with bortezomib resistance (Kumar & Rajkumar, 2008). In this regard, Badros et al. (2009) reported a phase I study of bortezomib and the approved HDAC inhibitor, vorinostat, in heavily pretreated relapsed/refractory MM patients. Sequential escalation of bortezomib at 1–1.3 mg/m^2 i.v. on days 1, 4, 8, and 11 was evaluated in combination with vorinostat at 100–500 mg p.o. daily for 8 days of each 21-day treatment cycle. The maximum-tolerated dose of vorinostat in this combination regimen was 400 mg daily. Of 23 MM patients treated, the overall response rate was 42%, including three partial responses among nine patients refractory to bortezomib. The most common grade 3 or greater toxicities for the combination therapy were myelosuppression, fatigue, and diarrhea. Despite the absence of a clear association between clinical responses and the PD parameters assessed in this study, the promising anti-myeloma efficacy observed in bortezomib-refractory patients is the basis for planned phase II/III studies in relapsed/refractory MM patients (Badros et al., 2009).

C. Single-Agent and Combination Therapies with Bortezomib in Waldenström's Macroglobulinemia

The effectiveness of bortezomib as a treatment for Waldenström's macroglobulinemia was first reported in 2005 (Dimopoulos et al., 2005). Ten patients with relapsed/refractory Waldenström's macroglobulinemia were treated with bortezomib using the standard dose regimen approved for MM. Six of these subjects achieved partial remission within a median time to disease progression of 1 month. The efficacy of bortezomib in Waldenström's macroglobulinemia was confirmed by two larger, multi-center, phase II trials, the NCI-Canada CTG study (Chen et al., 2007) and the WM-CTG study (Treon et al., 2007). In the former, 27 patients with pretreated or untreated Waldenström's macroglobulinemia were enrolled, with 26% achieving partial responses and 70% stable disease. Only one individual showed disease progression. Of this group, 74% developed new or worsening neuropathy, including five patients with grade 3 neuropathy (Chen et al., 2007). In the WM-CTG study, 27 Waldenström's macroglobulinemia patients, with all but one having relapsed/refractory disease, were treated with bortezomib. Overall responses were achieved in 85% of these patients, with 13 individuals experiencing major, and 10 minor, responses. Grade 3/4 neuropathy developed in 22% of these subjects (Treon et al., 2007).

Two trials investigating bortezomib combination therapy in Waldenström's macroglobulinemia have been reported. Twenty-three newly diagnosed Waldenström's macroglobulinemia patients were treated with bortezomib ($1.3 \, \text{mg/m}^2$) and dexamethasone (40 mg) on days 1, 4, 8, 11 and rituximab ($375 \, \text{mg/m}^2$) on day 11 on a 21-day cycle (Treon et al., 2009). Partial responses or better were achieved with 96% of the subjects, with 3 complete remissions, 2 near-complete remissions, 3 very good partial responses, 11 partial responses, and 3 minor responses. Eighteen of 23 patients (78%) remained disease free after 23 months. Sixteen subjects (50%) developed neuropathy, with 13 of these resolving to grade 1 or less within 6 months of treatment (Treon et al., 2009). These findings suggest that single-agent bortezomib and the bortezomib–dexamethasone–rituximab combination regimens are effective therapies for the treatment of Waldenström's macroglobulinemia. However, peripheral neuropathy may be dose limiting. It may be possible that weekly bortezomib administration schedules may help minimize the development of neuropathy in these patients.

D. Clinical Evaluation of Bortezomib in Additional Hematological and Solid Tumors as Monotherapy and in Combination with Standard-of-Care Agents

There have been several comprehensive reviews of phase I and II clinical findings with bortezomib in various solid and hematological cancers (Ludwig et al., 2005; Sterz et al., 2008; Yang et al., 2009). Although bortezomib displays significant preclinical benefits in multiple malignancies, its activity against solid tumors appears limited for reasons that are not completely understood. Bennett and Kirk (2008) speculated that, given the therapeutic index of bortezomib on the approved twice weekly clinical dosing regimen, the magnitude and duration of proteasome inhibition may be suboptimal for the treatment of solid tumors. Alternatively, the unique pathophysiology of immunoglobulin-secreting plasma cell tumors, such as MM, may sensitize them to proteasome inhibition more so than for other tumors.

Bortezomib monotherapy has been investigated clinically as a treatment for a wide range of solid tumors. The results were negative for breast (Engel et al., 2007; Yang et al., 2006), colon (Mackay et al., 2005), pancreatic (Alberts et al., 2005), renal cell (Davis et al., 2004), and urothelial (Rosenberg et al., 2008) carcinomas. Likewise, bortezomib was ineffective as a treatment for metastatic neuroendocrine tumors (Shah et al., 2004) and metastatic melanoma (Markovic et al., 2005). Partial responses were observed in only 1 of 65 patients with small-cell lung cancer (Lara et al., 2006), and 1 of 21 patients with soft-tissue sarcoma (Maki et al., 2005).

Bortezomib in combination with other chemotherapeutic agents has also been investigated clinically in this regard, but with disappointing results. The combinations included bortezomib with gemcitabine in pancreatic cancer (Alberts et al., 2005), bortezomib and temozolomide with radiotherapy for central nervous system tumors (Kubicek et al., 2009), bortezomib and capecitabine in breast cancer (Schmid et al., 2008), bortezomib and carboplatin in ovarian cancer (Aghajanian et al., 2005; Ramirez et al., 2008), bortezomib and docetaxel in hormone-refractory prostate cancer (Hainsworth et al., 2007), and bortezomib and irinotecan in colorectal, lung, and gastroesophageal cancers (Ryan et al., 2006).

Bortezomib was also investigated as a monotherapy and in combination with standard-of-care regimens as a treatment for non-small-cell lung cancer. Partial responses were observed in 8% of patients who received monotherapy and 9% of those receiving the combination therapy (Fanucchi et al., 2006), indicating a modest benefit of bortezomib, with no additional benefit when combined with docetaxel. Similarly, bortezomib in combination with cisplatin and gemcitabine as a first-line treatment of patients with non-small-cell lung cancer achieved a response rate of 38%, similar to that observed in advanced lung cancer patients treated with cisplatin and gemcitabine at higher doses

(Voortman et al., 2007). Bortezomib in combination with cetuximab yielded a 43% incidence of stable disease at 6 weeks in patients with Epidermal Growth Factor Receptor (EGFR)-expressing non-small-cell lung cancer or heavily pretreated head and neck cancers (Dudek et al., 2009).

Davies et al. (2009) conducted a trial of bortezomib in combination with carboplatin and gemcitabine in patients with chemotherapy-naive non-small-cell lung cancer (Davies et al. 2009). The disease control rate in this trial was 68% overall, with 23% partial responses and a 45% incidence of stable disease. After follow-up of more than 3 years, median overall survival was 11 months, with 1-year and 2-year survival rates being 47 and 19%, respectively. Median progression-free survival was 5 months, with a 1-year progression-free survival rate of 7%. These data are the most encouraging in suggesting a possible role for bortezomib in the treatment of specific solid tumors (Davies et al., 2009).

VI. Clinical Studies with "Next-Generation" Proteasome Inhibitors

Despite its toxicity profile and limited therapeutic index in humans, the clinical outcomes achieved with bortezomib monotherapy, and in combination with other agents, as treatment for MM, mantle cell lymphoma, and Waldenström's macroglobulinemia validate the proteasome as an important molecular target for the treatment of specific hematological human cancers. Although the toxicity profile of bortezomib can be managed in a clinical setting (Adams, 2003; Ludwig et al., 2005; Sterz et al., 2008), the toxicities observed are not inconsequential. The limitations imposed by these adverse effects are one major justification for pursuing the development of novel proteasome inhibitors that may display a therapeutic index that is superior to existing agents. The limited benefit observed with bortezomib in solid tumors has also prompted interest in the possibility that the next-generation proteasome inhibitors may have broader clinical potential. Moreover, bortezomib resistance in MM patients is a critical issue, necessitating a switch to alternative therapies. Several mechanisms of escape for bortezomib-mediated proteasome inhibition have been proposed. These include mutations or over-expression in the β5 subunit of the proteasome complex, thereby impairing bortezomib binding and inhibition (Oerlemans et al., 2008). It has also been suggested that bortezomib resistance may be due in part to an increased utilization by tumor cells of alternative pathways of protein degradation (the aggresomal pathway) (Kumar & Rajkumar, 2008) as noted above, thus bypassing the proteasome-ubiquitination pathway. Up-regulation of specific heat shock proteins, particularly Hsp27, has also been associated with bortezomib resistance in MM (Chauhan et al., 2003). Structurally and mechanistically distinct proteasome inhibitors may provide a means to bypass or limit the impact of the escape mechanisms associated with bortezomib resistance. In particular, the irreversibility of proteasome inhibition and/or differential enzyme-inhibitor kinetic off-rates may offer an additional means both of overcoming bortezomib resistance in MM and of expanding the therapeutic utility of proteasome inhibitors for a larger number of tumor types.

A. Carfilzomib

Carfilzomib (CFZ, PR-171), an irreversible proteasome inhibitor, entered clinical development in 2005 as a potential treatment for MM. It was also hoped this agent might be effective in those patients experiencing bortezomib resistance (Demo et al., 2007; Kuhn et al., 2007). In one study, 46 patients with relapsed and refractory MM received i.v. CFZ twice weekly on days 1, 2, 8, 9, 15, and 16 of a 28-day cycle (Jagannath et al., 2009). Clinical benefit was observed in 26% of evaluable patients, including partial responses in five patients and minor responses in five. The duration of the response for these clinical effects was 7.4 months. Peripheral neuropathy developed in less than 10% of the study participants, with one incidence of grade 3 in a patient with pre-existing grade 2 neuropathy.

In a follow-up study, 31 patients with relapsed MM, including 14 bortezomib-naive and 17 bortezomib-exposed subjects, received up to twelve 28-day cycles of CFZ (Vij et al., 2009). In the bortezomib-naive group, CFZ induced a partial response or better in 57% of the subjects, with a median duration of response of 8.6 months. For the bortezomib-exposed group, a partial response or better was observed in 18% of the group, with a median duration of response of greater than 8.5 months. Work continues on assessing the effectiveness of CFZ as a treatment for MM given the clinical activity and reduced incidence of peripheral neuropathy observed in this patient population.

B. NPI-0052

NPI-0052, also known as salinosporamide A, is an irreversible proteasome inhibitor currently in clinical development. Initial studies were launched in 2006. Phase I studies conducted in patients with solid tumors and lymphoma demonstrated dose-dependent PD inhibition of proteasome activity in peripheral blood mononuclear cells and a stabilization of disease for approximately 11 months (Aghajanian et al., 2008). Three phase I trials have been initiated with NPI-0052 monotherapy in patients with MM and solid tumors, as well as a study of NPI-0052 in combination with vorinostat, a histone deacetylase inhibitor, in patients with solid tumors (Bennett & Kirk, 2008). The results of a study with relapsed or refractory MM were reported recently (Hofmeister et al., 2009). In this trial, NPI-0052 was administered once weekly at doses of 0.025–0.7 mg/m^2 for 3 weeks in a 28-day cycle, as opposed to the twice weekly regimens employed for bortezomib. The maximum-tolerated dose has not yet been identified at the time of this report, but evidence for clinical benefit and the absence of neutropenia and peripheral neuropathy were observed in this patient population. Based upon these encouraging, albeit early, clinical observations, additional trials of NPI-0052 in combination with lenalidomide as a treatment for MM are being initiated (Hofmeister et al., 2009).

C. CEP-18770

The next-generation boronic acid proteasome inhibitor CEP-18770 entered the clinic in late 2007. A phase I study was conducted to assess its safety, pharmacokinetics, and the PDs in patients with solid tumors and lymphoma to establish a maximum-tolerated dose and the optimal regimen for proteasome inhibition (Marangon et al., 2009). While orally active in laboratory animals, in the clinical trial CEP-18770 was administered as a slow i.v. bolus on days 1, 4, 8, and 11 of a 21-day cycle, with dose escalation following a modified Fibonacci sequence starting from 0.1 mg/m^2. Blood samples were collected prior to drug administration and over a 48 h time course following the first day of administration, and before administration and on days 4, 8, and 11 of cycle one and prior to the starting day of the second cycle. The inhibition of the chymotrypsin-like activity of 20S proteosome was assessed in blood samples by a fluorogenic kinetic assay (Lightcap et al., 2000) similar to that used for bortezomib. Preliminary pharmacokinetic data obtained on day 1 of treatment showed Cmax and AUC$_{exp}$ values (mean ± SD) of 88 ± 43 ng/mL and 124 ± 59 ng/mL h and 177 ± 62 ng/mL and 384 ± 97 ng/mL h at doses of 0.4 and 0.6 mg/m^2, respectively, with an elimination half-life of approximately 3 days. CEP-18770 demonstrated a dose-related inhibition of chymotrypsin-like proteosome activity *ex vivo*, achieving approximately 40% peak inhibition at the dose of 0.6 mg/m^2 and approximately 57% inhibition at 1.8 mg/m^2. A maximum-tolerated dose for CEP-18770 was achieved in this study. Expansion of the study to include patients with relapsed/refractory MM is planned to investigate the efficacy of CEP-18770 in this group. To date, the data indicate that CEP-18770 displays a favorable overall safety profile with no significant peripheral neurotoxicity. Based upon these findings, an international, multicenter phase I/II trial of CEP-18770 monotherapy is being initiated in patients with relapsed and refractory MM.

VII. Conclusion

The clinical efficacy of bortezomib in MM and mantle cell lymphoma served both to validate the proteasome complex as a therapeutic target in oncology and to revolutionize the treatment of these B-cell malignancies. Advances in the discovery and clinical development of several chemically unique next-generation proteasome inhibitors with distinct mechanisms of action, pharmacological profiles, and therapeutic indices relative to bortezomib offer considerable possibilities for the future of cancer treatment. First, the potential efficacy of these new inhibitors, including CFZ, NPI-0052, and CEP-18770, in overcoming bortezomib resistance is suggested by preclinical and clinical results, suggesting that such drugs could have a major impact on the treatment of relapsed and refractory MM patients. Second, these new agents may make it possible to address whether proteasome inhibitors have broader therapeutic applications for the treatment of other hematological and solid tumors, either as single agents or in combination with standards of care therapies. The results for bortezomib in this regard have been generally disappointing. A question remains as to whether these clinical observations are bortezomib specific or characteristic of proteasome inhibitors as a class. Additional structurally and pharmacologically distinct classes of reversible and irreversible inhibitors with unique mechanisms of action against the proteasome, distinct off-target selectivity profiles, and efficacy achievable with alternative dosing regimens may help address these important questions. Third, although the toxicities of bortezomib-based therapies are generally manageable, the peripheral neuropathy, cardiovascular toxicities, and thrombocytopenia are limiting. Several "next-generation" inhibitors, including CFZ, NPI-0052, and CEP-18770, reportedly are less likely to induce peripheral neuropathy. The narrow therapeutic index of bortezomib and the liabilities associated with its peripheral neuropathy have limited the application of proteasome inhibitors as potential immunomodulatory agents for non-oncological indications, such as the management of inflammatory diseases (Bennett & Kirk, 2008). These non-oncological applications await further investigation with novel and chemically distinct inhibitors with more favorable therapeutic indices. The discovery and development of new inhibitors of the ubiquitin–proteasome–NF-κB pathway offers the potential to further revolutionize the treatment and management of cancer and possibly other conditions for which modulation of the ubiquitin–proteasome–NF-κB pathway may confer therapeutic benefit.

Conflict of Interest: The authors of this chapter are employees of Cephalon Inc, a biopharmaceutical company undertaking the clinical development of CEP-18770, a novel next-generation boronic acid proteasome inhibitor for use as an oncologic therapeutic agent.

References

Adams, J. (2003). The development of proteasome inhibitors as anticancer drugs. *Cancer Cell,* 5, 417–421.

Adams, J., Palombella, V. J., Sausville, E. A., Johnson, J., Destree, A., Lazarus, D. D., et al. (1999). Proteasome inhibitors: A novel class of potent and effective antitumor agents. *Cancer Research,* 59, 2615–2622.

Adams, J., & Stein, R. (1996). Novel inhibitors of the proteasome and their therapeutic use in inflammation. *Annual Reports in Medicinal Chemistry,* 31, 279–287.

Aghajanian, C., Dizon, D. S., Sabbatini, P., Raizer, J. J., Dupont, J., & Spriggs, D. R. (2005). Phase I trial of bortezomib and carboplatin in recurrent ovarian or primary peritoneal cancer. *Journal of Clinical Oncology,* 23, 5943–5949.

Aghajanian, C., Hamlin, P., Gordon, D. S., Hong, M., Naing, A., Younes, A., et al. (2008). Phase I study of the novel proteasome inhibitor NPI-0052 in patients with lymphoma and solid tumors. *Journal of Clinical Oncology,* 26, Supplement, #3574.

Aghajanian, C., Soignet, S., Dizon, D. S., Pien, C. S., Adams, J., Elliott, P. J., et al. (2002). A phase I trial of the novel proteasome inhibitor PS341 in advanced solid tumor malignancies. *Clinical Cancer Research,* 8, 2505–2511.

Ahn, K. S., Sethi, G., Chao, T. H., Neuteboom, S. T. C., Chaturvedi, M. M., Pallasino, M. A., et al. (2007). Salinosporamide A (NPI-0052) potentiates apoptosis, suppress osteoclastogenesis, and inhibits invasion through down-regulation of NF-κB-regulated gene products. *Blood,* 110, 2286–2295.

Alberts, S. R., Foster, N. R., Morton, R. F., Kugler, J., Schaefer, P., Wiesenfeld, M., et al. (2005). PS-341 and gemcitabine in patients with metastatic pancreatic adenocarcinoma: A North Central Cancer Treatment Group (NCCTG) randomized phase II study. *Annals of Oncology,* 16, 1654–1661.

Alexanian, R., Barlogie, B., & Tucker, S. (1990). VAD-based regimens as primary treatment for multiple myeloma. *American Journal of Hematology,* 33, 86–89.

Amiri, K. I., Horton, L. W., LaFleur, B. J., Sosman, J. A., & Richmond, A. (2004). Augmenting chemosensitivity of malignant melanoma tumors via proteasome inhibition; implications for bortezomib (Velcade™, PS-341) as therapeutic agent for malignant melanoma. *Cancer Research,* 64, 4912–4918.

Arastu-Kapur, S., Shenk, K., Parlati, F., & Bennett, M. K. (2008). Non-proteasomal targets of proteasome inhibitors bortezomib and carfilzomib. *Blood (ASH Annual Meeting Abstracts),* 112, #2657

Badros, A., Burger, A. M., Philip, S., Niesvizky, R., Kolla, S. S., Goloubeva, O., et al. (2009). Phase I study of vorinostat in combination with bortezomib for relapsed and refractory multiple myeloma. *Clinical Cancer Research,* 15, 5250–5257.

Baldwin, J. E. (1976). Rules for ring closure. *Journal of the Chemical Society, Chemical Communications,* 734–736.

Baritaki, S., Chapman, A., Yeung, K., Spandidos, D. A., Palladino, M., & Bonavida, B. (2009). Inhibition of epithelial to mesenchymal transition in metastatic prostate cancer cells by the novel proteasome inhibitor, NPI-0052: pivotal roles of Snail repression and RKIP induction. *Oncogene,* 28, 3573–3585.

Barlogie, B., Smith, L., & Alexanian, R. (1984). Effective treatment of advanced multiple myeloma refractory to alkylating agents. *New England Journal of Medicine,* 310, 1353–1356.

Belch, A., Kouroukis, C. T., Crump, M., Sehn, L., Gascoyne, R. D., Klasa, R., et al. (2007). A phase II study of bortezomib in mantle cell lymphoma: The National Cancer Institute of Canada Clinical Trials Group trial IND.150. *Annals of Oncology,* 18, 116–121.

Bennett, M. K., & Kirk, C. J. (2008). Development of proteasome inhibitors in oncology and autoimmune diseases. *Current Opinion in Drug Discovery & Development,* 11, 616–625.

Berenson, J. R., Yellin, O., Woytowitz, D., Flam, M. S., Cartmell, A., Patel, R., et al. (2009). Bortezomib, ascorbic acid and melphalan (BAM) therapy for patients with newly diagnosed multiple myeloma: An effective and well-tolerated frontline regimen. *European Journal of Haematology, 82,* 433–439.

Biehn, S. E., Moore, D. T., Voorhees, P. M., Garcia, R. A., Lehman, M. J., Dees, E. C., et al. (2007). Extended follow-up of outcome measures in multiple myeloma patients treated on a phase I study with bortezomib and pegylated liposomal doxorubicin. *Annals of Hematology, 86,* 211–216.

Bogner, C., Peschel, C., & Decker, T. (2006). Targeting the proteasome in mantle cell lymphoma: A promising therapeutic approach. *Leukemia and Lymphoma, 47,* 195–205.

Bold, R. J., Virudachalam, S., & Mcconkey, D. J. (2001). Chemosensitization of pancreatic cancer by inhibition of the 26S proteasome. *Journal of Surgical Research, 100,* 11–17.

Braccalenti, G., Pasqualinda, F., Gubbiotti, M., Cerroni, P., Falchi, L., Luzi, D., et al. (2007). Anti-tumour activity of bortezomib-pegylated liposomal doxorubicine association as salvage therapy in multiple myeloma patients. *Blood (ASH Annual Meeting Abstracts), 110, #4832.*

Bross, P. F., Kane, R., Farrell, A. T., Abraham, S., Benson, K., Brower, M. E., et al. (2004). Approval summary for bortezomib for injection in the treatment of multiple myeloma. *Clinical Cancer Research, 10,* 3954–3964.

Campbell, R. A., Sanchez, E., Steinberg, J. A., Baritaki, S., Gordon, M., Wang, C., et al. (2007). Antimyeloma effects of arsenic trioxide are enhanced by melphalan, bortezomib and ascorbic acid. *British Journal of Haematology, 138,* 467–478.

Cavo, M. (2006). Proteasome inhibitor bortezomib for the treatment of multiple myeloma. *Leukemia, 20,* 1341–1352.

Chauhan, D., Bianchi, G., & Anderson, K. C. (2008). Targeting the UPS as therapy in multiple myeloma. *BMC Biochemistry, 9* (Supplement 1): SI doi: 10.1186/147-209-9-SI-SI.

Chauhan, D., Catley, L., Li, G., Podar, K., Hideshima, T., Velankar, M., et al. (2005). A novel orally active proteasome inhibitor induces apoptosis in multiple myeloma cells with a mechanism distinct from bortezomib. *Cancer Cell, 8,* 407–419.

Chauhan, D., Li, G., Shringarpure, R., Podar, K., Yasuyuki, O., Hideshima, T., et al. (2003). Blockade of Hsp27 overcomes bortezomib/proteasome inhibitor PS-341 resistance in lymphoma cells. *Cancer Research, 63,* 6174–6177.

Chauhan, D., Singh, A., Brahmandam, M., Podar, K., Hideshima, T., Richardson, P., et al. (2008). Combination or proteasome inhibitors bortezomib and NPI-0052 trigger in vivo synergistic cytotoxicity in multiple myeloma. *Blood, 111,* 1654–1664.

Chen, C. I., Kouroukis, C. T., White, D., Voralia, M., Stadtmauer, E., Stewart, A. K., et al. (2007). Bortezomib is active in patients with untreated or relapsed Waldenstrom's macroglobulinemia: A phase II study of the National Cancer Institute of Canada Clinical Trials Group. *Journal of Clinical Oncology, 25,* 1570–1575.

Ciechanover, A. (1994). The ubiquitin-proteasome proteolytic pathway. *Cell, 79,* 13–21.

Ciolli, S., Leoni, F., Gigli, F., Rigacci, L., & Bosi, A. (2006). Low dose Velcade, thalidomide and dexamethasone (LD-VTD): An effective regimen for relapsed and refractory multiple myeloma patients. *Leukemia and Lymphoma, 47,* 171–173.

Concannon, C. G., Koehler, B. F., Reimertz, C., Murphy, B. M., Bonner, C., Thurow, N., et al. (2007). Apoptosis induced by proteasome inhibition in cancer cells: Predominant role of the p53/PUMA pathway. *Oncogene, 26,* 1681–1692.

Cusack, J. C. Jr., Liu, R., Houston, M., Abendroth, K., Elliott, P. J., Adams, J., et al. (2001). Enhanced chemosensitivity to CPT-11 with proteasome inhibitor PS-341: Implications for systemic nuclear factor-kappaB inhibition. *Cancer Research, 61,* 3535–3540.

Cusack, J. C., Liu, R., Xia, L., Chao, T. H., Pien, C., Niu, W., et al. (2006). NPI-0052 enhances tumoricidal response to conventional cancer therapy in a colon carcinoma model. *Clinical Cancer Research, 12,* 6758–6764.

Daniel, K. G., Kuhn, D. J., Kazi, A., & Dou, Q. P. (2005). Anti-angiogenic and anti-tumor properties of proteasome inhibitors. *Current Cancer Drug Targets, 5,* 529–541.

Davies, A. M., Chansky, K., Lara, P. N. Jr, Gumerlock, P. H., Crowley, J., Albain, K. S., et al.; and Southwest Oncology Group. (2009). Bortezomib plus gemcitabine/carboplatin as first-line treatment of advanced non-small cell lung cancer: A phase II Southwest Oncology Group Study (S0339). *Journal of Thoracic Oncology, 4,* 87–92.

Davis, N. B., Taber, D. A., Ansari, R. H., Ryan, C. W., George, C., Vokes, E. E., et al. (2004). Phase II trial of PS-341 in patients with renal cell cancer: A University of Chicago phase II consortium study. *Journal of Clinical Oncology, 22,* 115–119.

Deleu, S., Lemaire, M., Arts, J., Menu, E., Van Valckenborgh, E., Vande Broek, I., et al. (2009). Bortezomib alone or in combination with the histone deacetylase inhibitor JNJ-26481585: Effect on myeloma bone disease in the 5T2MM murine model of myeloma. *Cancer Research, 69,* 5307–5311.

Delic, J., Masdehors, P., Omura, S., Cosset, J. M., Dumont, J., Binet, J. L., et al. (1998). The proteasome inhibitor lactacystin induces apoptosis and sensitizes chemo- and radioresistant human chronic lymphocytic leukemia lymphocytes to TNF-alpha-initiated apoptosis. *British Journal of Cancer, 77,* 1103–1107.

Demo, S. A., Kirk, C. J., Aujay, M. A., Buchholz, T. J., Dajee, M., Ho, M. N., et al. (2007). Antitumor activity of PR-171, a novel irreversible inhibitor of the proteasome. *Cancer Research, 67,* 6383–6391.

Dimopoulos, M. A., Anagnostopoulos, A., Kyrtsonis, M. C., Castritis, E., Bitsaktsis, A., & Pangalis, G. A. (2005). Treatment of relapsed or refractory Waldenström's macroglobulinemia with bortezomib. *Haematologica, 90,* 1655–1658.

Dimopoulos, M. A., Spencer, A., Attal, M., Prince, H. M., Harousseau, J. L., Dmoszynska, A., et al. (2007). Lenalidomide plus dexamethasone for relapsed or refractory multiple myeloma. *New England Journal of Medicine, 357,* 2123–2132.

Dispenzieri, A. (2005). Bortezomib for myeloma—much ado about something. *New England Journal of Medicine, 352,* 2546–2548.

Dorsey, B. D., Iqbal, M., Chatterjee, S., Menta, E., Bernardini, R., Bernareggi, A., et al. (2008). Discovery of a potent, selective and orally active proteasome inhibitor for the treatment of cancer. *Journal of Medicinal Chemistry, 51,* 1068–1072.

Drexler, H. C. (1997). Activation of the cell death program by inhibition of proteasome function. *Proceedings of the National Academy of Sciences of the United States of America, 94,* 855–860.

Dudek, A. Z., Lesniewski-Kmak, K., Shehadeh, N. J., Pandey, O. N., Franklin, M., Kratzke, R. A., et al. (2009). Phase I study of bortezomib and cetuximab in patients with solid tumors expressing epidermal growth factor receptor. *British Journal of Cancer, 100,* 1379–1384.

Engel, R. H., Brown, J. A., Von Roenn, J. H., O'Regan, R. M., Bergan, R., Badve, S., et al. (2007). A phase II study of single agent bortezomib in patients with metastatic breast cancer: A single institution experience. *Cancer Investigation, 25,* 733–737.

Fanucchi, M. P., Fossella, F. V., Belt, R., Natale, R., Fidias, P., Carbone, D. P., et al. (2006). Randomized phase II study of bortezomib alone and bortezomib in combination with docetaxel in previously treated advanced non-small-cell lung cancer. *Journal of Clinical Oncology, 24,* 5025–5033.

Feling, R. H., Buchanan, G. O., Mincer, T. J., Kauffman, C. A., Jensen, P. R., & Fenical, W. (2003). Salinosporamide A: A highly cytotoxic proteasome inhibitor from a novel microbial source, a marine bacterium of the new genus *Salinospora*. *Angewandte Chemie (International ed. in English), 42,* 355–357.

Fels, D. R., Ye, J., Segan, A. T., Kridel, S. J., Spiotto, M., Olson, M., et al. (2008). Preferential cytotoxicity of bortezomib toward hypoxic tumor cells via over activation of endoplasmic reticulum stress pathways. *Cancer Research, 68,* 9323–9330.

Fenteany, G., Standaert, R. F., Lane, W. S., Choi, S., Corey, E. J., & Schreiber, S. L. (1995). Inhibition of proteasome activities and subunit-specific amino-terminal threonine modification by lactacystin. *Science, 268,* 725–731.

Fisher, R. I., Bernstein, S. H., Kahl, B. S., Djulbegovic, B., Robertson, M. J., de Vos, S., et al. (2006). Multicenter phase II study of bortezomib in patients with relapsed or refractory mantle cell lymphoma. *Journal of Clinical Oncology, 24,* 4867–4874.

Fribley, A., Zeng, Q., & Wang, C. Y. (2004). Proteasome inhibitor PS-341 induces apoptosis through induction of endoplasmic reticulum stress-reactive oxygen species in head and neck squamous cell carcinoma cells. *Molecular and Cellular Biology, 24,* 9695–9704.

Goy, A., Bernstein, S. H., Kahl, B. S., Djulbegovic, B., Robertson, M. J., de Vos, S., et al. (2009). Bortezomib in patients with relapsed or refractory mantle cell lymphoma: Updated time-to-event analyses of the multicenter phase 2 PINNACLE study. *Annals of Oncology, 20,* 520–525.

Groll, M., Berkers, C. R., Ploegh, H. L., & Ovaa, H. (2006). Crystal structure of the boronic acid-based proteasome inhibitor bortezomib in complex with the yeast 20S proteasome. *Structure, 14,* 451–456.

Groll, M., Ditzel, L., Lowe, J., Stock, D., Bochtler, M., Bartunik, H., et al. (1997). Structure of 20S proteasome from yeast at 2.4 Å resolution. *Nature, 386,* 463–471.

Groll, M., Huber, R., & Potts, B. C. (2006). Crystal structures of salinosporamide A (NPI-0052) and B (NPI-0047) in complex with the 20S proteasome reveal important consequences of β-lactone ring opening and a mechanism for irreversible binding. *Journal of the American Chemical Society, 128,* 5136–5141.

Groll, M., Kim, K. B., Kairies, N., Huber, R., & Crews, C. M. (2000). Crystal structure of epoxomicin: 20S proteasome reveals a molecular basis of α,β-epoxyketone proteasome inhibitors. *Journal of the American Chemical Society, 122,* 1237–1238.

Hainsworth, J. D., Meluch, A. A., Spigel, D. R., Barton, J. Jr, Simons, L., Meng, C., et al. (2007). Weekly docetaxel and bortezomib as first-line treatment for patients with hormone-refractory prostate cancer: A Minnie Pearl Cancer Research Network phase II trial. *Clinical Genitourinary Cancer, 5,* 278–283.

Hanada, M., Sugawara, K., Kaneta, K., Toda, S., Mishiyaa, Y., Tomita, K., et al. (1992). Epoxomicin, a new antitumor agent of microbial origin. *Journal of Antibiotics, 45,* 1746–1752.

Hideshima, T., Richardson, P., Chauhan, D., Palombella, V. J., Elliott, P. J., Adams, J., et al. (2001). The proteasome inhibitor PS-341 inhibits growth, induces apoptosis, and overcomes drug resistance in human multiple myeloma cells. *Cancer Research, 61,* 3071–3076.

Hideshima, T., Chauhan, D., Hayashi, T., Akiyama, M., Mitsiades, N., Mitsiades, C., Podar, K., Munshi, N. C., Richardson, P. G. & Anderson, K. C., (2003). Proteasome inhibitor PS-341 abrogates IL-6 triggered signaling cascades via caspase-dependent downregulation of gp130 in multiple myeloma. *Oncogene, 22,* 8386–8393.

Hoeller, D., & Dikic, I. (2009). Targeting the ubiquitin system in cancer therapy. *Nature, 458,* 438–444.

Hofmeister, C. C., Richardson, P., Zimmerman, T., Spear, M. A., Palladino, M. A., Longenecker, A. M., et al. (2009). Clinical trial of the novel structure proteasome inhibitor NPI-0052 in patients with relapsed and relapsed/refractory multiple myeloma. *Journal of Clinical Oncology, 27,* 15 Supplement, #8505.

Iqbal, M., Chatterjee, S., Kauer, J. C., Mallamo, J. P., Messina, P. A., Reiboldt, A., et al. (1996). Potent α-ketocarbonyl and boronic ester derived inhibitors of proteasome. *Bioorganic & Medicinal Chemistry Letters, 6,* 287–290.

Jagannath, S., Barlogie, B., Berenson, J. R., Siegel, D. S., Irwin, D., Richardson, P. G., et al. (2004). A phase 2 study of two doses of bortezomib in relapsed or refractory myeloma. *British Journal of Haematology, 127,* 165–172.

Jagannath, S., Barlogie, B., Berenson, J. R., Siegel, D. S., Irwin, D., Richardson, P. G., et al. (2008). Updated survival analyses after prolonged follow-up of the phase 2 multicenter CREST study of bortezomib in relapsed or refractory multiple myeloma. *British Journal of Haematology, 143,* 537–540.

Jagannath, S., Vij, R., Stewart, K., Somlo, G., Jakubowiak, A., Trudel, S., et al. (2009). Final results of PX-171-003-A0, part 1 of an open-label, single-arm, phase II study of carfilzomib (CFZ) in patients (pts) with relapsed and refractory multiple myeloma (MM). *Journal of Clinical Oncology, 27,* 15 Supplement, #8504.

Joazeiro, C. A., Anderson, K. C., & Hunter, T. (2006). Proteasome inhibitor drugs on the rise. *Cancer Res., 66,* 7840–7842.

Kane, R. C., Dagher, R., Farrell, A., Ko, C. W., Sridhara, R., Justice, R., et al. (2007). Bortezomib for the treatment of mantle cell lymphoma. *Clinical Cancer Research, 13,* 5291–5294.

Kane, R. C., Farrell, A. T., Sridhara, R., & Pazdur, R. (2006). United States Food and Drug Administration approval summary: Bortezomib for the treatment of progressive multiple myeloma after one prior therapy. *Clinical Cancer Research, 12,* 2955–2960.

Kirk, C. J., Jiang, J., Muchamuel, T., Dajee, M., Swinarski, D., Aujay, M., et al. (2008). The selective proteasome inhibitor Carfilzomib is well-tolerated in experimental animals with dose intensive administration. *Blood (ASH Annual Meeting Abstracts), 112,* #2765.

Kropff, M., Liebisch, P., Knop, S., Weisel, K., Wand, H., Gann, C. N., et al. (2009, March 10). DSMM XI study: Dose definition for intravenous cyclophosphamide in combination with bortezomib/dexamethasone for remission induction in patients with newly diagnosed myeloma. *Annals of Hematology, 88,* 1125–1130.

Kubicek, G. J., Werner-Wasik, M., Machtay, M., Mallon, G., Myers, T., Ramirez, M., et al. (2009). Phase I trial using proteasome inhibitor bortezomib and concurrent temozolomide and radiotherapy for central nervous system malignancies. *International Journal of Radiation Oncology, Biology, Physics, 74,* 433–439.

Kuhn, D. J., Chen, Q., Voorhees, P. M., Strader, J. S., Shenk, K. D., Sun, C. M., et al. (2007). Potent activity of carfilzomib, a novel, irreversible inhibitor of the ubiquitin-proteasome pathway, against pre-clinical models of multiple myeloma. *Blood, 110,* 3281–3290.

Kumar, S., Blade, J., San Miguel, R., Hajek, A., Nagler, P., Sonneveld, A., et al. (2007). Pegylated liposomal doxorubicin (PLD) in combination with bortezomib (B) may provide therapeutic advantage for high-risk multiple myeloma patients relapsing within 12 months of stem cell transplant. *Blood (ASH Annual Meeting Abstracts), 110,* #2730.

Kumar, S., & Rajkumar, S. V. (2008). Many facets of bortezomib resistance and susceptibility. *Blood, 112,* 2177–2178.

Lara, P. N. Jr, Chansky, K., Davies, A. M., Franklin, W. A., Gumerlock, P. H., Guaglianone, P. P., et al. (2006). Bortezomib (PS-341) in relapsed or refractory extensive stage small cell lung cancer: A Southwest Oncology Group phase II trial (S0327). *Journal of Thoracic Oncology, 1,* 996–1001.

LeBlanc, R., Catley, L. P., Hideshima, T., Lentzsch, S., Mitsiades, C. S., Mitsiades, N., et al. (2002). Proteasome inhibitor PS-341 inhibits human multiple myeloma cell growth in vivo and prolongs survival in a murine model. *Cancer Research, 62,* 4996–5000.

Lightcap, E. S., McCormack, T. A., Pien, C. S., Chau, V., Adams, J., & Elliott, P. J. (2000). Proteasome inhibition measurements: Clinical applications. *Clinical Chemistry, 46,* 673–683.

Ling, Y. H., Liebes, L., Jiang, J. D., Holland, J. F., Elliott, P. J., Adams, J., et al. (2003). Mechanisms of proteasome inhibitor PS-341-induced G2-M-phase arrest and apoptosis in human non-small cell lung cancer cell lines. *Clinical Cancer Research, 9,* 1145–1154.

Ludwig, H., Khayat, D., Giaccone, G., & Facon, T. (2005). Proteasome inhibition and its clinical prospects in the treatment of hematologic and solid malignancies. *Cancer, 104,* 1794–1807.

Ma, M. H., Yang, H. H., Parker, K., Manyak, S., Friedman, J. M., Altamirano, C., et al. (2003). The proteasome inhibitor PS-341 markedly enhances sensitivity of multiple myeloma tumor cells to chemotherapeutic agents. *Clinical Cancer Research, 9,* 1136–1144.

Macherla, V. R., Mitchell, S. S., Manam, R. R., Reed, K. A., Chao, T.-H., Nicholson, B., et al. (2005). Structure-activity relationship studies of salinosporamide A (NPI-0052), a novel marine derived proteasome inhibitor. *Journal of Medicinal Chemistry, 48,* 3684–3687.

Mackay, H., Hedley, D., Major, P., Townsley, C., Mackenzie, M., Vincent, M., et al. (2005). A phase II trial with pharmacodynamic endpoints of the proteasome inhibitor bortezomib in patients with metastatic colorectal cancer. *Clinical Cancer Research, 11,* 5526–5533.

Maki, R. G., Kraft, A. S., Scheu, K., Yamada, J., Wadler, S., Antonescu, C. R., et al. (2005). A multicenter phase II study of bortezomib in recurrent or metastatic sarcomas. *Cancer, 103,* 1431–1438.

Marangon, E., Sala, F., Brunelli, D., Sessa, C., O'Dall, E., Cereda, R., et al. (2009). Pharmaco-kinetics and pharmacodynamics of the new proteasome inhibitor CEP-18770. Preliminary results from a phase I study. *Proceedings Annual ASMS Conference,,* Philadelphia, PA, May 31–June 4. #452.

Markovic, S. N., Geyer, S. M., Dawkins, F., Sharfman, W., Albertini, M., Maples, W., et al. (2005). A phase II study of bortezomib in the treatment of metastatic malignant mela-noma. *Cancer, 103,* 2584–2589.

Miller, C. P., Ban, K., Dujka, M. E., McConkey, D. J., Munsell, M., Palladino, M., et al. (2007). NPI-0052, a novel proteasome inhibitor, induces caspase-8 and ROS-dependent apoptosis alone and in combination with HDAC inhibitors in leukemia cells. *Blood, 110,* 267–277.

Mitsiades, N., Mitsiades, C. S., Poulaki, V., Chauhan, D., Fanourakis, G., Gu, X., et al. (2002a). Molecular sequelae of proteasome inhibition in human multiple myeloma cells. *Proceedings of the National Academy of Sciences of the United States of America, 99,* 14374–14379.

Mitsiades, N., Mitsiades, C. S., Poulaki, V., Chauhan, D., Richardson, P. G., Hideshima, T., (2002b). Biological sequelae of NFkB blockade in multiple myeloma: Therapeutic applica-tions. *Blood, 99,* 4079–4086.

Mitsiades, N., Mitsiades, C. S., Richardson, P. G., Poulaki, V., Tai, Y. T., Chauhan, D., et al. (2003). The proteasome inhibitor PS-341 potentiates sensitivity of multiple myeloma cells to conventional chemotherapeutic agents: Therapeutic applications. *Blood, 101,* 2377–2380.

Muchamuel, T., Aujay, M., Bennet, M. K., Dajee, M., Demo, S., Kirk, C. J., et al. (2008). Pre-clinical pharmacology and in vitro characterization of PR-047, an oral inhibitor of the 20S proteasome. *Blood (ASH Annual Meeting Abstracts), 112,* #3671.

Nawrocki, S. T., Bruns, C. J., Harbison, M. T., Bold, R. J., Gotsch, B. S., Abbruzzese, J. L., et al. (2002). Effects of the proteasome inhibitor PS-341 on apoptosis and angiogenesis in orthotopic human pancreatic tumor xenografts. *Molecular Cancer Research, 1,* 1243–1253.

Nawrocki, S. T., Carew, J. S., Pino, M. S., Highshaw, R. A., Dunner, K. Jr, Huang, P., et al. (2005). Bortezomib sensitizes pancreatic cancer cells to endoplasmic reticulum stress-mediated apoptosis. *Cancer Research, 65,* 11658–11666.

O'Connor, O. A., Moskowitz, C., Portlock, C., Hamlin, P., Straus, D., Dumitrescu, O., et al. (2009). Patients with chemotherapy-refractory mantle cell lymphoma experience high response rates and identical progression-free survivals compared with patients with relapsed disease following treatment with single agent bortezomib: Results of a multicentre Phase 2 clinical trial. *British Journal of Haematology, 145,* 34–39.

Oerlemans, R., Franke, N. E., Assaraf, Y. G., Cloos, J., van Zantwijk, I., Berkers, C. R., et al. (2008). Molecular basis of bortezomib resistance: Proteasome subunit β5 (*PSMB5*) gene mutation and over expression of PSMB5 protein. *Blood, 112,* 2489–2499.

Omura, S., Matsuzaki, K., Fujimoto, T., Kosuge, K., Furuya, T., Fujita, S., et al. (1991). Structure of lactacystin, a new microbial metabolite which induces differentiation of neuroblastoma cells. *Journal of Antibiotics, 44,* 117–118.

Orlowski, R. Z., & Kuhn, D. J. (2008). Proteasome inhibitors in cancer therapy: Lessons from the first decade. *Clinical Cancer Research, 14,* 1649–1657.

Orlowski, R. Z., Nagler, A., Sonneveld, P., Bladé, J., Hajek, R., Spencer, A., et al. (2007). Randomized phase III study of pegylated liposomal doxorubicin plus bortezomib compared with bortezomib alone in relapsed or refractory multiple myeloma: Combination therapy improves time to progression. *Journal of Clinical Oncology, 25,* 3892–3901.

Orlowski, R. Z., Stinchcombe, T. E., Mitchell, B. S., Shea, T. C., Baldwin, A. S., Stahl, S., et al. (2002). Phase I trial of the proteasome inhibitor PS-341 in patients with refractory hematologic malignancies. *Journal of Clinical Oncology, 20,* 4420–4427.

Orlowski, R. Z., Voorhees, P. M., Garcia, R. A., Hall, M. D., Kudrik, F. J., Allred, T., et al. (2005). Phase 1 trial of the proteasome inhibitor bortezomib and pegylated liposomal doxorubicin in patients with advanced hematologic malignancies. *Blood, 105,* 3058–3065.

Peese, K. (2009). Orally bioavailable proteasome inhibitors: Preclinical development of PR-047, *Drug Discovery Today,* doi:10.1016/j.drudis.2009.06.005.

Pei, X. Y., Dai, Y., & Grant, S. (2004). Synergistic induction of oxidative injury and apoptosis in human multiple myeloma cells by the proteasome inhibitor bortezomib and histone deacetylase inhibitors. *Clinical Cancer Research, 10,* 3839–3852.

Pineda-Roman, M., Zangari, M., van Rhee, F., Anaissie, E., Szymonifka, J., Hoering, A., et al. (2008). VTD combination therapy with bortezomib-thalidomide-dexamethasone is highly effective in advanced and refractory multiple myeloma. *Leukemia, 22,* 1419–1427.

Piva, R., Ruggeri, B., Willliams, M., Costa, G., Tamagno, I., Ferrero, D., et al. (2008). CEP-18770: A novel orally-active proteasome inhibitor with a tumor-selective pharmacological profile competitive with bortezomib. *Blood, 111,* 2765–2775.

Podar, K., Raab, M. S., Zhang, J., McMillin, D., Breitkreutz, I., Tai, Y. T., et al. (2007). Targeting PKC in multiple myeloma: In vitro and in vivo effects of the novel, orally available small-molecule inhibitor enzastaurin (LY317615.HCl). *Blood, 109,* 1669–1677.

Rajkumar, S. V., Richardson, P. G., Hideshima, T., & Anderson, K. C. (2005). Proteasome inhibition as a novel therapeutic target in human cancer. *Journal of Clinical Oncology, 23,* 630–639.

Ramirez, P. T., Landen, C. N. Jr, Coleman, R. L., Milam, M. R., Levenback, C., Johnston, T. A., et al. (2008). Phase I trial of the proteasome inhibitor bortezomib in combination with carboplatin in patients with platinum- and taxane-resistant ovarian cancer. *Gynecologic Oncology, 108,* 68–71.

Reece, D. E., Rodriguez, G. P., Chen, C., Trudel, S., Kukreti, V., Mikhael, J., et al. (2008). Phase I-II trial of bortezomib plus oral cyclophosphamide and prednisone in relapsed and refractory multiple myeloma. *Journal of Clinical Oncology, 26,* 4777–4783.

Reeder, C. B., Reece, D. E., Kukreti, V., Chen, C., Trudel, S., Hentz, J., et al. (2009). Cyclophosphamide, bortezomib and dexamethasone induction for newly diagnosed multiple myeloma: High response rates in a phase II clinical trial. *Leukemia, 23,* 1337–1341.

Richardson, P. G., Barlogie, B., Berenson, J., Singhal, S., Jagannath, S., Irwin, D., et al. (2003). A phase 2 study of bortezomib in relapsed refractory myeloma. *New England Journal of Medicine, 348,* 2609–2617.

Richardson, P. G., Barlogie, B., Berenson, J., Singhal, S., Jagannath, S., Irwin, D. H., et al. (2006). Extended follow-up of a phase II trial in relapsed refractory multiple myeloma: Final time-to-event results from the SUMMIT trial. *Cancer, 106,* 1316–1319.

Richardson, P. G., Jagannath, S., Jakubowiak, A., Lonial, S., Raje, N., Alsina, M., et al. (2008). Lenalidomide, bortezomib, and dexamethasone in patients with relapsed or relapsed/

refractory multiple myeloma (MM): Encouraging response rates and tolerability with correlation of outcome and adverse cytogenetics in a phase II study. *Blood (ASH Annual Meeting Abstracts), 112, #1742.*

Richardson, P. G., Lonial, S., Jakubowiak, A., Jagannath, S., Raje, N. S., Avigan, D., et al. (2008). Lenalidomide, bortezomib, and dexamethasone in patients with newly diagnosed multiple myeloma: Encouraging efficacy in high risk groups with updated results of a phase I/II study. *Blood (ASH Annual Meeting Abstracts), 112, #92.*

Richardson, P. G., Mitsiades, C., Hideshima, T., & Anderson, K. C. (2006). Bortezomib: Proteasome inhibition as an effective anticancer therapy. *Annual Review of Medicine, 57,* 33–47.

Richardson, P. G., Sonneveld, P., Schuster, M. W., Irwin, D., Stadtmauer, E. A., Facon, T., et al. (2005). Bortezomib or high-dose dexamethasone for relapsed multiple myeloma. *New England Journal of Medicine, 352,* 2487–2498.

Richardson, P. G., Sonneveld, P., Schuster, M., Irwin, D., Stadtmauer, E. A., Facon, T., et al. (2007). Extended follow-up of a phase 3 trial in relapsed multiple myeloma: Final time-to-event results of the APEX trial. *Blood, 110,* 3557–3560.

Richardson, P. G., Xie, W., Mitsiades, C., Chanan-Khan, A. A., Lonial, S., Hassoun, H., et al. (2009). Single-agent bortezomib in previously untreated multiple myeloma: Efficacy, characterization of peripheral neuropathy, and molecular correlations with response and neuropathy. *Journal of Clinical Oncology, 27,* 3518–3525.

Ron, D., & Walters, P. (2007). Signal integration in the endoplasmic reticulum unfolded protein response. *Nature Reviews. Molecular Cell Biology, 8,* 519–529.

Rosenberg, J. E., Halabi, S., Sanford, B. L., Himelstein, A. L., Atkins, J. N., Hohl, R. J., et al.; and Cancer and Leukemia Group B. (2008). Phase II study of bortezomib in patients with previously treated advanced urothelial tract transitional cell carcinoma: CALGB 90207. *Annals of Oncology, 19,* 946–950.

Ruiz, S., Krupnik, Y., Keating, M., Chandra, J., Palladino, M., & McConkey, D. (2006). The proteasome inhibitor NPI-0052 is a more effective inducer of apoptosis than bortezomib in lymphocytes from patients with chronic lymphocytic leukemia. *Molecular Cancer Therapeutics, 5,* 1836–1843.

Russo, S. M., Tepper, J. E., Baldwin, A. S. Jr, Liu, R., Adams, J., Elliott, P., et al. (2001). Enhancement of radiosensitivity by proteasome inhibition: Implications for a role of NF-kappaB. *International Journal of Radiation Oncology, Biology, Physics, 50,* 183–193.

Ryan, D. P., O'Neil, B. H., Supko, J. G., Rocha Lima, C. M., Dees, E. C., Appleman, L. J., et al. (2006). A Phase I study of bortezomib plus irinotecan in patients with advanced solid tumors. *Cancer, 107,* 2688–2697.

Saito, S., Furuno, A., Sakurai, J., Sakamoto, A., Park, H.-R., Shin-ya, K., et al. (2009). Chemical genomics identifies the unfolded protein response as a target for selective cancer cell killing during glucose deprivation. *Cancer Research, 69,* 4225–4234.

Sanchez, E., Campell, R. A., Steinberg, J. A., Li, M., Chen, H., Bonavida, B., et al. (2008). The novel proteasome inhibitor CEP-18770 inhibits myeloma tumor growth in vitro and in vivo and enhances the anti-MM effects of melphalan. *Blood (ASH Annual Meeting Abstracts), 112, #843.*

San Miguel, J. F., Schlag, R., Khuageva, N. K., Dimopoulos, M. A., Shpilberg, O., Kropff, M., et al. (2008). Bortezomib plus melphalan and prednisone for initial treatment of multiple myeloma. *New England Journal of Medicine, 359,* 906–917.

Schmid, P., Kühnhardt, D., Kiewe, P., Lehnbauer-Dehm, S., Schippinger, W., Greil, R., et al. (2008). A phase I/II study of bortezomib and capecitabine in patients with metastatic breast cancer previously treated with taxanes and/or anthracyclines. *Annals of Oncology, 19,* 871–876.

Shah, M. H., Young, D., Kindler, H. L., Webb, I., Kleiber, B., Wright, J., et al. (2004). Phase II study of the proteasome inhibitor bortezomib (PS-341) in patients with metastatic neuroendocrine tumors. *Clinical Cancer Research, 10,* 6111–6118.

Sin, N., Kim, K. B., Elofsson, M., Meng, L., Auth, H., Kwok, B. H. B., et al. (1999). Total synthesis of the potent proteasome inhibitor epoxomicin: A useful tool for understanding proteasome biology. *Bioorganic & Medicinal Chemistry Letters, 9,* 2283–2288.

Singhal, S., Mehta, J., Desikan, R., Ayers, D., Roberson, P., Eddlemon, P., et al. (1999). Antitumor activity of thalidomide in refractory multiple myeloma. *New England Journal of Medicine, 341,* 1565–1571.

Sonneveld, P., Hajek, R., Nagler, A., Spencer, A., Bladé, J., Robak, T., et al. (2008). Combined pegylated liposomal doxorubicin and bortezomib is highly effective in patients with recurrent or refractory multiple myeloma who received prior thalidomide/lenalidomide therapy. *Cancer, 112,* 1529–1537.

Stapnes, C., Døskeland, A. P., Hatfield, K., Ersvær, E., Ryningen, A., Lorens, J. B., et al. (2007). The proteasome inhibitors bortezomib and PR-171 have antiproliferative and proapoptotic effects on primary human acute myeloid leukaemia cells. *British Journal of Haematology, 136,* 814–828.

Sterz, J., von Metzler, I., Hahne, J. C., Lamottke, B., Rademacher, J., Heider, U., et al. (2008). The potential of proteasome inhibitors in cancer therapy. *Expert Opinion on Investigational Drugs, 17,* 879–895.

Sunwoo, J. B., Chen, Z., Dong, G., Yeh, N., Bancroft, C. C., Suasville, E., et al. (2001). Novel proteasome inhibitor PS-341 inhibits activation of nuclear factor-κB, cell survival, tumor growth and angiogenesis in squamous cell carcinoma. *Clinical Cancer Research, 7,* 1419–1428.

Szokalska, A., Makowski, M., Nowis, D., Wilczynski, G. M., Kujawa, M., Wójcik, C., et al. (2009). Proteasome inhibition potentiates antitumor effects of photodynamic therapy in mice through induction of endoplasmic reticulum stress and unfolded protein response. *Cancer Research, 69,* 4235–4243.

Teicher, B. A., Ara, G., Herbst, R., Palombella, V. J., & Adams, J. (1999). The proteasome inhibitor PS-341 in cancer therapy. *Clinical Cancer Research, 5,* 2638–2645.

Terpos, E., Sezer, O., Croucher, P., & Dimopoulos, M. A. (2007). Myeloma bone disease and proteasome inhibition therapies. *Blood, 110,* 1098–1104.

Treon, S. P., Hunter, Z. R., Matous, J., Joyce, R. M., Mannion, B., Advani, R., et al. (2007). Multicenter clinical trial of bortezomib in relapsed/refractory Waldenstrom's macroglobulinemia: Results of WMCTG trial 03-248. *Clinical Cancer Research, 13,* 3320–3325.

Treon, S. P., Ioakimidis, L., Soumerai, J. D., Patterson, C. J., Sheehy, P., Nelson, M., et al. (2009). Primary therapy of Waldenström macroglobulinemia with bortezomib, dexamethasone, and rituximab: WMCTG clinical trial 05-180. *Journal of Clinical Oncology,,* doi:10.1200/JCO.2008.20.4677.

Vij, R., Wang, M., Orlowski, R., Stewart, A. K., Jagannath, S., Kukreti, V., et al. (2009). PX-171-004, a multicenter phase II study of carfilzomib (CFZ) in patients with relapsed myeloma: An efficacy update. *Journal of Clinical Oncology, 27(15 Supplement),* #8537.

Vinitsky, A., Michaud, C., Powers, J. C., & Orlowski, M. (1992). Inhibition of the chymotrypsin-like activity of the pituitary multi-catalytic proteinase complex. *Biochemistry, 31,* 9421–9428.

von Lilienfeld-Toal, M., Hahn-Ast, C., Furkert, K., Hoffmann, F., Naumann, R., Bargou, R., et al. (2008). A systematic review of phase II trials of thalidomide/dexamethasone combination therapy in patients with relapsed or refractory multiple myeloma. *European Journal of Haematology, 81,* 247–252.

von Metzler, I., Krebbel, H., Hecht, M., Manz, R. A., Fleissner, C., Mieth, M., et al. (2007). Bortezomib inhibits human osteoclastogenesis. *Leukemia, 21,* 2025–2034.

Voortman, J., Smit, E. F., Honeywell, R., Kuenen, B. C., Peters, G. J., van de Velde, H., et al. (2007). A parallel dose-escalation study of weekly and twice-weekly bortezomib in combination with gemcitabine and cisplatin in the first-line treatment of patients with advanced solid tumors. *Clinical Cancer Research, 13,* 3642–3651.

Wang, C. Y., Mayo, M. W., & Baldwin, A. S. Jr, (1996).TNF- and cancer therapy-induced apoptosis: Potentiation by inhibition of NF-kappaB. *Science, 274,* 784–87.

Weber, D. M., Chen, C., Niesvizky, R., Wang, M., Belch, A., Stadtmauer, E. A., et al. (2007). Lenalidomide plus dexamethasone for relapsed multiple myeloma in North America. *New England Journal of Medicine, 357,* 2133–2142.

Williams, S., Pettaway, C., Song, R., Papandreou, C., Logothetis, C., & McConkey, D. J. (2003). Differential effects of the proteasome inhibitor bortezomib on apoptosis and angiogenesis in human prostate tumor xenografts. *Molecular Cancer Therapeutics, 2,* 835–843.

Williams, S. A., & McConkey, D. J. (2003). The proteasome inhibitor bortezomib stabilizes a novel active form of p53 in human LNCaP-Pro5 prostate cancer cells. *Cancer Research, 63,* 7338–7344.

Williamson, M. J., Blank, J. L., Bruzzese, F. J., Cao, Y., Daniels, J. S., Dick, L. R., et al. (2006). Comparison of biochemical and biological effects of ML858 (salinosporamide A) and bortezomib. *Molecular Cancer Therapeutics, 5,* 3052–3061.

Wolf, J., Richardson, P. G., Schuster, M., LeBlanc, A., Walters, I. B., & Battleman, D. S. (2008). Utility of bortezomib retreatment in relapsed or refractory multiple myeloma patients: A multicenter case series. *Clinical Advances in Hematology & Oncology, 6,* 755–760.

Yang, C. H., Gonzalez-Angulo, A. M., Reuben, J. M., Booser, D. J., Pusztai, L., Krishnamurthy, S., et al. (2006). Bortezomib (VELCADE) in metastatic breast cancer: Pharmacodynamics, biological effects, and prediction of clinical benefits. *Annals of Oncology, 17,* 813–817.

Yang, H., Zonder, J. A., & Dou, Q. P. (2009). Clinical development of novel proteasome inhibitors for cancer treatment. *Expert Opinion on Investigational Drugs, 18,* 957–971.

Zhou, H. J., Aujay, M. A., Bennett, M. K., Dajee, M., Demo, S. D., Fang, Y., et al. (2009). Design and synthesis of an orally bioavailable and selective epoxyketone proteasome inhibitor (PR-047). *Journal of Medicinal Chemistry, 52,* 3028–3038.

John R. Atack

Department of Neuroscience, Johnson & Johnson Pharmaceutical Research and
Development, Turnhoutseweg 30, Beerse, B-2340, Belgium

Subtype-Selective GABA$_A$ Receptor Modulation Yields a Novel Pharmacological Profile: The Design and Development of TPA023

Abstract

TPA023 is a GABA$_A$ $\alpha2/\alpha3$ subtype-selective modulator which in pre-clinical species has anxiolytic-like activity but does not produce sedative-like properties and is without abuse potential. It has good oral bioavailability in rat and dog but not in rhesus monkey (respective oral bioavailability values

Advances in Pharmacology, Volume 57
© 2009 Elsevier Inc. All rights reserved.

1054-3589/08 $35.00
10.1016/S1054-3589(08)57004-9

of 36, 54, and 1%), and in all the three species the half-life after i.v. administration was relatively short (0.6–1.5 h). The plasma concentrations of TPA023 required to produce 50% receptor occupancy were 21–25, 19, and 9 ng/mL in rats, baboons, and humans, respectively. In man, TPA023 has a half-life of around 3–6 h when administered as an immediate release formulation, but exposure was more prolonged when it was formulated into a controlled release, gel extrusion module (GEM) tablet. *In vivo* metabolism was via *t*-butyl hydroxylation and N-deethylation. A drug-drug interaction study with itraconazole confirmed *in vitro* metabolic results implicating CYP3A enzymes as the major contributors to *in vivo* oxidative metabolism. The maximum tolerated doses in healthy, normal volunteers were 2 and 8 mg for the immediate-release and GEM formulations, respectively. A post hoc analysis of three separate Phase IIa studies, all of which were halted prematurely, showed that TPA023 reduced scores on the Hamilton Anxiety Scale to a significantly greater extent than placebo. In addition, TPA023 has recently been reported to produce a trend toward improved cognitive performance in a small group of schizophrenia patients. Collectively, these data demonstrate that the $\alpha2/\alpha3$-selective partial agonist efficacy of TPA023 translates into a novel pharmacological profile.

I. Introduction

Chlordiazepoxide (Librium®) and diazepam (Valium®) were introduced into clinical practice by Roche in the early 1960s (Sternbach, 1979) and heralded the introduction of a large number of other structurally related 1,4-benzodiazepines, including high-potency (high-affinity) benzodiazepines such as lorazepam, clonazepam, and alprazolam (Moroz, 2004). These benzodiazepines possess anxiolytic and hypnotic properties and are far safer than the barbiturates that they superseded (Ator, 2005). Although the benzodiazepines have anticonvulsant activity, the development of tolerance limits their clinical utility as antiepileptic drugs to the emergency room rather than as prophylactics (Haigh & Feely, 1988). In addition, benzodiazepines also produce myorelaxation and impair cognition, making them suitable, for example, as aids in performing endoscopic procedures and as premedications for general anesthesia (Bell, 2002).

In the mid-1970s, benzodiazepines went from being perceived as being safe and effective to being considered dangerous and addictive based on accounts of physical and psychological dependence (Lader, Tylee, & Donoghue, 2009). Nevertheless, benzodiazepines are still frequently prescribed, a practice that has been described as being analogous to watching pornography (Gorman, 2005) in so far as "If you ask a person at random if he watches pornography, he will vehemently deny it, but someone must because it is a billion dollar a year business. Similarly, if you ask a physician if they prescribe [benzodiazepines] he or she will say of course not ... Yet, like pornography, benzodiazepine prescriptions generate billions of dollars a year of revenue around the world, so somebody must be prescribing them." The continued use of benzodiazepines is presumably because they remain the drugs of choice as anxiolytics and hypnotics, given their overall efficacy and safety profiles.

For over 20 years the search has been underway for compounds that act via the benzodiazepine binding site of GABA$_A$ receptors and are anxioselective (i.e., anxiolytic but with a much reduced sedative liability). To date, no such agent has been approved for human use (Atack, 2003). The recognition that benzodiazepines interact with different subtypes of GABA$_A$ receptors, coupled to recent evidence that particular GABA$_A$ receptor subtypes are associated with specific aspects of the pharmacological actions of benzodiazepines (Rudolph & Mohler, 2006; Vicini & Ortinski, 2004), has stimulated renewed interest in this area. In this report, the rationale behind developing anxioselective compounds that target specifically the α2- and α3-subunit-containing GABA$_A$ receptors subtypes is reviewed. In addition, preclinical and clinical data for TPA023 (Atack, Wafford, et al., 2006; de Haas et al., 2007), also known as L-830982 (or L-000830982) and MK-0777 (Lewis et al., 2008), are summarized in this chapter.

A. GABA$_A$ Receptor Subtypes

GABA$_A$ receptors are comprised of five subunits derived from an extensive family of proteins including the α1-6, β1-3, γ1-3, δ, ε, θ, π subunits plus the structurally related, but pharmacologically distinct, ρ1-3 subunits that form the so-called GABA$_C$ receptors (Barnard et al., 1998; Olsen & Sieghart, 2008; Simon et al., 2004). The expression of these different proteins within the brain is heterogeneous (Fritschy & Möhler, 1995; Pirker, Schwarzer, Wieselthaler, Sieghart, & Sperk, 2000; Sperk, Schwarzer, Tsunashima, Fuchs, & Sieghart, 1997; Wisden et al., 1992), suggesting that different populations of GABA$_A$ receptors perform distinct functions within the central nervous system. As a corollary, drugs that selectively modulate the activity of particular GABA$_A$ receptor subtypes might possess novel pharmacological profiles (Olsen & Sieghart, 2009).

The majority of brain GABA$_A$ receptors are comprised of α, β, and γ subunits in a stoichiometry of 2:2:1 arranged in a αβαβγ sequence (Sieghart, 1995, 2006). The GABA binding site is at the interface of α and β subunits whereas the benzodiazepine site is found at the interface of α and γ2 subunits (Sarto-Jackson & Sieghart, 2008; Sieghart & Sperk, 2002). However, not all α and γ2 subunit combinations possess a benzodiazepine recognition site. Hence, although GABA$_A$ receptors containing β, γ2 plus either α1, α2, α3, or α5 subunits possess a binding site for classical benzodiazepines, such as diazepam, flunitrazepam, and lorazepam, analogous receptors containing α4 or α6 subunits do not. Accordingly, α1-, α2-, α3-, and α5-containing and α4- and α6-containing GABA$_A$ receptors correspond to the diazepam-sensitive and diazepam-insensitive receptor populations identified in native tissue using the imidazobenzodiazepine radioligand [^{3}H]Ro 15-4513 (Wong & Skolnick, 1992). Moreover, the lack of benzodiazepine sensitivity of α4- and α6-containing GABA$_A$ sites can be solely attributed to an arginine residue which replaces the histidine found in α1, α2, α3, and α5 subunits (Table I; Wieland, Lüddens, & Seeburg, 1992).

The lack of binding of classical benzodiazepines to α4- and α6-containing GABA$_A$ receptors highlights the importance of the α subunit in determining the pharmacology of the benzodiazepine binding site and has been exploited to produce transgenic mice that possess GABA$_A$ subunit populations that are insensitive to diazepam (Benson, Löw, Keist, Mohler, & Rudolph, 1998; Rudolph & Möhler, 2004, 2006). Thus, by systematically introducing α1H101R (Table I), α2H101R, α3H126R, or α5H105R mutations, mice are produced in which α1, α2, α3, or α5 GABA$_A$ receptor populations are rendered insensitive to classical benzodiazepines, such as diazepam. Accordingly, differences in the pharmacological phenotype produced by diazepam (or other benzodiazepine binding site ligands) in wild-type and point-mutated (knock-in) mice can be attributed to the specifically targeted subtype (Table II). Moreover, this approach can be extended to produce mice with more than one diazepam-insensitive, point-mutated GABA$_A$ receptor population, such as α1H101R/α2H101R animals (Knabl, Zeilhofer, Crestani, Rudolph, & Zeilhofer, 2009). These are loss-of-function studies in that they presume that the differences in diazepam-mediated behavior between wild-type mice and knock-in mice are due to the relevant subtype. In the future, it may be possible to cross single and double point-mutated mice (Knabl et al., 2009) to generate animals with a triple mutation (e.g., α1H101R/α2H101R/α3H126R mice) in which behaviors can be compared within the same animals before and after treatment with diazepam, thereby more directly defining the pharmacology of these different subtypes.

The information obtained with point-mutated, diazepam-insensitive mice, from mice in which specific α subunits have been deleted (knock-out mice) and from pharmacological studies with subtype-selective compounds, has been used to delineate which of the different α subunit-containing GABA$_A$ receptor populations are associated with specific aspects of benzodiazepine pharmacology. For example, α1-containing GABA$_A$ receptors are associated with sedation (McKernan et al., 2000; Mirza et al., 2008; Rowlett, Platt, Lelas, Atack, & Dawson, 2005; Rudolph et al., 1999), while spinal α2/α3 receptors are associated with analgesia (Knabl et al., 2008, 2009; Munro et al., 2008) and those containing an α5 subunit are related to aspects of cognition (Atack, Bayley, et al., 2006; Ballard et al., 2009;

TABLE I Comparison of the Mouse Sequences of GABA$_A$ Receptor α Subunits and Point-Mutated, Diazepam-Insensitive α1 Subunit[a]

Subunit	Residue	Sequence	Residue	Diazepam binding
α1	86	NNLMASKIWTPDTFFHNGKKSVAHNMTMPNK	116	✓
α2	86	NNLMASKIWTPDTFFHNGKKSVAHNMTMPNK	116	✓
α3	111	NNLLASKIWTPDTFFHNGKKSMAHNMTTPNK	141	✓
α4	84	NNMMVTKVWTPDTFFRNGKKSVSHNMTAPNK	114	✗
α5	90	NNLLASKIWTPDTFFHNGKKSIAHNMTTPNK	120	✓
α6	85	NLMNVSKIWTPDTFFRNGKKSIAHNMTTPNK	115	✗
α1H101R	86	NNLMASKIWTPDTFFRNGKKSVAHNMTMPNK	116	✗

[a] Modified from Benson et al. (1998).

TABLE II   Simplified Overview to Illustrate the Principle Behind the Use of Point-Mutated Mice to Define Which GABA$_A$ Subtypes Are Associated with Specific Pharmacological Features of Diazepam[a]

Mouse	Diazepam-induced behaviors	Conclusions
Wild type	A + B + C + D	Normal profile
α1H101R	B + C + D	α1 receptors mediate behavior A
α2H101R	A + C + D	α2 receptors mediate behavior B
α3H126R	A + B + D	α3 receptors mediate behavior C
α5H105R	A + B + C	α5 receptors mediate behavior D

[a] It should be noted that although this table indicates which particular behaviors, hypothetically designated A, B, C, and D, may be solely attributed to a single GABA$_A$ subtype, in reality the situation is more complicated. For example, although sedation may be primarily associated with the α1 subtype, it is conceivable that sedation-like effects may be mediated via other subtypes if occupancy at those other subtypes is sufficient (e.g., Savić et al., 2008). Nevertheless, these data form the conceptual framework for the development of subtype-selective compounds.

Chambers et al., 2003; Cheng et al., 2006; Collinson et al., 2002; Crestani et al., 2002; Dawson et al., 2006; Harris et al., 2008). However, the specific GABA$_A$ subtype(s) associated with the anxiolytic properties of benzodiazepines is/are less clear. Hence, studies with knock-in and knock-out mice suggest that the α2 rather than the α3 subtype is responsible for the anxiolysis produced by diazepam (Löw et al., 2000; Yee et al., 2005), whereas pharmacological evidence using either an α3-selective inverse agonist (α3IA; Atack et al., 2005) or an α3-selective agonist (TP003; Dias et al., 2005) implicates the α3 subtype. Nevertheless, with the notable exceptions of TP003 and α3IA, the affinity and efficacy of compounds acting at the α2 and α3 subtypes generally track each other with most having a similar affinity for, and intrinsic efficacy at, α2- and α3-containing GABA$_A$ receptors (Atack, 2009).

B. Concept of Selective Efficacy Versus Selective Affinity

Based on the hypothesis that selective modulation of α2- and/or α3-relative to α1-containing GABA$_A$ receptors should result in a compound that retains anxiolytic efficacy yet has a much reduced sedation liability, Merck Sharp and Dohme (the UK division of Merck & Co., Inc.) commenced a program to identify and optimize such compounds. The initial approach was to search for compounds with subtype-selective affinity. However, when that proved unsuccessful, the strategy changed to identifying compounds with selective efficacy (Atack, 2009). Described below are the concepts and relative merits of the selective affinity versus selective efficacy approaches (Atack, 2005).

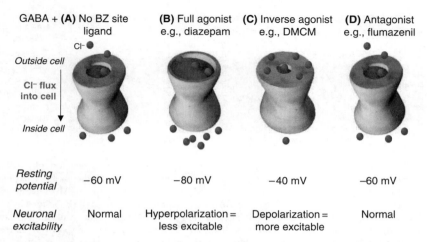

	GABA + **(A)** No BZ site ligand	**(B)** Full agonist e.g., diazepam	**(C)** Inverse agonist e.g., DMCM	**(D)** Antagonist e.g., flumazenil
Resting potential	−60 mV	−80 mV	−40 mV	−60 mV
Neuronal excitability	Normal	Hyperpolarization = less excitable	Depolarization = more excitable	Normal

FIGURE I   Schematic representation of the effects of a benzodiazepine site agonist, inverse agonist, and antagonist on GABA$_A$ receptor function. (A). In the absence of any ligand at the benzodiazepine binding site, GABA binds to the receptor allowing chloride ions to flow into the cell. (B). An agonist at the benzodiazepine binding site enhances the effects of GABA, increasing the chloride flux into the cell resulting in a hyperpolarization of the membrane potential. (C). In contrast to an agonist, an inverse agonist at the benzodiazepine site reduces rather than increases the GABA-mediated chloride flux, causing a partial depolarization of the membrane potential, which consequently increases neuronal excitability. (D). A benzodiazepine site antagonist, such as flumazenil (Ro 15-1788), has no effect on GABA receptor function and therefore does not affect the membrane potential. Although for simplicity, benzodiazepine site agonists and inverse agonists are shown as increasing the pore size, this is incorrect since these compounds actually increase and decrease, respectively, the probability of GABA-induced channel open events, effectively increasing and decreasing the apparent affinity of the GABA$_A$ receptor for GABA.

The binding of compounds at the benzodiazepine recognition site can allosterically modulate the binding of GABA such that a compound with agonist efficacy at this site enhances the effects of GABA by increasing the channel opening frequency, but not the single-channel conductance or channel opening duration, thereby increasing chloride flux and causing hyperpolarization of the membrane resting potential (Fig. 1). In contrast, an inverse agonist does the opposite, decreasing GABA-induced chloride flux thereby producing a partial depolarization of the membrane potential. On the other hand, an antagonist may bind with very high affinity to this recognition site but it has no effect on GABA-mediated chloride flux (Fig. 1). For example, the prototypic benzodiazepine site antagonist flumazenil (Ro 15-1788; Hunkeler et al., 1981) binds with very high affinity (~1 nM) to α1-, α2-, α3-, and α5-containing GABA$_A$ receptors yet has minimal *in vivo* effects (Bonetti et al., 1982). This inactivity of a benzodiazepine site antagonist is in marked contrast to GABA recognition site antagonists, such as bicuculline, which

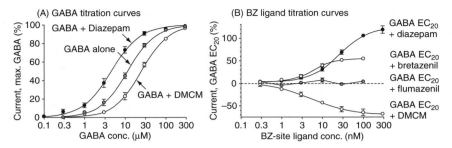

FIGURE 2 (A). Electrophysiological measurement of current as a function of GABA concentration in the absence and presence of a fixed concentration of either benzodiazepine site agonist (diazepam) or inverse agonist (DMCM) in recombinant human GABA$_A$ receptors containing α3, β3, and γ2 subunits. The GABA concentration–effect curve (EC$_{50}$ for GABA alone = 11 μM) is leftward-shifted by an agonist (EC$_{50}$ = 4.5 μM) and rightward-shifted by an inverse agonist (EC$_{50}$ = 25 μM), corresponding to an increase or decrease, respectively, in the apparent GABA affinity. (B). Electrophysiological measurement of current as a function of benzodiazepine site ligand concentration using either a full agonist (diazepam), partial agonist (bretazenil), full inverse agonist (DMCM), or antagonist (flumazenil, Ro 15-1788) in the presence of a fixed, EC$_{20}$-equivalent concentration of GABA.

block the inhibitory effects of GABA and are therefore convulsant. It should be noted that the designation of compounds acting at the benzodiazepine site as agonists, inverse agonists, or antagonists is historical, with such compounds being more correctly described as positive-, negative-, or neutral allosteric modulators, respectively. Nevertheless, for the sake of convenience, the older nomenclature will be used throughout the chapter.

The efficacy of benzodiazepine site ligands is measured electrophysiologically in terms of their modulatory effects on GABA-induced currents (Fig. 2A). Thus, in the presence of a benzodiazepine site agonist, such as diazepam, there is a leftward shift in the GABA concentration–effect curve such that for any given submaximal concentration of GABA, the GABA-induced current is increased (Fig. 2A). The extent of the increase in the GABA-induced current varies as a function of the GABA concentration with, for example, a greater modulation being observed when using an EC$_{20}$ compared to an EC$_{80}$. On the other hand, an inverse agonist does the opposite, causing a rightward shift in the GABA concentration–effect curve (Fig. 2A). While this results in benzodiazepine site agonists increasing and inverse agonist decreasing the apparent affinity of the GABA$_A$ receptor for GABA, mechanistically an agonist increases and inverse agonist decreases the probability of a channel opening event once GABA binds. Importantly, a benzodiazepine site antagonist, such as flumazenil, will not alter the GABA-concentration–effect curve indicating that despite being bound to the GABA$_A$ receptor, the antagonist does not produce the agonist- or inverse agonist-induced allosteric changes that affect receptor function. In other words, a benzodiazepine antagonist does not affect the function of the GABA$_A$ receptor and therefore, by itself, has no functional consequences. However, because it does occupy the binding site, a benzodiazepine site antagonist can be used to block the effects of an agonist or inverse agonist. Thus, flumazenil is used clinically for the treatment of benzodiazepine overdose (Votey, Bosse, Bayer, & Hoffman, 1991; Weinbroum, Flaishon, Sorkine, Szold, & Rudick, 1997).

To assess the intrinsic efficacy of a benzodiazepine site ligand, the effects of different ligand concentrations are studied using a fixed GABA concentration, such as the GABA EC$_{20}$ (Fig. 2B). In these studies, an agonist produces a dose-dependent potentiation and an inverse agonist an attenuation of the GABA EC$_{20}$, with the maximal extent of these changes corresponding to the intrinsic efficacy of the compound. Between the extremes of a full agonist and a full inverse agonist, respective examples of which are diazepam and DMCM, there is a full spectrum of efficacy profiles, including partial agonists (such as bretazenil; Fig. 2B), antagonists (such as flumazenil), and partial inverse agonists (e.g., FG 7142). In recombinant systems expressing a β, γ2 and either an α1, α2, α3, or α5 subunit, these kinds of concentration–effect curves are constructed to examine the efficacy of benzodiazepine site ligands at the α1, α2, α3, and α5 GABA$_A$ receptor subtypes.

To selectively target a specific GABA$_A$ receptor subtype, such as α3 versus α1, it is theoretically possible to design compounds which, although they have the same intrinsic efficacy at these subtypes, have a higher affinity for the α3 compared to the α1 subunit. Using this approach, the higher affinity at the α3 subtype means that at non-saturating concentrations, more α3-containing receptors will be occupied relative to the α1 subtype, although some effects may still be exerted through the latter. For instance, at a compound concentration of 10 nM and assuming α1 and α3 affinities of 30 and 3 nM, respectively (Fig. 3A), α3 receptor occupancy will be 75% whereas only 25% of the α1 subtype will be occupied, resulting in most of

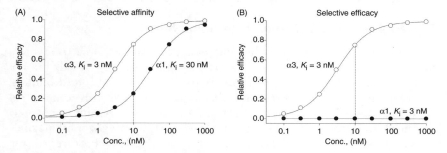

FIGURE 3 Schematic representation of the effects of compounds with α3 versus α1 selective affinity or selective efficacy on the GABA currents produced by a GABA EC$_{20}$ equivalent as measured in recombinant α1- and α3-containing GABA$_A$ receptors.

the *in vivo* efficacy being mediated via the α3 subtype. In contrast, using the selective efficacy approach, a compound might bind with equivalent affinity at the α1 and α3 subtypes but if the compound is an antagonist at the α1 subtype it will exert no effect at this receptor subtype, even at very high levels of occupancy (Fig. 3B). In this case, a compound concentration of 10 nM would produce 75% occupancy at both the α1 and α3 subtypes, yet no effect would be exerted through the α1-containing subtype. Indeed, even at a compound concentration of 1,000 nM, where there is essentially complete occupancy of both the α1 and α3 subtypes, such an agent would not affect GABA function at the α1 subtype.

The binding and efficacy profiles of hypothetical α2/α3 binding-selective and α2/α3 efficacy-selective compounds are illustrated in Fig. 4. A binding-selective compound relies upon the fact that it has higher affinity for particular subtypes, resulting in greater occupancy of these subtypes *in vivo*. Thus, despite the fact that the compound may have equivalent efficacy at the four different GABA$_A$ receptor subtypes, selectivity is achieved *in vivo* based on preferential occupancy (Fig. 4A). Alternatively, an efficacy-selective compound may have equivalent affinity at each of the GABA$_A$ subtypes, but with efficacy at only certain subtypes (Fig. 4B). In this case, *in vivo* occupancy at each subtype is comparable but since antagonism at certain subtypes has no effect on GABA$_A$ receptor function, *in vivo* effects are only exerted via subtypes at which the compound is an agonist. Between these two extremes, there are multiple permutations of compounds with various degrees of binding and/or efficacy selectivity. For example, a compound may be a full agonist at some subtypes and partial agonist at others, or a partial agonists at some subtypes and weak partial agonists at others (Fig. 4C), or may have some binding and some efficacy selectivity (Fig. 4D).

II. Identification of TPA023

A. Origins of the Triazolophthalazine Series

The initial approach to achieving subtype selectivity was to identify compounds with higher affinity at the α2 and/or α3 relative to the α1 subtypes. The aim was to find compounds with 50- to 100-fold binding selectivity as this degree of selective affinity is achievable with compounds binding at the α5 subtype (Quirk et al., 1996). By screening the Merck chemical collection, a low-affinity (1.4–6.4 µM) 2,3-dihydrophthalazine-1,4-dione compound was identified (Carling et al., 2004). Features of this molecule were combined (Fig. 5) with aspects of a compound described in the literature (Compound 80; Tarzia et al., 1988) and which resembles the triazolopyridazine CL 218,872 (Lippa, Coupet et al., 1979). The resulting compound (Compound 10, Carling et al., 2004) has much higher affinity than the screening hit (16–280 nM vs. 1.4–6.4 μM) and it displays a modest (approximately sevenfold) α3 versus α1 binding selectivity (Fig. 5D). Replacement of the aryl ring of the C-6 benzyloxy group with a 2-pyridyl group, as well as increasing the hydrophobicity around the phthalazine core, resulted in a molecule (Compound 62, Carling et al., 2004; Compound 3, Carling et al., 2005; Compound 1, Russell et al., 2005) that possesses anxiolytic-like activity in the rat elevated plus maze (EPM; Carling et al., 2004). This compound has only a threefold to sixfold higher affinity at the α2/α3 compared to α1 subtypes (Fig. 5E) but possesses good pharmacokinetic properties in rat, with a half-life of 1 h, an oral bioavailability of 33%, and a C_{max} of 179 ng/mL following a 3 mg/kg oral dose (Carling et al., 2004). Further efforts failed to yield a lead with sufficiently high affinity and α2/α3 binding selectivity, either from the triazolophthalazine series or from a number of structurally diverse chemical series (Fig. 6).

B. α3 Efficacy-Selective Compounds

The starting point in the development of efficacy-selective compounds was the triazolophthalazine compound shown in Fig. 5E. This compound has a modest (sixfold) α3 versus α1 binding selectivity but a similar, partial agonist efficacy at both subtypes (Fig. 5E). The replacement of the [2.2.2]-bicyclic ring system (Fig. 7A) with a pendant phenyl group increases the affinity and efficacy without any α3 versus α1 efficacy selectivity (Fig. 7B; Compound 11; Carling et al., 2005). Retaining the 3,7-diphenyl substituents, but replacing the 2-pyridyl group with a 1,2,4-triazole, is well tolerated and does not greatly affect affinity while introducing a modest degree of α3 efficacy selectivity (Fig. 7C; Compound 12; Carling et al., 2005). Replacement of the 7-phenyl group with cyclohexyl, cyclopentyl, or cyclobutyl (Compounds 13, 14, and 15, respectively; Carling et al., 2005) has only a modest effect on affinity but a marked decrease in agonist efficacy at both the α1 and α3 subtypes. Although the latter compound (Fig. 7D, MRK-067; Compound I, Hsieh, Lin, & Matuszewski, 2004; TP13, McCabe et al., 2004; Compound 15, Carling et al., 2005; TP123, Ator, 2005) was taken forward, preclinical toxicity issues related to glutathione incorporation into the 3-phenyl ring (see later) limited its further development. Fluorination of the 3-phenyl ring does not markedly affect either affinity or efficacy but greatly reduces metabolism at this site (see later). Thus, the 2,6-difluorophenyl compound (Fig. 7F), designated MRK-409 (Atack, Wafford, et al., 2009; also known as MK-0343, de Haas et al., 2008), was progressed into man.

Affinity

Efficacy

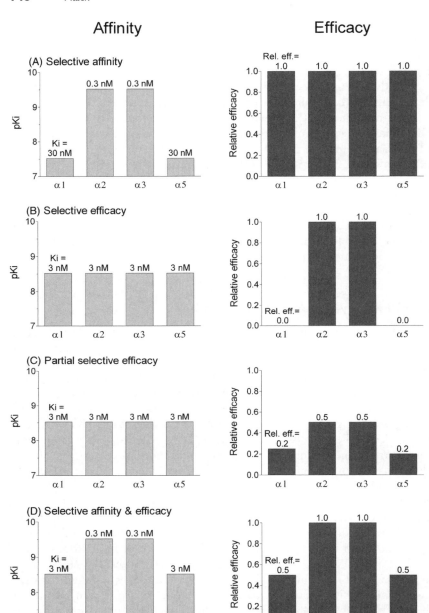

(A) Selective affinity

(B) Selective efficacy

(C) Partial selective efficacy

(D) Selective affinity & efficacy

The observations that reducing the size of the 7-substituent does not greatly affect affinity but does reduce efficacy were further explored by introducing a *tert*-butyl group at the 7-position. This produces a compound (Fig. 7G; Compound 16, Carling et al., 2005) which displays antagonism at the α1 subtype. However, the metabolic instability of the 3-phenyl ring precluded its further development. Fluorination at the 2- and 5-positions of the 3-phenyl ring resulted in L-838417 (Fig. 7H) which retains the affinity and α1 antagonism and α3 partial agonism of Compound 16. While L-838417 proved a useful laboratory tool (McKernan et al., 2000), pharmacokinetic issues prevented it being progressed further (Scott-Stevens, Atack, Sohal, & Worboys, 2005). The 2-fluorophenyl and 2-ethyl-1,2,4-triazole analog of Compound 16 resulted in the development candidate TPA023 (Fig. 7I; Atack, Wafford, et al., 2006; Compound 17, Carling et al., 2005), also known as MK-0777 (Lewis et al., 2008), L-830982, and L-000830982. The key determinants of the structure–activity relationship of TPA023 are summarized in Fig. 8.

III. Preclinical Features of TPA023 _____

A. *In Vitro* Binding and Efficacy

The *in vitro* properties of the lead triazolopyridazine compound TPA023, as well as the structurally related analogs MRK-067, MRK409, MRK-696, and L-838417 are shown in Fig. 9. The affinity of each for the different subtypes of human recombinant GABA$_A$ receptors are essentially the same and there is no subtype selectivity. The affinities of

---

FIGURE 4 Hypothetical binding and efficacy profiles of compounds with various selectivity profiles. (A). Compound A has α2/α3 selective affinity (binding selectivity), with affinity for the α2 and α3 subtypes ($K_i = 0.3$ nM), being 100-fold higher compared to the α1 and α5 subtypes ($K_i = 30$ nM), but it is a full agonist at each subtype, with an efficacy relative to a prototypic non-selective agonist, such as chlordiazepoxide, of 1.0. *In vivo*, Compound A exerts its selectivity by virtue of the fact that it will have greater occupancy at the α2/α3 compared to α1 and α5 subtypes. (B). Compound B has α2/α3 efficacy selectivity in that is has equivalent affinity for all four subtypes ($K_i = 3$ nM) but only has efficacy at the α2 and α3 subtypes, at which it is a full agonist, whereas it is an antagonist at the α1 and α5 subtypes. Consequently, even though Compound B occupies the α1, α2, α3, and α5 subtypes to an equivalent extent *in vivo*, it will only modulate GABA function at the α2 and α3 subtypes and will have no effect on the functioning of the α1 and α5 subtypes. (C) Compound C has partially selective efficacy in that although it has efficacy at each of the four subtypes, it has greater efficacy at the α2/α3 compared to α1 and α5 subtypes. (D) Compound D has a degree of α2/α3 binding and efficacy selectivity. Numbers above each bar represent either K_i (nM) or efficacy relative to a non-selective prototypic benzodiazepine agonist, such as chlordiazepoxide.

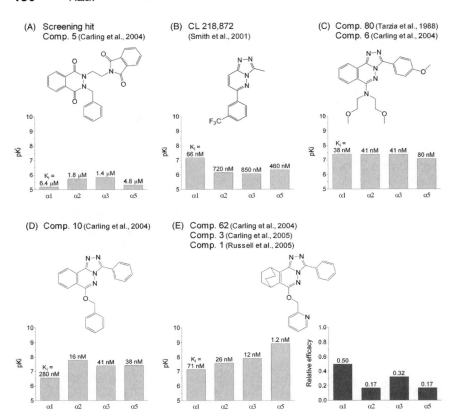

FIGURE 5   The triazolopyridazine series was initially pursued to achieve α2/α3 versus α1 binding selectivity. Features of a screening hit (A) were combined with aspects of the literature compounds CL 218,872 (B) and a triazolophthalazine (C; Compound 80, Tarzia et al., 1988). The resulting lead compound (D; Compound 10, Carling et al., 2004) displayed increased affinity relative to the screening hit. This affinity was improved further by replacing the aryl ring of the C-6 benzyloxy group with a 2-pyridyl group. Introduction of the [2.2.2]-bicyclic ring structure around the core increased hydrophobicity and, although affinity was decreased, agonist efficacy increased (E; Compound 62, Carling et al., 2004; Compound 3, Carling et al., 2005; Compound 1, Russell et al., 2005).

MRK-067 (0.09–0.20 nM) and MRK-696 (0.11–0.22 nM) are slightly higher than those of either MRK-409 (0.21–0.40 nM) or TPA023 (0.19–0.41 nM), which in turn are slightly higher than those of L-838417 (0.67–2.3 nM). The affinities at recombinant GABA$_A$ receptors are similar to those observed for native, rat cerebellum or spinal cord receptors for MRK-067 (0.08–0.18 nM), MRK-409 (0.27–0.28 nM), MRK-696 (0.19–0.39 nM), L-838417 (0.9–1.3 nM), and TPA023 (0.32–0.33 nM; Atack, Wafford, et al., 2006).

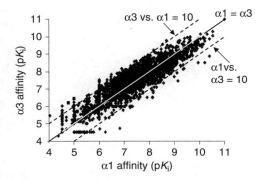

FIGURE 6   Scatter plot showing the $\alpha3$ affinity (pK_i) plotted as a function of the $\alpha1$ affinity for over 3000 compounds derived from approximately 10 different chemical series (including the triazolophthalazines). Very few compounds had $\alpha3$ versus $\alpha1$ selectivity > 10, with none having selectivity of > 100-fold. Based on these data, the decision was made to move away from designing compounds with selective affinity for $\alpha2/\alpha3$ subtypes and instead target $\alpha2/\alpha3$ efficacy-selectivity.

All five compounds display higher efficacy at $\alpha2$- and/or $\alpha3$-containing receptors compared to the $\alpha1$ subtype. However, whereas MRK-067, MRK-409, and MRK-696 are weak partial agonists at the $\alpha1$ subtype, L-838417 and TPA023 are $\alpha1$ antagonists. Efficacy at the $\alpha5$ subtype is more variable in that it is similar to the $\alpha2/\alpha3$ efficacy for L-838417 but lower than the $\alpha2$ and/or $\alpha3$ efficacy for MRK-067, MRK-409, MRK-696, and TPA023, with negligible (i.e., antagonist) $\alpha5$ efficacy being observed for the latter compound. Overall, the intrinsic efficacy of TPA023 was weaker than the other compounds, being only 21% of that of a full agonist. Accordingly, this compound is characterized as a weak $\alpha3$ partial agonist.

B. Selection of Development Candidates

Preclinical studies identified MRK-067 as having a non-sedating anxiolytic profile. While this lead progressed into development it was ultimately found to be genotoxic in an *in vitro* rat hepatocyte alkaline elution toxicity assay. This toxicity is thought due to formation of a reactive arene oxide intermediate (Fig. 10) which, with the use of different recombinant cytochrome P450 enzyme preparations, was found to be mediated via CYP1A1/2. This was consistent with the observation that 25% of a MRK-067 dose administered to rat is excreted as glutathione conjugates. In addition, the genotoxicty of MRK-067 in an *in vitro* alkaline elution assay was increased in hepatocytes prepared from rats treated with β-naphthoflavone (β-NF), a known inducer of

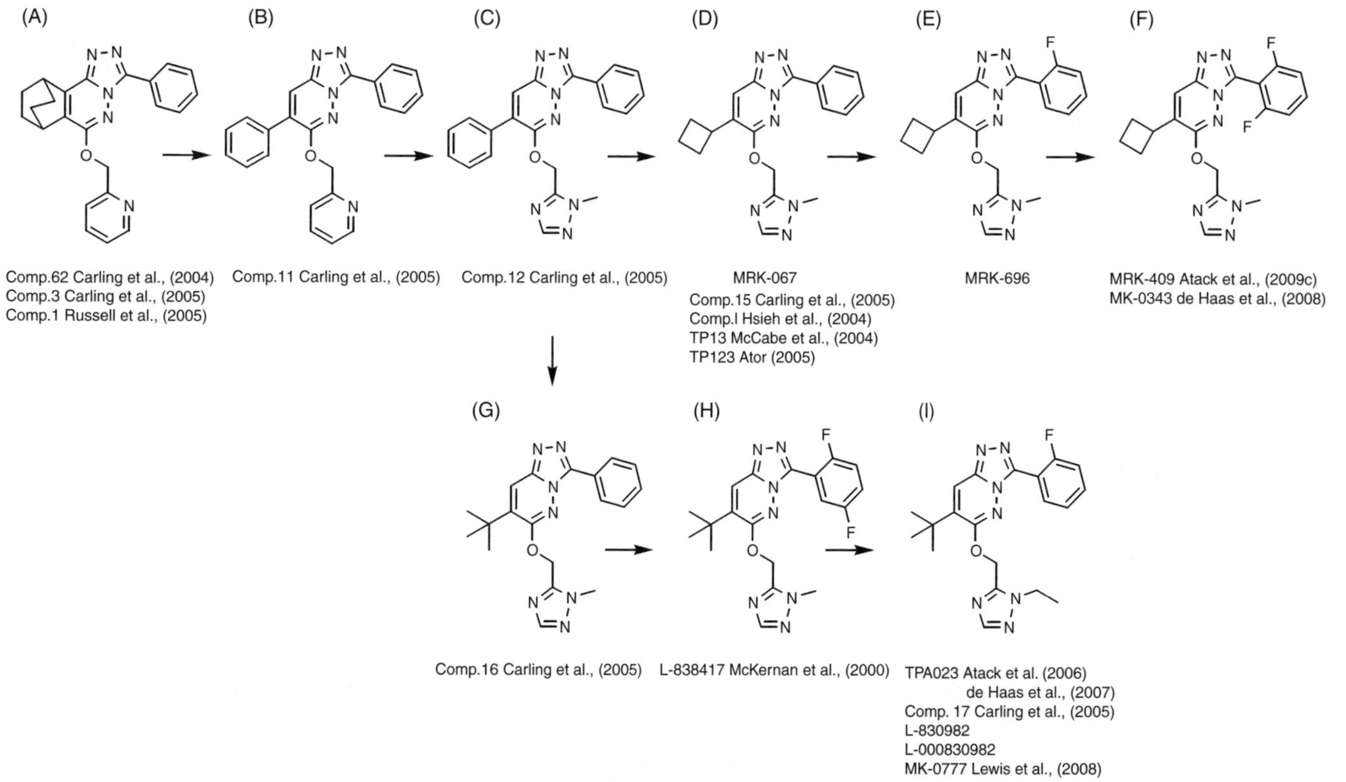

FIGURE 7 Summary of the identification of key compounds in the triazolopyridazine series originating from the [2.2.2]-bicyclic starting compound (62, Carling et al., 2004; Compound 3, Carling et al., 2005; see also Fig. 5E).

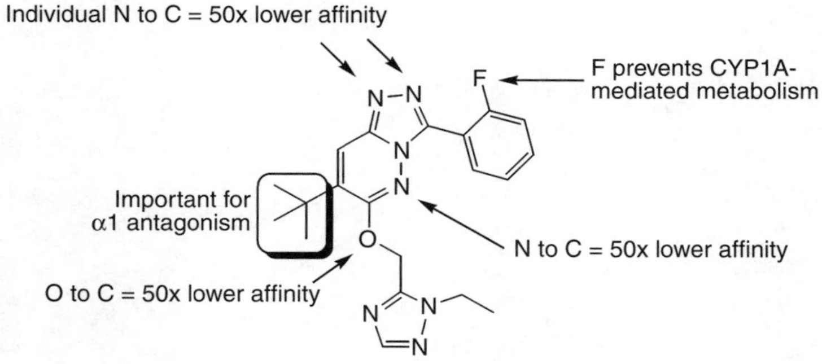

FIGURE 8   Key features of the structure–activity relationship of TPA023.

CYP1A expression. As a consequence, the turnover of compounds was measured in normal and β-NF-induced rat liver microsomes with, for example, the turnover of MRK-067 increasing from ~20% in normal rat liver microsomes to > 90% in β-NF-induced microsomes.

Using the β-NF-induced microsome assay it was found that fluorination of the pendant 3-phenyl ring reduced CYP1A-mediated metabolism. This observation was consistent with homology models of CYP1A2 that showed increasing the bulk of the phenyl group should restrict access to the enzyme active site. More specifically, it was found that the increase in the *in vitro* turnover in β-NF-induced compared to normal rat liver microsomes was not as great for the 2-fluorophenyl analog, MRK-696, relative to the unsubstituted MRK-067 whereas the 2,6-difluorophenyl analog MRK-409 had similar rates of turnover in normal and β-NF-induced rat liver microsomes. Accordingly, MRK-409, also known as MK-0343 (de Haas et al., 2008), which has a preclinical non-sedating anxiolytic profile very similar to MRK-067, was selected for further development and progressed into man. Surprisingly, this compound causes sedation in man (Atack, Wafford, et al., 2009). This was rationalized as being due to the fact that although MRK-409 has relatively low efficacy at the α1 subtype this is, nevertheless, sufficient to cause sedation since humans appear to be particularly sensitive to even weak partial agonist activity at this subtype. These data therefore defined the requirement for no efficacy at the α1 subtype. This, together with the desire to have a compound with no increased turnover in β-NF-induced relative to normal rat microsomes, highlighted TPA023 as a lead for further development. It should also be noted that introduction of a *t*-butyl at the C-7 position and a 2-ethyl group on the 1,2,4 triazole substituent at the C-6 position provides CYP3A4-mediated metabolic soft spots that divert metabolism away from the C-3 phenyl group.

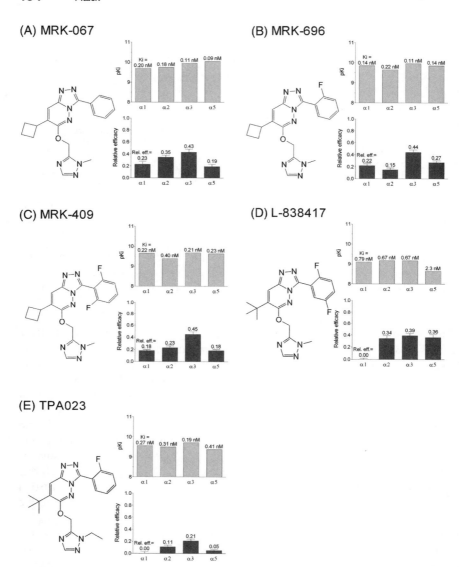

FIGURE 9 Structure and *in vitro* affinity and efficacy of TPA023 and related compounds. Affinities were measured using a competition radioligand ([³H]flumazenil) binding assay and are plotted as pK_i. The values above the bars represent the affinity in nano molars. Efficacy was measured using whole-cell patch clamp electrophysiology. These data are expressed relative to the non-selective full agonist chlordiazepoxide which, by definition, has an efficacy of 1.0 at each subtype. The α1, α2, α3, and α5 labels refer to recombinant human GABA$_A$ receptors containing β3 and γ2 subunits plus either an α1, α2, α3, or α5 subunit stably expressed in mouse fibroblast L(tk⁻) cells.

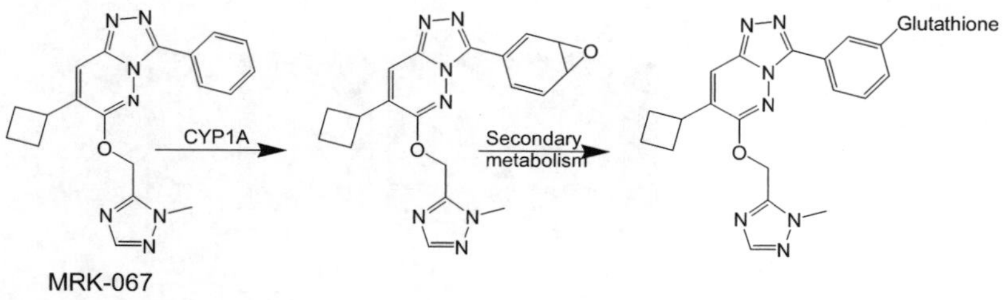

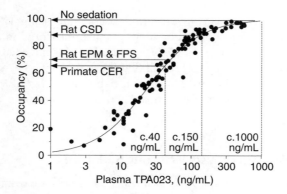

FIGURE 10 Overview of the metabolism of MRK-067. The formation of an arene oxide reactive intermediate is associated with metabolism by CYP1A. Secondary metabolism resulted in the formation of glutathione conjugates, the excretion of which, in rat, accounts for 25% of the administered dose.

C. In Vivo Receptor Occupancy

When administered orally to rats, TPA023 displays good receptor occupancy, being maximal within 0.5 h (Atack, Wafford, et al., 2006). This agrees well with the plasma T_{max} values observed in more detailed pharmacokinetic analyses (see below), suggesting that brain drug concentrations do not lag behind plasma concentrations. The dose of TPA023 resulting in 50% occupancy of rat brain GABA$_A$ receptors was 0.42 mg/kg, with the corresponding plasma concentration being 25 ng/mL (Fig. 11).

FIGURE 11 Rat brain TPA023 GABA$_A$ receptor occupancy expressed as a function of plasma drug concentration. Each data point represents a single rat in which occupancy was measured using a [^{3}H]flumazenil *in vivo* binding assay (Atack, Wafford, et al., 2006) and trunk blood collected for measurement of plasma drug concentrations. Arrows indicate the level of occupancy at the minimum effective dose in either the primate (squirrel monkey) conditioned emotional response (CER; 65% occupancy) or rat elevated plus maze and fear-potentiated startle (EPM and FPS; both 70%) or conditioned suppression of drinking (CSD; 88%) assays (Atack, Wafford, et al., 2006). The corresponding plasma drug concentrations for this range of occupancies (65–88%) is also shown (40–150 ng/mL).

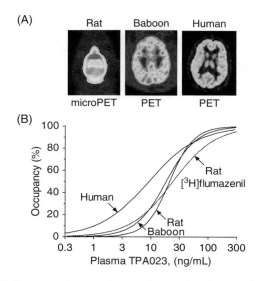

FIGURE 12 (A) Representative pseudocolor images showing the distribution of [^{11}C] flumazenil binding in horizontal sections of rat, baboon, and human brain as measured using microPET in the rat (Atack et al., 2007) or PET for baboon and human. (B) Plasma–occupancy relationship derived from the rat microPET and baboon and human PET studies. Dashed line shows plasma–occupancy curve derived from rat brain using an *in vivo* [^{3}H]flumazenil binding assay (see Fig. 11). Data modified from Atack, Fryer, et al. (2009).

In addition to measuring rat brain occupancy using [^{3}H]flumazenil ($EC_{50} = 25$ ng/mL, Fig. 11), occupancy was also measured in rat, baboon, and man using [^{11}C]flumazenil PET (Fig. 12). The plasma–occupancy curves derived from these experiments reveal that the plasma EC_{50} values measured using [^{11}C]flumazenil in rat (21 ng/mL), baboon (19 ng/mL), and human (9 ng/mL) were similar to those measured in rat using the *in vivo* [^{3}H] flumazenil binding assay (25 ng/mL).

D. Preclinical Anxiolysis Without Sedation

TPA023 was tested in a variety of rodent and primate behavioral assays (Atack, Wafford, et al., 2006). It is efficacious in both unconditioned (rat EPM) and conditioned (rat fear-potentiated startle (FPS), rat conditioned suppression of drinking (CSD), and primate conditioned emotional response (CER)) models of anxiety, with the minimal effective doses required for efficacy in these assays corresponding to occupancy values ranging from 65 to 88% (Atack, Wafford, et al., 2006). The corresponding plasma drug concentrations ranged from 40 to 150 ng/mL (Fig. 11). TPA023 is also efficacious in the mouse pentylenetetrazole-induced seizure model,

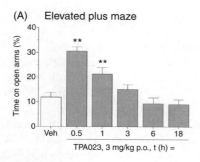
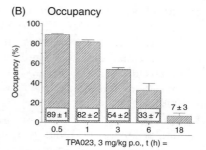

FIGURE 13 The time course of the anxiolytic response in the elevated plus maze test corresponds to the duration of receptor occupancy. Rats were administered TPA023 (3 mg/kg p.o. in 0.5% methyl cellulose) and at various times thereafter (0.5, 1, 3, 6, or 18 h) tested on the elevated plus maze. After the 5 min trial, alternate animals were taken and occupancy measured using an *in vivo* [^{3}H]flumazenil binding assay. Values shown are means $\pm$ SEM ($n = 18$ for plus maze and $n = 9$ for occupancy data).

providing full seizure protection at a dose of 10 mg/kg i.p. (84% occupancy), with the ED$_{50}$ for protection against tonic convulsions (1.4 mg/kg i.p.) corresponding to around 50% occupancy.

The anxiolytic-like effect of TPA023 in the EPM tracked the extent of receptor occupancy (Fig. 13). Hence, a significant anxiolytic-like response is observed 0.5 and 1 h after administration of 3 mg/kg p.o., at which times the respective occupancy values were 89 and 82%. However, by 3 h after administration, occupancy had fallen to 54% and there was no longer a significant enhancement of plus maze performance.

TPA023 produces no overt signs of sedation, ataxia, and/or myorelaxation in either the mouse rotarod, rat chain-pulling or squirrel monkey lever pressing assays, even at doses corresponding to $\geq 99\%$ occupancy (Atack, Wafford, et al., 2006). In mice, the partial inverse agonist FG 7142 induces clonic seizure activity in animals pre-treated for 7 days with the non-selective full agonist triazolam. However, no such FG-7142-precipitated withdrawal signs are observed in mice pre-treated with TPA023. Moreover, after 7 days of pre-treatment with the full agonist triazolam, switching to TPA023 does not precipitate any signs of withdrawal (Atack, Wafford, et al., 2006).

E. TPA023 Has a Much Reduced Abuse Potential

The abuse potential of non-selective, full agonist benzodiazepine site ligands remains a concern (Ator, 2005; Griffiths & Weert, 1997). It is not clear whether the rewarding properties of benzodiazepines are due to specific GABA$_A$ receptor subtypes, although the $\alpha3$ subtype-selective agonist TP003 (Dias et al., 2005) has a much reduced abuse potential relative to non-selective full agonists (Fischer et al., 2009). MRK-067 produces a degree of self-administration in baboons that is greater than vehicle but not as great as lorazepam (Ator, 2005). On the other hand, the self-administration of TPA023 does not differ significantly from vehicle (Ator, 2005), even at a dose corresponding to essentially full occupancy as measured using the [^{11}C]flumazenil PET assay (Fig. 14). Hence, TPA023 does not appear to have abuse potential in baboons (Ator, Atack, Hargreaves, Burns, & Dawson, 2009).

In the rat drug-discrimination assay TPA023 produces interoceptive cues that permit discriminative training (Kohut & Ator, 2008) but it does not generalize to lorazepam in the baboon whereas MRK-067 (TPA123) displays partial generalization. On the other hand, the α1-preferring zolpidem and zaleplon both produce lorazepam-like responding (Ator, 2005). While these data suggest that the interoceptive cues

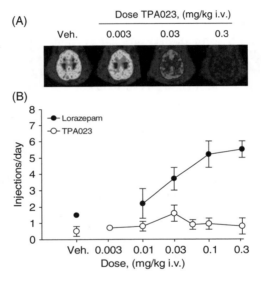

FIGURE 14 TPA023 shows no tendency to be self-administered in baboons even at doses associated with complete occupancy. (A). Representative images of baboon brain [^{11}C] flumazenil uptake, as measured using PET, at i.v. doses of 0.003, 0.03, and 0.3 mg/kg TPA023. There is a dose-dependent inhibition of [^{11}C]flumazenil binding corresponding to a dose related increase in occupancy, with 0.3 mg/kg producing essentially 100% occupancy. The baboons used for the PET studies were a different cohort from those used for self-administration studies. (B). Self-administration with various doses (0.003–0.3 mg/kg, i.v.) of TPA023. Baboons trained to self-administer cocaine also self-administer lorazepam in a dose-dependent manner, self-injecting on average approximately six out of a total of eight possible injections/day. In contrast, substitution of cocaine with TPA023 produces rates of responding that are not significantly different from vehicle even at a dose (0.3 mg/kg i.v.) that results in complete occupancy of baboon brain GABA$_A$ receptors. Data modified from Ator et al. (2009).

associated with lorazepam may be associated with the α1 subtype, it is also possible that the reduced or negligible generalization to lorazepam of TPA023 and MRK-067 may be related to their lower α2/α3 efficacy in comparison to lorazepam.

In addition to possessing negligible abuse potential, and to not generalizing to the non-selective full agonist lorazepam, TPA023 does not appear to show signs of physical dependence, as demonstrated by the lack of overt signs of withdrawal after multiple administrations to mice (Atack, Wafford, et al., 2006). There is also no evidence of TPA023 producing physical dependence in baboons treated for 1 month with TPA023 at 32 mg/kg/day delivered i.g. as a suspension at a rate of 600 mL/day. This produces a plasma concentration in the region of 60 ng/mL that, based on a plasma EC_{50} concentration of 19 ng/mL (Fig. 12), corresponds to a receptor occupancy of approximately 85% (Ator et al., 2009). In addition, the non-selective partial inverse agonist FG 7142 precipitates signs of withdrawal (seizure activity) in mice treated for 7 days with the non-selective full agonist triazolam but not in mice given TPA023 for 7 days. Furthermore, TPA023 does not precipitate withdrawal signs in mice treated for 7 days with triazolam (Atack, Wafford, et al., 2006).

IV. Preclinical Metabolism and Pharmacokinetics of TPA023

A. Pharmacokinetics in Rat, Dog, and Rhesus Monkey

Displayed in Fig. 15 are the plasma pharmacokinetics of TPA023 in rat, dog, and rhesus monkey. With respect to i.v. kinetics, rat and dog show moderate clearance, with respective clearance rates (26 and 13 mL/min/kg)

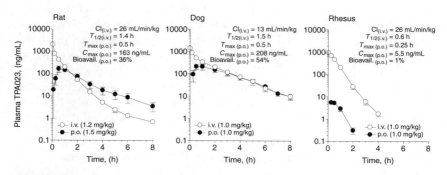

FIGURE 15 Pharmacokinetics of TPA023 in male Sprague–Dawley rats, female beagle dogs, and male rhesus monkeys. Values shown are mean $\pm$ SEM ($n = 3$).

representing about one-third of liver blood flow in each species. In contrast, clearance in the rhesus monkey (26 mL/min/kg) was relatively high in that it represents around two-thirds of liver blood flow. Given these moderate to high clearance rates, along with the low volume of distribution in each species (ranging from 0.9 to 1.4 L/kg), the half-life in all of these species is relatively short (0.6–1.5 h).

Following oral administration to rats (1.5 mg/kg) and dogs (1.0 mg/kg), TPA023 is rapidly absorbed ($T_{max} = 0.5$ h). The bioavailability following this route of administration is 36% in rats and 54% in dogs, and total exposures are 343 and 714 ng.h/mL, respectively, indicating that in rats and dogs TPA023 is well absorbed. In contrast, the systemic exposure in rhesus monkeys was very low following oral administration of 1.0 mg/kg with an AUC_{0-inf} of 6 ng.h/mL and oral bioavailability is 1%. This poor exposure is probably the consequence of a high rate of first-pass metabolism, as reflected by the relatively high clearance in this species.

B. *In Vitro* Metabolism of TPA023

The metabolism of TPA023 was examined *in vitro* using rat, dog, rhesus monkey, and human liver microsomes. Following incubation, the metabolites were assessed by liquid chromatography and mass spectrometry with the initial tentative identifications confirmed by subsequent synthesis of each metabolite. The predominant metabolites produced by human microsomes were the alcohol (M1) and free triazole (M2) (Fig. 16), and both of these metabolites were also produced by liver microsomes derived from rat, dog, and rhesus monkey, with these latter species also yielded metabolites representing further oxidation of the M1 metabolite. Finally, oxidation of the pendant 2-fluorophenyl group was observed following incubation of TPA023 with dog and rhesus monkey microsomes.

Selective antibodies and chemical inhibitors were used to examine the contribution of different P-450 enzymes to the metabolism of TPA023 in human liver microsomes (Ma, Polsky-Fisher, Vickers, Cui, & Rodrigues, 2007). Both the *t*-butyl hydroxylation and the N-deethylation reactions were substantially inhibited by CYP3A-specific antibodies and inhibitors. More specific analyses revealed that CYP3A4 played a major role in TPA023 metabolism while CYP3A5 also played a role, but primarily at higher concentrations of compound. These data were confirmed in experiments in which TPA023 was incubated with human recombinant P450 proteins (Ma et al., 2007).

C. *In Vivo* Metabolism of TPA023 in Preclinical Species

Following oral administration of 3 mg/kg TPA023, the M1 and M2 metabolites were the major species observed in rat plasma, with their

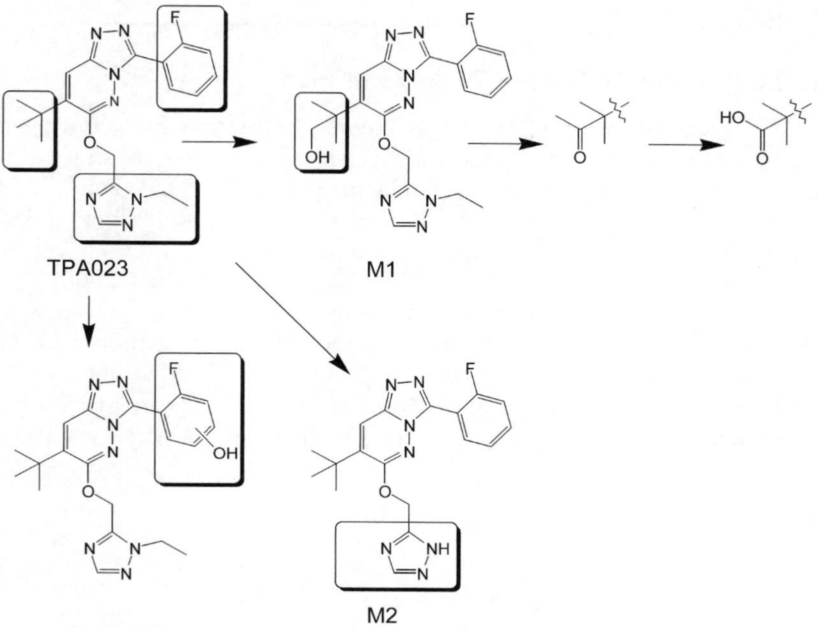

FIGURE 16 Scheme summarizing the metabolites produced *in vitro* by the incubation of TPA023 with rat, dog, rhesus monkey, and human liver microsomes. The major metabolites produced by human microsomes were the alcohol (M1) and free triazole (M2). Rat, dog, and rhesus monkey microsomes also produced these metabolites as well as metabolites representing further oxidation of the alcohol as well as oxidation of the pendant 2-fluorophenyl group, although this metabolite was not produced by rat microsomes.

kinetics following those of TPA023. However, although C_{max} metabolite concentrations were 25–35% of TPA023, M1 and M2 both displayed very poor blood–brain barrier penetration. Hence, although the brain to plasma ratio for TPA023 was in the region of 0.3–0.5, the corresponding values for the M1 and M2 metabolites were in the region of 0.02. In addition to the M1 and M2 metabolites, the metabolite containing both the alcohol and the free triazole was also detected, as were the further oxidation species of the M1 metabolite. However, none of these metabolites were detected in brain. In summary, despite the fact that the M1 metabolite has an affinity for the GABA$_A$ receptor (0.16–0.51 nM) comparable to TPA023 (0.19–0.41 nM), while the M2 metabolite has an affinity (6.4–22 nM) that is approximately 25- to 50-fold lower than the parent, the virtual absence of these metabolites in brain suggests it is unlikely they contribute to the *in vivo* pharmacological actions of TPA023.

V. Human Studies

A. In Vivo Metabolism of TPA023 in Man

The metabolism of TPA023 was studied in humans by following the recovery of radioactivity in urine and feces for 7 days after the oral administration of [^{14}C]TPA023 as part of a 3.0 mg dose of TPA023 (Fig. 17). The kinetics of plasma radioactivity followed those of total plasma TPA023 concentrations, with the T_{max} being 2.0 h, the mean ($\pm$SD) $C_{max} = 28 \pm 3$ ng/mL, and an apparent half-life of 6.7 h (Polsky-Fisher et al., 2006).

After 7 days the total radioactivity recovered in the urine and feces was 83%, with the majority (53%) in the urine. The most abundant urinary metabolites were the t-butyl hydroxyl (M11, Fig. 17; **M1**, Fig. 16) and triazolopyridazine N1-glucuronide (M5), representing 14 and 10% of the total dose, respectively. In addition, the glucuronide of O-dealkyl TPA023

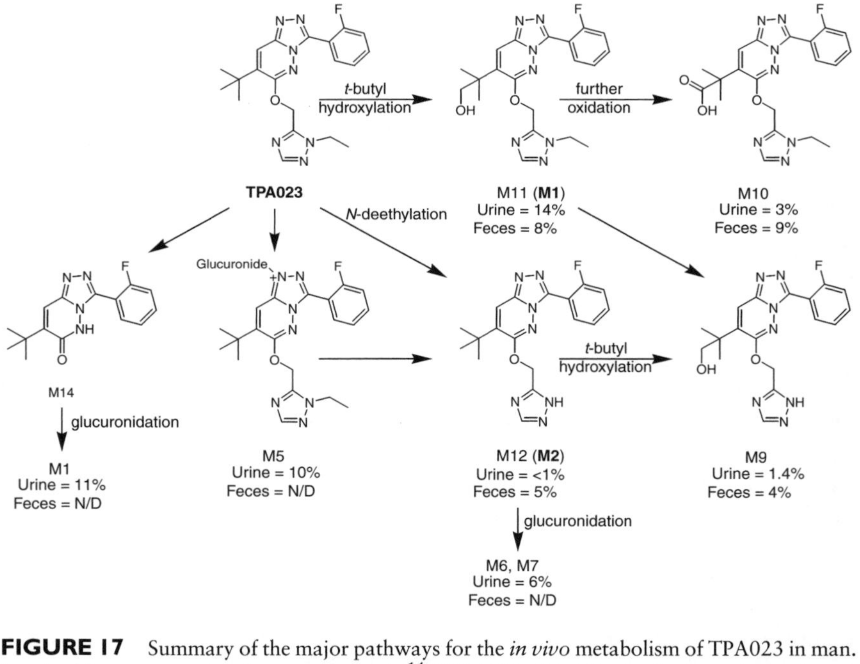

FIGURE 17 Summary of the major pathways for the *in vivo* metabolism of TPA023 in man. Five healthy young male volunteers received [^{14}C]TPA023 (99 μCi) as a single total oral dose of 3.0 mg TPA023 (given as a solution in 10% propylene glycol). Urine, feces, and plasma were collected at various intervals over the following 7 days and samples were analyzed by LC-MS/MS (Polsky-Fisher et al., 2006). N/D = Not detected. The numbering of metabolites is consistent with published data (Polsky-Fisher et al., 2006) with **M1** and **M2** referring to the metabolites described in Fig. 16.

(M1) was found, accounting for 11% of the total dose, and, following deethylation, glucuronidation on the triazole group (M6, M7) accounted for a further 6% of the dose. Hence, in the urine, TPA023 is cleared primarily by oxidative metabolism via the *t*-butyl hydroxylation and *N*-deethylation routes identified in human, rat, dog, and rhesus monkey microsomes.

The five major metabolites identified in feces were the *t*-butyl hydroxylation product M11, which comprises 8% of the total dose, the carboxylic acid M10 that derived from the further oxidation of M11 (9%), the *N*-deethylated metabolite (M12, Fig. 17 or **M2**, Fig. 16; 5%), the combined *t*-butyl hydroxyl-*N*-desethyl metabolite (M9; 4%), and a fluorophenyl ring hydroxylated metabolite (M13), which is unique to the feces but only comprised a relatively minor proportion of the total dose (1%).

B. Human Pharmacokinetics

Following oral administration of single doses ranging from 0.05 to 3 mg, TPA023 is rapidly absorbed from immediate release tablets with a T_{max} of approximately 2 h (Fig. 18A). The exposure is dose-dependent, with the C_{max} being linearly related to the dose (Fig. 18A, inset). Preclinical data show that TPA023 has a relatively short half-life, ranging from 0.6 to 1.5 h in rats, dogs, and rhesus monkey (Fig. 15) and consistent with it has a fairly short half-life in young, healthy males of between 3.3 and 5.2 h (Table III). The half-life is slightly longer in the elderly (7 h) and at corresponding doses the C_{max} and total exposures are about 25 and 50% greater in the elderly compared to young volunteers (Table III).

By delivering TPA023 using an Enterion® capsule, it was ascertained that its formulation into slow-release tablets would produce a sustained absorption phase. For this purpose, TPA023 was encapsulated in an insoluble outer coating into which holes were drilled using a laser to form a gel extrusion module (GEM; Juang & Storey, 2003). The plasma kinetics of the GEM formulation of TPA023 are considerably altered relative to the immediate release tablet formulation (Fig. 18B). Single-ascending dose studies of the GEM formulation revealed that the compound displays dose-proportional exposure as judged by not only C_{max} (inset, Fig. 18C) but also the area under the curve.

In vitro metabolic studies using human liver microsomes suggest that CYP3A enzymes play an important role in the oxidative metabolism of TPA023 (Ma et al., 2007). This was confirmed *in vivo* in a drug–drug interaction study in which the pharmacokinetics of the 0.25 mg immediate release formulation of TPA023 were studied in the absence and presence of itraconazole, a CYP3A4 inhibitor. These data showed (Fig. 18D) that in the presence of itraconazole there is a 1.5-fold increase in the C_{max} and a 4.5-fold increase in total human plasma TPA023 exposure as measured by the area under the time–concentration curve (Polsky-Fisher et al., 2006).

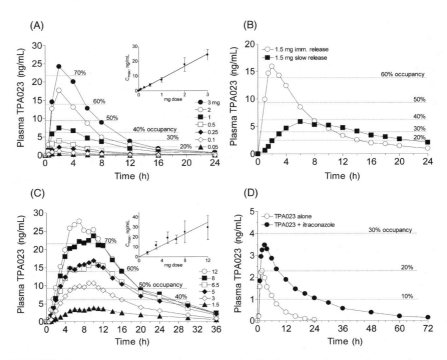

FIGURE 18   Pharmacokinetics of TPA023 in healthy human volunteers. (A). Single-dose pharmacokinetics following oral administration of various doses (0.05–3.0 mg) of an immediate release (IR) formulation ($n = 6$/dose group). (B). Comparison of the kinetics of 1.5 mg doses of TPA023 formulated either an immediate release, or slow-release, gel extrusion module (GEM) tablets ($n = 6$/dose group). (C). The plasma kinetics of TPA023 when administered as the controlled release (GEM) formulation either twice a day (doses of 1.5, 3.0, 5.0, and 6.5 mg) or once a day (8 and 12 mg). (D). Effects of the CYP3A4 inhibitor itraconazole (2×100 mg) on the pharmacokinetics of TPA023 (0.25 mg immediate release formulation) in healthy male and female subjects. The values shown are mean, $n = 12$, in a double-blind crossover study. The dashed lines indicate the plasma concentrations of TPA023 required to give the specified level of occupancy. The occupancy estimations are based on a human plasma EC_{50} of 9 ng/mL (Fig. 12).

The plasma pharmacokinetics following single doses of 1.5 mg of the GEM formulation of TPA023 were compared in fasted and high-fat breakfast fed subjects. The ratio of the C_{max} and AUC values under fed and fasted conditions were 1.07 and 0.99, respectively, demonstrating no marked food effects on single doses of TPA023.

Based on the human TPA023 plasma concentration–occupancy curve (Fig. 12), the estimated occupancy values at different plasma concentrations were superimposed onto the pharmacokinetic plots (Fig. 18). In the single-ascending dose with the immediate release formulation (Fig. 18A), a 3 mg dose achieves peak plasma concentrations ($\sim$25 ng/mL) corresponding to around 70% occupancy. Similarly, the peak plasma concentrations achieved

TABLE III Summary of Pharmacokinetic Properties and Adverse Events for TPA023 When Administered Orally to Healthy Human Volunteers

Immediate release—single dose, healthy young men

Dose (mg)	N=	T_{max} (h)	C_{max} (ng/mL)	$T_{1/2}$ (h)	Dizziness	Motor in coordination	Loss of concentration	Headache	Altered perception
Placebo	16	–	–		–	–	–	2	–
0.05	6	1.7	0.5 ± 0.1	3.4	–	–	–	3	–
0.1	6	1.8	1.1 ± 0.3	3.3	–	–	–	1	–
0.25	6	2.0	2.2 ± 0.4	3.7	–	–	–	1	–
0.50	6	2.0	3.9 ± 1.0	3.4	–	–	–	1	–
1.0	6	2.2	7.4 ± 1.6	4.7	–	–	–	1	–
2.0	6	2.0	18 ± 5	5.0	5	–	3	–	–
3.0	6	2.3	24 ± 4	5.2	4	5	1	1	4
3.0[a]	5	2.0	28 ± 3	6.7	2	–	–	–	–

Immediate release—single dose, healthy elderly men and women

Dose (mg)	N=	T_{max} (h)	C_{max} (ng/mL)	$T_{1/2}$ (h)	Dizziness	Light headedness	Drowsiness/sleepiness
Placebo	12	–	–		–	–	2
0.5	12	2.1	5.6 ± 0.8	6.5	–	–	–
1.0	12	2.1	11 ± 3	6.8	3	1	–
1.5	12	–	16 ± 4	–	3	4	5
2.0	12	–	21 ± 5	–	1	–	8

Immediate vs. controlled release (gel extrusion module—GEM) formulation

Dose (mg)	N=	T_{max} (h)	C_{max} (ng/mL)	$T_{1/2}$ (h)	Dizziness	Headache
1.5 IR	16	–	–	–	3	–
1.5 GEM	16	–	–	–	–	1

(Continued)

TABLE III (*Continued*)

Controlled release (GEM) formulation—multiple dose study

Dose (mg)	N =	T_{max} (h)	C_{max} (ng/mL)	$T_{1/2}$ (h)	Headache	Drowsiness	Dizziness	Violent dreams	Strange/vivid dreams
Placebo	12	–	–	–	3	–	2	1	2
1.5 b.i.d.	6	–	4.1 ± 1.5	–	2	–	–	–	–
3.0 b.i.d.	5	–	12 ± 4	–	1	1	1	–	–
5 b.i.d.	6	–	19 ± 6	–	4	5	–	–	3
6.5 b.i.d.	6	–	18 ± 4	–	–	1	2	4	–
8 q.d.	6	–	25 ± 11	–	1	–	3	–	–
12 q.d.	6	–	30 ± 12	–	–	2	3	–	–

N/A = not applicable, N/D = not determined.

[a]This was an ADME study in which [^{14}C]TPA023 was administered along with TPA023 for a total dose of 3 mg as an oral solution.

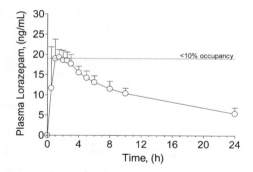

FIGURE 19 Plasma lorazepam concentrations following a single 2 mg oral dose administered to healthy normal volunteers. Values shown are mean ±SD ($n = 12$; data redrawn from de Haas et al., 2007). The estimate of occupancy is based upon the fact that 1.5–2.5 h after a single, 2 mg dose of lorazepam, occupancy is <10% (Atack, Fryer, et al., 2009). Terminal half-life is approximately 7 h (de Haas et al., 2007), consistent with previous reports of 11–17 h (Greenblatt et al., 1988; Blin et al., 1999).

with single 8 and 12 mg doses of the controlled release (GEM) formulation at ~25 ng/mL also corresponded to an occupancy of 70% or greater. In comparison, a single 2 mg dose of lorazepam produces peak plasma concentrations of approximately 20 ng/mL (Fig. 19; de Haas et al., 2007), similar to previous published data of 18–33 ng/mL (Blin et al., 1999; Greenblatt, Harmatz, Dorsey, & Shader, 1988). However, single doses of either 1 or 2 mg lorazepam produce only very low levels of receptor occupancy (<10%; Lingford-Hughes, Wilson, Feeney, Grasby, & Nutt, 2005; Atack, Fryer, et al., 2009) and, in general, the non-selective classical benzodiazepines, such as alprazolam, clonazepam, diazepam, midazolam, as well as the α1 subtype-preferring zolpidem, produce either sedation or sleep at receptor occupancy values of 15–30% (Abadie et al., 1996; Fujita et al., 1999; Pauli, Farde, Halldin, & Sedvall, 1991; Shinotoh et al., 1989; Videbæk et al., 1993). Hence, TPA023 is able to achieve levels of receptor occupancy in man that are much greater than those required for non-selective or α1-preferring benzodiazepine site ligands to produce sedation and/or sleep. This indicates that at comparable levels of occupancy, TPA023 has a much reduced sedation liability in comparison to diazepam, lorazepam, alprazolam, or zolpidem.

C. Tolerability of TPA023 in Normal Volunteers

1. Immediate Release Formulation

TPA023 was well tolerated in single oral doses of the immediate release formulation up to 2.0 mg and multiple oral doses up to 2.0 mg t.i.d. The dose-limiting adverse events observed at 3.0 mg are dizziness, altered perception, and motor incoordination (Table III).

Dizziness was also observed in two out of the five subjects receiving [^{14}C]TPA023 in a solution of 3 mg TPA023 total dose for an ADME study (Polsky-Fisher et al., 2006). The adverse events observed in the elderly were similar to those in the young, although there was a greater degree of drowsiness and sleepiness in the elderly as compared to the younger subjects (Table III).

2. Controlled Release (GEM) Formulation

At oral doses of 1.5 and 3 mg of the GEM formulation b.i.d., TPA023 was very well tolerated, although more adverse events, including headache, drowsiness, and strange or vivid dreams, were reported at a dose of 5 mg b.i.d. Overall, the 5 and 6.5 mg b.i.d. doses were considered to be reasonably well tolerated, although altered dreams were observed at a dose of 6.5 mg b.i.d., with some subjects reporting violent dreams (Table III). However, it should be noted that these adverse events were also observed in subjects receiving placebo. With once-a-day oral administration, the 8 mg dose was well tolerated, with mild dizziness being the most frequent adverse event. In contrast, the 12 mg dose was poorly tolerated, with moderate levels of dizziness reported along with disturbances in balance and coordination that were collectively considered to be dose limiting. Consequently, a dose of 8 mg q.d. was considered to be the maximum tolerated dose for the controlled release (GEM) formulation. In a separate, multiple, titrated-dose study in healthy young subjects, GEM-formulated TPA023 was escalated from 3, 5, 8, 10 through to 13 mg b.i.d. All the subjects successfully escalated from 3 to 5 mg b.i.d., with most tolerating well 7 days of doses of either 8 or 10 mg b.i.d. A dose of 13 mg was not well tolerated by some subjects.

D. Pharmacodynamic Effects of TPA023 in Normal Volunteers

The pharmacodynamic effects of TPA023 (0.5 and 1.5 mg immediate release formulation) were compared to those of lorazepam (2 mg) in healthy males volunteers (de Haas et al., 2007; data summarized in Table IV). In this study the 0.5 mg and 1.5 mg doses give C_{max} values in the region of 5 and 13 ng/mL, respectively, with T_{max} at 2–2.5 h. Lorazepam displays a C_{max} of approximately 19 ng/mL and T_{max} at 1.5 h (Fig. 19).

Using the visual analog scale of alertness, lorazepam produces subjective sedative effects whereas TPA023 does not (Table IV). There is a similar dissociation between lorazepam and TPA023 with regard to saccadic eye movements. Hence, lorazepam affects not only saccadic peak velocity but also saccadic latency and inaccuracy, whereas TPA023 only alters peak velocity (Fig. 20A) and has no effect on saccadic latency or inaccuracy (Table IV). Furthermore, lorazepam alters body posture, as measured by the extent of body sway with the eyes either open or shut

TABLE IV Comparison of the Pharmacodynamic Effects of TPA023 and Lorazepam in Healthy Male Volunteers

	TPA023		
	0.5 mg	*1.5 mg*	*2 mg Lorazepam*
	Sedation		
VAS alertness	↔	↔	↓
Saccadic eye movements			
Peak velocity	↓↓	↓↓↓	↓↓↓
Latency	↔	↔	↑↑↑
Inaccuracy	↔	↔	↑↑↑
	Posture		
Body sway—eyes open	↔	↔	↑↑↑
Body sway—eyes closed	↔	↔	↑↑↑
	Cognitive performance		
Word recognition	↔	↔	↓
Picture recognition	↔	↔	↓

↓, ↓↓, ↓↓↓ = significantly decreased by $p<0.05$, $p<0.01$, and $p<0.001$, respectively.
↑↑↑ = significantly increased by $p<0.001$

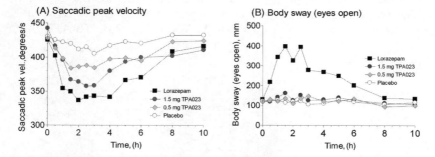

FIGURE 20   Pharmacodynamic effects of TPA023 in man. Healthy young male volunteers ($n = 12$) participated in a double-blind, 4-period crossover study in which each subject received four treatments; placebo, TPA023 (0.5 and 1.5 mg single-dose immediate release formulation) or lorazepam (2 mg single dose). Responses measured were (A) saccadic eye movement peak velocity and (B) body sway (eyes open). Whereas lorazepam has a marked effect on both parameters, TPA023 gives a dose-dependent effect on saccadic eye movement peak velocity but does not affect body sway. Data redrawn from de Haas et al. (2007) with error bars omitted for clarity.

and impairs performance on word and picture recognition tasks of cognition while TPA023 does not significantly affect performance in any of these assays (Table IV and Fig. 20B). These effects of lorazepam on alertness, postural stability, and memory are similar to those reported for other non-selective benzodiazepine site ligands such as diazepam, flurazepam, lormetazepam, triazolam, temazepam, and zopiclone (discussed in de Haas et al., 2007). Furthermore, TPA023 differs from the non-selective partial agonist bretazenil which also affects alertness, saccadic eye movements, and posture (Van Stevenick et al., 1996). Hence, in this regard, and despite suggestions that TPA023 causes sedation in man (Rogawski, 2006), TPA023 differentiated itself from non-selective full and partial agonists, suggesting a novel pharmacodynamic profile.

E. Anxiolytic Efficacy of TPA023 in Man

The efficacy of TPA023 relative to lorazepam was evaluated at Columbia University in healthy male volunteers using a CO_2-induced anxiety model (http://nyspi.org/AR2002-03/divs/Therapeutics-c.html; accessed on October 16, 2009), although no results from this study have been reported. This experiment was followed by a number of Phase II studies examining the efficacy of TPA023 in generalized anxiety disorder (GAD). However, during the course of these clinical trials it was found that the compound causes cataract formation in rodents following long-term administration, and accordingly the Phase II studies were terminated prior to completion. Nonetheless, pooling of the limited clinical efficacy data that were accumulated before termination suggests an anxiolytic-like effect of TPA023 (Fig. 21). Thus, TPA023

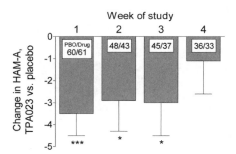

FIGURE 21 Indication of anxiolytic efficacy of TPA023 in GAD. The data show the difference in the Hamilton Anxiety (HAM-A) score in subjects given TPA023 compared to placebo. At week 1 the average change in the HAM-A score is 3.5 points greater in the TPA023 group as compared placebo. These data are an analysis of three separate, two-arm, flexible-dose (1.5–4.5 mg b.i.d. or 3–8 mg b.i.d.), Phase II studies using the extended-release (GEM) formulation of TPA023. All of these studies were terminated prematurely due to the formation of cataracts during long-term rodent toxicity tests. Numbers within each bar indicate the number of subjects in the placebo (PBO) and TPA023 (drug) groups, respectively. Error bars represent SEM, *, and *** $= p < 0.05$ and $p < 0.001$, respectively.

decreases the Hamilton-A score to a significantly greater extent than placebo at weeks 1, 2, and 3 in the 4-week study. While the difference is not significant at week 4, this is probably due, in part, to the relatively small number of subjects completing these trials (36 on placebo and 33 on TPA023).

F. TPA023 in Schizophrenia

Non-selective, benzodiazepine site full agonists alone have little effect on the core symptoms of schizophrenia (Hollister, 1981; Volz, Khorsand, Gillies, & Leucht, 2007; Wolkowitz & Pickar, 1992). However, an open-label study of the non-selective partial agonist bretazenil suggests antipsychotic efficacy for such compounds (Delini-Stula & Berdah-Tordjman, 1996), suggesting that compounds with efficacy and/or selectivity profiles different from non-selective full agonists may have clinical utility in this disorder.

It is conceivable that the sedating properties of classical benzodiazepine anxiolytics may mask any beneficial effects mediated by other GABA$_A$ subtypes. Hence, a compound that modulates GABA$_A$ receptors but is relatively non-sedating may permit relatively high levels of occupancy at subtypes that may be involved in the pathophysiology of schizophrenia. More specifically, agonism at the α2 and/or α3 subtypes might play a role in schizophrenia. Evidence supporting a possible beneficial effect of certain types of benzodiazepine site agonists in the treatment of schizophrenia includes the fact that the α2 subtype is located on the initial axon initial segment of the large pyramidal neurons, presumably exerting an inhibitory influence on their output (Lewis, Hashimoto, & Volk, 2005). Furthermore, there is an increased expression of α2-containing GABA$_A$ receptors in the axon initial segment in the portmortem dorsolateral prefrontal cortex of subjects with schizophrenia (Volk et al., 2002), which may reflect a compensatory response to a loss of GABA input from the chandelier cell axon terminals (Lewis et al., 2005). Accordingly, an enhancement of the function of the α2-containing GABA$_A$ receptors in schizophrenia has been hypothesized to restore some of the loss of synchronization of cortical output that is thought to occur in schizophrenia and might underlie deficits in working memory function (Lewis et al., 2005). Such findings suggest a GABA$_A$ α2 subtype-selective agonist might improve cognitive function in schizophrenia.

In addition to the α2 subtype, mice lacking the α3 subunit display a deficit in sensorimotor gating, which is a characteristic of schizophrenia, as judged by an appreciable attenuation in the pre-pulse inhibition of an auditory startle response (Yee et al., 2005). As this deficit is normalized by the dopamine D2-receptor antagonist haloperidol, α3 knock-out mice appear to display a hyperdopaminergic phenotype (Yee et al., 2005).

Taken together these findings have led to the hypothesis that selectively enhancing the function of α3-containing GABA$_A$ receptors may be an effective strategy for the treatment of schizophrenia (Möhler, 2007).

TPA023 was evaluated in a small, 15-subject trial to evaluate its efficacy as a treatment for the cognitive deficits associated with schizophrenia (Lewis et al., 2008). Although TPA023 has no effect on Brief Psychiatric Rating Scale scores, there is a tendency for it to improve performance in each of the AX Continuous Performance (Fig. 22), N-back, and Preparing to Overcome Prepotency tasks. Because of the small sample size, this study was under-powered, making it not possible to conclusively establish efficacy in this regard. In addition, EEG measurements made during the Preparing to Over-come Prepotency task reveal a trend toward increased frontal area gamma band power in TPA023- compared to placebo-treated subjects. This finding is consistent with the hypothesis that enhanced signaling through the α2 subtype may improve cognitive impairments associated with the dysfunction of the dorsolateral prefrontal cortex in schizophrenia subjects (Akbarian, 2008; Lewis et al., 2008).

It should be noted that because TPA023 displays only weak partial agonist efficacy at the α2 and α3 subtypes it will produce only a relatively modest modulation of α2- and/or α3-containing GABA$_A$ receptors. This relatively low level of intrinsic efficacy may be insufficient to fully test whether

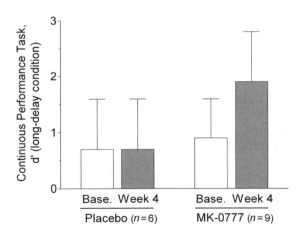

FIGURE 22   Trend for TPA023 to increase performance in the Continuous Performance Task in a small population of schizophrenia subjects. Patients received either placebo ($n = 6$) or TPA023 ($n = 9$) over a 4-week period. The TPA023 was administered b.i.d. at a dose of 3 mg during week 1, 5 mg during week 2, and 8 mg during weeks 3 and 4. Performance on the AX Continuous Performance, N-back, and Preparing to Overcome Prepotency tasks was assessed prior to (baseline) or 4 weeks after treatment with either placebo or TPA023. Performance on the Continuous Performance Task was identical at baseline (base.) and after 4 weeks of placebo (mean ± SD = 0.7 ± 0.9) whereas with the TPA023-treated subjects there was an increase from 0.9 ± 0.7 to 1.9 ± 0.9. Data redrawn from Lewis et al. (2008).

such a modulation of GABAergic function is sufficient to robustly increase cognitive performance in a small population of schizophrenia patients. Accordingly, the effects of TPA023 are currently being evaluated in a larger group of subjects as part of the National Institute of Mental Health-sponsored Treatment Units for Research on Neurocognition and Schizophrenia (TURNS) (ClinicalTrials.gov identifier NCT00505076; October 16).

G. Additional Clinical Studies

TPA023 (under the designation L-000830982) has also been evaluated at the Center for Human Drug Research as a treatment for Essential Tremor (http://www.trialregister.nl/trialreg/admin/rctview.asp?TC=414; accessed on October 16, 2009). To date, no results from this work have been published.

VI. Additional Anxioselective and Other GABA$_A$ Receptor Modulators

Clinical and preclinical data point to the potential for α2/α3 selective GABA$_A$ modulators, such as TPA023, to be anxioselective. However, studies with other compounds have yielded conflicting findings (e.g., ocinaplon, DOV 51892, and adipiplon), whereas other agents (e.g., NS11394 and TPA023B) have provided data consistent with this hypothesis. The *in vitro* affinity and efficacy of these compounds are summarized in Fig. 23.

A. Ocinaplon and DOV 51892

Although data from point-mutated transgenic mice and subtype-selective GABA$_A$ modulators suggest strongly that α1 subtype agonist activity must be avoided to eliminate sedation, data reported on ocinaplon, DOV 15982 and, possibly, CL-218,872 highlight that the hypothesis that "α1 = sedation" is probably an over simplification. Hence, ocinaplon (also known as CL 273,547 and DOV 273,547; Vanover & Barrett, 1994) is a pyrazolopyrimidine with a higher efficacy at the α1 compared to α2, α3, and α5 subtypes (Fig. 23A; Lippa et al., 2005). In a subsequent publication, this α1-selective efficacy was somewhat diminished (Berezhnoy et al., 2008) but more importantly the absolute efficacy at α1-containing GABA$_A$ receptors approaches that of a full agonist. Despite this marked α1 agonist efficacy, ocinaplon is anxioselective in rats and primates with, for example, a 32-fold separation between anxiolytic-like and sedative-like doses in rhesus monkey (Lippa et al., 2005). In a clinical trial conducted in patients with GAD a dose of 240 mg/day ocinaplon produces a reduction in the Hamilton Anxiety Scale that is significantly greater than placebo without causing

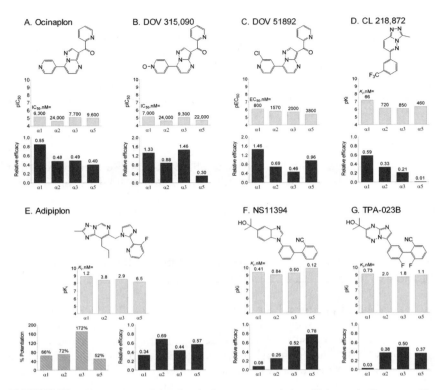

FIGURE 23 Comparison of the chemical structure, and the affinity and efficacy profiles of a variety of GABA$_A$ receptor subtype-selective compounds with novel pharmacological profiles. Illustrated in the upper panel are the affinities expressed as pIC$_{50}$, pEC$_{50}$, or pK$_i$, with the value above each bar representing the affinity in nanomolars. The lower panel shows the relative efficacy at each GABA$_A$ receptor subtype. The binding affinity of each compound was assessed using [³H]flumazenil radioligand binding, with data being expressed either as IC$_{50}$ (ocinaplon and DOV 315,090: Berezhnoy et al., 2008) or K$_i$ values (CL 218,872, adipiplon, NS11394, and TPA023B: Smith et al., 2001, Krause et al., 2007; Mirza et al., 2008; Atack, Hallett, et al., 2009). In the case of DOV 51892, the binding affinity at the different GABA$_A$ receptor subtypes has not been reported, and therefore the functional affinity (EC$_{50}$) is illustrated. However, the functional affinity (ranging from 0.8 to 3.8 μM) is comparable to the binding affinity, IC$_{50}$ of 1.5 μM, of DOV 51892 at rat cerebellar membranes (Popik et al., 2006). Efficacy data are expressed relative to either diazepam for ocinaplon, DOV 315,090, DOV 51892, and NS11394 (Lippa et al., 2005; Popik et al., 2006; Berezhnoy et al., 2008; Mirza et al., 2008), relative to lorazepam for adipiplon (Krause et al., 2007) or relative to chlordiazepoxide for TPA023B (Atack, Hallett, et al., 2009). For all compounds except CL 218,872, efficacy was measured electrophysiologically. Efficacy data for CL 218,872 was assessed using a [³⁶Cl] flux assay and is expressed relative to chlordiazepoxide (Smith et al., 2001). In this assay, the partial agonist efficacies of CL 218,872 at the α1(0.59) and α3 (0.21) subtypes are similar to those reported using electrophysiological assays (Wafford, Whiting, & Kemp, 1993).

appreciable sedation (Lippa et al., 2005). Ultimately, clinical studies of ocinaplon were halted due to elevations in liver function tests.

The lack of sedation reported for ocinaplon cannot be due to the pharmacological effects being exerted by the major metabolite DOV 315,090, since this compound has even greater α1 efficacy than the parent compound (Fig. 23B) (Berezhnoy et al., 2008). The fact that α1 subtype efficacy is not necessarily associated with sedation is further emphasized by findings with DOV 51892, a structural analog of ocinaplon (Chen, Yang, & Tobak, 2008). Whereas ocinaplon is nearly a full agonist at the α1 subtype, DOV 51892 has greater α1 efficacy and may be classified as a super-agonist at this subtype (Fig. 23C; Basile, Lippa, & Skolnick, 2006; Popik et al., 2006). Moreover, DOV 51892 is a full agonist at α5- and a partial agonist at the α2- and α3-containing GABA$_A$ receptors. Despite the fact that DOV 51892 is an α1 super-agonist, it is an anxiolytic without causing pronounced motor effects or myorelaxation in preclinical species (Popik et al., 2006).

The observation that α1 efficacy is not associated with sedation is unrelated to the fact that both ocinaplon and DOV 51892 are pyrazolo-pyrimidine structures since similar effects have been reported with the triazolopyridazine CL-218,872 (Fig. 23D). The differential affinity of this compound for high- and low-affinity binding sites in rat brain is the basis for the original description of the heterogeneity of benzodiazepines sites, the so-called Type I and Type II (also known as BZ$_1$ and BZ$_2$ or ω1 and ω2) benzodiazepine binding sites (Klepner, Lippa, Benson, Sano, & Beer, 1979; Lippa, Coupet, et al., 1979; Lippa, Critchett, et al., 1979). Subsequently, it became apparent that the Type I benzodiazepine sites correspond to GABA$_A$ receptors containing an α1 subunit whereas the Type II binding sites comprise the combined population of α2-, α3-, and α5-containing GABA$_A$ receptors (Sieghart, 1995). Despite being α1-preferring, CL 218,872 was initially reported to produce anxiolysis, and anticonvulsant activity, in the absence of the sedation (Lippa, Coupet, et al., 1979; Lippa, Meyerson, & Beer, 1982), although the anxioselective nature of CL 218,872, particularly its non-sedating properties, was not observed by others (File, Pellow, & Wilks, 1985; McElroy, Fleming, & Feldman, 1985; Oakley, Jones, & Straughan, 1984). Nevertheless, the preclinical and clinical data with ocinaplon and DOV 51892 remain paradoxical as both have a marked degree of α1 efficacy (Fig. 23) yet neither produces overt sedation. In contrast, zolpidem, which like CL 218,872 is also α1-preferring, is used clinically as a hypnotic rather than as an anxiolytic (Benavides et al., 1988). One possible explanation for the lack of concordance between the apparent effect of ocinaplon and DOV 51892 at the α1 subtype and their clinical profile is that the *in vitro* measurement of intrinsic efficacy at recombinant GABA$_A$ receptors may not reflect the *in vivo* response (Chen et al., 2008).

B. Adipiplon

While ocinaplon and DOV 51892 highlight uncertainties over the role of the α1 subtype in mediating anxiolytic and/or sedative properties of GABA$_A$ receptors modulators, the hypnotic properties of the putative α3-selective compound adipiplon (NG2-73) raises issues about the potential role of the α3 subtype in sedation. Adipiplon is a triazolopyrimidine that is claimed to be α3-preferring (Krause et al., 2007) based on the fact that it produces a much greater potentiation of the current evoked by 2.5 µM GABA at α3- compared to α1-, α2-, or α5-containing GABA$_A$ receptors (Krause et al., 2007) (Fig. 23E, lower left panel). However, the relatively non-selective benzodiazepines lorazepam, triazolam, diazepam, and alprazolam also produced a much greater potentiation of GABA-induced currents at the α3 compared to α1, α2, and α5 subtypes (Krause et al., 2007) such that when efficacy is expressed relative to lorazepam, adipiplon loses its apparent α3 selectivity (Fig. 23E, lower right panel). Similarly, the intrinsic efficacy profile of adipiplon is that of a non-selective partial agonist when expressed relative to either diazepam or alprazolam rather than lorazepam. Therefore, when efficacy is expressed relative to a non-selective benzodiazepine rather than as a per cent potentiation, adipiplon does not appear to be α3-preferring but rather appears more as a non-selective partial agonist.

Adipiplon is a potent sedative hypnotic in rats (Rajachandran et al., 2007) with a minimum effective oral dose of 0.6 mg/kg p.o. corresponding to a plasma concentration of 2.6 ng/mL (Rajachandran et al., 2007). In a transient insomnia model in healthy volunteers, a 1 mg dose of adipiplon produces a 42% reduction in the latency to persistent sleep at a dose equivalent to a plasma C_{max} of 2.1 ng/mL, although the compound has a relatively short half-life of around ~1 h in man (Sprenger et al., 2007). In subsequent clinical studies, a number of undesirable next-day effects occurred which may be related to the bilayer tablet formation used to improve its plasma pharmacokinetics. Subsequently, the clinical development of adipiplon was terminated (press release, July 13, 2008; www.neurogen.com). A structurally related compound, NDT 9530021 (Anonymous, 2007), is described as having a similar efficacy profile to adipiplon (Kehne et al., 2007) and has potent anxiolytic and anticonvulsant properties (Kehne et al., 2007; Smith et al., 2007). Another analog, NG2-83, is reported to produce a marked anxiolytic response in the rhesus monkey with a minimum effective dose 100-fold lower than that which produced sedation (Anonymous, 2008).

C. Additional α2/α3 Efficacy-Selective Compounds

Preclinical data for the benzimidazole NS11394 indicates it has greater efficacy at the α2 and α3 compared to α1 subtype, making it similar to TPA023 and TPA023B in this regard (Figs. 9E, 23F, and 23G) (Mirza et al.,

2008; Munro et al., 2008). NS11394 is also a potent anxiolytic in rodent anxiety models but with a much reduced side-effect profile as compared to conventional benzodiazepines as regards sedation, ethanol interaction, and ataxia (Mirza et al., 2008). Furthermore, this compound produces robust analgesia in a variety of spontaneous and inflammatory pain models (Munro et al., 2008). However, NS11394 also has appreciable efficacy at the α5 subtype, which may be associated with memory impairment noted in mice and rats (Mirza et al., 2008).

A follow-up compound to TPA023, designated TPA023B, has been described (Atack, Hallett, et al., 2009; Kohut & Ator, 2008; Van Laere et al., 2008). An imidazotriazine (Fig. 23G) related to NS 2710 (Russell et al., 2006; Atack, 2009), TPA023B shares some structural similarities with NS11394 (Fig. 23F). A single oral dose of 1.5 mg produces receptor occupancy of around 50% at 5 and 24 h later (Van Laere et al., 2008), consistent with the plasma pharmacokinetics of this compound (Atack, Hallett, et al., 2009). As this level of occupancy is achieved without pronounced sedation (Van Laere et al., 2008), in this respect TPA023B is similar to TPA023. Nevertheless, TPA023B differs from TPA023 in possessing greater intrinsic efficacy (compare Fig. 9E and 23G) and in relation to the drug-discrimination paradigm (Kohut & Ator, 2008). In this assay, rats can be trained to discriminate TPA023 but not TPA023B, which is surprising as the greater intrinsic efficacy of TPA023B compared to TPA023 suggests that the interoceptive cues produced by the former would be greater than the latter.

D. Additional GABA$_A$ Modulators

Two additional compounds, AZD6280 and AZD7325, the structures and *in vitro* and *in vivo* properties of which remain unknown, are currently under clinical evaluation by AstraZeneca. The safety and tolerability of AZD6280 in being evaluated in Phase I studies whereas AZD7325 is being evaluated for proof of concept in two Phase II studies for efficacy in GAD, one assessing AZD7325 versus placebo (ClinicalTrials.gov identifier NCT00808249) and another assessing AZD7325 versus placebo and lorazepam (ClinicalTrials.gov identifier NCT00807937). Although the mechanism of action of these compounds has not been reported, the fact that the receptor occupancy of each compound has been assessed in man using [^{11}C]flumazenil PET studies suggests they act through the benzodiazepine binding site.

VII. Conclusion

TPA023 is a triazolopyridazine that binds with equivalent affinity to α1-, α2-, α3-, and α5-containing GABA$_A$ receptors subtypes but preferentially potentiates the effects of GABA at the α2 and α3 subtypes, being without efficacy at the α1- or α5-containing receptors. Preclinical studies demonstrate that TPA023 has anxiolytic efficacy in rodent and primate models without causing sedation, myorelaxation, or ataxia. Furthermore, TPA023 displays no abuse liability in baboons nor are there any pronounced signs of drug withdrawal after 1 month of continuous administration. Although the half-life of TPA023 is relatively short in laboratory animals (0.6–1.5 h), it is longer in humans, especially when administered in an extended-release capsule. TPA023 displays good receptor occupancy in man and has pharmacodynamic effects on saccadic eye movement and body posture that differentiate it from lorazepam. These data are consistent with its reduced sedation liability. Post hoc analysis of three Phase II studies that were terminated early due to preclinical toxicity suggests that TPA023 may have anxiolytic efficacy in GAD. More recently, data suggest that TPA023 may be useful in the treatment of cognitive deficits in schizophrenia (Lewis et al., 2008). The data of Lewis and colleagues represent an elegant, hypothesis-driven approach to the development of novel therapeutics for schizophrenia based on a rationale derived from histological examination of cortical neuronal circuitry in schizophrenia. These findings indicate a potential for subtype-selective $GABA_A$ modulators to have unique pharmacological properties, and therefore novel clinical profiles.

Acknowledgments

The author wishes to acknowledge the numerous people within the Merck Research Laboratories who contributed to the work described in the present manuscript. These contributors include the author's former colleagues in the Departments of Molecular and Cellular Biology, Biochemistry, Medicinal Chemistry, and Drug Metabolism and Pharmacokinetics at the Neuroscience Research Centre, Harlow, United Kingdom, as well as in the Department of Pharmaceutical Research and Development, Hoddesdon, United Kingdom, the Departments of Drug Metabolism and Imaging Research at West Point, Pennsylvania, and the Department of Clinical Pharmacology, Blue Bell, Pennsylvania.

Conflict of Interest: Dr. Atack was formerly an employee of Merck & Co., Inc., but no longer has any financial holdings or considerations related to that employment and has no other conflicts of interest.

References

Abadie, P., Rioux, P., Scatton, B., Zarifian, E., Barré, L., Patat, A. et al. (1996). Central benzodiazepine receptor occupancy by zolpidem in the human brain as assessed by positron emission tomography. *European Journal of Pharmacology, 295,* 35–44.

Akbarian, S. (2008). Editorial—Restoring GABAergic signaling and neuronal synchrony in schizophrenia. *American Journal of Psychiatry, 165,* 1507–1509.

Anonymous. (2007). NME digest. *Drug News & Perspectives, 20,* 635–642.

Anonymous. (2008). Psychopharmacologic drugs. *Drug Data Report, 30,* 482–489.

Atack, J. R. (2003). Anxioselective compounds acting at the GABA$_A$ receptor benzodiazepine binding site. *Current Drug Targets—CNS and Neurological Disorders, 2*, 213–232.

Atack, J. R. (2005). The benzodiazepine binding site of GABA$_A$ receptors as a target for the development of novel anxiolytics. *Expert Opinion on Investigational Drugs, 14*, 601–618.

Atack, J. R. (2009). GABA$_A$ receptor subtype-selective modulators. I. α2/α3-selective agonists as non-sedating anxiolytics. *Current Topics in Medicinal Chemistry*, in press.

Atack, J. R., Bayley, P. J., Seabrook, G. R., Wafford, K. A., McKernan, R. M., & Dawson, G. R. (2006). L-655,708 enhances cognition in rats but is not proconvulsant at a dose selective for α5-containing GABA$_A$ receptors. *Neuropharmacology, 51*, 1023–1029.

Atack, J. R., Fryer, T. D., Burns, H. D., Scott-Stevens, P., Gibson, R., Beech, J. S., et al. (2009). Benzodiazepine binding site occupancy by the novel GABA$_A$ receptor subtype-selective drug 7-(1,1-dimethylethyl)-6-(2-ethyl-2H-1,2,4-triazol-3-ylmethoxy)-3-(2-fluorophenyl)-1,2,4-triazolo[4,3-b]pyridazine (TPA023) in rats, primates and man. *Journal of Pharmacology and Experimental Therapeutics*, in press.

Atack, J. R., Hallett, D., Tye, S., Wafford, K. A., Ryan, C., Sanabria-Bohórquez, S. M., et al. (2009) Preclinical and clinical pharmacology of TPA023B, A GABA$_A$ receptor α2/α3 subtype-selective agonist. *Journal of Psychopharmacology*, in press

Atack, J. R., Hutson, P. H., Collinson, N., Marshall, G., Bentley, G., Moyes, C., et al. (2005). Anxiogenic properties of an inverse agonist selective for α3 subunit-containing GABA$_A$ receptors. *British Journal of Pharmacology, 144*, 357–366.

Atack, J. R., Scott-Stevens, P., Beech, J. S., Fryer, T. D., Hughes, J. L., Cleij, M. C., et al. (2007). Comparison of lorazepam [7-chloro-5-(2-chlorophenyl)-1,3-dihydro-3-hydroxy-2H-1,4-benzodiazepin-2-one] occupancy of rat brain γ-aminobutyric acid$_A$ receptors measured using in vivo [^{3}H]flumazenil (8-fluoro 5,6-dihydro-5-methyl-6-oxo-4H-imidazo[1,5-a][1,4]benzodiazepine-3-carboxylic acid ethyl ester) binding and [^{11}C]flumazenil micropositron emission tomography. *Journal of Pharmacology and Experimental Therapeutics, 320*, 1030–1037.

Atack, J. R., Wafford, K. A., Street, L. J., Dawson, G. R., Tye, S., McKernan, R. M., et al. (2009). MRK-409, a GABA$_A$ receptor subtype-selective agonist, is a non-sedating anxiolytic in preclinical species but causes sedation in man. *Journal of Psychopharmacology*, in press.

Atack, J. R., Wafford, K. A., Tye, S. J., Cook, S. M., Sohal, B., Pike, A., et al. (2006). TPA023 [7-(1,1-dimethylethyl)-6-(2-ethyl-2H-1,2,4-triazol-3-ylmethoxy)-3-(2-fluorophenyl)-1,2,4-triazolo[4,3-b]pyridazine], an agonist selective for α2- and α3-containing GABA$_A$ receptors, is a non-sedating anxiolytic in rodents and primates. *Journal of Pharmacology and Experimental Therapeutics, 316*, 410–422.

Ator, N. A. (2005). Contributions of GABA$_A$ receptor subtype selectivity to abuse liability and dependence potential of pharmacological treatments for anxiety and sleep disorders. *CNS Spectrums, 10*, 31–39.

Ator, N. A., Atack, J. R., Hargreaves, R. J., Burns, H. D., & Dawson, G. R. (2009). Reducing abuse liability of GABA$_A$/benzodiazepine ligands via selective efficacy at α$_1$ and α$_{2/3}$ subtypes. Submitted.

Ballard, T. M., Knoflach, F., Prinssen, E., Borroni, E., Vivian, J. A., Basile, J., et al. (2009). RO4938581, a novel cognitive enhancer acting at GABA$_A$ α5 subunit-containing receptors. *Psychopharmacology, 202*, 207–223.

Barnard, E. A., Skolnick, P., Olsen, R. W., Mohler, H., Sieghart, W., Biggio, G., et al. (1998). International Union of Pharmacology. XV. Subtypes of γ-aminobutyric acid$_A$ receptors: Classification on the basis of subunit structure and receptor function. *Pharmacological Reviews, 50*, 291–313.

Basile, A. S., Lippa, A. S., & Skolnick, P. (2006). GABA$_A$ receptor modulators as anxioselective anxiolytics. *Drug Discovery. Today, 3*, 475–481.

Bell, G. D. (2002). Premedication, preparation, and surveillance. *Endoscopy, 34*, 2–12.

Benavides, J., Peny, B., Dubois, A., Perrault, G., Morel, E., Zivkovic, B., et al. (1988). In vivo interaction of zolpidem with central benzodiazepine (BZD) binding sites (as labeled by [^{3}H]Ro 15-1788) in the mouse brain. Preferential affinity of zolpidem for the ω_1 (BZD$_1$) subtype. *Journal of Pharmacology and Experimental Therapeutics, 245,* 1033–1041.

Benson, J. A., Löw, K., Keist, R., Mohler, H., & Rudolph, U. (1998). Pharmacology of recombinant γ-aminobutyric acid$_A$ receptors rendered diazepam-insensitive by point-mutated α-subunits. *FEBS Letters, 431,* 400–404.

Berezhnoy, D., Gravielle, M. C., Downing, S., Kostakis, E., Basile, A. S., Skolnick, P., et al. (2008). Pharmacological properties of DOV 315,090, an ocinaplon metabolite. *BMC Pharmacology, 8,* 11.

Blin, O., Jacquet, A., Callamand, S., Jouve, E., Habib, M., Gayraud, D., et al. (1999). Pharmacokinetic-pharmacodynamic analysis of mnesic effects of lorazepam in healthy volunteers. *British Journal of Clinical Pharmacology, 48,* 510–512.

Bonetti, E. P., Pieri, L., Cumin, R., Schaffner, R., Pieri, M., Gamzu, E. R., et al. (1982). Benzodiazepine antagonist Ro 15-1788: Neurological and behavioral effects. *Psychopharmacology, 78,* 8–18.

Carling, R. W., Madin, A., Guiblin, A., Russell, M. G. N., Moore, K. W., Mitchinson, A., et al. (2005). 7-(1,1-Dimethylethyl)-6-(2-ethyl-2*H*-1,2,4-triazol-3-ylmethoxy)-3-(2-fluorophenyl)-1,2,4-triazolo[4,3-*b*]pyridazine: A functionally selective γ-aminobutyric acid$_A$ (GABA$_A$) α2/α3-subtype selective agonist that exhibits potent anxiolytic activity but is not sedating in animal models. *Journal of Medicinal Chemistry, 48,* 7089–7092.

Carling, R. W., Moore, K. W., Street, L. J., Wild, D., Isted, C., Leeson, P. D., et al. (2004). 3-Phenyl-6-(2-pyridyl)methyloxy-1,2,4-triazolo[3,4-*a*]phthalazines and analogues: High-affinity γ-aminobutyric acid-A benzodiazepine receptor ligands with α2, α3, and α5-subtype binding selectivity over α1. *Journal of Medicinal Chemistry, 47,* 1807–1822.

Chambers, M. S., Atack, J. R., Broughton, H. B., Collinson, N., Cook, S., Dawson, G. R., et al. (2003). Identification of a novel, selective GABA$_A$ α5 receptor inverse agonist which enhances cognition. *Journal of Medicinal Chemistry, 46,* 2227–2240.

Chen, Z., Yang, J., & Tobak, A. (2008). Designing new treatments for depression and anxiety. *IDrugs, 11,* 189–197.

Cheng, V. Y., Martin, L. J., Elliott, E. M., Kim, J. H., Mount, H. T. J., Taverna, F. A., et al. (2006). α5GABA$_A$ receptors mediate the amnestic but not sedative-hypnotic effects of the general anesthetic etomidate. *Journal of Neuroscience, 26,* 3713–3720.

Collinson, N., Kuenzi, F. M., Jarolimek, W., Maubach, K. A., Cothliff, R., Sur, C., et al. (2002). Enhanced learning and memory and altered GABAergic synaptic transmission in mice lacking the α5 subunit of the GABA$_A$ receptor. *Journal of Neuroscience, 22,* 5572–5580.

Crestani, F., Keist, R., Fritschy, J.-M., Benke, D., Vogt, K., Prut, L., et al. (2002). Trace fear conditioning involves hippocampal α5 GABA$_A$ receptors. *Proceedings of the National Academy of Sciences of the United States of America, 99,* 8980–8985.

Dawson, G. R., Maubach, K. A., Collinson, N., Cobain, M., Everitt, B. J., MacLeod, A. M., et al. (2006). An inverse agonist selective for α5 subunit-containing GABA$_A$ receptors enhances cognition. *Journal of Pharmacology and Experimental Therapeutics, 316,* 1335–1345.

de Haas, S. L., de Visser, S. J., van der Post, J. P., de Smet, M., Schoemaker, R. C., Rijnbeek, B., et al. (2007). Pharmacodynamic and pharmacokinetic effects of TPA023, a GABA$_A$ α$_{2,3}$ subtype-selective agonist, compared to lorazepam and placebo in healthy volunteers. *Journal of Psychopharmacology, 21,* 374–383.

de Haas, S. L., de Visser, S. J., van der Post, J. P., Schoemaker, R. C., van Dyck, K., Murphy, M. G., et al. (2008). Pharmacodynamic and pharmacokinetic effects of MK-0343, a GABA$_A$ α$_{2,3}$ subtype selective agonist, compared to lorazepam and placebo in healthy male volunteers. *Journal of Psychopharmacology, 22,* 24–32.

Delini-Stula, A., & Berdah-Tordjman, D. (1996). Antipsychotic effects of bretazenil, a partial benzodiazepine agonist in acute schizophrenia—A study group report. *Journal of Psychiatric Research, 30,* 239–250.

Dias, R., Sheppard, W. F. A., Fradley, R. L., Garrett, E. M., Stanley, J. L., Tye, S. J., et al. (2005). Evidence for a significant role of α3-containing GABA$_A$ receptors in mediating the anxiolytic effects of benzodiazepines. *Journal of Neuroscience, 25,* 10682–10688.

File, S. E., Pellow, S., & Wilks, L. (1985). The sedative effects of CL 218,872, like those of chlordiazepoxide, are reversed by benzodiazepine antagonists. *Psychopharmacology (Berlin), 85,* 295–300.

Fischer, B. D., Atack, J. R., Platt, D. M., Pike, A., Reynolds, D. S., Dawson, G. R., et al. (2009). Evaluation of the role of GABA$_A$ receptors containing α3 subunits in the therapeutic and unwanted side effects of benzodiazepine-type drugs in monkeys. Submitted.

Fritschy, J.-M., & Möhler, H. (1995). GABA$_A$-receptor heterogeneity in the adult rat brain: Differential regional and cellular distribution of seven major subunits. *Journal of Comparative Neurology, 359,* 154–194.

Fujita, M., Woods, S. W., Verhoeff, N. P. L. G., Abi-Dargham, A., Baldwin, R. M., Zoghbi, S. S., et al. (1999). Changes of benzodiazepine receptors during chronic benzodiazepine administration in humans. *European Journal of Pharmacology, 368,* 161–172.

Gorman, J. K. (2005). Benzodiazepines: Taking the good with the bad and the ugly. *CNS Spectrums, 10,* 14–15.

Greenblatt, D. J., Harmatz, J. S., Dorsey, C., & Shader, R. I. (1988). Comparative single-dose kinetics and dynamics of lorazepam, alprazolam, prazepam, and placebo. *Clinical Pharmacology and Therapeutics, 44,* 326–334.

Griffiths, R. R., & Weerts, E. M. (1997). Benzodiazepine self-administration in humans and laboratory animals—implications for problems of long-term use and abuse. *Psychopharmacology, 134,* 1–37.

Haigh, J. R. M., & Feely, M. (1988). Tolerance to the anticonvulsant effect of benzodiazepines. *Trends In Pharmacological Sciences, 9,* 361–366.

Harris, D., Clayton, T., Cook, J., Sahbaie, P., Halliwell, R. F., Furtmüller, R., et al. (2008). Selective influence on contextual memory: Physiochemical properties associated with selectivity of benzodiazepine ligands at GABA$_A$ receptors containing the α5 subunit. *Journal of Medicinal Chemistry, 51,* 3788–3803.

Hollister, L. E. (1981). Benzodiazepines—an overview. *British Journal of Clinical Pharmacology, 11,* 117S–119S.

Hsieh, J. Y.-K., Lin, L., & Matuszewski, B. K. (2004). A semi-automated 96-well solid phase extraction and high performance liquid chromatographic determination of a selective GABA-A receptor agonist in human and rat plasma using fluorescence detection. *Journal of Liquid Chromatography & Related Technologies, 27,* 2329–2341.

Hunkeler, W., Möhler, H., Pieri, L., Polc, P., Bonetti, E. P., Cumin, R., et al. (1981). Selective antagonists of benzodiazepines. *Nature, 290,* 514–516.

Juang, R. H., & Storey, D. (2003). Correlation of characteristics of gel extrusion module (GEM) tablet formulation and drug dissolution rate. *Journal of Controlled Rrelease, 89,* 375–385.

Kehne, J. E., McCloskey, T. C., Peterson, S., Near, K., Bradshaw, E., Natoli, J., et al. (2007). IV. Further pharmacological exploration of α3-subunit preferring GABA$_A$ receptor partial allosteric activators: Evidence for anxiolysis and reduced sedative tolerance of NDT 9530021. Program No. AAA21. 2007 Neuroscience Meeting Planner. San Diego, CA: *Society for Neuroscience* Online.

Klepner, C. A., Lippa, A. S., Benson, D. I., Sano, M. C., & Beer, B. (1979). Resolution of two biochemically and pharmacologically distinct benzodiazepine receptors. *Pharmacology, Biochemistry and Behavior, 11,* 457–462.

Knabl, J., Witschi, R., Hösl, K., Reinold, H., Zeilhofer, U. B., Ahmadi, S., et al. (2008). Reversal of pathological pain through specific spinal GABA$_A$ receptor subtypes. *Nature, 451,* 330–334.

Knabl, J., Zeilhofer, U. B., Crestani, F., Rudolph, U., & Zeilhofer, H. U. (2009). Genuine antihyperalgesia by systemic diazepam revealed by experiments in GABA$_A$ receptor point-mutated mice. *Pain, 141*, 233–238.

Kohut, S. J., & Ator, N. A. (2008). Novel discriminative stimulus effects of TPA023B, subtype-selective γ-aminobutyric-acid$_A$/benzodiazepine modulator: Comparisons with zolpidem, lorazepam, and TPA023. *Pharmacology Biochemistry & Behavior, 90*, 65–73.

Krause, J. E., Matchett, M., Crandall, M., Yu, J., Baltazar, C., Brodbeck, R. M., et al. (2007). I. Preclinical characterization in vitro of NG2-73 as a potent and selective partial allosteric activator of GABA$_A$ receptors with predominant efficacy at the α3 subunit. Program No. AAA26. 2007 Neuroscience Meeting Planner. San Diego, CA: Society for Neuroscience Online.

Lader, M., Tylee, A., & Donoghue, J. (2009). Withdrawing benzodiazepines in primary care. *CNS Drugs, 23*, 19–34.

Lewis, D. A., Cho, R. Y., Carter, C. S., Eklund, K., Forster, S., Kelly, M. A., et al. (2008). Subunit-selective modulation of GABA type A receptor neurotransmission and cognition in schizophrenia. *American Journal of Psychiatry, 165*, 1585–1593.

Lewis, D. A., Hashimoto, T., & Volk, D. W. (2005). Cortical inhibitory neurons and schizophrenia. *Nature Reviews Neuroscience, 6*, 312–324.

Lingford-Hughes, A., Wilson, S. J., Feeney, A., Grasby, P. G., & Nutt, D. J. (2005). A proof-of-concept study using [^{11}C]flumazenil PET to demonstrate that pagoclone is a partial agonist. *Psychopharmacology, 180*, 789–791.

Lippa, A., Czobor, P., Stark, J., Beer, B., Kostakis, E., Gravielle, M., et al. (2005). Selective anxiolysis produced by ocinaplon, a GABA$_A$ receptor modulator. *Proceedings of the National Academy of Sciences of the United States of America, 102*, 7380–7385.

Lippa, A. S., Coupet, J., Greenblatt, E. N., Klepner, C. A., & Beer, B. (1979). A synthetic non-benzodiazepine ligand for benzodiazepine receptors: A probe for investigating neuronal substrates of anxiety. *Pharmacology, Biochemistry and Behavior, 11*, 99–106.

Lippa, A. S., Critchett, D., Sano, M. C., Klepner, C. A., Greenblatt, E. N., Coupet, J., et al. (1979) Benzodiazepine receptors: Cellular and behavioral characteristics. *Pharmacology, Biochemistry and Behavior, 10*, 831–843.

Lippa, A. S., Meyerson, L. R., & Beer, B. (1982). Molecular substrates of anxiety: Clues from the heterogeneity of benzodiazepine receptors. *Life Sciences, 31*, 1409–1417.

Löw, K., Crestani, F., Keist, R., Benke, D., Brünig, I., Benson, J. A., et al. (2000). Molecular and neuronal substrate for the selective attenuation of anxiety. *Science, 290*, 131–134.

Ma, B., Polsky-Fisher, S. L., Vickers, S., Cui, D., & Rodrigues, A. D. (2007). Cytochrome P450 3A-dependent metabolism of a potent and selective γ-aminobutyric acid$_{A\alpha2/3}$ receptor agonist in vitro: Involvement of cytochrome P450 3A5 displaying biphasic kinetics. *Drug Metabolism and Disposition: The Biological Fate of Chemicals, 35*, 1301–1307.

McCabe, C., Shaw, D., Atack, J. R., Street, L. J., Wafford, K. A., Dawson, G. R., et al. (2004). Subtype-selective GABAergic drugs facilitate extinction of mouse operant behaviour. *Neuropharmacology, 46*, 171–178.

McElroy, J. F., Fleming, R. L., & Feldman, R. S. (1985). A comparison between chlordiazep-oxide and CL 218,872-a synthetic nonbenzodiazepine ligand for benzodiazepine receptors on spontaneous locomotor activity in rats. *Psychopharmacology (Berlin), 85*, 224–226.

McKernan, R. M., Rosahl, T. W., Reynolds, D. S., Sur, C., Wafford, K. A., Atack, J. R., et al. (2000). Sedative but not anxiolytic properties of benzodiazepines are mediated by the GABA$_A$ receptor α1 subtype. *Nature Neuroscience, 3*, 587–592.

Mirza, N. R., Larsen, J. S., Mathiasen, C., Jacobsen, T. A., Munro, G., Erichsen, H. K., et al. (2008). NS11394 [3'-[5-(1-hydroxy-1-methyl-ethyl)-benzoimidazol-1-yl]-biphenyl-2-car-bonitrile], a unique subtype-selective GABA$_A$ receptor positive allosteric modulator: In vitro actions, pharmacokinetic properties and in vivo anxiolytic efficacy. *Journal of Pharmacology and Experimental Therapeutics, 327,* 954–968.

Möhler, H. (2007). Molecular regulation of cognitive functions and developmental plasticity: Impact of GABA$_A$ receptors. *Journal of Neurochemistry, 102,* 1–12.

Moroz, G. (2004). High-potency benzodiazepines: Recent clinical results. *Journal of Clinical Psychiatry, 65*(Suppl 5), 13–18.

Munro, G., Lopez-Garcia, J. A., Rivera-Arconada, I., Erichsen, H. K., Nielsen, E. Ø., Larsen, J. S., et al. (2008). Comparison of the novel subtype-selective GABA$_A$ receptor-positive allosteric modulator NS11394 [3′-[5-(1-hydroxy-1-methyl-ethyl)-benzoimidazol-1-yl]-biphenyl-2-carbonitrile] with diazepam, zolpidem, bretazenil, and gaboxadol in rat models of inflammatory and neuropathic pain. *Journal of Pharmacology and Experimental Therapeutics, 327,* 969–981.

Oakley, N. R., Jones, B. J., & Straughan, D. W. (1984). The benzodiazepine receptor ligand CL218,872 has both anxiolytic and sedative properties in rodents. *Neuropharmacology, 23,* 797–802.

Olsen, R. W., & Sieghart, W. (2008). International Union of Pharmacology. LXX. Subtypes of γ-aminobutyric acid$_A$ receptors: Classification on the basis of subunit composition, pharmacology, and function. Update. *Pharmacological Reviews, 60,* 243–260.

Olsen, R. W., & Sieghart, W. (2009). GABA$_A$ receptors: Subtypes provide diversity of function and pharmacology. *Neuropharmacology, 56,* 141–148.

Pauli, S., Farde, L., Halldin, C., & Sedvall, G. (1991). Occupancy of the central benzodiazepine receptors during benzodiazepine treatment determined by PET. *European Neuropsychopharmacology, 1,* 229–231.

Pirker, S., Schwarzer, C., Wieselthaler, A., Sieghart, W., & Sperk, G. (2000). GABA$_A$ receptors: Immunocytochemical distribution of 13 subunits in the adult brain. *Neuroscience, 101,* 815–850.

Polsky-Fisher, S. L., Vickers, S., Cui, D., Subramanian, R., Arison, B. H., Agrawal, N. G. B., et al. (2006). Metabolism and disposition of a potent and selective GABA-A$_{α2/3}$ receptor agonist in healthy male volunteers. *Drug Metabolism and Disposition: The Biological Fate of Chemicals, 34,* 1004–1011.

Popik, P., Kostakis, E., Krawczyk, M., Nowak, G., Szewczyk, B., Krieter, P., et al. (2006). The anxioselective agent 7-(2-chloropyridin-4-yl)pyrazolo-[1,5-*a*]-pyrimidin-3-yl](pyridin-2-yl)methanone (DOV 51892) is more efficacious than diazepam at enhancing GABA-gated currents at α$_1$ subunit-containing GABA$_A$ receptors. *Journal of Pharmacology and Experimental Therapeutics, 319,* 1244–1252.

Quirk, K., Blurton, P., Fletcher, S., Leeson, P., Tang, F., Mellilo, D., et al. (1996). [^{3}H] L-655,708, a novel ligand selective for the benzodiazepine site of GABA$_A$ receptors which contain the α5 subunit. *Neuropharmacology, 35,* 1331–1335.

Rajachandran, L., McCloskey, T. C., Chock, M., Gambini-Elwood, D., Xie, L., & Kehne, J. H. (2007). II. Preclinical characterization in vivo of NG2-73, an α3-subunit preferring GABA$_A$ receptor partial allosteric activator, as a sedative-hypnotic agent with an improved side effect profile relative to zolpidem. Program No. AAA23. 2007 Neuroscience Meeting Planner. San Diego, CA: Society for Neuroscience. Online.

Rogawski, M. A. (2006). Diverse mechanisms of antiepileptic drugs in the development pipeline. *Epilepsy Research, 69,* 273–294.

Rowlett, J. K., Platt, D. M., Lelas, S., Atack, J. R., & Dawson, G. R. (2005). Different GABA$_A$ receptor subtypes mediate the anxiolytic, abuse-related, and motor effects of benzodiazepine-like drugs in primates. *Proceedings of the National Academy of Sciences of the United States of America, 102,* 915–920.

Rudolph, U., & Möhler, H. (2004). Analysis of GABA$_A$ receptor function and dissection of the pharmacology of benzodiazepines and general anesthetics through mouse genetics. *Annual Review of Pharmacology and Toxicology, 44,* 475–498.

Rudolph, U., & Möhler, H. (2006). GABA-based therapeutic approaches: GABA$_A$ receptor subtype functions. *Current Opinion in Pharmacology, 6,* 18–23.

Rudolph, U., Crestani, F., Benke, D., Brünig, I., Benson, J. A., Fritschy, J.-M., et al. (1999). Benzodiazepine actions mediated by specific γ-aminobutyric acid$_A$ receptor subtypes. *Nature, 401,* 796–800.

Russell, M. G. N., Carling, R. W., Atack, J. R., Bromidge, F. A., Cook, S. M., Hunt, P., et al. (2005). Discovery of functionally selective 7,8,9,10-tetrahydro-7,10-ethano-1,2,4-triazolo [3,4-*a*]phthalazines as GABA$_A$ receptor agonists at the α3 subunit. *Journal of Medicinal Chemistry, 48,* 1367–1383.

Russell, M. G. N., Carling, R. W., Street, L. J., Hallett, D. J., Goodacre, S., Mezzogori, E., et al. (2006). Discovery of imidazo[1,2-*b*][1,2,4]triazines as GABA$_A$ α2/3 subtype selective agonists for the treatment of anxiety. *Journal of Medicinal Chemistry, 49,* 1235–1238.

Sarto-Jackson, I., & Sieghart, W. (2008). Assembly of GABA$_A$ receptors. *Molecular Membrane Biology, 25,* 302–310.

Savić, M. M., Huang, S., Furtmüller, R., Clayton, T., Huck, S., Obradović, D. I., et al. (2008). Are GABA$_A$ receptors containing α5 subunits contributing to the sedative properties of benzodiazepine site agonists? *Neuropsychopharmacology, 33,* 332–339.

Scott-Stevens, P., Atack, J. R., Sohal, B., & Worboys, P. (2005). Rodent pharmacokinetics and receptor occupancy of the GABA$_A$ receptor subtype selective benzodiazepine site ligand L-838417. *Biopharmaceutics and Drug Disposition, 26,* 13–20.

Shinotoh, H., Iyo, M., Yamada, T., Inoue, O., Suzuki, K., Itoh, T., et al. (1989). Detection of benzodiazepine receptor occupancy in the human brain by positron emission tomography. *Psychopharmacology, 99,* 202–207.

Sieghart, W. (1995). Structure and pharmacology of γ-aminobutyric acid$_A$ receptor subtypes. *Pharmacological Reviews, 47,* 181–234.

Sieghart, W. (2006). Structure, pharmacology, and function of GABA$_A$ receptor subtypes. *Advances in Pharmacology, 54,* 231–263.

Sieghart, W., & Sperk, G. (2002). Subunit composition, distribution and function of GABA$_A$ receptor subtypes. *Current Topics in Medicinal Chemistry, 2,* 795–816.

Simon, J., Wakimoto, H., Fujita, N., Lalande, M., & Barnard, E. A. (2004). Analysis of the set of GABA$_A$ receptor genes in the human genome. *Journal of Biological Chemistry, 279,* 41422–41435.

Smith, A. J., Alder, L., Silk, J., Adkins, C., Fletcher, A. E., Scales, T., Kerby, J., Marshall, G., Wafford, K. A., McKernan, R. M., & Atack, J. R. (2001). Effect of a subunit on allosteric modulation of ion channel function in stably expressed human recombinant g-aminobutyric acid$_A$ receptors determined using ^{36}Cl ion flux. *Molecular Pharmacology, 59,* 1108–1118.

Smith, K. D., Srivastava, A. K., Kehne, J. H., Rajachandran, L., Xu, Y., Maynard, G., et al. (2007). V. Further pharmacological exploration of α3-subunit preferring GABA$_A$ receptor partial allosteric activator sedative-hypnotics: Anticonvulsant activity of NDT 9530021 in rats. Program No. AAA24. 2007 Neuroscience Meeting Planner. San Diego, CA: Society for Neuroscience. Online.

Sperk, G., Schwarzer, C., Tsunashima, K., Fuchs, K., & Sieghart, W. (1997). GABA$_A$ receptor subunits in the rat hippocampus I: Immuncytochemical distribution of 13 subunits. *Neuroscience, 80,* 987–1000.

Sprenger, K. J., Aneiro, L., Fung, L., Liu, Y., Changchit, A., Rajachandran, L., et al. (2007). III. Clinical trial data demonstrating sedative-hypnotic efficacy of the α3-subunit preferring GABA$_A$ receptor partial allosteric activator, NG2-73: Translational validity of pharmacokinetic/pharmacodynamic (PK/PD) relationships derived from preclinical studies. Program No. AAA17. 2007 Neuroscience Meeting Planner. San Diego, CA: Society for Neuroscience Online.

Sternbach, L. H. (1979). The benzodiazepine story. *Journal of Medicinal Chemistry*, 22, 1–7.

Tarzia, G., Occelli, E., Toja, E., Barone, D., Corsico, N., Gallico, L., et al. (1988). 6-(Alkylamino)-3-aryl-1,2,4-triazolo[3,4-a]phthalazines. A new class of benzodiazepine receptor ligands. *Journal of Medicinal Chemistry*, 31, 1115–1123.

Van Laere, K., Bormans, G., Sanabria-Bohórquez, S. M., de Groot, T., Dupont, P., De Lepeleire, I., et al. (2008). In vivo characterization and dynamic receptor occupancy imaging of TPA023B, an α2/α3/α5 subtype selective γ-aminobutyric acid-A partial agonist. *Biological Psychiatry*, 64, 153–161.

Vanover, K. E., & Barrett, J. E. (1994). Evaluation of the discriminative stimulus effects of the novel sedative-hypnotic CL 284,846. *Psychopharmacology*, 115, 289–296.

Van Steveninck, A. L., Gieschke, R., Schoemaker, R. C., Roncari, G., Tuk, B., Pieters, M. S. M., et al. (1996). Pharmacokinetic and pharmacodynamic interactions of bretazenil and diazepam with alcohol. *British Journal of Clinical Pharmacology*, 41, 565–573.

Vicini, S., & Ortinski, P. (2004). Genetic manipulations of GABA$_A$ receptor in mice make inhibition exciting. *Pharmacology and Therapeutics*, 103, 109–120.

Videbæk, C., Friberg, L., Holm, S., Wammen, S., Foged, C., Andersen, J. V., et al. (1993). Benzodiazepine receptor equilibrium constants for flumazenil and midazolam determined in humans with the single photon emission computer tomography tracer [^{123}I]iomazenil. *European Journal of Pharmacology*, 249, 43–51.

Volk, D. W., Pierri, J. N., Fritschy, J. M., Auh, S., Sampson, A. R., & Lewis, D. A. (2002). Reciprocal alterations in pre- and postsynaptic inhibitory markers at chandelier cell inputs to pyramidal neurons in schizophrenia. *Cereberal Cortex*, 12, 1063–1070.

Volz, A., Khorsand, V., Gillies, D., & Leucht, S. (2007). Benzodiazepines for schizophrenia (Review). *Cochrane Database of Systematic Reviews*, 1, CD006391.

Votey, S. R., Bosse, G. M., Bayer, M. J., & Hoffman, J. R. (1991). Flumazenil: A new benzodiazepine antagonist. *Annals of Emergency Medicine*, 20, 181–188.

Wafford, K., Whiting, P. J., & Kemp, J. A. (1993). Differences in affinity and efficacy of benzodiazepine receptor ligands at recombinant γ-aminobutyric acid$_A$ receptor subtypes. *Molecular Pharmacology*, 43, 240–244.

Weinbroum, A. A., Flaishon, R., Sorkine, P., Szold, O., & Rudick, V. (1997). A risk-benefit assessment of flumazenil in the management of benzodiazepine overdose. *Drug Safety*, 17, 181–196.

Wieland, H. A., Lüddens, H., & Seeburg, P. H. (1992). A single histidine in GABA$_A$ receptors is essential for benzodiazepine agonist binding. *Journal of Biological Chemistry*, 267, 1426–1429.

Wisden, W., Laurie, D. J., Monyer, H., & Seeburg, P. H. (1992). The distribution of 13 GABA$_A$ receptor subunit mRNAs in the rat brain. I. Telencephalon, diencephalon, mesencephalon. *Journal of Neuroscience*, 12, 1040–1062.

Wolkowitz, O. M., & Pickar, D. (1992). Benzodiazepines in the treatment of schizophrenia: A review and reappraisal. *American Journal of Psychiatry*, 148, 714–726.

Wong, G., & Skolnick, P. (1992). High affinity ligands for "diazepam-insensitive" benzodiazepine receptors. *European Journal of Pharmacology. Molecular Pharmacology Section*, 225, 63–68.

Yee, B. K., Keist, R., von Boehmer, L., Studer, R., Benke, D., Hagenbuch, N., et al. (2005). A schizophrenia-related sensorimotor deficit links α3-containing GABA$_A$ receptors to a dopamine hyperfunction. *Proceedings of the National Academy of Sciences of the United States of America*, 102, 17154–17159.

Nicholas A. DeMartinis[*,†], Jayesh Kamath[†], and Andrew Winokur[†]

[*]Neuroscience Research Unit, Pfizer, Inc., Eastern Point Rd., Groton, Connecticut 06340

[†]Department of Psychiatry, University of Connecticut School of Medicine, Farmington, Connecticut 06030-6415

New Approaches for the Treatment of Sleep Disorders

Abstract

Epidemiological studies have established that sleep disorders are common and often untreated. Besides having a negative impact on overall health, these conditions can significantly disrupt normal daily functions. While a number of drugs are employed in the treatment of sleep disorders, safety, tolerability, and variable efficacy limit their utility. Clinical developments in the area have been facilitated especially by advances in neurobiology and neuropharmacology. In this regard, a wide array of neuroactive substances has been found to be responsible for regulating sleep and

Advances in Pharmacology, Volume 57
1054-3589/08 $35.00
10.1016/S1054-3589(08)57005-0

wakefulness. Advances in the understanding of neurotransmitter and hormone receptor mechanisms and classifications have led to new opportunities for developing novel therapeutics for treating sleep disorders. Provided in this report is an overview of some of the more prevalent sleep disorders, including narcolepsy, insomnia, obstructive sleep apnea syndrome, and restless legs syndrome, with a summary and critique of medications used to treat these conditions. For each disorder, information is provided on recent approaches taken to develop novel therapeutics based on laboratory findings relating to the underlying biological abnormalities associated with the condition, in addition to approaches that leverage existing therapeutics to develop new treatment options for patients. Significant advances in the future await a better understanding of the underlying pathophysiology of these conditions and of the neurobiological alterations associated with these disorders. It is hoped that some of the research directions described herein will stimulate additional research in this area and thereby help foster the discovery of novel agents for treating major sleep disorders.

I. Introduction

Sleep Disorders Medicine is a relatively young discipline that has undergone significant advances in recent years. These include the striking growth in accredited clinical sleep centers and board certified sleep specialists who provide skilled care to individuals suffering with various types of sleep disorders. In addition, there has been an explosive growth in the number of basic science discoveries elucidating neurobiological mechanisms involved in the regulation of sleep and waking states and progress in clarifying the pathophysiology of the more common sleep disorders. While a number of drugs are employed in the treatment of sleep disorders, safety, tolerability, and variable efficacy limit their utility. Provided in this report is an overview of some of the more prevalent sleep disorders, including narcolepsy, insomnia, obstructive sleep apnea syndrome (OSAS), and restless legs syndrome (RLS), with a summary and critique of medications used to treat these conditions. For each disorder, information is provided on recent approaches taken to develop novel therapeutics based on laboratory findings relating to the underlying biological abnormalities associated with the condition, in addition to approaches that leverage existing therapeutics to develop new treatment options for patients.

Sleep difficulties have been recognized by astute clinicians from antiquity. In around 400 BC, Hippocrates provided one of the earliest accounts of severe clinical depression, which he referred to as melancholy, by describing a woman who "although she did not take to bed, she suffered from insomnia, loss of appetite..." (Akiskal & Akiskal, 2007). An association between sleep disturbances and many psychiatric and somatic disorders has been apparent for millennia. However, the technology needed to investigate sleep alterations has been available only since the development of polysomnography (PSG) in the 1950s. Since then, Sleep Disorders Medicine has experienced a dynamic, accelerating growth. Clinical developments in the area have been facilitated especially by advances in neurobiology and neuropharmacology. In this regard, a wide array of neuroactive substances has been found to be responsible for regulating sleep and wakefulness. Advances in the understanding of neurotransmitter and hormone receptor mechanisms and classifications have provided new opportunities for developing novel therapeutics for treating sleep disorders.

Epidemiological studies have established the prevalence of various sleep disorders. Besides having a negative impact on overall health, these conditions can significantly disrupt normal daily functions. For example, disruption of sleep can result in absenteeism from school or work, declines in mental and physical performance, and accidents. Sleep disorders also represent significant risk factors for the development of a variety of medical and psychiatric conditions. While a number of medications are commonly used to treat sleep disorders, there remains a significant need for safer and more effective treatment options.

In the following review, emphasis is placed on four sleep disorders: insomnia, narcolepsy, RLS, and OSAS. Included are discussions of current therapies and their limitations, along with an assessment of approaches being taken to develop new drugs to treat these conditions.

II. Narcolepsy

A. Clinical Background

Narcolepsy is a chronic, but not progressive, sleep disorder that has a typical onset in the late teens or early twenties. It has a reported prevalence of about 0.5% in the United States, with between 150,000 and 250,000 individuals having a confirmed diagnosis at any given time (Dauvilliers et al., 2003). It is believed, however, that the diagnosis is often missed. Narcolepsy is characterized by excessive daytime sleepiness (EDS), manifest by sleep attacks that are often described as irresistible. As a consequence of the chronic excessive sleepiness, and the frequent episodes of sleep attacks, many patients experience significant disruptions in daily functions. In 1880, Gelineau provided the original description of this syndrome, although earlier accounts of patients suffering with this disorder can be found in the literature (Guilleminault & Bassiri, 2005). While stimulant medications have been the drugs of choice for treating this condition, modafinil is now the preferred choice.

I. Clinical Syndrome

Narcolepsy is characterized by a constellation of symptoms that includes EDS, periodic sleep attacks, and episodes of cataplexy, which involve the sudden loss of muscle tone typically brought on by intense emotion, such as fear, anger, or even vigorous laughter (Guilleminault & Fromherz, 2005). Cataplexy is experienced by at least two-thirds of patients with narcolepsy. It may involve a diffuse distribution of muscle atonia or may be more discretely localized, so as to be manifested by sagging of the jaw or buckling of the knees. While the presence of excessive sleepiness and cataplexy the most prevalent and characteristic features of narcolepsy, other commonly observed symptoms include sleep paralysis, where an individual experiences a transient inability to move his/her muscles while awakening. This symptom lasts for approximately 60 s before voluntary muscle control returns. Other symptoms include hypnagogic or hypnopompic hallucinations. These involve sensory experiences while falling to, or waking from, sleep. They can take the form of unusual and disturbing or frightening visual perceptions. While sleep paralysis and hypnagogic or hypnopompic hallucinations can occasionally be experienced by individuals who do not have narcolepsy, they occur together and with much greater frequency and regularity in narcoleptics.

There is a tendency for narcolepsy to be familial, with its presence in a first-degree relative increasing significantly the risk for developing the disorder (Billiard et al., 1994; Mignot, 1998). However, most often narcolepsy is sporadic, without a clear familial basis. Evidence for this is provided by the fact that, in 16 monozygotic twin pairs with at least one twin having confirmed narcolepsy, only 4 of these pairs were found to be concordant for the disorder (Mignot, 1998). This suggests that variables apart from strictly genetic risk factors are responsible for the development of narcolepsy. Among these factors are environmental exposures and immune system dysfunctions. While narcolepsy is typically designated as a disorder of excessive sleepiness, the nighttime sleep of patients with narcolepsy is generally characterized by disruptions in sleep continuity.

The diagnosis of narcolepsy is based on clinical findings supported by objective laboratory tests. Typically, a patient being evaluated for narcolepsy will undergo an overnight PSG evaluation. While the findings from this study do not establish the diagnosis of narcolepsy, they are used, in large measure, to rule out the presence of other primary sleep disorders that might account for EDS. These would include OSAS and periodic leg movements. The PSG assessment may help document the presence of disturbed sleep maintenance and may yield a characteristic finding of short latency to the appearance of the first episode of rapid eye movement (REM) sleep. Referred to as REM latency, it is usually 60–90 min in normal individuals, but only 15 min in those with narcolepsy. Following the overnight PSG, a second study is usually conducted to help document the diagnosis of narcolepsy objectively. To this end, the multiple sleep latency test (MSLT) is conducted the day after the PSG. For the MSLT, the patient is asked to arise at around 7:00 AM and be out of bed for a couple of hours. At around 9:00 AM the patient is asked to return to bed in a quiet, darkened room and is instructed to "Try to fall asleep." The patient is still monitored with the PSG montage and is given a 20 min opportunity to fall asleep. After the 20 min nap opportunity, the patient is then asked to be out of bed and active until the next nap opportunity 2 h later. A total of four or five nap opportunities of 20 min each are conducted as part of the MSLT. Thus, during the testing day, nap opportunities may be offered at 9:00 AM, 11:00 AM, 1:00 PM, 3:00 PM, and possibly 5:00 PM. The latency to fall asleep at each nap opportunity is determined by an analysis of the sleep recording. If the patient fails to fall asleep during a given nap opportunity, a score of 20 min is assigned for the sleep latency value. The average time to fall asleep across the four or five nap opportunities is calculated to identify the mean sleep latency value for the MSLT. A mean sleep latency value of <8 min represents significant EDS and is used as an objective measure to support the diagnosis of narcolepsy. For each of the nap opportunities in which a patient does fall asleep, an assessment is made as to whether the patient entered REM sleep during that nap opportunity. The documentation of two REM onsets during the course of the four or five nap opportunities is further support for the diagnosis. A variation of the MSLT, the maintenance of wakefulness test (MWT), is employed to document the efficacy of drugs or drug candidates as treatments for narcolepsy. In the MWT, the patient is again studied on the day following an overnight PSG, with four or five 20-min test sessions during the day offered at 2-h intervals. However, for the MWT, the patient is placed in an erect position in a comfortable recliner in a quiet room with low illumination and instructed to "Try to stay awake." For this test, the mean time before falling asleep is calculated as an assessment of the patient's ability to remain awake. The change in duration of wakefulness from baseline is determined after administration of a test substance to determine its efficacy as a treatment for narcolepsy.

Another laboratory measure of narcolepsy is the human leukocyte antigen (HLA class II antigen system). In 1984, it was reported that 100% of patients with narcolepsy were positive for HLA DR2 (Juji, Satake, Honda, & Doi, 1984). The HLA gene, which is located on the short arm of chromosome 6, is known to play an important role in the recognition and processing of foreign antibodies. More recent studies have shown that DR15-DQ6 (DR2-DQw1 subtype) is strongly associated with narcolepsy (Honda & Matsuki, 1990). An association of HLA positive typing with cataplexy has been repeatedly demonstrated (Mignot et al., 1997). The International Classification of Sleep Disorders-2 (ICSD-2; 2005) indicates that positive typing for the HLA DBQI*0602 or the DR2 subtypes are strongly associated findings in narcoleptics. Another laboratory test for narcolepsy that is included in the ICSD-2 (2005) criteria involves low cerebrospinal fluid (CSF) levels of hypocretin-1 ($<$110 pg/ml). The role of the hypocretin/orexin peptide family in the pathophysiology of narcolepsy is discussed in more detail later.

2. Pathophysiology Relevant to Drug Development

Many of the defining clinical features of narcolepsy, including the appearance of sleep attacks, as opposed to simply daytime sleepiness, cataplexy, sleep paralysis, and hypnagogic hallucinations might be associated with and characterized by a breakthrough of elements of REM sleep into the daytime waking hours (Dement et al., 1966). For example, muscle atonia, which is regulated by lower brainstem regions, has long been recognized as one of the essential physiological changes associated with REM sleep. While this hypothesis is probably overly simplistic and fails to explain all of the complex clinical aspects of narcolepsy, it does provide a theoretical physiological framework to understand this disorder.

Additional ground-breaking work on the pathophysiology of narcolepsy was based on studies with a canine model of the condition conducted at the Sleep Disorders Center at Stanford University during the 1970s. Certain species of dogs were noted to display behavioral manifestations of cataplexy. In work on Dobermans and Labrador retrievers, both of which demonstrate cataplexy, a series of crossbreedings led to the development of animals with a well-established autosomal recessive genetic basis for their behavior (Foutz et al., 1979; Mignot et al., 1991). These narcoleptic dog strains also demonstrate a pattern of hypersomnolence. Subsequently, the *canacr*-1 gene was identified to be responsible for the transmission of narcoleptic features in these animals (Hungs et al., 2001; Mignot et al., 1993). This gene is a mutated form of the hypocretin receptor 2 gene (Hctr 2). Supporting this association was the finding that preprohypocretin knockout mice also demonstrate behavioral changes reminiscent of those observed in narcoleptic patients (Chemelli et al., 1999). Together these reports drew attention to a possible role for the hypocretin/orexin system in the pathophysiology of narcolepsy. While human gene abnormalities related to the hypocretin system appear to be rare (Mignot, 2005), approximately 85–90% of narcoleptics with cataplexy have low or undetectable levels of hypocretin-1 in their CSF (Nishino et al., 2000; Nishino et al., 2001). Moreover, postmortem brain studies reveal reductions in both hypocretin-1 and hypocretin-2 in tissues obtained from individuals diagnosed with narcolepsy (Peyron et al., 2000; Thannickal et al., 2000). Laboratory animal studies indicate that hypocretin/orexin neurons are localized in the lateral hypothalamus, with projections to many regions of the cerebral cortex, limbic, and lower brainstem regions. The hypocretin/orexin system has been shown to activate a host of transmitter systems in the central nervous system (CNS), including those associated with noradrenergic, dopaminergic, sertonergic, histaminergic, and cholinergic pathways (Taheri et al., 2002; Willie et al., 2001). Thus, the recently demonstrated reduction in hypocretin-1 in patients with narcolepsy may provide an important clue as to the reason for the profound changes in alertness and sleep–wake patterns characteristic of this condition.

3. Current Treatments

Apart from the pharmacological approaches for treating narcolepsy, behavioral treatments are employed in the management of this disorder. These include measures to regulate the sleep–wake schedule to improve consolidation of nighttime sleep, as well as the use of structured daytime naps to reduce the potential impact and functional problems caused by unintended, but impossible to resist, sleep attacks (Zvonkina & Black, 2008). Additionally, counseling interventions, diet, exercise, and instructions to be cautious about driving are all potential important components of the overall management strategy.

For several decades, CNS stimulants, such as dextroamphetamine and methylphenidate, were the mainstays for the pharmacological treatment of narcolepsy (Nishino & Mignot, 2008). These drugs were often effective in reducing daytime sleepiness and are still often employed for treating this symptom. The stimulants are less reliable, however, in controlling cataplectic attacks. As stimulants are known to enhance monoaminergic transmission in brain, it is not surprising that they maintain arousal and enhance vigilance. However, these actions are also associated with adverse effects that can be annoying and potentially serious (Nishino & Mignot, 2008). Most troubling are the cardiovascular side effects. Other difficulties encountered with these drugs include anxiety, insomnia, and abuse potential, although narcolepsy patients do not demonstrate a high likelihood to abuse these compounds (Guilleminault & Fromherz, 2005). In recent years modafinil has become the first-line treatment for symptoms of EDS in patients with narcolepsy. This drug has been on the market in France for this purpose since the mid-1980s and had been available in the United States since the late 1990s (Nishino, 2008). Modafinil is very effective in reducing daytime sleepiness in patients with narcolepsy and is also approved for treating EDS secondary to obstructive sleep apnea and to shift work induced insomnia. While for some patients modafinil is less effective than the stimulants (Bastuji & Jouvet, 1988; Dauvilliers et al., 2002), it is safe, well tolerated, and has a low abuse potential, making it the preferred medication for most. While modafinil reduces daytime sleepiness, it has yet to be proven efficacious as a treatment for cataplexy. Because of its relatively short half-life (9–14 h), many patients take a second dose of modafinil later in the day to maintain efficacy (Wong et al., 1998). Armodafinil, the R-enantiomer of mod-afinil, was recently approved for the same indications as modafinil. With a longer half-life (10–15 h) than modafinil, armodafinil may be taken only once a day (Wong et al., 1999). The mechanism of action of modafinil and armodafinil in reducing excessive sleepiness remains unknown, although several possibilities have been proposed (Nishino, 2008). While in general modafinil is thought to modulate brain dopa-mine systems, the mechanism of this effect is yet to be elucidated (Ballon & Feifel, 2006; Minzenberg & Carter, 2008).

Numerous approaches have been taken to treat the cataplexy asso-ciated with narcolepsy (Morgenthaler et al., 2007). As described in the practice parameters for the treatment of narcolepsy by the American Academy of Sleep Medicine, drugs employed to treat cataplexy symptoms include the tricyclic antidepressants, selective serotonin reuptake inhibi-tors (SSRIs), venlaxine, and reboxetine (Morgenthaler et al., 2007). Some treatment options for daytime sleepiness mentioned in this report include the monoamine oxidase (MAO) inhibitor selegiline and ritanserin, a 5-HT_2 receptor antagonist. Sodium oxybate, also known as γ-hydroxy-butyrate, was recently approved as a treatment for cataplexy, daytime sleepiness, and disrupted nighttime sleep (Broughton & Mamelak, 1979; Lammers et al., 1993; Pardi & Black, 2006; Scharf et al., 1985). Use of sodium oxybate is limited, however, by the fact that patients must take a second dose during the night to facilitate sleep consolidation. Also, sodium oxybate, which is known by some as the "date rape" drug, carries a black box warning about abuse potential. To minimize abuse, its distribution must be carefully monitored. Accordingly, although sodium oxybate is effective in treating symptoms of narcolepsy, it is unlikely to be generally used for this purpose.

B. Narcolepsy Drug Development Background

1. Drug Development Issues and Challenges

Because narcolepsy is a relatively uncommon disorder, it is difficult to recruit appropriate subjects for clinical trials who are not being effectively treated with current medications. Additionally, the market for drugs to treat narcolepsy is limited. Nonetheless, compounds that are able to counter the symptoms of narcolepsy can be useful in treat-ing other conditions, with opportunities for approval for other indications.

For example, there are a number of disorders characterized by sleepiness or fatigue that may respond to drugs such as modafinil, mak-ing the market for such agents much more clinically meaningful and lucrative.

C. Mechanisms in Development

A review of narcolepsy clinical trials activity (ClinicalTrials.gov) reveals a lack of such studies using drugs with novel mechanisms of action. Nonetheless, new approaches are being taken as described below.

1. Histamine H3 Receptor Antagonists

Histamine is a neurotransmitter known to promote wakefulness and vigilance (Szabadi, 2006). The brain histamine system innervates the tuberomammillary nucleus (TMN) of the hypothalamus and projects diffusely to various regions of the cerebral cortex where it interacts with histamine H1 receptors (Haas & Panula, 2003). As histamine H1 receptor antagonists, classical antihistamines are sedating (Tashiro et al., 2002).

The histamine H3 receptor is located presynaptically, with its activation inhibiting the release of histamine and other neurotransmitters (Clapham & Kilpatrick, 1992; Gemkow et al., 2009; Schlicker et al., 1993). Accordingly, blockade of this site enhances the release of a host of substances known to maintain arousal and vigilance. For this reason, efforts are underway to develop histamine H3 receptor antagonists as treatments for a number of CNS disorders, including narcolepsy. Among them is GSK-189254, which is currently undergoing Phase 2 clinical trials in patients with narcolepsy (ClinicalTrials.Gov NCT00366080). Preclinical work demonstrated that GSK-189254 is active in the rat novel object recognition paradigm and increases wakefulness in rats and mice (Dean et al., 2006). Another histamine H3 receptor antagonist that has undergone clinical trials is JNJ-17216498. Laboratory animal studies revealed that this compound reduces the number of cataplectic episodes in narcoleptic animal models. A Phase 2 clinical trial with narcoleptic patients was initiated in November 2006 and listed as terminated in December 2007 (ClinicalTrials.Gov NCT00424931). However, no results from this study have yet been published. While it remains unknown whether blockage of histamine H3 receptor antagonists dampens symptoms of narcolepsy, preclinical results have tended to support the theory that such agents may be of value in treating this condition. Indeed, there are now data indicating that the histaminergic system interacts with hypocretin/orexin pathways in the maintenance of wakefulness and arousal (Cortese et al., 2008; Soya et al., 2008). This lends further support to the notion that facilitation of histaminergic transmission might help overcome the reduction in hypocretin/orexin activity that appears to be a key component of the pathophysiology of narcolepsy.

2. Hypocretin/Orexin Replacement Therapy

In light of the fact that the hypocretin/orexin system appears to be deficient in patients with narcolepsy, efforts are underway to develop drugs that will directly activate the receptors for these substances. While early preclinical studies have yielded mixed results, enthusiasm for this approach remains high (Nishino et al., 2003; Yoshida et al., 2003). A study listed on ClinicalTrials.gov involves intranasal administration of Orexin A to 15 patients with narcolepsy and 15 healthy controls in a crossover design employing a single administration of Orexin A and of placebo. Outcome measures are to include sleep recordings and assessments of the cytokine system and neurocognitive function. This study is currently listed as ongoing but no longer recruiting participants.

3. Enhancement of Dopaminergic Neurotransmission

The CNS catecholamine systems have long been thought to play important roles in the maintenance of wakefulness and vigilance (Mendelson, 2001; Siegel, 2004; Stenberg, 2007; Tamakawa et al., 2006). To exploit this possibility, studies are being conducted with ADX-N05 (formerly YKP10A), a compound shown to be a weak inhibitor of dopamine uptake, with effects on norepinephrine or serotonin (http://www.biomedicine.org/medicine-technology-1/Addrenex-Pharmaceuticals-Expands-Product-Pipeline-by-Licensing-New-Drug-to-Treat-Narcolepsy-4357-2/) (Gordon et al., 1998). While the precise mechanism of action of ADX-N05 remains unknown, responses noted in clinical studies indicate a profile reminiscent of dopamine reuptake inhibitors such as nomifensine and bupropion (Amsterdam et al., 2002). In a small, pilot study, moderate doses of YKP10A appeared to display antidepressant properties, although it was acknowledged that the trial was not adequately powered to produce statistically significant findings. In a preclinical study to evaluate its potential in narcolepsy, the responses to ADX-N05 were compared to those elicited by dextroamphetamine, modafinil, and saline in mice (Hasan et al., 2009). A variety of electroencephalographic (EEG) and behavioral assessments, along with an evaluation of the effects of these drugs on brain gene expression, were conducted. The results indicate that ADX-N05 (YKP10A) enhances wakefulness, although its effects on the other endpoints differed from those induced by the dextroamphetamine and modafinil. Phase 2 trials in narcolepsy are reportedly planned for ADX-N05.

4. Thyrotropin Releasing Hormone Analogs

Thyrotropin releasing hormone (TRH) is believed to play a role in the regulation of arousal (Gary et al., 2003). Evidence for this is provided by the finding that animals pretreated with CNS depressants, such as ethanol or barbiturates, and then treated with TRH experience a significantly reduced sleeping time and no hypothermia. Moreover, direct administration of TRH in the dorsal hippocampus of hibernating ground squirrels results in full physiological and behavioral reversal of the hibernation state. Studies with TRH and a TRH analog (Montirelin, CG-3703) in canine narcolepsy and mouse models found these agents diminish hypersomnolence (are wake promoting) and reduce episodes of cataplexy (Kotorii et al., 2009; Nishino et al., 1997; Riehl et al., 2000). It has also been found that TRH directly activates hypocretin neurons (Gonzalez et al., 2009) and that the response to it is diminished in orexin knockout mice. Taken together these data support the notion that a TRH analog may be of benefit in the treatment of narcolepsy.

D. Narcolepsy Summary and Future Directions

There are a number of pharmacological options available for the treatment of key symptoms of narcolepsy, including EDS and cataplexy. While narcolepsy can be extremely incapacitating, many patients experience significant symptomatic relief with these medications. Nonetheless, treatment of this condition is not optimal from the standpoint of efficacy and safety. Most troubling is the fact that there is no safe and convenient medication that reduces both excessive sleepiness and cataplexy. These issues are being addressed experimentally with the development of histamine H3 receptor antagonists and of agents that activate the hypocretin/orexin, catecholamine, and TRH systems. Obstacles slowing the development of drugs for treating narcolepsy include the market size and a limited patient population for clinical trials.

III. Obstructive Sleep Apnea _____

A. Clinical Background

OSAS is characterized by transient interruptions in air flow during sleep that are secondary to an obstruction at some point in the nasal–oropharyngeal pathway. Those with OSAS experience frequent arousals and shifts from deeper to lighter stages of sleep. Such individuals can ultimately develop symptoms of EDS, which may be quite severe. Medical disabilities, in particular those related to the cardiovascular system, can result from OSAS.

1. Clinical Syndrome

In the nineteenth century, Charles Dickens created a character, Pickwick, displaying symptoms, including obesity and profound daytime sleepiness, associated today with OSAS. The Dickens portrayal led to the description of this syndrome as Pickwickian. Other early descriptions of patients with symptoms of OSAS were provided by physicians such as

Dr. William Hill in the late nineteenth century and Sir William Osler in the early twentieth century (Fairbanks, 1987). Utilizing modern PSG techniques, it has been possible to make a more objective assessment of physiological findings characteristic of this condition, providing the foundation for the current concepts and definitions of this disorder (Guilleminault et al., 2005).

An apneic event is, by definition, an episode of obstruction of air flow during sleep lasting more than 10 s and typically with duration of 20–30 s or longer (Fairbanks, 1987). An hypopneic event also involves an interruption of flow in the airway secondary to an obstruction that lasts for less than 10 s. Patients with OSAS are unable to adequately ventilate during sleep. This phenomenon is especially prominent during slow wave sleep (SWS), when muscle tone is markedly reduced, and during REM sleep, a period characterized by muscle atonia (Veasey, 2003). A consequence of the loss of muscle tone involves the reduction in tone of palatal, lingual, and pharyngeal muscles, which can lead to a significant risk for the collapse of airway patency. The dilator effect of the pharyngeal muscles, and the protrusive effect of the genioglossus muscles, may consequently be inadequate for maintaining airway patency sufficient for normal airflow (Levitzky, 2008; Pack, 1994). These developments may lead to a measurable reduction in oxyhemoglobin saturation and a consequent decline in ventilation of the CNS. When brainstem chemoreceptors detect this change in oxyhemoglobin concentration, they stimulate an arousal response in higher brain centers, triggering a shift from a deep phase of sleep (SWS or REM) to a light phase, enabling the individual to make an effort to restore airway patency (Fairbanks, 1987; Ondze, Espa, Dauvilliers, Billiard & Besset, 2003). During the obstructive phase of an apneic event, the individual continues to make efforts at respiration, albeit these are ineffective because of the airway obstruction. In contrast, someone with a disorder characterized by central apneic events makes no respiratory effort because of the lack of respiratory drive. For a person with OSAS, the termination of an apneic event is typically marked by a loud grunting sound, often coupled with a change in body position, in an effort to clear the airway. While this arousal and successful termination of the obstructive event is essential for survival, sleep continuity is disrupted, and there is a loss of, or interference with, elements of sleep believed to be critically involved in the restorative aspects of sleep. As a consequence, individuals with OSAS often develop profound symptoms of EDS, the symptom most likely to lead them to seek medical assistance (Cheshire et al., 1992). Another factor that causes patients to seek evaluation at a Sleep Disorders Center is a spouse or bed partner who observes repeated episodes of cessation of breathing during sleep and who becomes alarmed enough by these observations to insist on a medical evaluation.

Epidemiological studies of the prevalence of OSAS has suggested that of those between the ages of 30 and 60, about 4% of males and 2% of females

TABLE I   Clinical Manifestations of Obstructive Sleep Apnea

Excessive daytime sleepiness
Loud snoring
Obesity
Morning headaches
Personality changes and irritability
Enuresis
Sexual impotence

display clinically verifiable symptoms of OSAS (Young et al., 1993). Studies indicate both age and gender-related risks factors for the development of this condition (Young et al., 2004). Other risk factors include snoring, obesity, a thick neck, and retrognathia (Fairbanks, 1987). Patients with OSAS typically are unaware of the repeated episodes of hypoxia-induced obstructive events they are experiencing throughout the night. The most common symptom associated with OSAS is EDS, although a number of other symptoms are associated with this disorder as well (Table I) (Moran, 1987; Pack, 1994). EDS can functionally impair those with OSAS. There can be a reduction of cognitive ability leading to poor work performance and an increased risk for motor vehicle accidents, which can be fatal (Cheshire et al., 1992; Pack, 1994; Van Dongen et al., 2003). There are also important long-term health consequences associated with OSAS. These represent a significant component of the important public health consequences of this disorder if it is not diagnosed and treated appropriately. In particular, the hypoventilation during sleep leads to the development of pulmonary hypertension, which can increase cardiac load and evolve into systemic hypertension (Peker et al., 2000; Phillips & Somers, 2000; Shahar et al., 2001). Those with OSAS are also at significantly increased risk for developing fatal cardiac arrhythmias (Phillips & Somers, 2000). These sequelae make it imperative to diagnose OSAS as early as possible and to initiate sustained treatment for the condition.

The diagnosis of OSAS is based on a thorough medical history, which often includes the spouse or bed partner as a key informant, and an extensive physical examination that includes careful evaluation of essential components of the airway, including nares, mouth, tongue, tonsils, and pharynx (Moran, 1987; Guilleminault & Bassiri, 2005). A definitive diagnosis is based, in part, on the results of an overnight PSG evaluation (Table II). Based on the results of the overnight sleep study, an apnea–hypopnea index (AHI) is determined, with a delineation of obstructive events per hour noted. By convention, an AHI of >5/h is considered mild OSAS, whereas >15 events/h is indicative of clinically significant OSAS. The diagnostic sleep study also involves determination of the extent of oxyhemoglobin desaturations occurring during the episodes of obstruction of the airway. A second sleep study night is often performed

TABLE II PSG Variables Assessed in the Diagnosis of OSAS[a]

---

* EEG activity—to determine the presence of sleep, specific sleep stages, stage shifts, and occurrence of arousals from sleep
* Electrooculogram—to document eye movements during sleep and to identify the presence of REM
* Nasal and oral air flow monitors—to document periods of cessation of airflow, indicating an apneic or hypopneic event
* Electrocardiogram tracing—to identify the presence of cardiac arrythmias
* Thoracic monitoring of respiratory effort—to document sustained effort during apneic events
* Electromyogram (submental placement)—to document the presence of muscle atonia during the REM sleep phase
* Arterial oxygen saturation—to document episodes of oxyhemoglobin desaturation and the extent of desaturation during apneic events
* Electromyogram—anterior tibialis muscles—to document the presence of periodic limb movements and to determine the relationship of arousals to apneic/hypopneic events vs. periodic limb movements of sleep

---

[a] Abbreviations: PSG, polysomnographic; OSAS, obstructive sleep apnea syndrome; EEG, electroencephalographic; REM, rapid eye movement.

to evaluate the efficacy of nasal continuous positive airway pressure (CPAP) in controlling apneic events and in maintaining adequate oxygenation.

2. Pathophysiology Relevant to Drug Development

While awake, a balance exists between forces on the airway tending to reduce the capacity of the lumen and the tonic maintenance of patency. The former is generated primarily from inspiratory effort attributable to the thoracic musculature and the latter by the upper airway dilator musculature, particularly involving a group of approximately 20 muscles that constitute the pharyngeal dilator group (Levitzky, 2008). Of particular relevance for preclinical models is the genioglossus dilator muscle which operates under the control of the hypoglossal nerve (Pack, 1994; Schwab et al., 2005). Muscle tone, including that provided to the upper airway, is reduced during SWS, and muscle atonia is a characteristic feature of REM sleep. This establishes a situation where collapse of the airway can occur, leading to apneic events. Thus, these events are most likely to occur during the REM phase of sleep. A number of other factors can influence significantly the likelihood of obstructive events, including retrognathia or micrognathia, enlarged tonsils and adenoids, and enlarged pharyngeal tissues. The likelihood of developing OSAS is enhanced even further in obese individuals with one or more of these risk factors (Fairbanks, 1987; Pack, 1994).

The CNS mechanisms involved in regulating respiration are complex, with a detailed discussion of them beyond the scope of this report. Numerous neurotransmitters play a role in the brainstem regulation of upper

TABLE III   Neurochemicals in the Brain Stem Motor Nuclei of the Upper Airway
Dilator Muscles (Veasey, 2003)

Glycine
Glutamate
Acetylcholine
Norepinephrine
Serotonin
Substance P
Thyrotropin releasing hormone
Vasopressin
Oxytocin
Hypocretin/orexin

airway dilator motoneurons (Table III) (Veasey, 2003). Among the wide
array of relevant neuroactive substances, likely to play roles in modulating upper airway dilator muscle activity, serotonin appears to be particularly important, especially with respect to its effects on the hypoglossal
nucleus and genioglossus dilator muscle. Serotonin has for some time
been known to play an important role in sleep, with its brainstem effects
being reduced during SWS and REM sleep (Jouvet, 1999). With respect
to OSAS, studies suggest that 5-HT excites upper airway dilator motoneurons (Fenik & Veasey, 2003). As this influence declines during SWS
and REM sleep, pretreatment of upper airway dilator motoneurons with
serotonin reduces sleep-dependent suppression of upper airway dilator
activity (Jelev et al., 2001). Of the 14 distinct serotonin receptor subtypes
(Barnes & Sharp, 1999; Hannon & Hoyer, 2008), serotonin 2a appears
to predominate on the hypoglossal nerve (Veasey, 2003). The English
bulldog, an animal model of obstructive sleep apnea, has been the subject of studies aimed at defining the contribution of serotonin dysfunction to this disorder (Hendricks et al., 1987). It has been found that
administration of serotonin agonists markedly reduces obstructive sleep-
disordered breathing events (Veasey et al., 1999), suggesting such agents
might represent a novel approach for the treatment of this condition
(Veasey, 2001).

3. Current Treatments

A variety of strategies are employed for treating patients with OSAS
(Buysse, 2007; Jayaraman et al., 2008; Veasey, 2001; Veasey et al.,
2006). Since, because of gravitational forces, apneic events appear to
be most common when individuals sleep on their backs, positional
therapy is sometimes employed. This involves sewing a tennis ball or
some other object into the back of the pajama tops to prevent sleep on
the back. Weight loss is another approach to managing this condition as
are some surgical interventions. With regard to the latter, examples

include uvulopalatopharyngoplasty, uvulopalatopharyngoglossoplasty and tonsillectomy, and adenoidectomy (Fujita, 1987). However, surgical procedures carry their own risk of morbidity and mortality. Another approach is use of a mandibular advancement splint, a dental appliance (Sanders, 1987). The splint helps move the mandible forward, maintaining a patent upper airway during sleep. This approach is most effective for some with milder forms of OSAS.

By far the most frequently employed treatment for OSAS is CPAP (Grunstein, 2005). With a CPAP apparatus the airway is essentially splinted open during sleep, preventing obstructive events during sleep. CPAP has been shown to reduce the AHI and prevent episodes of oxyhemoglobin desaturations. It has been demonstrated that CPAP reduces EDS, and therefore neurocognitive dysfunction, and reduces the development of cardiovascular problems (Bradley & Floras, 2003; Pepperell et al., 2002; White et al., 2002). In spite of its effectiveness, patient compliance is a significant problem with CPAP therapy because it is cumbersome and inconvenient to use (Jones & Morrell, 2008; Weaver et al., 1997).

Various approaches have been taken in selecting medications for treating OSAS. Included have been drugs to stimulate the central ventilatory drive, REM suppressant agents, serotonergic agents to improve airway patency, and drugs to offset symptoms of excessive sleepiness (Veasey et al., 2005; Veasey et al., 2006). Examples of agents used to increase the central ventilatory drive are methylxanthines such as aminophylline and theophylline; opioid antagonists such as naloxone, doxapram; a potassium channel blocker; and nicotine, a central stimulant. Overall, the ventilatory stimulants display only limited efficacy as treatment for OSAS. The use of REM suppressant agents is based on the fact that apneic episodes are typically most abundant during REM sleep, when muscle atonia is especially predominant. The tricyclic antidepressant protriptyline, which is a potent, selective norepinephrine reuptaker inhibitor known to suppress REM sleep, has been employed for this purpose. Additionally, clonidine, an α_2-adrenoceptor agonist that inhibits REM sleep, has been examined as well. However, the results of trials with clonidine did not support its use for this purpose. A few OSAS clinical studies have been performed using the SSRIs fluoxetine and paroxetine. While some degree of reduction in AHI was reported with this approach, the overall results were disappointing (Veasey et al., 2006).

Mirtazapine is a norepinephrine α_2-adrenoceptor antagonist, a histamine H1 receptor antagonist, and a serotonin-2 and serotonin-3 receptor antagonist that at low doses reduces apneic events and increases genioglossus activity in a rat model of OSAS (Berry et al., 2005; Carley & Radulovacki, 1999). In a single case study, mirtazapine significantly lowered the AHI in an 82-year-old male with OSAS (Castillo et al., 2004). It has been reported that administration of mirtazapine produces excessive daytime somnolence and significant weight gain in some patients (Veasey et al., 2006). These effects would be particularly troublesome for those with OSAS.

The use of nasal sprays containing corticosteroids may help minimize airway obstructive events associated with pronounced nasal airway blockade. Finally, modafinil has been approved for treating EDS in patients with OSAS and armodafinil is being studied in this regard (Black & Hirshkowitz, 2005; Hirshkowitz et al., 2007; Kingshott et al., 2001; Schwartz et al., 2003).

B. Obstructive Sleep Apnea Drug Development Background

1. Endpoints and Study Design

The testing of any new drug candidate for the treatment of OSAS must begin with careful PSG-based assessments of sleep-related respiratory patterns in the trial subjects. Thus, for any new candidate compound, it is necessary to demonstrate a significant reduction in AHI and in the number and extent of episodes of oxyhemoglobin desaturations. Assessment of improvement in symptoms of EDS, based on laboratory measures such as the MSLT and on self-report scales, is also needed. More extended measures of treatment impact should document improvement in neurocognitive function and a reduction in the development of cardiovascular disorders.

2. Drug Development Issues and Challenge

Because of the complex nature of respiratory function during sleep, and the various factors that may influence the development of obstructive events in the airway, it is difficult to predict the possible effectiveness of a particular pharmacological approach for the treatment of OSAS.

C. Mechanisms in Development

1. Histamine H3 Receptor Antagonists

It has been known for decades that histamine H1 receptor antagonists are sedating, indicating a role for this transmitter in the sleep–wake cycle. Because the presynaptically localized histamine H3 receptor controls the release of histamine and other neurotransmitters, its inhibition enhances the release of these agents, resulting in activating, arousing effects (Gemkow et al., 2009). MK-0249, a histamine H3 receptor antagonist, is currently undergoing clinical trials in comparison with, in randomized fashion, modafinil or placebo in patients with OSAS on CPAP therapy as a treatment for EDS (ClinicalTrials.gov NCT00620659).

2. AMPA Glutamate Receptor Agonists

As glutamate is the major excitatory neurotransmitter in the CNS, activation of glutamate receptors should induce arousal and maintain wakefulness. Ampakines, which are glutamate AMPA receptor agonists, have been examined for their ability to influence respiration. In this regard, CX1739, an AMPA receptor agonist, is reported to reverse opioid-induced respiratory depression in laboratory animals (Cortex Pharmaceuticals press release). It has also been announced that CX1739 has been approved for a clinical trial as treatment for moderate to severe OSAS (http://sleeposition.blogspot.com/2009/07/cortex-cx1739-sleep-apnea.html).

3. Serotonin Modulating Combination Drug

In a company report, BTG Pharmaceuticals announced the development of a combination product, BGC20-0166, containing two marketed drugs known to modify serotonergic activity. The two agents are fluoxetine, an SSRI, and ondansetron, a serotonin 3 (5-HT_3) receptor antagonist. The 5-HT_3 receptor antagonists are reported to reduce sleep-related apnea in rats and REM sleep-disordered breathing in the English bulldog model of obstructive sleep apnea (Veasey et al., 2001). In a study described at the 2009 American Thoracic Society Meeting, 17 patients with obstructive sleep apnea were randomized to treatment with the combination of fluoxetine 10 mg daily and ondansetron 24 mg daily or placebo for 28 days. Patients receiving the fluoxetine/ondansetron combination demonstrated a 40% reduction in AHI at day 28, with no significant alterations in sleep (Prasad et al., 2009). The company announced it will soon initiate a second Phase 2 clinical trial with BGC20-0166 in patients with mild to moderate OSAS (http://www.btgplc.com/BTGDevelopmentProgrammes/230/BGC200166.html).

4. TRH Receptor Agonists

TRH is highly concentrated in regions of the brainstem, including the nucleus tractus solitarius, where it is co-localized with serotonin and, in some cases, substance P as well (Hokfelt et al., 1975). Autoradiographic localization studies revealed that TRH receptors are highly and discretely localized in the rat dorsal vagal complex in areas known to regulate motoneurons involved in respiratory control (Manaker & Rizio, 1989). In an *in vitro* study of rat hypoglossal motoneurons, TRH enhanced the excitability of hypoglossal motoneurons by both directly causing a depolarization and also by decreasing membrane conductance, thereby lowering the threshold for repetitive firing (Bayliss et al., 1992). Based on such findings, a TRH analog patent (US Patent 5968932) was issued claiming the use of CG-3703 (montirelin) as a treatment for OSAS. Support for this patent application involved studies conducted with the English bulldog model of sleep apnea. In these experiments, montirelin treatment induced a 50% reduction in sleep-disordered breathing, while total sleep time was preserved. To date, there have been no reported findings from clinical studies on the efficacy of TRH analogs for treating OSAS.

D. Obstructive Sleep Apnea Summary and Future Directions

Obstructive sleep apnea is a common disorder which affects both the quality of life and cardiovascular health. While there is a wide array of treatment approaches for OSAS, each is limited in terms of efficacy, safety, or patient compliance. Thus, the overall impact of current pharmacotherapies for OSAS is quite modest. Exploitation of novel pharmacological mechanisms for managing this condition holds the promise of producing safe and effective drugs for the treatment of this important sleep disorder.

IV. Insomnia

A. Clinical Background

Insomnia is characterized by difficulty initiating sleep, maintaining sleep, or poor quality sleep that negatively affects quality of life with varying degrees of severity. While up to half of the United States population may report occasional episodes of insomnia with little or no significant impairment of function, a core group of 10–15% of adults experience symptoms of chronic insomnia (Zammit, 2007). International studies suggest that 7–37% of the population suffers from insomnia in Western countries (Leger & Poursain, 2005; Zammit, 2007). The most common pattern of insomnia involves waking during the night or experiencing poor quality sleep that is nonrestorative, although patterns of difficulty falling asleep or early awakening are nearly as common. Difficulty in falling asleep and early awakening are common symptoms of major depression, one of the more frequent causes of secondary insomnia. The term primary insomnia designates a group of patients that have no other identifiable medical reason for having sleep problems. Besides major depression, other causes of secondary insomnia include anxiety disorders, chronic pain and pain syndromes such as fibromyalgia, and shift work sleep disorder. A study of the natural course of insomnia found that three out of four subjects initially reporting insomnia experienced at least 1 year of ongoing symptoms, and nearly half continued to experience insomnia through the entire 3-year reporting period (Morin et al., 2009). The course of insomnia was more likely to be persistent in women and older adults. Women experience insomnia at greater rates than men (Lindberg et al., 1997) and are more likely to have co-morbid psychiatric conditions that are responsible for the insomnia (Kessler et al., 1993). Despite its high prevalence, few people seek treatment for insomnia. A 2005 survey found that only 14% of those reporting insomnia sought medical treatment in the United States (NSF 2005 Sleep in America Poll), and low rates of treatment seeking have been observed despite patient recognition of the presence and impact of insomnia symptoms (Leger & Poursain, 2005). This suggests that developing new treatment options that address patient concerns about seeking treatment has potential for substantial public health impact.

The functional impacts of insomnia are probably the best understood consequences of disorder because they are readily apparent to both the patient and his or her friends and family. Common daytime symptoms such as fatigue, excessive sleepiness, and concentration difficulties can result in decreased productivity at work and at home, absenteeism, and poor quality work output (Bolge et al., 2009; Roth et al., 2006). In addition, the impact of insomnia on overall health, and on specific medical conditions, is evident from investigations demonstrating negative effects on cardiac disease (Sarsour et al., 2009), glucose control (Vgontzas et al., 2009), obesity, mental health (LeBlanc et al., 2007), and increased health-care costs (Pollack et al., 2009).

For many years the benzodiazepines were the most widely prescribed drugs for the treatment of insomnia. Currently, nonbenzodiazepine hypnotics that act selectively at GABA-A receptor subtypes, are the preferred treatments (see Chapter 4). The efficacy of the benzodiazepines and non-benzodiazepine hypnotics have been demonstrated in many randomized controlled clinical trials (Dundar et al., 2004; Smith et al., 2002), with the most common positive endpoint being a decreased latency to persistent sleep (LPS) and increased sleep efficiency/total sleep time.

Ramelteon, a melatonin receptor agonist, has also been approved as a treatment for this condition. A melatonin receptor 1 and 2 (MT1 and MT2) agonist, ramelteon has been shown to decrease the latency to persistent sleep at 8 and 16 mg doses compared with placebo, with no increase in total sleep time (Reynoldson, Elliott & Nelson, 2008). The most frequent adverse effects associated with its use are headache, somnolence, fatigue, nausea, dizziness, and insomnia, with an overall incidence of these effects being similar to that of placebo. Maintenance of efficacy, as well as long-term safety and tolerability, was demonstrated for ramelteon during 6-month (Mayer et al., 2009) and 12-month (Richardson et al., 2009) clinical trials. It has been found to be free of rebound insomnia and of effects on motor activity, and it does not impair cognition. Its lack of abuse potential makes ramelteon the only nonscheduled FDA-approved hypnotic.

For many, current hypnotics offer a reasonable risk–benefit ratio (Schutte-Rodin et al., 2008). However, some do not respond adequately to these compounds or exhibit tolerance to their therapeutic effects. Additionally, the need for new options for managing insomnia is illustrated by problems with tolerability, including daytime sedation, and cognitive and psychomotor side effects (Bixler et al., 1987; Kales, 1980). Additional risks include the potential for developing dependence and the risk for abnormal behaviors, such as engaging in complex activities while sleeping. These risks may be greater for the pediatric and elderly populations, for which there are few treatment alternatives. In addition, many are reluctant to routinely use a hypnotic with controlled substance status. While ramelteon has minimized this concern, some do not respond to this agent, or experience side effects that preclude its continued use.

It has become increasingly clear that there is a broader range of targets when treating insomnia beyond the need to decrease sleep latency and increase sleep efficiency. For example, agents designed to influence SWS, which is involved in memory consolidation and related to the restorative quality of sleep, may prove to be more efficacious than current therapies (Wafford & Ebert, 2008). A number of mechanistic approaches are now being examined to design agents that act to influence SWS in this way.

B. Insomnia Drug Development Background

Hypnotic efficacy is assessed by determining the effect of the test agent on the induction and maintenance of sleep utilizing PSG, subjective and global clinical sleep rating scales, and sleep diary endpoints (Morin, 2003). There is also value in addressing unmet medical needs by targeting SWS and by examining the impact on those aspects of quality of life most affected by insomnia (Ohayon, 2005). While the former can be assessed with standard PSG techniques, addressing the restorative qualities of sleep requires the development of new measurement techniques that are scientifically validated and acceptable to regulatory agencies. A major challenge for insomnia drug development is competition from a host of less expensive, but generally effective, generic agents. Thus, approval of new drugs in this area requires definitive evidence of efficacy and safety advantages over existing medications.

C. Mechanisms in Development

I. γ-Aminobutyric Acid

As the predominant inhibitory neurotransmitter, the amino acid γ-aminobutyric acid (GABA) is involved in the modulation of sleep and waking (Mendelson, 2001; Siegel, 2004). It is not surprising, therefore, that GABA receptors have been key targets for drugs used to treat insomnia. GABA is found in high concentrations throughout the neuroaxis, including the brainstem, reticular activating system, limbic regions, and cerebral cortex. GABA is utilized both by interneurons and by neurons projecting to distant brain regions. For example, in the reticular activating system GABA interneurons exert modulatory effects on glutamate excitatory neurons, and in the thalamic reticular nucleus GABA is inhibitory on projection systems to cortical regions that facilitate the development of the synchronous activity of SWS. In the posterior hypothalamus, GABA exerts inhibitory effects during SWS on the TMN, modulating the effects of histamine, an activating agent. While GABA acts through both GABA-A and GABA-B receptor subtypes, approved hypnotic agents work solely through attachment to the GABA-A site. A ligand-gated ion channel, the GABA-A receptor, controls the neuronal influx of chloride ion, resulting in hyperpolarization of the postsynaptic membrane. A variety of drugs allosterically modify the GABA-A receptor, making it more responsive to GABA. Included in this group are the benzodiazepines, ethanol, and the barbiturates. The nonbenzodiazepine hypnotics, such as zolpidem, zaleplon, and eszopiclone, attach selectively to a subclass of benzodiazepine-sensitive GABA-A receptors. GABA-A receptor subtypes are based on the stoichiometry of the subunit combination of this pentameric receptor site. Efforts are now underway to develop agents that interact even more selectively with GABA-A receptor subtypes, both as full and partial agonists, in an attempt to identify hypnotics and anxiolytics with greater efficacy and safety (see Chapter 4).

There are a number of nonbenzodiazepine products in development that target the α_1 subunit of the GABA-A receptor. Included are indiplon and new formulations of existing compounds, such as a transmucosal formulation of zolpidem, an inhaled formulation of zaleplon (AZ-007), and a new formulation of eszopiclone aimed at improving tolerability (SEP-0227018). While demonstrating improvements in total sleep time, LPS, latency to sleep onset, wake after sleep onset (WASO), and sleep quality in immediate release and sustained release formulations (Lydiard et al., 2006; Marrs, 2008), indiplon has faced challenges to regulatory approval in the United States because of concerns about the sustained release formulation and its efficacy relative to current treatments. The transmucosal formulation of zolpidem has been evaluated in two Phase 3 studies with a focus on middle of the night (MOTN) awakening. A 3.5 mg dose significantly reduced latency to sleep onset after MOTN awakenings, improved sleep quality, next-day alertness ratings, WASO, and number of awakenings as compared to placebo (Roth et al., 2009). Rebound effects on sleep were not noted (Rosenberg et al., 2009) in this study. An earlier crossover study reported that transmucosal zolpidem was efficacious on a number of sleep parameters at 1.75 and 3.5 mg as well (Roth et al., 2008).

The development of AZ-007 (an inhaled formulation of zaleplon) has included a Phase 1 pharmacokinetics study that revealed a median time to peak venous concentration (T_{max}) of 1.6 min and onset of sedation at 2 min. Sepracor, the manufacturer of ezopiclone, has announced that its alternate formulation, SEP-0227018 is currently being evaluated in a Phase 2 trial.

Gabapentin and pregabalin are calcium channel $\alpha_2\delta$-subunit modulators, which are believed to exert their insomnia-relevant pharmacological effects primarily through indirect impact on GABA neurotransmission. Gabapentin modulates neuronal calcium flux through actions on the $\alpha_2\delta$ subunit of voltage-gated calcium channels, increasing synaptic GABA concentrations and GABA turnover (Czapinski et al., 2005). These effects appear most likely to mediate its impact on sleep, although there may be indirect effects through downstream modulation of monoamine neurotransmitters involved in sleep physiology. Pregabalin shares similar mechanisms of action with gabapentin, although it is more potent as reflected by its lower dose in clinical use (200–600 mg/day vs. 900–2,400 mg/day for gabapentin). In healthy subjects, treatment with gabapentin titrated to 1,800 mg/day over a week was associated with significant increases in SWS percentage, with no effect on other PSG variables (Foldvary-Schaefer et al., 2002). Single-dose gabapentin at 300 and 600 mg has been found to decrease awakenings, increase sleep efficiency, and decrease Stage 1 sleep in healthy control subjects (Bazil, Battista, & Basner, 2005); gabapentin dosed at 600 mg was associated with increased SWS, decreased arousals, and decreased REM sleep. The effect of pregabalin on sleep physiology has been examined in healthy subjects compared with alprazolam in a randomized, blinded, crossover trial (Hindmarch et al., 2005). Subjects received each of the following treatments for 3-day treatment periods with a 7-day washout: pregabalin 150 mg, alprazolam 1 mg, or placebo. Treatment with pregabalin was associated with increased SWS, increased Stage 4 sleep, reduction in sleep latency, reduced REM duration, and decreased number of awakenings. PD200390 is a calcium channel $\alpha_2\delta$-subunit modulator which was being developed for insomnia with a focus on WASO. Its development was discontinued in early 2009, and no other drugs with this mechanism were under development at the time of this writing.

2. Serotonergic System

It has been known for years that serotonin enhances wakefulness by enhancing the activity of the reticular activating system (Rothballer, 1957). Serotonergic neurons in the dorsal raphe nucleus project widely to the hypothalamus, thalamus, basal ganglia, and cerebral cortex, and stimulation of 5-HT$_{2a}$ receptors mediates the activating effect (Abrams et al., 2005). Moreover, two 5-HT$_{2a}$ receptor antagonists approved for major depression are known to improve sleep as well. Thus, the antidepressant nefazodone increases sleep efficiency, decreases the number of awakenings, and increase the percentage of REM sleep in patients with major depression. This contrasts with many other antidepressants which are known to disrupt sleep architecture (Rush et al., 1998). Likewise, the antidepressant mirtazapine, a 5-HT_{2a} receptor antagonist, decreases sleep latency, increases sleep efficiency, and reduces WASO in patients with major depression (Winokur et al., 2003). While these results would seem to support the development of these drugs as treatments for insomnia, these agents have other effects that could influence their utility in this regard. However, the mixed $5\text{-HT}_{2a}/5\text{-HT}_{2c}$ receptor antagonist ritanserin increases SWS in healthy subjects, in poor sleepers (Viola et al., 2002), and in preclinical models (Dugovic, 1992), leading to efforts to develop more specific agents as treatments for insomnia (Teegarden et al., 2008). The potential benefits of this approach as compared to existing agents include a decreased risk for dependence, fewer adverse psychomotor effects, and the likelihood that such compounds would not be classified as controlled substances.

The 5-HT_{2a} receptor antagonists currently in development for insomnia include eplivanserin, pimavanserin, and esmirtazepine, a stereoisomer of the antidepressant mirtazepine. Volinanserin, pruvanserin, and APD125 are 5-HT_{2a} receptor antagonists that have been abandoned as potential treatments for this condition at present. Of compounds with this mechanism, eplivanserin has advanced the furthest through the drug development process, having successfully completed a large Phase 3 development program. The results of these studies have been filed with regulatory authorities and it has the potential to be approved for marketing within the next year. Eplivanserin has been demonstrated to improve sleep maintenance insomnia, with a significant reduction in WASO and the number of nocturnal awakenings (NAWs) noted for up to 12 weeks. In the Epilong trial (Cowen—28th Annual Health Care Conference, 18 March 2008, Slides 22–25, http://en.sanofi-aventis.com/binaries/08-03-18_Cowen_Slide_EN_tcm28-19536.pdf), >1,000 sleep maintenance insomnia patients received either eplivanserin 5 mg or placebo, with patient reported outcome measures of NAW and WASO. Patients receiving 5 mg eplivanserin reported greater reductions in NAW compared to placebo at weeks 6 (–0.99 vs. –0.66) and 12 (–1.08 vs. –0.74) and significant reduction in WASO compared to placebo at weeks 6 (–47.8 vs. –33.7 min) and 12 (–53.3 vs. 39.8 min). Similar results were obtained in a 6-week study using PSG endpoints rather than patient reports. In this case, patients receiving 5 mg of eplivanserin demonstrated significantly greater reductions in NAW compared to placebo at weeks 6 (–2.72 vs. –0.97) and 12 (–2.91 vs. –1.09) and a significant reduction in WASO compared to placebo at weeks 6 (–24.8 vs. –18.4 min) and 12 (–25.7 vs. –22.1 min).

Pimavanserin (ACP-103) is a potent and selective serotonin 5-HT_{2A} inverse agonist in development for Parkinson's disease psychosis and insomnia. In a clinical study, healthy older subjects were randomized to one of five treatment arms, including placebo and four different doses (1, 2.5, 5, and 20 mg) of pimavanserin (PR Newswire, 19 April 2006, http://www.prnewswire.com/cgi-bin/stories.pl?ACCT=104&STORY=/www/story/04-19-2006/0004342825&EDATE=). The PSG assessments revealed that once-daily administration of 5 and 20 mg induced statistically significant increases in SWS. Adverse events were mild to moderate in nature and comparable across the placebo and pimavanserin-treated groups. The company has not announced specific plans for moving development of this compound forward for insomnia at the time of this writing.

Esmirtazepine (Org 50081) is currently in Phase 3 development for treatment of insomnia. Results from Phase 2 studies have not been formally presented, but a company press release in January 2002 stated that "Investigated dosages of the Org 50081 compound showed positive and robust results on multiple sleep parameters such as total sleep time and wakefulness after sleep onset. A statistically significant shorter time to sleep onset was demonstrated in Org 50081 treatment groups compared to placebo." The sponsor has completed one Phase 3 trial and has five ongoing Phase 3 trials in adults and elderly subjects with chronic insomnia at the time of this writing.

3. Melatonin System

Melatonin is a peptide hormone released from the pineal gland during the dark phase of the circadian cycle (Turek & Gillette, 2004). Its release is regulated by light signals received by melanopsin-containing cells in the retina. The absence of light signals results in release of melatonin into the CSF and circulatory system. Melatonin, through interactions with melatonin MT1, MT2, and MT3 receptors, coordinates a wide range of physiological processes linked to the circadian cycle. It has been demonstrated in human studies that melatonin decreases sleep latency and increases sleep efficiency when administered in the early evening (Stone, Turner, Mills, & Nicholson, 2000). Studies in those with insomnia have yielded mixed results, with variability in outcomes attributed to dose, time of melatonin administration relative to the circadian cycle, and target populations (Turek & Gillette, 2004; Feeney et al., 2009). Melatonin causes a shift in circadian rhythms in healthy subjects (Lewy et al., 1996), with most studies on the use of melatonin for jet lag demonstrating benefit (Herxheimer & Petrie, 2002).

It has been suggested that MT1 receptors mediate the sleep promoting effects of melatonin, while MT2 receptors mediate the circadian phase-shifting effects. Ramelteon, a melatonin receptor agonist, shows a 1,000-fold greater selectivity for MT1 over MT2 receptors (Reynoldson et al., 2008). While it would seem this agent would be best for treating initial insomnia, it is also being examined for potential beneficial effects in managing disturbances in circadian rhythm. The apparent absence of adverse psychomotor effects and potential for abuse also make melatonin agonists an attractive alternative to conventional therapies in the treatment of insomnia.

Tasimelteon is a melatonin MT1 and MT2 agonist being developed as a treatment for circadian rhythm sleep disorders and insomnia. Clinical studies have been completed examining the efficacy of tasimelteon to reduce sleep disruption and promote circadian readjustment. The results indicated that tasimelteon improves sleep onset and sleep maintenance without next-day residual effects (Rajaratnam et al., 2009). It has also been found to shift the intrinsic circadian rhythm as measured by production of melatonin.

Tasimelteon has also been evaluated in a Phase 3 study with PSG endpoints, in which patients with chronic initial insomnia were randomized to receive either 20 or 50 mg of tasimelteon or placebo over the course of 4 weeks. Both doses of the study drug demonstrated significant improvement in LPS compared to placebo; mean LPS improved by 45.0 min in the 20 mg group, 46.4 min in the 50 mg group, and 28.3 min in the placebo group on nights 1 and 8 of treatment. Similar improvements were observed in the data from nights 22 and 29 of treatment. There were no significant effects of the drug on total sleep time in this study. It is expected that a second Phase 3 trial in chronic insomnia would be required to pursue approval for that indication.

4. Histamine System

The basic sleep physiology of histamine has been discussed above with regard to narcolepsy drug development. Histamine exerts its actions in brain through histamine H1, H2, and H3 receptors. Antihistaminic agents, including compounds used in cough–cold preparations, are frequently sedating, primarily because of their blockade of histamine H1 sites (Haas & Panula, 2003). Indeed, nonselective histamine antagonists, such as diphenhydramine, are often used off-label for the treatment of insomnia because of their sedating effects, although these compounds interact with a host of transmitter systems, making it impossible to attribute the effects on sleep on histamine receptor blockade alone. For example, diphenhydramine is less desirable as a choice for treatment of insomnia in older populations because its anticholinergic muscarinic effects increase the potential for cognitive impairment in this population. Thus, selective histamine H1 receptor antagonists could effect medications for the treatment of insomnia in terms of both safety and efficacy.

Doxepin, a tricyclic antidepressant, has a very high affinity, and some selectivity, for histamine H1 receptors in comparison with other neurotransmitter receptors (Cusack et al., 1994). Because of this, doxepin is undergoing clinical trails as a treatment for insomnia at doses much lower than those used to treat depression. Doxepin, at doses approximately one-quarter of those used to treat depression, was examined in a controlled trial for insomnia using PSG endpoints (Hajak et al., 2001). In this study, patients with primary insomnia received from 25 to 50 mg of doxepin or placebo for 4 weeks and subsequently observed over a 2-week washout phase. Doxepin significantly increased sleep efficiency in assessments on Night 1 and Night 28 as compared to placebo. Although there were no significant changes in sleep latency, the subjects did not exhibit abnormal sleep latency at baseline. Global improvement of these patients was significantly improved during the first night of treatment, and patient-rated sleep quality ($p <$ or $= 0.001$) and working ability ($p <$ or $= 0.005$) was significantly enhanced over the study treatment period. Rebound in sleep parameters was not observed, although it was reported that the doxepin group had significantly more patients with severe rebound insomnia. Low-dose doxepin was evaluated in three Phase 3 studies for treatment of insomnia and one for study in transient insomnia. A crossover design with 2-day treatment periods examined the effect of 1 mg, 3 mg, 6 mg of doxepin and placebo in subjects with chronic insomnia. PSG revealed significant improvements in WASO, total sleep time, and overall sleep efficiency for each doxepin dose compared with placebo (Roth et al., 2007). Tolerability was comparable to placebo, with no cognitive or next-day residual effects. A similar study in an elderly population had comparable results (Scharf et al., 2008). In both of these studies, improvements in sleep efficiency were observed even through the last third of sleep time, suggesting this treatment could address the need for hypnotic options that address middle and late insomnia.

Doxepin efficacy for chronic insomnia was also examined in a Phase 3 placebo-controlled 12-week trial of 1 and 3 mg in elderly adults and a Phase 2 placebo-controlled 5-week trial of 3 and 6 mg in adults, with PSG assessments on nights 1 and week 12 of treatment. A combined analysis of the results from these studies (Lankford et al., 2009) revealed improved total sleep time and percentage of time asleep in the final hours of sleeping time, with no significant effects on cognitive measures in the first hour of waking. A study examining a 6 mg dose in a healthy subject model of transient insomnia found significantly improved WASO on night one for each dose, from 17 min for the 1 mg dose in the elderly subject study to 40 min for the 6 mg dose in the transient insomnia study. There was no significant difference in number of awakenings at any dose of doxepin, suggesting that low-dose doxepin helps maintain sleep with minimal impact on arousability.

5. Orexin/Hypocretin System

While orexin/hypocretin agonists are the focus for treating narcolepsy, antagonists of this system are being examined as therapies for insomnia. Almorexant (ACT-078573) is an orally active orexin receptor antagonist of OX1 and OX2 receptors. This compound has been demonstrated to increase nonREM and REM sleep in rats and induces somnolence and increases surrogate markers of REM sleep in dogs (Brisbare-Roch et al., 2007). Also reported was the finding that human subjects taking almorexant display subjective and objective electrophysiological signs of sleep, with subjective alertness returning to baseline approximately 6 h after 400 mg and approximately 10 h after 1,000 mg. EEG assessments revealed a dose-dependent reduction in latency to Stage 2 sleep at 200 mg and higher. No signs of cataplexy were observed in individuals taking this agent. A Phase 2 single-dose, two-way crossover study was conducted in patients with insomnia comparing almorexant 50, 100, 200, and 400 mg versus placebo (Roecker & Coleman, 2008). The results revealed dose-dependent increases in sleep efficiency, decreased WASO, and LPS at doses of 100 mg or higher. No next-day performance impairment was observed with any of the doses tested. Almorexant is currently being evaluated in a Phase 3 trial comparing 100 and 200 mg doses to zolpidem 10 mg and placebo over a 16-day treatment period. Efficacy endpoints include PSG (WASO and LPS) and subjective sleep measures.

Another orexin antagonist, GW649868, is in development as a treatment for insomnia. Its hypnotic effects were assessed in two randomized, double-blind, placebo-controlled crossover studies (Bettica et al., 2009). The Phase 1 study assessed the PSG effects of 30 and 60 mg SB-649868 in healthy male subjects, and the Phase 2 study evaluated the PSG effects of 10, 30, and 60 mg in male subjects with a diagnosis of primary insomnia. The agent was administered after dinner at 90 min before bed time in both studies. It was found that SB-649868 significantly reduced LPS and WASO and increased total sleep time compared to placebo. There were no findings of next-day residual effects.

D. Insomnia Summary and Future Directions

Advances in understanding of the basic neurobiology of sleep and wakefulness are yielding an increasing number of potential drug targets for the treatment of insomnia. While progress has been slower in understanding the pathophysiology of primary insomnia, the increased numbers of clinical studies aimed at evaluating new mechanisms for this condition offer an opportunity to address this issue. Although currently available therapy has a reasonable risk–benefit profile for many, there is a continuing need for new treatments that do not produce adverse psychomotor effects, nighttime arousal or behavioral symptoms, or dependence and abuse potential. With regard to efficacy, clinical needs include effectiveness in treating middle and late insomnia, improving SWS, and diminishing non-restorative sleep. A safe agent with these characteristics would be highly competitive in the current generic market, as it would address symptoms that are poorly managed with current agents and in turn enhance functioning and quality of life.

V. Restless Leg Syndrome

A. Clinical Background

I. Clinical Syndrome

RLS is a sensorimotor neurological disorder characterized by an uncontrollable and distressing urge to move the legs and sometimes the arms. This compulsion is usually accompanied by deep, unpleasant, and discomforting sensations in these limbs, such as creeping, crawling, tingling, or itching (Allen et al., 2003b). These symptoms are partially relieved by movement of the affected limb. These symptoms, which are triggered by rest when sufferers are in sedentary or reclining positions, are particularly intense at night, causing significant sleep impairment (Allen et al., 2003b). Sleep disruption and its negative impact on quality of life are the main reasons patients seek treatment for this condition (Allen & Early, 2001). It is estimated that RLS affects about 5–10% of the general population in Western countries (Phillips et al., 2000). It is more prevalent in the elderly and in females (Rothdach et al., 2000; Ulfberg, Nystrom, Carter, & Edling, 2001). Approximately 75% of patients with moderate to severe RLS report difficulties with sleep initiation, maintenance, or awakenings (Allen & Early, 2001). Population-based studies suggest an increased risk of hypertension and coronary artery disease in patients with RLS (Javaheri, 2008; Sforza et al., 1999).

From a pathophysiological perspective, the condition can be divided into primary or idiopathic and secondary RLS. Common causes of secondary RLS include iron deficiency, pregnancy, and uremia associated with renal failure (O'Keeffe et al., 1994; Manconi et al., 2004; Rijsman et al., 2004). It is known that RLS occurs in those with rheumatoid arthritis or fibromyalgia and can be comorbid in patients with peripheral neuropathy or radiculopathy (Ondo & Jankovic, 1996; Polydefkis et al., 2000; Rijsman & de Weerd, 1999; Walters et al., 1996). Symptoms of the disorder can be caused or exacerbated by a variety of medications and other agents. Included in this group are dopamine receptor antagonists, antidepressants, antihistamines, alcohol, caffeine, and nicotine (Picchietti & Winkelman, 2005; Winkelmann et al., 2001).

As for treatment, RLS-related symptoms are placed into one of three categories reflecting the increasing severity of the disorder: intermittent, daily, or refractory to treatment (Silber et al., 2004). Dopamine receptor agonists are the only approved treatments for RLS, although other drug classes have been used (Trenkwalder et al., 2008).

2. Pathophysiology Relevant to Drug Development

Very little is known about the pathophysiology of RLS. Research is focused on anatomical localization of RLS pathways, defects in neurotransmitter systems, and defects in iron metabolism. Results of neuroimaging, neuroanatomical, and neurophysiological studies show involvement of several brain structures in RLS. This includes the cerebral cortex, basal ganglia, thalamus, A11 neurons, substantia nigra, brainstem nuclei, and spinal cord (Paulus et al., 2007a; Paulus et al., 2007b; Wetter et al., 2004). Neuroimaging studies point to a functional impairment of dopaminergic pathways in these areas, resulting, in part, disinhibition of subcortical brain regions (Paulus et al., 2007b; Wetter et al., 2004).

The central pathophysiological theory of RLS involves dysfunction of descending inhibitory pathways resulting in a reduction of inhibition at the spinal level (Paulus et al., 2007b). Indeed, it appears that a dysfunction of dopaminergic systems plays a central role in the pathophysiology of RLS (Allen, 2007). This hypothesis is supported by the observation that dopamine agonists are very efficacious treatments for this condition (Trenkwalder et al., 2008). However, there is also evidence that modifications of other neurotransmitters, including opioids, GABA, glutamate, serotonin, and norepinephrine, and of their interactions with dopamine systems are responsible for particular symptoms of RLS (Paulus et al., 2007b). Thus, for example, it is proposed that the endogenous opioid system contributes significantly to the pain and unpleasant sensations associated with RLS (Paulus et al., 2007b). Supporting the contribution of nondopaminergic systems is the finding that pharmacological interventions that modify the activity of these other neurotransmitter pathways are effective in treating certain symptoms of this disorder (Trenkwalder et al., 2008).

Deficiencies in iron metabolism have also been linked to changes in the dopamine system (Allen, 2004) as iron is a required cofactor in dopamine biosynthesis, and iron-deprived rats display altered dopamine levels, and dopamine receptor and transporter number and function (Erikson et al., 2000; Erikson et al., 2001). Laboratory animal and human imaging studies suggest that decreased availability of iron in the substantia nigra disrupts cell function and reduces dopaminergic activity in this brain region (Allen, 2007).

Dopamine systems are major targets for drug development because of efficacy and side-effect problems associated with dopamine agonists (Trenkwalder et al., 2008). However, efforts are also underway to develop agents that interact with the other neurotransmitter systems that appear to be involved in RLS (Trenkwalder et al., 2008). Beyond this, consideration is being given to examining the safety and efficacy of agents that interact with either adenosine 2A receptors or the $\alpha_2\delta$ subunit of voltage-gated calcium channels (Sills, 2006).

3. Current Treatments

Treatment of RLS secondary to iatrogenic or substance-related causes involves removal of the offending agents, such as antipsychotics or antidepressants (Picchietti & Winkelman, 2005; Winkelmann et al., 2001). In those with iron deficiency as the primary cause of RLS, iron supplementation is the first-line treatment (Earley et al., 2004). If RLS symptoms persist despite these treatments, other approaches are considered. For these patients, and those with idiopathic RLS, long-term symptom management is generally required.

At present, medications based on the dopamine system are considered the drugs of choice for RLS. This includes both direct-acting dopamine receptor agonists and agents that enhance dopamine transmission in brain (Trenkwalder et al., 2008). Levodopa (L-DOPA)/carbidopa and L-DOPA/benserazide are administered to increase dopamine levels in the CNS. L-DOPA is converted to dopamine (Conti et al., 2007). Typically it is administered with peripherally acting DOPA decarboxylase inhibitors such as carbidopa or benserazide to increase the amount of L-DOPA that reaches the brain (Silber et al., 2004). L-DOPA treatment must be intermittent because of the risk of developing the augmentation phenomenon, which involves worsening of RLS symptoms (Garcia-Borreguero et al., 2007).

There are two general classes of dopamine receptor agonists, ergolines and nonergolines (Trenkwalder et al., 2008). At present, the nonergolines are considered the frontline therapy for RLS (Silber et al., 2004). These include ropirinole and pramipexole, the only FDA-approved treatments for RLS in the United States. The ergolines that could be employed are carbergoline and bromocriptine. Pergolide, an egoline once used for the treatment of Parkinson's disease, was removed from the US market in 2007 because of concerns about valvular heart disease risk associated with this agent (Lanier, 2003). Indeed, use of the ergolines as a group is limited and requires special monitoring due to the risk of cardiac valvular fibrosis and other fibrotic side effects (Horvath et al., 2004).

The dopamine agonists employed to treat RLS interact with dopamine D1, D2, or D3 receptors (Kvernmo et al., 2008). Within this group receptor subtype selectivity varies, as does full and partial agonism at each site. Evidence to date suggests that activation of dopamine D2 receptors is most important with regard to treating the symptoms of RLS (Kvernmo et al., 2008). Both ropinirole and pramipexole are full agonists at D2 receptors and have high affinity for the D3 receptor subtype, and both have a higher affinity for the D3 receptor than for the D2 (Kvernmo et al., 2008; Walters et al., 2004; Winkelman et al., 2006).

Second-line treatments for RLS include anticonvulsants, opioids, benzodiazepines, and sedative hypnotics (Trenkwalder et al., 2008). Gabapentin is the most frequently employed anticonvulsant for the treatment of RLS. Other anticonvulsants used for this indication include carbamazepine, valproic acid, and topiramate. As the mechanisms of action of these anticonvulsants vary, their effectiveness in treating symptoms of RLS reveals little about the underlying pathology.

Opioids currently considered in the treatment of RLS include oxycodone, tramadol, and methadone (Trenkwalder et al., 2008). Among the benzodiazepines and hypnotics employed to treat this condition are clonazepam, zolpidem, and temazepam (Trenkwalder et al., 2008).

4. Unmet Needs

Very little is known about the etiology and pathophysiology of RLS. As a consequence, most of the current treatment options are not intended to modify the disease, but rather to provide symptom relief. Unfortunately, these drugs carry the risk of significant side effects, and many do not provide complete relief of symptoms (Trenkwalder et al., 2008).

Agents such as L-DOPA/carbidopa have been associated with rebound and the risk of the development of augmentation (Guilleminault et al., 1993). Rebound is the worsening of symptoms of RLS at the end of a treatment period, resulting in late-night or morning recurrence of symptoms. Rebound is characterized by wearing off of the medication effect or tolerance (Winkelman et al., 2007). Augmentation is a more serious side effect. It entails the development of symptoms earlier in the day and/or an increase in the severity of symptoms (Garcia-Borreguero et al., 2007). One explanation for augmentation is that these drugs shift the circadian timing of the appearance of RLS symptoms to an earlier time of the day (Garcia-Borreguero et al., 2004). It has also been claimed that augmentation is due to a reduction in the number of dopamine D2 receptors relative to D1 receptors and an increase in dopamine levels (Paulus & Trenkwalder, 2006). Although less common and less severe than rebound, augmentation can also occur with direct-acting dopamine receptor agonists (Trenkwalder et al., 2008). Additionally, the ergoline dopamine receptor agonists are associated with cardiac valvular and other fibrotic side effects requiring close cardiopulmonary monitoring (Horvath et al., 2004).

The use of opioids, benzodiazepines, and other hypnotics is restricted because of their abuse potential, the risk of respiratory depression, and other side effects such as sedation and cognitive impairment (Trenkwalder et al., 2008). Additionally, many of these second-line agents do not treat all aspects of RLS symptomatology. Consequently, these drugs are often used only as adjunctive agents with dopamine agonists.

B. Restless Leg Syndrome Drug Development Background

1. Study Design and End Points

The eligibility criteria for an RLS study are designed to exclude those with secondary RLS, with other primary sleep disorders, and with medical or psychiatric conditions that will confound the assessment of RLS symptomatology (e.g., movement disorders). Patients also must meet a specific symptomatic threshold. The International Restless Legs Scale (IRLS) is used to establish subject eligibility (Allen et al., 2003a).

The primary efficacy assessment when examining the RLS response to drugs or test agents includes assessment of symptomatology. The IRLS rating scale is used frequently for this purpose. Assessment of sleep is often a co-primary efficacy assessment, although it may be considered a major secondary efficacy assessment instead. Sleep is studied using questionnaires such as Pittsburgh Sleep Quality Index (Buysse et al., 1989) or Medical Outcomes Study sleep scale (Hays et al., 2005). Sleep diary assessments are frequently included to gather objective data on a daily basis (Monk et al., 1994). This includes data on total sleep time and wake time after sleep onset. Daytime sleepiness is evaluated using the Epworth Sleepiness Scale (Johns, 1991) and the sudden onset of sleep scale (Hobson et al., 2002). Comprehensive studies include actigraphy or PSG, with a focus on specific PSG variables such as the periodic limb movements during sleep index (Zucconi et al., 2006).

Other secondary efficacy assessments include pain and quality of life. This is accomplished with general questionnaires or with the RLS pain scale (Kushida et al., 2009) and the RLS quality of life scale (Qol-RLS) (Kohnen et al., 2007). Compound safety and tolerability assessments should include quantitative evaluation of augmentation with the Augmentation Severity Rating Scale (Garcia-Borreguero et al., 2007).

2. Drug Development Issues and Challenges

Limited knowledge of RLS pathophysiology remains the major barrier to the development of drugs to treat this condition (Paulus et al., 2007b). Current drug development strategies are based primarily on known pharmacological mechanisms or involve extensions of those mechanisms. In a few cases, anecdotal evidence or exploration of mechanisms of effective agents, such as gabapentin, is providing clues for new approaches for treating RLS.

The disorder frequently occurs in the context of other general medical conditions, and its clinical presentation is often complicated by comorbidities (Ondo & Jankovic, 1996; Polydefkis et al., 2000; Rijsman & de Weerd, 1999; Walters et al., 1996). Additionally, it can be difficult to distinguish between primary and secondary RLS and to differentially diagnose it from other sleep disorders. These issues present significant challenges for designing clinical trials aimed at identifying agents that are effective in treating this condition.

As augmentation can occur relatively late during treatment, long-term studies may be required to identify its incidence with a particular agent.

C. Mechanisms in Development

1. Strategies Targeting the Dopamine System

The dopamine system remains a major target for RLS drug development because of the proven efficacy of dopamine agonists in treating this disorder. Several new agents are being examined to reduce or eliminate the side effects associated with current dopamine agonists without compromising efficacy.

a. Alternate Delivery Systems   Two dopamine agonists are undergoing investigation as a patch application. It is thought that maintenance of stable blood levels may minimize the risk for augmentation and rebound. The rotigotine patch is currently under investigation in several large-scale controlled trials (Stiasny-Kolster et al., 2004). An ergot derivative, rotigotine is a dopamine D3/D2/D1 agonist. It is also under investigation as a nasal spray (ClinicalTrials.gov Identifier # NCT00389831).

The lisuride patch has displayed efficacy in one small, proof-of-principle study (Benes, 2006). A nonergoline, lisuride, is an agonist at dopamine D2/D3/D4 sites and a partial agonist at dopamine D1 receptors.

b. Differential Dopamine Receptor Selectivity   Strategies under preliminary investigation include partial agonism at dopamine D2 receptors (aplindore) (ClinicalTrials.gov Identifier # NCT00626418) (Heinrich et al., 2006) as well as D2 agonism/D1 partial agonism (dihydroergocriptine) (Tergau, Wischer, Wolf, & Paulus, 2001).

c. Other Approaches for Enhancing Dopaminergic Activity   A strategy under investigation entails selective inhibition (nitisinone) of an enzyme involved in the metabolism of tyrosine, the precursor dopamine. It is hypothesized that inhibition of this enzyme, hydroxyphenylpyruvate dioxygenase, will result in a stable increase in brain dopamine levels because of an increase in tyrosine availability (http://www.synosia.com/press/2008/synosia_20081211.html) (Santra & Baumann, 2008).

2. Strategies Involving Mixed Monoamine Modulation

Bupropion, a dopamine and norepinephrine reuptake inhibitor, is under investigation as a treatment for RLS (ClinicalTrials.gov Identifier #

NCT00621571) (Lee et al., 2009). Bupropion is about twice as potent an inhibitor of dopamine reuptake as of norepinephrine uptake.

Safinamide, a selective and reversible MAO-B inhibitor and a dopamine and noradrenaline uptake inhibitor, is being investigated as a possible therapy for RLS (http://newron.emperor-design.com/uploads/SafinamideRL-SPressReleaseFinal110105.pdf). Its blockade of voltage-sensitive sodium/calcium channels and inhibition of glutamate release may also play a role in its mechanism of action (Fariello, 2007).

3. Inhibition of Voltage-Gated Calcium Channels

Gabapentin has been used off-label to treat RLS (Trenkwalder et al., 2008). After years of uncertainty, it now appears that the mechanism of action of gabapentin is inhibition of voltage-gated calcium channels containing the $\alpha_2\delta$ subunit (Sills, 2006). Two agents from this class, pregabalin (Sommer et al., 2007) and gabapentin enacarbil (Kushida et al., 2009), are under investigation as treatments for RLS.

Pregabalin is a gabapentin analog and is virtually identical to it in terms of its mechanism of action therapeutic profile (Sills, 2006). A prodrug of gabapentin, gabapentin enacarbil, is designed to display greater bioavailability and a better pharmacokinetic profile than gabapentin (Cundy et al., 2008).

4. Other Mechanisms

Adenosine A_{2A} receptors are selectively localized in the basal ganglia. These receptors play an important role in modulating glutamatergic regulation of GABAergic and enkephalergic neurons (Jenner et al., 2009). Basal ganglia neurons are involved in the pathophysiology of RLS (Paulus et al., 2007b). It is hypothesized that reducing striatopallidal neuronal activity by blocking adenosine A_{2A} receptors will diminish RLS symptoms. To examine this theory, adenosine A_{2A} receptor antagonists, such as istradefylline, are being developed as novel treatment options for RLS (ClinicalTrials.gov Identifier # NCT00199446).

Preliminary studies, case reports, or anecdotal evidence suggest that clonidine, an α-adrenergic agonist (Wagner et al., 1996) and amantadine, an NMDA antagonist (Evidente et al., 2000) are effective in the treatment of RLS. Botulinum toxin (ClinicalTrials.gov Identifier # NCT00479154), levetiracetam, an indirect modulator of GABAergic neurotransmission (ClinicalTrials.gov Identifier # NCT00247364), and sequential compression devices (ClinicalTrials.gov Identifier # NCT00479531) are also under investigation as treatments for this condition. Table IV provides a summary of new drug treatment approaches under development for RLS.

TABLE IV   Mechanisms or Delivery Systems in Development for Treatment of RLS[a]

Mechanisms/delivery systems	References/ClinicalTrial.gov Identifier
Strategies targeting the dopamine system	
Alternate delivery systems	
Rotigotine transdermal patch	Stiasny-Kolster et al. (2004)
Lisuride transdermal patch	Benes (2006)
Rotigotine nasal spray	NCT00389831
Differential dopamine receptor selectivity	
Aplindore (D2 partial agonism)	NCT00626418; Heinrich et al. (2006)
Dihydroergocriptine (D2 agonism/D1 partial agonism)	Tergau et al. (2001)
Other mechanisms targeting the dopamine system	
Nitisinone (Hydroxyphenylpyruvate dioxygenase enzyme inhibition)	http://www.synosia.com/press/2008/synosia_20081211.html; Santra and Baumann (2008)
Strategies involving mixed monoamine modulation	
Bupropion (dopamine/norepinephrine reuptake inhibition)	NCT00621571; Lee et al. (2009)
Sulfinamide (reversible monoamine oxidase inhibition/dopamine-norepinephrine reuptake inhibition/blockade of voltage-sensitive calcium/sodium channels)	http://newron.emperor-design.com/uploads/SafinamideRLSPressReleaseFinal110105.pdf; Fariello (2007)
Inhibition of voltage-gated calcium channels	
Pregabalin	Sommer et al. (2007)
Gabapentin encarbil (prodrug of gabapentin)	Kushida et al. (2009)
Other Mechanisms	
Istradefylline (adenosine A_2A receptor antagonism)	NCT00199446; Jenner et al. (2009)
Clonidine (α-adrenergic agonism)	Wagner et al. (1996)
Amantadine (NMDA antagonism)	Evidente et al. (2000)
Levetiracetam (anticonvulsant)	NCT00247364
Botulinum toxin	NCT00479154
Sequential compression devices	NCT00479531

[a] Abbreviations: RLS, restless legs syndrome.

D. Summary and Future Directions

While the dopaminergic approach for treating RLS is reasonable given the proven efficacy of dopamine receptor agonist for treating this condition, other targets may emerge as more is learned about the underlying neuropathology. Indeed, several nondopaminergic strategies are already being pursued (Trenkwalder et al., 2008). It is possible that some of these nondopaminergic approaches may target specific symptomatic aspects of RLS more effectively than dopaminergic agents. Future research efforts should consider combination strategies with the aim of identifying agents that improve efficacy and reduce side effects when given together. There also need to be larger head to head studies in an attempt to identify subpopulations of patients benefiting more from particular drugs or mechanisms of action. Finally, new pathophysiological and genetic insights may reveal disease-modifying treatment regimens that could supplant the current therapies aimed at treating symptoms only.

VI. Conclusion

Given their prevalence, sleep disorders exact a significant toll in terms of suffering, impaired functioning, and as risk factors for the development of significant medical or psychiatric disorders. Provided in this report are descriptions of the current treatment options for insomnia, narcolepsy, RLS, and obstructive sleep apnea. While a number of drugs are employed to treat each of these conditions, all are limited with respect to efficacy and tolerability. Significant advances in the future await a better understanding of the underlying pathophysiology of these conditions and of the neurobiological alterations associated with these disorders. It is hoped that some of the research directions described herein will stimulate additional research in this area and thereby help foster the discovery of novel agents for treating major sleep disorders.

Acknowledgments

We appreciate the skilled assistance of Pamela Guilbeault in the preparation of this manuscript. We gratefully acknowledge the support of the Dr. Manfred J. Sakel Distinguished Chair in Psychiatry (to AW) for assistance in the preparation of this manuscript.

Disclosure/Conflict of Interest: Dr. DeMartinis has been a full-time employee of Pfizer, Inc., which markets gabapentin and pregabalin, for the past 3 years and has Pfizer stock holdings. He has no other financial relationships or financial holdings with any of the commercial entities with interests discussed in this publication.

Over the past 3 years, Dr. Kamath served as principal investigator for clinical trials studies carried out at the University of Connecticut Health Center for studies funded by Cephalon, Sanofi-Sythelabo, Wyeth, Bristol Myers Sqibb, and Eli Lilly. Funding for the conduct of these clinical trials was paid to the University of Connecticut Health Center.

Over the past 3 years, Dr. Kamath served on the speaker's bureau for Pfizer, Astra-Zeneca, Bristol Myers Sqibb, and Eli Lilly and was paid for promotional speaking. None of these activities involved products that were discussed in this chapter.

Dr. Winokur served as a paid consultant for Schering-Plough Pharmaceuticals with regard to the development of esmirtazapine (ORG 50081) for the indication of primary insomnia. Dr. Winokur also served as principal investigator for a clinical trial funded by Schering-Plough Pharmaceuticals to evaluate the safety and tolerability of esmirtazapine (ORG 50081) in the treatment of insomnia in elderly individuals with primary insomnia. Funding for the conduct of this clinical trial was paid to the University of Connecticut Health Center. Dr. Winokur is a member of TRH Therapeutics, LLP, which holds an approved patent for the use of TRH and TRH analogs for the treatment of idiopathic cancer-related fatigue (US Patent No 7462595). Dr. Winokur was also involved in the filing of US Patent No 5968932 which claims the use of the TRH analog CG-3703 (montirelin) by Grünenthal GmbH for the treatment of OSAS on behalf of Grünenthal GmbH and the University of Pennsylvania.

Dr. Winokur served as a paid consultant for Pfizer Pharmaceuticals for participating in a meeting to discuss the potential for developing pregabalin for the indication of generalized anxiety disorder. Over the past 3 years, Dr. Winokur served as a paid consultant for the Food and Drug Administration to participate in several Advisory Committee Meetings for the Psychopharmacologic Drugs Division. Finally, Dr. Winokur served as principal investigator for clinical trial studies carried out at the University of Connecticut Health Center for studies funded by Sepracor, Pfizer, Sanofi-Synthelabo, Astro-Zeneca, Merck, and Lundbeck.

References

Abrams, J. K., Johnson, P. L., Hay-Schmidt, A., Mikkelsen, J. D., Shekhar, A., & Lowry, C. A. (2005). Serotonergic systems associated with arousal and vigilance behaviors following administration of anxiogenic drugs. *Neuroscience*, *133*(4), 983–997.

Akiskal, H. S., & Akiskal, K. K. (2007). In search of Aristotle: Temperament, human nature, melancholia, creativity and eminence. *Journal of Affective Disorders*, *100*(1–3), 1–6.

Allen, R. (2004). Dopamine and iron in the pathophysiology of restless legs syndrome (RLS). *Sleep Medicine*, *5*(4), 385–391.

Allen, R. P. (2007). Controversies and challenges in defining the etiology and pathophysiology of restless legs syndrome. *American Journal of Medicine*, *120*(1 Suppl 1), S13–S21.

Allen, R. P., & Earley, C. J. (2001). Restless legs syndrome: A review of clinical and pathophysiologic features. *Journal of Clinical Neurophysiology*, *18*(2), 128–147.

Allen, R. P., Kushida, C. A., & Atkinson, M. J. (2003a). Factor analysis of the International Restless Legs Syndrome Study Group's scale for restless legs severity. *Sleep Medicine*, *4*(2), 133–135.

Allen, R. P., Picchietti, D., Hening, W. A., Trenkwalder, C., Walters, A. S., & Montplaisi, J. (2003b). Restless legs syndrome: Diagnostic criteria, special considerations, and epidemiology. A report from the restless legs syndrome diagnosis and epidemiology workshop at the National Institutes of Health. *Sleep Medicine*, *4*(2), 101–119.

Amsterdam, J. D., Brunswick, D. J., & Hundert, M. (2002). A single-site, double-blind, placebo-controlled, dose-ranging study of YKP10A—a putative, new antidepressant. *Progress in Neuro-Psychopharmacology and Biological Psychiatry*, *26*(7–8), 1333–1338.

Ballon, J. S., & Feifel, D. (2006). A systematic review of modafinil: Potential clinical uses and mechanisms of action. *Journal of Clinical Psychiatry*, *67*(4), 554–566.

Barnes, N. M., & Sharp, T. (1999). A review of central 5-HT receptors and their function. *Neuropharmacology*, *38*(8), 1083–1152.

Bastuji, H., & Jouvet, M. (1988). Successful treatment of idiopathic hypersomnia and narcolepsy with modafinil. *Progress in Neuro-Psychopharmacology and Biological Psychiatry*, *12*(5), 695–700.

Bayliss, D. A., Viana, F., & Berger, A. J. (1992). Mechanisms underlying excitatory effects of thyrotropin-releasing hormone on rat hypoglossal motoneurons in vitro. *Journal of Neurophysiology*, *68*(5), 1733–1745.

Bazil, C. W., Battista, J., & Basner, R. C. (2005). Gabapentin improves sleep in the presence of alcohol. *Journal of Clinical Sleep Medicine*, *1*(3), 284–287.

Benes, H. (2006). Transdermal lisuride: Short-term efficacy and tolerability study in patients with severe restless legs syndrome. *Sleep Medicine, 7*(1), 31–35.

Berry, R. B., Koch, G. L., & Hayward, L. F. (2005). Low-dose mirtazapine increases genioglossus activity in the anesthetized rat. *Sleep, 28*(1), 78–84.

Bettica, P. U., Squassante, L., Groeger, J. A., Gennery, B., & Dijk, D. (2009). Hypnotic effects of SB-649868, an orexin antagonist, and zolpidem in a model of situational insomnia. *Sleep* (Abstract Supplement), *32*, A40.

Billiard, M., Pasquie-Magnetto, V., Heckman, M., Carlander, B., Besset, A., Zachariev, Z., et al. (1994). Family studies in narcolepsy. *Sleep, 17*(8 Suppl), S54–S59.

Bixler, E. O., Kales, A., Brubaker, B. H., & Kales, J. D. (1987). Adverse reactions to benzodiazepine hypnotics: Spontaneous reporting system. *Pharmacology, 35*(5), 286–300.

Black, J. E., & Hirshkowitz, M. (2005). Modafinil for treatment of residual excessive sleepiness in nasal continuous positive airway pressure-treated obstructive sleep apnea/hypopnea syndrome. *Sleep, 28*(4), 464–471.

Bolge, S. C., Doan, J. F., Kannan, H., & Baran, R. W. (2009). Association of insomnia with quality of life, work productivity, and activity impairment. *Quality of Life Research, 18*(4), 415–422.

Bradley, T. D., & Floras, J. S. (2003). Sleep apnea and heart failure: Part II: Central sleep apnea. *Circulation, 107*(13), 1822–1826.

Brisbare-Roch, C., Dingemanse, J., Koberstein, R., Hoever, P., Aissaoui, H., Flores, S., et al. (2007). Promotion of sleep by targeting the orexin system in rats, dogs and humans. *Nature Medicine, 13*(2), 150–155.

Broughton, R., & Mamelak, M. (1979). The treatment of narcolepsy-cataplexy with nocturnal gamma-hydroxybutyrate. *Canadian Journal of Neurological Sciences, 6*(1), 1–6.

Buysse, B. (2007). Treatment effects of sleep apnea: Where are we now? *European Respiratory Review, 16*(106), 146–168.

Buysse, D. J., Reynolds, C. F., 3rd, Monk, T. H., Berman, S. R., & Kupfer, D. J. (1989). The Pittsburgh Sleep Quality Index: A new instrument for psychiatric practice and research. *Psychiatry Research, 28*(2), 193–213.

Carley, D. W., & Radulovacki, M. (1999). Mirtazapine, a mixed-profile serotonin agonist/antagonist, suppresses sleep apnea in the rat. *American Journal of Respiratory and Critical Care Medicine, 160*(6), 1824–1829.

Castillo, J. L., Menendez, P., Segovia, L., & Guilleminault, C. (2004). Effectiveness of mirtazapine in the treatment of sleep apnea/hypopnea syndrome (SAHS). *Sleep Medicine, 5*(5), 507–508.

Chemelli, R. M., Willie, J. T., Sinton, C. M., Elmquist, J. K., Scammell, T., Lee, C., et al. (1999). Narcolepsy in orexin knockout mice: Molecular genetics of sleep regulation. *Cell, 98*(4), 437–451.

Cheshire, K., Engleman, H., Deary, I., Shapiro, C., & Douglas, N. J. (1992). Factors impairing daytime performance in patients with sleep apnea/hypopnea syndrome. *Archives of Internal Medicine, 152*(3), 538–541.

Clapham, J., & Kilpatrick, G. J. (1992). Histamine H3 receptors modulate the release of [3H]-acetylcholine from slices of rat entorhinal cortex: Evidence for the possible existence of H3 receptor subtypes. *British Journal of Pharmacology, 107*(4), 919–923.

Conti, C. F., de Oliveira, M. M., Andriolo, R. B., Saconato, H., Atallah, A. N., Valbuza, J. S., et al. (2007). Levodopa for idiopathic restless legs syndrome: Evidence-based review. *Movement Disorders, 22*(13), 1943–1951.

Cortese, S., Konofal, E., & Lecendreux, M. (2008). Alertness and feeding behaviors in ADHD: Does the hypocretin/orexin system play a role? *Medical Hypotheses, 71*(5), 770–775.

Cundy, K. C., Sastry, S., Luo, W., Zou, J., Moors, T. L., & Canafax, D. M. (2008). Clinical pharmacokinetics of XP13512, a novel transported prodrug of gabapentin. *Journal of Clinical Pharmacology, 48*(12), 1378–1388.

Cusack, B., Nelson, A., & Richelson, E. (1994). Binding of antidepressants to human brain receptors: Focus on newer generation compounds. *Psychopharmacology (Berlin)*, *114*(4), 559–565.

Czapinski, P., Blaszczyk, B., & Czuczwar, S. J. (2005). Mechanisms of action of antiepileptic drugs. *Current Topics in Medicinal Chemistry*, *5*(1), 3–14.

Dauvilliers, Y., Billiard, M., & Montplaisir, J. (2003). Clinical aspects and pathophysiology of narcolepsy. *Clinical Neurophysiology*, *114*(11), 2000–2017.

Dauvilliers, Y., Neidhart, E., Billiard, M., & Tafti, M. (2002). Sexual dimorphism of the catechol-O-methyltransferase gene in narcolepsy is associated with response to modafinil. *Pharmacogenomics J*, *2*(1), 65–68.

Dean, D., Apps, J., Bamford, M., Bamford, M., Davies, S., Harriss, L., Medhurst, A., Panchal, T., Parr, C., Sehmi, S., et al. (2006). *A novel series of histamine H3 antagonists*, Paper presented at the XIXth International Symposium on Medicinal Chemistry, Istanbul, Turkey, p 195.

Dement, W., Rechtschaffen, A., & Gulevich, G. (1966). The nature of the narcoleptic sleep attack. *Neurology*, *16*(1), 18–33.

Dugovic, C. (1992). Functional activity of 5-HT2 receptors in the modulation of the sleep/wakefulness states. *Journal of Sleep Research*, *1*(3), 163–168.

Dundar, Y., Dodd, S., Strobl, J., Boland, A., Dickson, R., & Walley, T. (2004). Comparative efficacy of newer hypnotic drugs for the short-term management of insomnia: A systematic review and meta-analysis. *Human Psychopharmacology*, *19*(5), 305–322.

Earley, C. J., Heckler, D., & Allen, R. P. (2004). The treatment of restless legs syndrome with intravenous iron dextran. *Sleep Medicine*, *5*(3), 231–235.

Erikson, K. M., Jones, B. C., & Beard, J. L. (2000). Iron deficiency alters dopamine transporter functioning in rat striatum. *Journal of Nutrition*, *130*(11), 2831–2837.

Erikson, K. M., Jones, B. C., Hess, E. J., Zhang, Q., & Beard, J. L. (2001). Iron deficiency decreases dopamine D1 and D2 receptors in rat brain. *Pharmacology, Biochemistry and Behavior*, *69*(3–4), 409–418.

Evidente, V. G., Adler, C. H., Caviness, J. N., Hentz, J. G., & Gwinn-Hardy, K. (2000). Amantadine is beneficial in restless legs syndrome. *Movement Disorders*, *15*(2), 324–327.

Fairbanks, D. (1987). Snoring: An overview with historical perspectives. In D. Fairbanks, S. Fujita, T. Ikematsu, & F. B. Simmons (Eds.), *Snoring and obstructive sleep apnea* (pp. 1–18). New York: Raven Press.

Fariello, R. G. (2007). Safinamide. *Neurotherapeutics*, *4*(1), 110–116.

Feeney, J., Birznieks, G., Scott, C., Torres, R., Welsch, C., Baroldi, P., Polymeropoulos, M., & Walsh, J. (2009). Melatonin agonist improves sleep in primary insomnia characterized by difficulty falling asleep. *Sleep* (Abstract Supplement), *32*, A43.

Fenik, P., & Veasey, S. C. (2003). Pharmacological characterization of serotonergic receptor activity in the hypoglossal nucleus. *American Journal of Respiratory and Critical Care Medicine*, *167*(4), 563–569.

Foldvary-Schaefer, N., De Leon Sanchez, I., Karafa, M., Mascha, E., Dinner, D., & Morris, H. H. (2002). Gabapentin increases slow-wave sleep in normal adults. *Epilepsia*, *43*(12), 1493–1497.

Foutz, A. S., Mitler, M. M., Cavalli-Sforza, L. L., & Dement, W. C. (1979). Genetic factors in canine narcolepsy. *Sleep*, *1*(4), 413–421.

Fujita, S. (1987). Pharyngeal surgery for management of snoring and obstructive sleep apnea. In D. Fairbanks, S. Fujita, T. Ikematsu, & F. B. Simmons (Eds.), *Snoring and obstructive sleep apnea* (pp. 101–128). New York: Raven Press.

Garcia-Borreguero, D., Allen, R. P., Kohnen, R., Hogl, B., Trenkwalder, C., Oertel, W., et al. (2007). Diagnostic standards for dopaminergic augmentation of restless legs syndrome: Report from a World Association of Sleep Medicine-International Restless Legs Syndrome Study Group consensus conference at the Max Planck Institute. *Sleep Medicine*, *8*(5), 520–530.

Garcia-Borreguero, D., Larrosa, O., Granizo, J. J., de la Llave, Y., & Hening, W. A. (2004). Circadian variation in neuroendocrine response to L-dopa in patients with restless legs syndrome. *Sleep, 27*(4), 669–673.

Gary, K. A., Sevarino, K. A., Yarbrough, G. G., Prange, A. J., Jr., & Winokur, A. (2003). The thyrotropin-releasing hormone (TRH) hypothesis of homeostatic regulation: Implications for TRH-based therapeutics. *Journal of Pharmacology and Experimental Therapeutics, 305*(2), 410–416.

Gemkow, M. J., Davenport, A. J., Harich, S., Ellenbroek, B. A., Cesura, A., & Hallett, D. (2009). The histamine H3 receptor as a therapeutic drug target for CNS disorders. *Drug Discovery Today, 14*(9–10), 509–515.

Gonzalez, J. A., Horjales-Araujo, E., Fugger, L., Broberger, C., & Burdakov, D. (2009). Stimulation of orexin/hypocretin neurons by thyrotropin-releasing hormone. *Journal of Physiology, 587*(Pt 6), 1179–1186.

Gordon, R., Bernard, P., Pack, E., Lee, K., & Choi, Y. M. (1998). Pharmacological profile of YKP10A: A novel antidepressant. *Society for Neuroscience Abstract 583*, 24.

Grunstein, R. (2005). Continuous positive airway pressure treatment for obstructive sleep apnea-hypopnea syndrome. In M. H. Kryger, T. Roth, & W. C. Dement (Eds.), *Principles and practice of sleep medicine* (pp. 1066–1080). Philadelphia: Elsevier, Saunders.

Guilleminault, C., & Bassiri, A. (2005). Clinical features and evaluation of obstructive sleep apnea-hypopnea syndrome and the upper airway resistance syndrome. In M. Kryger, T. Roth, & W. C. Dement (Eds.), *Principles and practice of sleep medicine* (pp. 1043–1052). Philadelphia: Elsevier, Saunders.

Guilleminault, C., Cetel, M., & Philip, P. (1993). Dopaminergic treatment of restless legs and rebound phenomenon. *Neurology, 43*(2), 445.

Guilleminault, C., & Fromherz, S. (2005). Narcolepsy: Diagnosis and management. In M. H. Kryger, T. Roth, & W. C. Dement (Eds.), *Principles and practice of sleep medicine* (4th ed., pp. 780–790). Philadelphia: Elsevier, Saunders.

Haas, H., & Panula, P. (2003). The role of histamine and the tuberomammillary nucleus in the nervous system. *Nature Reviews Neuroscience, 4*(2), 121–130.

Hajak, G., Rodenbeck, A., Voderholzer, U., Riemann, D., Cohrs, S., Hohagen, F., et al. (2001). Doxepin in the treatment of primary insomnia: A placebo-controlled, double-blind, polysomnographic study. *Journal of Clinical Psychiatry, 62*(6), 453–463.

Hannon, J., & Hoyer, D. (2008). Molecular biology of 5-HT receptors. *Behavioural Brain Research, 195*(1), 198–213.

Hasan, S., Pradervand, S., Ahnaou, A., Drinkenburg, W., Tafti, M., & Franken, P. (2009). How to keep the brain awake? The complex molecular pharmacogenetics of wake promotion. *Neuropsychopharmacology, 34*(7), 1625–1640.

Hays, R. D., Martin, S. A., Sesti, A. M., & Spritzer, K. L. (2005). Psychometric properties of the Medical Outcomes Study Sleep measure. *Sleep Medicine, 6*(1), 41–44.

Heinrich, J. N., Brennan, J., Lai, M. H., Sullivan, K., Hornby, G., Popiolek, M., et al. (2006). Aplindore (DAB-452), a high affinity selective dopamine D2 receptor partial agonist. *European Journal of Pharmacology, 552*(1–3), 36–45.

Hendricks, J. C., Kline, L. R., Kovalski, R. J., O'Brien, J. A., Morrison, A. R., & Pack, A. I. (1987). The English bulldog: A natural model of sleep-disordered breathing. *Journal of Applied Physiology, 63*(4), 1344–1350.

Herxheimer, A., & Petrie, K. J. (2002). Melatonin for the prevention and treatment of jet lag. *Cochrane Database of Systematic Reviews*, (2), CD001520.

Hindmarch, I., Trick, L., & Ridout, F. (2005). A double-blind, placebo- and positive-internal-controlled (alprazolam) investigation of the cognitive and psychomotor profile of pregabalin in healthy volunteers. *Psychopharmacology (Berlin), 183*(2), 133–143.

Hirshkowitz, M., Black, J. E., Wesnes, K., Niebler, G., Arora, S., & Roth, T. (2007). Adjunct armodafinil improves wakefulness and memory in obstructive sleep apnea/hypopnea syndrome. *Respiratory Medicine, 101*(3), 616–627.

Hobson, D. E., Lang, A. E., Martin, W. R., Razmy, A., Rivest, J., & Fleming, J. (2002). Excessive daytime sleepiness and sudden-onset sleep in Parkinson disease: A survey by the Canadian Movement Disorders Group. *JAMA, 287*(4), 455–463.

Hokfelt, T., Fuxe, K., Johansson, O., Jeffcoate, S., & White, N. (1975). Thyrotropin releasing hormone (TRH)-containing nerve terminals in certain brain stem nuclei and in the spinal cord. *Neuroscience Letters, 1*(3), 133–139.

Honda, Y., & Matsuki, K. (1990). Genetic aspects of narcolepsy. In M. J. Thorpy (Ed.), *Handbook of sleep disorders* (pp. 217–234). New York: Marcel Dekker, Inc.

Horvath, J., Fross, R. D., Kleiner-Fisman, G., Lerch, R., Stalder, H., Liaudat, S., et al. (2004). Severe multivalvular heart disease: A new complication of the ergot derivative dopamine agonists. *Movement Disorders, 19*(6), 656–662.

Hungs, M., Fan, J., Lin, L., Lin, X., Maki, R. A., & Mignot, E. (2001). Identification and functional analysis of mutations in the hypocretin (orexin) genes of narcoleptic canines. *Genome Research, 11*(4), 531–539.

Javaheri, S. (2008). Sleep dysfunction in heart failure. *Current Treatment Options in Neurology, 10*(5), 323–335.

Jayaraman, G., Sharafkhaneh, H., Hirshkowitz, M., & Sharafkhaneh, A. (2008). Pharmacotherapy of obstructive sleep apnea. *Therapeutic Advances in Respiratory Disease, 2*(6), 375–386.

Jelev, A., Sood, S., Liu, H., Nolan, P., & Horner, R. L. (2001). Microdialysis perfusion of 5-HT into hypoglossal motor nucleus differentially modulates genioglossus activity across natural sleep-wake states in rats. *Journal of Physiology, 532*(Pt 2), 467–481.

Jenner, P., Mori, A., Hauser, R., Morelli, M., Fredholm, B. B., & Chen, J. F. (2009). Adenosine, adenosine A 2A antagonists, and Parkinson's disease. *Parkinsonism & Related Disorders, 15*(6), 406–413.

Johns, M. W. (1991). A new method for measuring daytime sleepiness: The Epworth sleepiness scale. *Sleep, 14*(6), 540–545.

Jones, M., & Morrell, M. J. (2008). Sleep and breathing disorders in adults. In S. Pandi-Permal, J. C. Verster, J. M. Monti, M. Lader, & S. Z. Langer (Eds.), *Sleep disorders: Diagnosis and therapeutics* (pp. 526–535). London: Informa Health Care.

Jouvet, M. (1999). Sleep and serotonin: An unfinished story. *Neuropsychopharmacology, 21*(2 Suppl), 24S–27S.

Juji, T., Satake, M., Honda, Y., & Doi, Y. (1984). HLA antigens in Japanese patients with narcolepsy. All the patients were DR2 positive. *Tissue Antigens, 24*(5), 316–319.

Kales, A. (1980). Benzodiazepine hypnotics: Carryover effectiveness, rebound insomnia, and performance effects. *NIDA Research Monograph,* (33), 61–69.

Kessler, R. C., McGonagle, K. A., Swartz, M., Blazer, D. G., & Nelson, C. B. (1993). Sex and depression in the National Comorbidity Survey. I: Lifetime prevalence, chronicity and recurrence. *Journal of Affective Disorders, 29*(2–3), 85–96.

Kingshott, R. N., Vennelle, M., Coleman, E. L., Engleman, H. M., Mackay, T. W., & Douglas, N. J. (2001). Randomized, double-blind, placebo-controlled crossover trial of modafinil in the treatment of residual excessive daytime sleepiness in the sleep apnea/hypopnea syndrome. *American Journal of Respiratory and Critical Care Medicine, 163*(4), 918–923.

Kohnen, R., Allen, R. P., Benes, H., Garcia-Borreguero, D., Hening, W. A., Stiasny-Kolster, K., et al. (2007). Assessment of restless legs syndrome—methodological approaches for use in practice and clinical trials. *Movement Disorders, 22* Suppl 18, S485–494.

Kotorii, N., Okuro, M., Okuro, M., Matsummura, M., Anegawa, E., Takahashi, T., et al. (2009). Effects of thyrotropin-releasing hormone analogs in the narcoleptic model mouse. *Sleep, 32*(Supplement), A241.

Kushida, C. A., Becker, P. M., Ellenbogen, A. L., Canafax, D. M., & Barrett, R. W. (2009). Randomized, double-blind, placebo-controlled study of XP13512/GSK1838262 in patients with RLS. *Neurology, 72*(5), 439–446.

Kvernmo, T., Houben, J., & Sylte, I. (2008). Receptor-binding and pharmacokinetic properties of dopaminergic agonists. *Current Topics in Medicinal Chemistry, 8*(12), 1049–1067.

Lammers, G. J., Arends, J., Declerck, A. C., Ferrari, M. D., Schouwink, G., & Troost, J. (1993). Gammahydroxybutyrate and narcolepsy: A double-blind placebo-controlled study. *Sleep, 16*(3), 216–220.

Lanier, W. L. (2003). Additional insights into pergolide-associated valvular heart disease. *Mayo Clinic Proceedings, 78*(6), 684–686.

Lankford, A., Jochelson, P., & Durrence, H. H. (2009). *Effects of doxepin 1, 3, and 6 mg on sleep efficiency by hour from two long-term trials of chronic insomnia.* Presented at the American Psychiatric Association 2009 Annual Meeting, San Francisco, CA, May 16–21.

LeBlanc, M., Beaulieu-Bonneau, S., Merette, C., Savard, J., Ivers, H., & Morin, C. M. (2007). Psychological and health-related quality of life factors associated with insomnia in a population-based sample. *Journal of Psychosomatic Research, 63*(2), 157–166.

Lee, J. J., Erdos, J., Wilkosz, M. F., LaPlante, R., & Wagoner, B. (2009). Bupropion as a possible treatment option for restless legs syndrome. *The Annals of Pharmacotherapy, 43*(2), 370–374.

Leger, D., & Poursain, B. (2005). An international survey of insomnia: Under-recognition and under-treatment of a polysymptomatic condition. *Current Medical Research and Opinion, 21*(11), 1785–1792.

Levitzky, M. G. (2008). Using the pathophysiology of obstructive sleep apnea to teach cardiopulmonary integration. *Advances in Physiology Education, 32*(3), 196–202.

Lewy, A. J., Ahmed, S., & Sack, R. L. (1996). Phase shifting the human circadian clock using melatonin. *Behavioural Brain Research, 73*(1–2), 131–134.

Lindberg, E., Janson, C., Gislason, T., Bjornsson, E., Hetta, J., & Boman, G. (1997). Sleep disturbances in a young adult population: Can gender differences be explained by differences in psychological status? *Sleep, 20*(6), 381–387.

Lydiard, R. B., Lankford, D. A., Seiden, D. J., Landin, R., Farber, R., & Walsh, J. K. (2006). Efficacy and tolerability of modified-release indiplon in elderly patients with chronic insomnia: Results of a 2-week double-blind, placebo-controlled trial. *Journal of Clinical Sleep Medicine, 2*(3), 309–315.

Manaker, S., & Rizio, G. (1989). Autoradiographic localization of thyrotropin-releasing hormone and substance P receptors in the rat dorsal vagal complex. *Journal of Comparative Neurology, 290*(4), 516–526.

Manconi, M., Govoni, V., De Vito, A., Economou, N. T., Cesnik, E., Casetta, I., et al. (2004). Restless legs syndrome and pregnancy. *Neurology, 63*(6), 1065–1069.

Marrs, J. C. (2008). Indiplon: A nonbenzodiazepine sedative-hypnotic for the treatment of insomnia. *The Annals of Pharmacotherapy, 42*(7), 1070–1079.

Mayer, G., Wang-Weigand, S., Roth-Schechter, B., Lehmann, R., Staner, C., & Partinen, M. (2009). Efficacy and safety of 6-month nightly ramelteon administration in adults with chronic primary insomnia. *Sleep, 32*(3), 351–360.

Mendelson, W. B. (2001). Neurotransmitters and sleep. *Journal of Clinical Psychiatry, 62 Suppl 10*, 5–8.

Mignot, E. (1998). Genetic and familial aspects of narcolepsy. *Neurology, 50*(2 Suppl 1), S16–S22.

Mignot, E. (2005). Narcolepsy: Pharmacology, pathophysiology, and genetics. In M. H. Kryger, T. Roth, & W. C. Dement (Eds.), *Principles and practice of sleep medicine* (pp. 761–779). Philadelphia: Elsevier, Saunders.

Mignot, E., Hayduk, R., Black, J., Grumet, F. C., & Guilleminault, C. (1997). HLA Class II studies in 509 narcoleptic patients. *Sleep Research, 26*, 433.

Mignot, E., Nishino, S., Sharp, L. H., Arrigoni, J., Siegel, J. M., Reid, M. S., et al. (1993). Heterozygosity at the canarc-1 locus can confer susceptibility for narcolepsy: Induction of cataplexy in heterozygous asymptomatic dogs after administration of a combination of drugs acting on monoaminergic and cholinergic systems. *Journal of Neuroscience, 13*(3), 1057–1064.

Mignot, E., Wang, C., Rattazzi, C., Gaiser, C., Lovett, M., Guilleminault, C., et al. (1991). Genetic linkage of autosomal recessive canine narcolepsy with a mu immunoglobulin heavy-chain switch-like segment. *Proceedings of the National Academy of Sciences of the United States of America, 88*(8), 3475–3478.

Minzenberg, M. J., & Carter, C. S. (2008). Modafinil: A review of neurochemical actions and effects on cognition. *Neuropsychopharmacology, 33*(7), 1477–1502.

Monk, T. H., Reynolds, C. F., 3rd, Kupfer, D. J., Buysse, D. J., Coble, P. A., Hayes, A. J., et al. (1994). The Pittsburgh sleep diary. *Journal of Sleep Research, 3,* 111–120.

Moran, W., Jr. (1987). Table 1 Obstructive sleep apnea: Diagnosis by history, physical exam, and special studies. In D. Fairbanks, S. Fujito, T. Ikematsum, & F. B. Simmon (Eds.), *Snoring and obstructive sleep apnea.* New York: Raven Press.

Morgenthaler, T. I., Kapur, V. K., Brown, T., Swick, T. J., Alessi, C., Aurora, R. N., et al. (2007). Practice parameters for the treatment of narcolepsy and other hypersomnias of central origin. *Sleep, 30*(12), 1705–1711.

Morin, C. M. (2003). Measuring outcomes in randomized clinical trials of insomnia treatments. *Sleep Medicine Reviews, 7*(3), 263–279.

Morin, C. M., Belanger, L., LeBlanc, M., Ivers, H., Savard, J., Espie, C. A., et al. (2009). The natural history of insomnia: A population-based 3-year longitudinal study. *Archives of Internal Medicine, 169*(5), 447–453.

National Sleep Foundation. (2005). Summary Findings of the 2005 Sleep in America poll. http://www.sleepfoundation.org/sites/default/files/2005_summary_of_findings.pdf.

Nishino, S. (2008). Modafinil and neuropharmacology of narcolepsy. In S. Pandi-Permal, J. C., Verster, J. M. Monti, M. Lader, & S. Z. Langer (Eds.), *Sleep disorders: Diagnosis and therapeutics* (pp. 597–607). London: Informa Health Care.

Nishino, S., Arrigoni, J., Shelton, J., Kanbayashi, T., Dement, W. C., & Mignot, E. (1997). Effects of thyrotropin-releasing hormone and its analogs on daytime sleepiness and cataplexy in canine narcolepsy. *Journal of Neuroscience, 17*(16), 6401–6408.

Nishino, S., Fujiki, N., Yoshido, Y., & Mignot, E. (2003). The effects of hypocretin-1 (Orexin A) in hypocretin receptor 2 gene mutated and hypocretin ligand-deficient narcoleptic dogs. *Sleep, 26*(supplement), A287.

Nishino, S., & Mignot, E. (2008). Wake-promoting medications: Basic mechanisms and pharmacology. In M. Kryger, T. Roth, & W. C. Dement (Eds.), *Principles and practice of sleep medicine* (4th ed., pp. 418–434). Philadelphia: Elsevier.

Nishino, S., Ripley, B., Overeem, S., Lammers, G. J., & Mignot, E. (2000). Hypocretin (orexin) deficiency in human narcolepsy. *Lancet, 355*(9197), 39–40.

Nishino, S., Ripley, B., Overeem, S., Nevsimalova, S., Lammers, G. J., Vankova, J., et al. (2001). Low cerebrospinal fluid hypocretin (Orexin) and altered energy homeostasis in human narcolepsy. *Annals of Neurology, 50*(3), 381–388.

Ohayon, M. M. (2005). Prevalence and correlates of nonrestorative sleep complaints. *Archives of Internal Medicine, 165*(1), 35–41.

O'Keeffe, S. T., Gavin, K., & Lavan, J. N. (1994). Iron status and restless legs syndrome in the elderly. *Age and Ageing, 23*(3), 200–203.

Ondo, W., & Jankovic, J. (1996). Restless legs syndrome: Clinicoetiologic correlates. *Neurology, 47*(6), 1435–1441.

Pack, A. I. (1994). Obstructive sleep apnea. *Advances in Internal Medicine, 39,* 517–567.

Pardi, D., & Black, J. (2006). gamma-Hydroxybutyrate/sodium oxybate: Neurobiology, and impact on sleep and wakefulness. *CNS Drugs, 20*(12), 993–1018.

Paulus, W., Dowling, P., Rijsman, R., Stiasny-Kolster, K., & Trenkwalder, C. (2007a). Update of the pathophysiology of the restless-legs-syndrome. *Movement Disorders, 22 Suppl 18*, S431–439.

Paulus, W., Dowling, P., Rijsman, R., Stiasny-Kolster, K., Trenkwalder, C., & de Weerd, A. (2007b). Pathophysiological concepts of restless legs syndrome. *Movement Disorders, 22*(10), 1451–1456.

Paulus, W., & Trenkwalder, C. (2006). Less is more: Pathophysiology of dopaminergic-therapy-related augmentation in restless legs syndrome. *Lancet Neurology, 5*(10), 878–886.

Peker, Y., Hedner, J., Kraiczi, H., & Loth, S. (2000). Respiratory disturbance index: An independent predictor of mortality in coronary artery disease. *American Journal of Respiratory and Critical Care Medicine, 162*(1), 81–86.

Pepperell, J. C., Ramdassingh-Dow, S., Crosthwaite, N., Mullins, R., Jenkinson, C., Stradling, J. R., et al. (2002). Ambulatory blood pressure after therapeutic and subtherapeutic nasal continuous positive airway pressure for obstructive sleep apnoea: A randomised parallel trial. *Lancet, 359*(9302), 204–210.

Peyron, C., Faraco, J., Rogers, W., Ripley, B., Overeem, S., Charnay, Y., et al. (2000). A mutation in a case of early onset narcolepsy and a generalized absence of hypocretin peptides in human narcoleptic brains. *Nature Medicine, 6*(9), 991–997.

Phillips, B., Young, T., Finn, L., Asher, K., Hening, W. A., & Purvis, C. (2000). Epidemiology of restless legs symptoms in adults. *Archives of Internal Medicine, 160*(14), 2137–2141.

Phillips, B. G., & Somers, V. K. (2000). Neural and humoral mechanisms mediating cardiovascular responses to obstructive sleep apnea. *Respiration Physiology, 119*(2–3), 181–187.

Picchietti, D., & Winkelman, J. W. (2005). Restless legs syndrome, periodic limb movements in sleep, and depression. *Sleep, 28*(7), 891–898.

Pollack, M., Seal, B., Joish, V. N., & Cziraky, M. J. (2009). Insomnia-related comorbidities and economic costs among a commercially insured population in the United States. *Current Medical Research and Opinion, 25*(8), 1901–1911.

Polydefkis, M., Allen, R. P., Hauer, P., Earley, C. J., Griffin, J. W., & McArthur, J. C. (2000). Subclinical sensory neuropathy in late-onset restless legs syndrome. *Neurology, 55*(8), 1115–1121.

Prasad, B., Radulovacki, M., Olopade, C., Herdegen, J., & Carley, J. Y. (2009). *Single-blind, placebo-controlled study of the efficacy and safety of ondansetron and fluoxetine in patients with obstructive sleep apnea syndrome Abstract #7101*. Paper presented at the American Thoracic Society 2009 International Conference, San Diego, CA.

Rajaratnam, S. M., Polymeropoulos, M. H., Fisher, D. M., Roth, T., Scott, C., Birznieks, G., et al. (2009). Melatonin agonist tasimelteon (VEC-162) for transient insomnia after sleep-time shift: Two randomised controlled multicentre trials. *Lancet, 373*(9662), 482–491.

Reynoldson, J. N., Elliott, E., Sr., & Nelson, L. A. (2008). Ramelteon: A novel approach in the treatment of insomnia. *The Annals of Pharmacotherapy, 42*(9), 1262–1271.

Richardson, G. S., Zammit, G., Wang-Weigand, S., & Zhang, J. (2009). Safety and subjective sleep effects of ramelteon administration in adults and older adults with chronic primary insomnia: A 1-year, open-label study. *Journal of Clinical Psychiatry, 70*(4), 467–476.

Riehl, J., Honda, K., Kwan, M., Hong, J., Mignot, E., & Nishino, S. (2000). Chronic oral administration of CG-3703, a thyrotropin releasing hormone analog, increases wake and decreases cataplexy in canine narcolepsy. *Neuropsychopharmacology, 23*(1), 34–45.

Rijsman, R. M., & de Weerd, A. W. (1999). Secondary periodic limb movement disorder and restless legs syndrome. *Sleep Medicine Reviews, 3*(2), 147–158.

Rijsman, R. M., de Weerd, A. W., Stam, C. J., Kerkhof, G. A., & Rosman, J. B. (2004). Periodic limb movement disorder and restless legs syndrome in dialysis patients. *Nephrology (Carlton), 9*(6), 353–361.

Roecker, A. J., & Coleman, P. J. (2008). Orexin receptor antagonists: Medicinal chemistry and therapeutic potential. *Current Topics in Medicinal Chemistry*, *8*(11), 977–987.

Rosenberg, R., Roehrs, T., Singh, N., Steinberg, F., & Roth, T. (2009). Absence of rebound effects with low-dose zolpidem tartrate sublingual lozenge 3.5 mg prn use: Preliminary analysis. *Sleep* (Abstract Supplement), *32*, A282.

Roth, T., Hull, S. G., Lankford, D. A., Rosenberg, R., & Scharf, M. B. (2008). Low-dose sublingual zolpidem tartrate is associated with dose-related improvement in sleep onset and duration in insomnia characterized by middle-of-the-night (MOTN) awakenings. *Sleep*. *31*(9), 1277–1284.

Roth, T., Jaeger, S., Jin, R., Kalsekar, A., Stang, P. E., & Kessler, R. C. (2006). Sleep problems, comorbid mental disorders, and role functioning in the national comorbidity survey replication. *Biological Psychiatry*, *60*(12), 1364–1371.

Roth, T., Rogowski, R., Hull, S., Schwartz, H., Koshorek, G., Corser, B., et al. (2007). Efficacy and safety of doxepin 1 mg, 3 mg, and 6 mg in adults with primary insomnia. *Sleep*, *30*(11), 1555–1561.

Roth, T., Rosenberg, R., Seiden, D., Singh, N., Steinberg, F., Sakai, S., et al. (2009). As-needed treatment of insomnia following MOTN awakening: Clinical efficacy of low dose zolpidem tartrate sublingual lozenge. *Sleep* (Abstract Supplement), *32*, A282.

Rothballer, A. B. (1957). The effect of phenylephrine, methamphetamine, cocaine, and serotonin upon the adrenaline-sensitive component of the reticular activating system. *Electroencephalography and Clinical Neurophysiology*, *9*(3), 409–417.

Rothdach, A. J., Trenkwalder, C., Haberstock, J., Keil, U., & Berger, K. (2000). Prevalence and risk factors of RLS in an elderly population: The MEMO study. Memory and morbidity in Augsburg elderly. *Neurology*, *54*(5), 1064–1068.

Rush, A. J., Armitage, R., Gillin, J. C., Yonkers, K. A., Winokur, A., Moldofsky, H., et al. (1998). Comparative effects of nefazodone and fluoxetine on sleep in outpatients with major depressive disorder. *Biological Psychiatry*, *44*(1), 3–14.

Sanders, M. (1987). Nonsurgical management of snoring and obstructive sleep apnea. In D. Fairbanks, S. Fujita, T. Ikematsu, & F. B. Simmons (Eds.), *Snoring and obstructive sleep apnea* (pp. 79–100). New York: Raven Press.

Santra, S., & Baumann, U. (2008). Experience of nitisinone for the pharmacological treatment of hereditary tyrosinaemia type 1. *Expert Opinion on Pharmacotherapy*, *9*(7), 1229–1236.

Sarsour, K., Morin, C. M., Foley, K., Kalsekar, A., & Walsh, J. K. (2009). Association of insomnia severity and comorbid medical and psychiatric disorders in a health plan-based sample: Insomnia severity and comorbidities. *Sleep Medicine*, [Epub ahead of print] Available online 1 May 2009.

Scharf, M., Rogowski, R., Hull, S., Cohn, M., Mayleben, D., Feldman, N., et al. (2008). Efficacy and safety of doxepin 1 mg, 3 mg, and 6 mg in elderly patients with primary insomnia: A randomized, double-blind, placebo-controlled crossover study. *Journal of Clinical Psychiatry*, *69*(10), 1557–1564.

Scharf, M. B., Brown, D., Woods, M., Brown, L., & Hirschowitz, J. (1985). The effects and effectiveness of gamma-hydroxybutyrate in patients with narcolepsy. *Journal of Clinical Psychiatry*, *46*(6), 222–225.

Schlicker, E., Fink, K., Detzner, M., & Gothert, M. (1993). Histamine inhibits dopamine release in the mouse striatum via presynaptic H3 receptors. *Journal of Neural Transmission. General Section*, *93*(1), 1–10.

Schutte-Rodin, S., Broch, L., Buysse, D., Dorsey, C., & Sateia, M. (2008). Clinical guideline for the evaluation and management of chronic insomnia in adults. *Journal of Clinical Sleep Medicine*, *4*(5), 487–504.

Schwab, R., Kuna, S. T., & Reemers, J. E. (2005). Anatomy and physiology of upper airway obstruction. In M. H. Kryger, T. Roth, & W. C. Dement (Eds.), *Principles and practice of sleep medicine* (pp. 983–1000). Philadelphia: Elsevier, Saunders.

Schwartz, J. R., Hirshkowitz, M., Erman, M. K., & Schmidt-Nowara, W. (2003). Modafinil as adjunct therapy for daytime sleepiness in obstructive sleep apnea: A 12-week, open-label study. *Chest*, *124*(6), 2192–2199.

Sforza, E., Nicolas, A., Lavigne, G., Gosselin, A., Petit, D., & Montplaisir, J. (1999). EEG and cardiac activation during periodic leg movements in sleep: Support for a hierarchy of arousal responses. *Neurology, 52*(4), 786–791.

Shahar, E., Whitney, C. W., Redline, S., Lee, E. T., Newman, A. B., Javier Nieto, F., et al. (2001). Sleep-disordered breathing and cardiovascular disease: Cross-sectional results of the Sleep Heart Health Study. *American Journal of Respiratory and Critical Care Medicine, 163*(1), 19–25.

Siegel, J. M. (2004). The neurotransmitters of sleep. *Journal of Clinical Psychiatry, 65 Suppl 16*, 4–7.

Silber, M. H., Ehrenberg, B. L., Allen, R. P., Buchfuhrer, M. J., Earley, C. J., Hening, W. A., et al. (2004). An algorithm for the management of restless legs syndrome. *Mayo Clinic Proceedings, 79*(7), 916–922.

Sills, G. J. (2006). The mechanisms of action of gabapentin and pregabalin. *Current Opinion in Pharmacology, 6*(1), 108–113.

Smith, M. T., Perlis, M. L., Park, A., Smith, M. S., Pennington, J., Giles, D. E., et al. (2002). Comparative meta-analysis of pharmacotherapy and behavior therapy for persistent insomnia. *American Journal of Psychiatry, 159*(1), 5–11.

Sommer, M., Bachmann, C. G., Liebetanz, K. M., Schindehutte, J., Tings, T., & Paulus, W. (2007). Pregabalin in restless legs syndrome with and without neuropathic pain. *ACTA Neurologica Scandinavica, 115*(5), 347–350.

Soya, A., Song, Y. H., Kodama, T., Honda, Y., Fujiki, N., & Nishino, S. (2008). CSF histamine levels in rats reflect the central histamine neurotransmission. *Neuroscience Letters, 430*(3), 224–229.

Stenberg, D. (2007). Neuroanatomy and neurochemistry of sleep. *Cellular and Molecular Life Science, 64*(10), 1187–1204.

Stiasny-Kolster, K., Kohnen, R., Schollmayer, E., Moller, J. C., & Oertel, W. H. (2004). Patch application of the dopamine agonist rotigotine to patients with moderate to advanced stages of restless legs syndrome: A double-blind, placebo-controlled pilot study. *Movement Disorders, 19*(12), 1432–1438.

Stone, B. M., Turner, C., Mills, S. L., & Nicholson, A. N. (2000). Hypnotic activity of melatonin. *Sleep, 23*(5), 663–669.

Szabadi, E. (2006). Drugs for sleep disorders: Mechanisms and therapeutic prospects. *British Journal of Clinical Pharmacology, 61*(6), 761–766.

Taheri, S., Zeitzer, J. M., & Mignot, E. (2002). The role of hypocretins (orexins) in sleep regulation and narcolepsy. *Annual Review of Neuroscience, 25*, 283–313.

Tamakawa, Y., Karashima, A., Koyama, Y., Katayama, N., & Nakao, M. (2006). A quartet neural system model orchestrating sleep and wakefulness mechanisms. *Journal of Neurophysiology, 95*(4), 2055–2069.

Tashiro, M., Mochizuki, H., Iwabuchi, K., Sakurada, Y., Itoh, M., Watanabe, T., et al. (2002). Roles of histamine in regulation of arousal and cognition: Functional neuroimaging of histamine H1 receptors in human brain. *Life Sciences, 72*(4–5), 409–414.

Teegarden, B. R., Al Shamma, H., & Xiong, Y. (2008). 5-HT(2A) inverse-agonists for the treatment of insomnia. *Current Topics in Medicinal Chemistry, 8*(11), 969–976.

Tergau, F., Wischer, S., Wolf, C., & Paulus, W. (2001). Treatment of restless legs syndrome with the dopamine agonist alpha-dihydroergocryptine. *Movement Disorders, 16*(4), 731–735.

Thannickal, T. C., Moore, R. Y., Nienhuis, R., Ramanathan, L., Gulyani, S., Aldrich, M., et al. (2000). Reduced number of hypocretin neurons in human narcolepsy. *Neuron, 27*(3), 469–474.

Trenkwalder, C., Hening, W. A., Montagna, P., Oertel, W. H., Allen, R. P., Walters, A. S., et al. (2008). Treatment of restless legs syndrome: An evidence-based review and implications for clinical practice. *Movement Disorders, 23*(16), 2267–2302.

Turek, F. W., & Gillette, M. U. (2004). Melatonin, sleep, and circadian rhythms: Rationale for development of specific melatonin agonists. *Sleep Medicine, 5*(6), 523–532.

Ulfberg, J., Nystrom, B., Carter, N., & Edling, C. (2001). Restless legs syndrome among working-aged women. *European Neurology, 46*(1), 17–19.

Van Dongen, H. P., Maislin, G., Mullington, J. M., & Dinges, D. F. (2003). The cumulative cost of additional wakefulness: Dose-response effects on neurobehavioral functions and sleep physiology from chronic sleep restriction and total sleep deprivation. *Sleep, 26*(2), 117–126.

Veasey, S., Strollo, Jr, P. J., Atwood, Jr. C. W., & Sanders, M. H. (2005). Medical therapy for obstructive sleep apnea-hypopnea syndrom. In M. H. Kryger, T. Roth, & W. C. Dement (Eds.), *Principles and practice of sleep medicine* (pp. 1053–1065). Philadelphia: Elsevier, Saunders.

Veasey, S. C. (2001). Pharmacotherapies for obstructive sleep apnea: How close are we? *Current Opinion in Pulomnary Medicine, 7*(6), 399–403.

Veasey, S. C. (2003). Serotonin agonists and antagonists in obstructive sleep apnea: Therapeutic potential. *American Journal of Respiratory Medicine, 2*(1), 21–29.

Veasey, S. C., Chachkes, J., Fenik, P., & Hendricks, J. C. (2001). The effects of ondansetron on sleep-disordered breathing in the English bulldog. *Sleep, 24*(2), 155–160.

Veasey, S. C., Fenik, P., Panckeri, K., Pack, A. I., & Hendricks, J. C. (1999). The effects of trazodone with L-tryptophan on sleep-disordered breathing in the English bulldog. *American Journal of Respiratory and Critical Care Medicine, 160*(5 Pt 1), 1659–1667.

Veasey, S. C., Guilleminault, C., Strohl, K. P., Sanders, M. H., Ballard, R. D., & Magalang, U. J. (2006). Medical therapy for obstructive sleep apnea: A review by the Medical Therapy for Obstructive Sleep Apnea Task Force of the Standards of Practice Committee of the American Academy of Sleep Medicine. *Sleep, 29*(8), 1036–1044.

Vgontzas, A. N., Liao, D., Pejovic, S., Calhoun, S., Karataraki, M., & Bixler, E. O. (2009). Insomnia with objective short sleep duration is associated with type 2 diabetes: A population-based study. *Diabetes Care,* 2009 Jul 29. [Epub ahead of print].

Viola, A. U., Brandenberger, G., Toussaint, M., Bouhours, P., Paul Macher, J., & Luthringer, R. (2002). Ritanserin, a serotonin-2 receptor antagonist, improves ultradian sleep rhythmicity in young poor sleepers. *Clinical Neurophysiology, 113*(3), 429–434.

Wafford, K. A., & Ebert, B. (2008). Emerging anti-insomnia drugs: Tackling sleeplessness and the quality of wake time. *Nature Reviews Drug Discovery, 7*(6), 530–540.

Wagner, M. L., Walters, A. S., Coleman, R. G., Hening, W. A., Grasing, K., & Chokroverty, S. (1996). Randomized, double-blind, placebo-controlled study of clonidine in restless legs syndrome. *Sleep, 19*(1), 52–58.

Walters, A. S., Ondo, W. G., Dreykluft, T., Grunstein, R., Lee, D., & Sethi, K. (2004). Ropinirole is effective in the treatment of restless legs syndrome. TREAT RLS 2: A 12-week, double-blind, randomized, parallel-group, placebo-controlled study. *Movement Disorders, 19*(12), 1414–1423.

Walters, A. S., Wagner, M., & Hening, W. A. (1996). Periodic limb movements as the initial manifestation of restless legs syndrome triggered by lumbosacral radiculopathy. *Sleep, 19*(10), 825–826.

Weaver, T. E., Kribbs, N. B., Pack, A. I., Kline, L. R., Chugh, D. K., Maislin, G., et al. (1997). Night-to-night variability in CPAP use over the first three months of treatment. *Sleep, 20*(4), 278–283.

Wetter, T. C., Eisensehr, I., & Trenkwalder, C. (2004). Functional neuroimaging studies in restless legs syndrome. *Sleep Medicine, 5*(4), 401–406.

White, J., Cates, C., & Wright, J. (2002). Continuous positive airways pressure for obstructive sleep apnoea. *Cochrane Database of Systematic Reviews,* Issue 2, Art. No.: CD001106.

Willie, J. T., Chemelli, R. M., Sinton, C. M., & Yanagisawa, M. (2001). To eat or to sleep? Orexin in the regulation of feeding and wakefulness. *Annual Review of Neuroscience, 24,* 429–458.

Winkelman, J. W., Allen, R. P., Tenzer, P., & Hening, W. (2007). Restless legs syndrome: Nonpharmacologic and pharmacologic treatments. *Geriatrics, 62*(10), 13–16.

Winkelman, J. W., Sethi, K. D., Kushida, C. A., Becker, P. M., Koester, J., Cappola, J. J., et al. (2006). Efficacy and safety of pramipexole in restless legs syndrome. *Neurology, 67*(6), 1034–1039.

Winkelmann, J., Schadrack, J., Wetter, T. C., Zieglgansberger, W., & Trenkwalder, C. (2001). Opioid and dopamine antagonist drug challenges in untreated restless legs syndrome patients. *Sleep Medicine, 2*(1), 57–61.

Winokur, A., DeMartinis, N. A., 3rd, McNally, D. P., Gary, E. M., Cormier, J. L., & Gary, K. A. (2003). Comparative effects of mirtazapine and fluoxetine on sleep physiology measures in patients with major depression and insomnia. *Journal of Clinical Psychiatry, 64*(10), 1224–1229.

Wong, Y. N., King, S. P., Laughton, W. B., McCormick, G. C., & Grebow, P. E. (1998). Single-dose pharmacokinetics of modafinil and methylphenidate given alone or in combination in healthy male volunteers. *Journal of Clinical Pharmacology, 38*(3), 276–282.

Wong, Y. N., Simcoe, D., Hartman, L. N., Laughton, W. B., King, S. P., McCormick, G. C., et al. (1999). A double-blind, placebo-controlled, ascending-dose evaluation of the pharmacokinetics and tolerability of modafinil tablets in healthy male volunteers. *Journal of Clinical Pharmacology, 39*(1), 30–40.

Yoshida, Y., Fujiki, N., Maki, R. A., Schwarz, D., & Nishino, S. (2003). Differential kinetics of hypocretins in the cerebrospinal fluid after intracerebroventricular administration in rats. *Neuroscience Letters, 346*(3), 182–186.

Young, T., Palta, M., Dempsey, J., Skatrud, J., Weber, S., & Badr, S. (1993). The occurrence of sleep-disordered breathing among middle-aged adults. *New England Journal of Medicine, 328*(17), 1230–1235.

Young, T., Skatrud, J., & Peppard, P. E. (2004). Risk factors for obstructive sleep apnea in adults. *JAMA, 291*(16), 2013–2016.

Zammit, G. K. (2007). The prevalence, morbidities, and treatments of insomnia. *CNS & Neurological Disorders Drug Targets, 6*(1), 3–16.

Zucconi, M., Ferri, R., Allen, R., Baier, P. C., Bruni, O., Chokroverty, S., et al. (2006). The official World Association of Sleep Medicine (WASM) standards for recording and scoring periodic leg movements in sleep (PLMS) and wakefulness (PLMW) developed in collaboration with a task force from the International Restless Legs Syndrome Study Group (IRLSSG). *Sleep Medicine, 7*(2), 175–183.

Zvonkina, V., & Black, J. E. (2008). Pharmacological treatment of narcolepsy. In S. Pandi-Permal, J. C. Verster, J. M. Monti, M. Lader, & S. Z. Langer (Eds.), *Sleep disorders: Diagnosis and therapeutics* (pp. 587–596). London: Informa Health Care.

Jerry R. Colca and Rolf F. Kletzien

Metabolic Solutions Development Company, 125 S. Kalamazoo Mall #202,
Kalamazoo, Michigan 49007

Current and Emerging Strategies for Treating Dyslipidemia and Macrovascular Disease

Abstract

Statins, inhibitors of hydroxymethylglutaryl CoA (HMG-CoA) reductase, have been in clinical use for over 20 years. The widespread use of these agents has left doubt of the efficacy of cholesterol-lowering therapy to prevent cardiovascular disease. In spite of the widespread use of these agents and the successful lowering of circulating cholesterol together with reduction of cardiovascular-related deaths, there is consensus that further improvements in therapy are needed. Cardiovascular disease remains a major cause of premature death and continues to exert an extensive drain on the health-care costs. This chapter

Advances in Pharmacology, Volume 57
1054-3589/08 $35.00
10.1016/S1054-3589(08)57006-2

outlines some of the emerging strategies for discovering and developing novel treatments of dyslipidemia and macrovascular disease. Mechanisms considered include alternate ways to lower total cholesterol through inhibition of synthesis, limitation of absorption, or recycling. Other approaches include the modification of circulating forms of cholesterol and changes in gene expression at the key sites of storage, utilization, and pathology. The next successful strategy will likely be one that works well in concert with existing statins.

I. Introduction

The main goal of cholesterol lowering therapies is to aid in the prevention of cholesterol deposition in blood vessels, a contributing factor for atherosclerosis, progressive vascular disease, heart attacks, and stroke. While there are many factors involved in the vascular pathology that may predispose to cardiovascular disease including elevated blood pressure (see Chapter 8 by Taylor and Abdel-Rahman, this volume) and inflammatory events, there is little doubt that elevated circulating cholesterol, as well as overall cholesterol metabolism, plays a significant role. The role of elevated circulating cholesterol in cardiovascular disease was first addressed in individuals with extreme familial hypercholesterolemia. Today, as a result of large clinical studies with the statins, treatment has been expanded to those with moderately elevated level of cholesterol, with almost all those at risk for the development of cardiovascular disease being treated with statins. Reviewed in this chapter are the current and emerging strategies to exploit what is now known about cholesterol-modifying treatments for developing new therapies to reduce cardiovascular morbidity and mortality. Particular emphasis is placed on approaches aimed at decreasing cholesterol synthesis, absorption, and transport ("reverse transport"). The development of new treatments having broader effects on the more common dyslipidemia found in general metabolic disease is also considered.

Steinberg (2006) has reviewed the discovery of the "statins," inhibitors of hydroxymethylglutaryl CoA (HMG-CoA) reductase, and how long-term clinical trials with them have removed any doubt about the importance of circulating cholesterol in cardiovascular disease. Before the discovery of these drugs, there was considerable controversy about the significance of the role of circulating cholesterol in the pathology associated with cardiovascular disease, and about the possible risks of interfering pharmacologically with a metabolic pathway that is essential for life. Such concerns were reinforced when initial attempts to reduce cholesterol synthesis with MER/29 (tripananol) was associated with significant toxicities, including cataracts and blindness. Although the MER/29-induced toxicities were ultimately traced to the accumulation of demonstrol resulting from the inhibition of its conversion to cholesterol, safety concerns raised by the clinical experience with this drug slowed exploration of alternative approaches for regulating cholesterol biosynthesis pathway. Thus, while the first HMG-CoA reductase inhibitor was identified in the mid-1970s (Endo, Tsujita, Kuroda, & Tanzawa, 1977), fear about potential side effects prevented the clinical development of this chemical class. Rather, lovastatin (Mevacor) was the first drug with this mechanism of action to be tested clinically. The initial studies were small and involved only high-risk patients with extremely elevated cholesterol. In 1987 lovastatin was the first drug of this class approved for human use. Subsequently, six other "statins" were developed and marketed. With the development of new molecules and few concerns about safety, clinical trials were undertaken in larger populations, including those with moderately elevated circulating cholesterol. This drug class is now used extensively as outcome studies demonstrate they reduce significantly the cardiovascular mortality associated with high levels of circulating cholesterol levels (Hebert, Gaziano, Chan, & Hennekens, 1997; Simes et al., 2002). Their usage has also increased because price reductions associated with the launch of generic products. While some side effects of statins are known (Joy & Hegele, 2009), none significantly restrict their use. Nonetheless, because of the growing evidence that lower levels of circulating low-density lipoprotein (LDL) cholesterol is better for cardiovascular health, efforts are underway to develop novel cholesterol synthesis inhibitors.

Cholesterol absorption from the intestine has for some time been a target for lipid-lowering treatments. This approach applies to both the cholesterol derived from the diet and that which is recycled through the bile. The resin cholestyramine was first introduced in 1957. The aim was to bind bile salts which, in turn, diverts hepatic cholesterol to the production of new bile salts. Approaches to reduce the absorption of cholesterol include modification of intestinal transport mechanisms (Huff, Pollex, & Hegele, 2006; Iqbal & Hussain, 2009).

As circulating cholesterol is packaged in lipoprotein particles before entering the bloodstream, cholesterol lowering might be achieved by limiting the synthesis of these storage particles. Efforts have been made to affect the ability of cholesterol to be packaged in LDL particles by modifying the transcription of selected lipoproteins.

Cholesterol is carried in the circulation in chylomicrons, vLDL (very low-density lipoprotein), LDL, and HDL (high-density lipoprotein). Each particle has its own function. The HDL cholesterol, often referred to as "good cholesterol," appears to play an important role in regulating the cholesterol that resides in cells in the vessel wall. Because low circulating levels of HDL cholesterol are associated with poor cardiovascular outcomes

(Lewis & Rader, 2005), approaches are being taken to attempt to elevate it. One approach is to counter the ways circulating HDL is reduced in disease. One way that HDL levels are lowered is through the action of cholesterol ester transfer protein (CETP) (de Grooth et al., 2004). This enzyme promotes the transfer of cholesterol to more atherogenic LDL particles in exchange for triacylglycerols. Therefore, inhibition of CETP should increase circulating HDL cholesterol. While this approach has been examined in human trials, it does not seem to translate into clinical benefit (Kastelein et al., 2007).

In the present chapter, emphasis is placed on new approaches for reducing circulating levels of cholesterol (Fig. 1). Any newly developed drug should work in concert with statins to yield the most optimal results in the treatment of dyslipidemia. Those desiring an overview of human cholesterol metabolism in general are urged to consult a recent review of this topic (Charlton-Menys & Durrington, 2008).

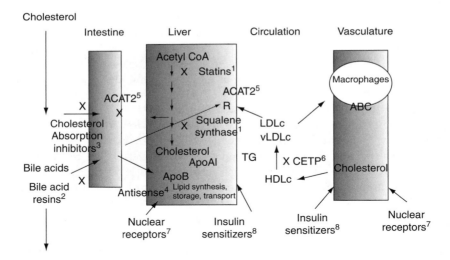

FIGURE 1   Site of action of various treatment strategies for dyslipidemia. Cholesterol synthesis (1) can be inhibited early in the process (HMG-CoA reductase) or at a later branch (squalene synthase) point leaving the synthesis of nonsteroidal pathways intact. Bile acid-binding resins (2) have been used to in effect eliminate cholesterol carbon and force the liver to put more of the synthesized cholesterol into new bile acids. Absorption of cholesterol (dietary and recycled) can also be inhibited by a direct effect on enterocyte transport mechanisms (3 and 5). Antisense inhibition of apoB limits productions of atherogenic lipoprotein particles (4). Inhibition of CETP (6) results in increased circulating HDL. Various nuclear receptor activators (7) and insulin-sensitizing agents (8) have multiple effects of peripheral tissues (including macrophages) that include lipid handling as well anti-inflammatory properties. See text for details.

It is critical to find additional therapeutic options for reducing the growing morbidity and mortality associated with macrovascular disease. To reduce health-care costs significantly, such therapies must be broadly effective and not limited to specific types of dyslipidemia. The heart disease and stroke statistics for 2009 (Lloyd-Jones et al., 2009) reveal that in 2006 (the last year for which adequate statistics are available), in spite of widespread use of statins, cardiovascular disease still accounts for 34.2% of all deaths in the United States, with myocardial infarcts and stroke being the major culprits.

II. Mechanisms of Action

A. Cholesterol Synthesis Inhibition

The statins are the first, and thus far only, class of successfully marketed cholesterol synthesis inhibitors. As reviewed by Steinberg (2006), the original molecules were fungal metabolites discovered empirically in an assay unrelated to a specific biochemical mechanism. As it turned out that the lead molecule ML-236B is an inhibitor of HMG-CoA reductase, a rate-limiting enzyme in cholesterol biosynthesis, this mechanism was the basis of the commercially successful members of this class (Table I). While the original clinical trials with the statins were limited to individuals with familial hypercholesterolemia, it is now known these agents have broader applications, being useful also for those with moderately elevated circulating cholesterol. Indeed, studies suggest that the statins can significantly reduce cardiovascular events in healthy men and women considered to have normal LDL cholesterol levels but elevated levels of a circulating marker of inflammation (Ridker et al., 2008). Because of the increased use of statins, most other therapeutics employed for the treatment or prevention of cardiovascular disease are likely be taken in combination with them. The efforts to reduce cholesterol concentrations even further are also stimulating the study of new ways to inhibit cholesterol synthesis.

TABLE I Most Common Statins in Current Clinical Use

Generic name	Trade name	Generic available
Lovastatin	Mevacor	Yes
Simvastatin	Zocor	Yes
Pravastatin	Pravachol	Yes
Fluvastatin	Lescol	No
Atorvastatin	Lipitor	No
Rosuvastatin	Crestor	No

One of the novel approaches for reducing cholesterol synthesis is through inhibition of squalene synthase. As HMG-CoA reductase inhibitors affect cholesterol synthesis early in the pathway, there is the potential for an accumulation of HMG-CoA. Furthermore, inhibition of the reductase limits production of important substrates, such as ubiquinone, farnesol, and prenylated proteins, that are constituents of other biochemical processes. By contrast, because squalene synthase occurs later in cholesterol biosynthesis, inhibition of this enzyme would not affect these other pathways (Fig. 1).

Novel 3′-substituted quinuclidines that inhibit the liver microsomal squalene synthase were first identified over a decade ago (McTaggart et al., 1996). As predicted, treatment of rats with these compound, unlike with a statin, results in a decrease in the synthesis of cholesterol without the inhibition of the incorporation of labeled mevalonate into ubiquinone. Hiyoshi et al. (2000) selected as a lead the squalene synthase inhibitor ER-28448 [5-{N-[2-butenyl-3-(2-methoxyphenyl)]-N-methylamino}-1,1-penthylidenebis(phosphonic acid) trisodium salt] after screening agents in a microsomal assay, in isolated hepatocytes, and in animal studies with rats and monkeys. Their results indicate this compound is more potent in lowering cholesterol in rhesus monkeys than the statins, and also displayed less potential to damage the liver. Subsequent work suggests that ER-28448, in addition to lowering circulating cholesterol levels, may also lower triglycerides by inhibiting fatty acid synthesis secondary to an increase in cellular farnesol (Hiyoshi et al., 2003).

The squalene synthase inhibitor that has undergone the most extensive investigation is Lapaquistat (TAK 475; (1-{[[(3R,5S)-7-chloro-5-(2,3-dimethoxyphenyl)-1-(3-hydroxy-2,2-dimethylpropyl)-2-oxo-1,2,3,5-tetra-hydro-4,1-benzoxazepin-3-yl]acetyl}piperidin-4-yl) acetic acid). Although the published data on this agent is limited (Bays et al., 2007; Davidson et al., 2007), it is notable the data were sufficient for proceeding to Phase III clinical trails, suggesting safety and efficacy in humans. However, Takeda announced suspension of this program in 2008 because the compounds reportedly displayed no significant advantages over currently marketed products.

B. Cholesterol Absorption

The pool of circulating cholesterol is replenished by de novo synthesis and by its absorption from dietary sources and from the enterohepatic circulation of existing stores. Several approaches are being undertaken to examine ways to reduce cholesterol accumulation from these sources.

While bile acid sequestrants, such as cholestyramine, do not inhibit cholesterol absorption, they cause depletion by reducing bile salt reabsorption. The reduction in bile acid recycling upregulates cholesterol 7-α-hydroxylase, thereby diverting cholesterol into bile acids, and upregulates the LDL receptor delivering more cholesterol to the liver. Other examples of bile acid sequestrants are colestipol, colestilan, colextran, and colesevelam (Aldridge & Ito, 2001). These resins are generally considered safe because they work solely in the intestine and do not enter the general circulation.

Compounds have been developed to directly interfere with the absorption of cholesterol by intestinal enterocytes. Ezetimide is the first commercial success of this class (Rosenblum et al., 1998). It localizes in the intestinal brush border and inhibits cholesterol absorption without reducing the absorption of fat-soluble vitamins (van Heek & Davis, 2002). It was also found that the ability of ezetimibe to inhibit cholesterol absorption depends on the activity of the Niemann–Pick C1Like 1 (NPC1L1) channels in the enterocyte brush border (Altmann et al., 2004). Indeed, Garcia-Calvo et al. (2005) demonstrated that binding of ezetimide to the intestinal membranes depends upon the expression of NPC1L1, confirming these channels are a component of the mechanism of action. With this information, one might conclude that decreasing the expression of the NPC1L1 protein is a way to decrease cholesterol absorption. It is interesting to note that the expression of NPC1L1 may also be affected by both dietary lipids and by synthetic peroxisome proliferator-activated receptor (PPAR) ligands.

Studies have been undertaken to examine the use of naturally occurring plant sterols to compete for cholesterol absorptive mechanism(s). Increasing dietary plant phytosterols, such as sitosterol and campesterol, moderately lowers cholesterol levels. Because ingestion of these molecules may also result in a reduction of the absorption of other fat-soluble nutrients, this approach remains controversial (Weingartner, Bohm, & Laufs, 2009).

C. Lipoprotein Particle Construction

Once cholesterol is synthesized, absorbed or reabsorbed, it must be esterified and packaged into lipoprotein particles. There are two Acyl-CoA cholesteryl acyl transferases (ACAT; also known as sterol O-acyltransferase) enzymes located in the endoplasmic reticulum that play an important role in this process. Because ACAT2 knockout mice appear to be protected against vascular lesions, inhibition of ACAT2 may be an effective approach for regulating levels of circulating cholesterol (Rudel, Lee, & Parini, 2005). ACAT in the eneterocyte plays a role in the absorption of cholesterol, that is, once cholesterol is taken up by the NPC1L1 channel, it must be esterified before it is transferred into the circulatory system. A similar process is necessary before hepatic secretion of cholesterol in the form of a lipoprotein particle. To be safely effective, it is believed a therapeutic must be selective for ACAT2 over ACAT1 to decrease atherogenic plasma lipoproteins without interfering with key cellular functions. It has been demonstrated that such selectivity is achievable (Lada et al., 2004). Indeed laboratory animal data with pactimide demonstrate both a reduction in cholesterol absorption and secretion of VLDL from the liver (Kitayama, Koga, Inaba, & Fujioka, 2006). However, two large clinical trials with pactimide failed to demonstrate clinical utility, and even suggested a potential negative outcome versus placebo (Meuwese et al., 2009).

Use of an antisense inhibitor (Isis 301012) of apolipoprotein B (apoB) in normal volunteers with mild dyslipidemia results in a significant dose-dependent reduction in circulating apoB (up to 50%) and in LDL cholesterol (up to 35%) (Kastelein et al., 2006). This effect is maintained over a 3-month period. Clinical studies are continuing to examine the potential of Isis 301012 (Mipomersen) as a treatment for hypercholesterolemia and coronary heart disease.

D. Regulation of HDL–CETP

Inasmuch as HDL is a universal acceptor lipoprotein for cholesterol efflux from cells, it plays an important role in removing excess cholesterol from peripheral tissues to maintain homeostasis. CETP is responsible for the transfer of cholesterol ester from HDL to LDL and vLDL. Triglyceride is exchanged from vLDL and LDL to HDL in the process, an important feature in determining the circulation half-life of HDL (Lewis & Rader, 2005). The process of reverse cholesterol transport is completed when cholesterol transferred to LDL is subsequently removed from the circulation by the liver through specific LDL receptors. However, under circumstances where the liver fails to adequately remove the LDL, the pool of potentially atherogenic LDL and vLDL is increased. The interest in targeting CETP for therapeutic intervention is based on the notion that its inhibition would elevate HDL levels. The idea for this came originally from human genetic studies, with CETP deficiency found to result in greatly elevated levels of HDL (Barter & Kastelein, 2006). Studies with laboratory animals supported the hypothesis with the discovery that rodents lacking the enzyme are generally resistant to atherosclerosis, and that introduction of a transgene expressing CETP makes laboratory mice more susceptible to atherosclerosis (Barter & Kastelein, 2006). While these and other results stimulated drug discovery based on this mechanism, progress was slow. This is because the active site resembles a hydrophobic clam shell, making it extremely difficult to identify highly selective CETP inhibitors. Nevertheless, CETP inhibitors have resulted from these efforts.

Important clinical information has emerged from human studies conducted with two experimental CETP inhibitors. Both JTT-705 and torceptrapib increase circulating HDL levels, with larger HDL particle sizes and decreased apoA1 catabolism (Brousseau et al., 2004; Kuivenhoven et al., 2005). Torceptrapib has a pronounced effect on HDL levels, with a 50% increase over that elicited by concomitant statin treatment (Brousseau et al.,

2004). JTT-705 (also known as R1658) has a smaller, but significant effect, with a 28% increase in HDL levels above that obtained with statin treatment alone (Kuivenhoven et al., 2005). Torceptrapib development has been discontinued owing to no demonstrable benefit and a possible increased incidence of cardiovascular disease (Kastelein et al., 2007). This was a completely unexpected development. However, in retrospect it is notable that reports of its elevating blood pressure suggested it may have off target effects unrelated to CETP inhibition (Tall, Yvan-Charvet, & Wang, 2007). Development of JTT-705 has continued, with results of a 4-week Phase II trial revealing blood pressure effects no different from placebo, and no drug-related cardiovascular adverse events (Steiner, Kastelein, Kallend, & Stroes, 2008).

The effect of torceptrapib on the progress of cardiovascular disease and its termination as a clinical candidate has left open the question as to whether CETP is proatherogenic in man and whether this enzyme represents a desirable pharmacological target for raising HDL. Thus, more consideration is being given to the possibility that interfering with the normal process of reverse cholesterol transport may have significant adverse consequences. Consideration should be given to targeting other pathways that may be more amenable to more physiological manipulation. In this regard, there is a growing appreciation that insulin resistance is highly correlated with low levels of circulating HDL cholesterol in humans (Lewis & Rader, 2005). Results from clinical studies with insulin-sensitizing agents reveal they are capable of elevating circulating HDL cholesterol (Berhanu et al., 2006; Goldberg et al., 2005) and, in at least one trial, cardiovascular events were reduced (Erdmann et al., 2007). Thus, targeting pathways involved in insulin sensitivity for elevating HDL may be a safer therapeutic approach than inhibiting reverse cholesterol transport.

E. Nuclear Receptors (α, δ, γ)

Fibrate drugs have been employed for more than 40 years to lower lipid levels. In recent years, it was discovered that these agents exert their effects by binding to and activating the transcription factor PPARα (Issemann, Prince, Tugwood, & Green, 1993). This results in the increased expression of the enzymatic machinery needed to metabolize fatty acids. These drugs have been used primarily to lower circulating triglycerides, especially when they are elevated. While in some cases these agents may have additional effects on cholesterol, they can be combined with statin for combination therapy to ensure this response.

There have been several reviews published on PPAR-related transcription factors as well as the liver X receptor (LXR) transcription factor, both of which regulate lipid transport (Barbier et al., 2002; Li & Glass, 2004). Compounds activating these transcription factors have pleiotropic effects on cholesterol

TABLE II Nuclear Receptors Targeted as Potential Treatments of Dyslipidemia

Receptor	Key tissues	Effects	Example ligands
PPARα	Liver, macrophages	Lipid synthesis; anti-inflammatory	Fibrates
PPARδ	Liver, macrophages	Lipid synthesis; anti-inflammatory	GW501516
PPARγ	Liver, macrophages	Lipid synthesis; anti-inflammatory	Rosiglitazone
LXR	Liver, macrophages	Cholesterol transport, metabolism	GW3965; WAY-252623 (LXR-623)

metabolism, not only because of regulation of hepatic gene expression, including those involved in producing proteins involved in cholesterol absorption and trafficking, but also because of effects in macrophages that regulate the handling of lipid by these cells. Additional effects in the macrophages include the inhibition of inflammatory responses that can affect lesion development and vascular pathology (Rigamonti, Chinetti-Gbaguidi, & Staels, 2008). A new approach in these areas has been to search for selective activators of a host of transcription factors (Feldman, Lambert, & Henke, 2008). Selective modulation of these receptors may make it possible to more optimally increase positive effects of these agents, such as lowering lipids and improving insulin sensitivity. Shown in Table II are the nuclear receptors that are being evaluated as potential targets for treatment of dyslipidemia.

One of the most ambitious new discovery efforts for treating dyslipidemia involves the LXR receptor. Interest in this approach is based on the observation that activation of LXR receptors (e.g., with oxysterols) controls absorption of cholesterol, mediates the efflux of cholesterol form macrophages, and promotes reverse cholesterol transport. Undesirable effects of LXR activation include increases in circulating triglycerides and hepatic steatosis. It is possible that some of these negative effects occur through activation of the LXRα form expressed in the liver. If so, synthetic ligands that selectively activate LXRβ may display an improved clinical profile (Joseph & Tontonoz, 2003). An example of such an agent is WAY-252623, a nonsteroidal partial LXR agonist. Quinet et al. (2009) recently compared this compound to a statin in several animal species, including the cynomolgus monkeys. Treatment with the compound reduced atherosclerotic lesions in mice and lowered cholesterol levels in the primates. The reduction of LDL cholesterol in the primates occurred with an increased expression of target genes for cholesterol transport (ABCA1/G1) in peripheral blood cells. Moreover, the reduction in circulating cholesterol in these primates was greater than that observed with a statin. However, the test agent also increases hepatic lipid accumulation, possibly limiting enthusiasm for this approach.

F. Insulin Sensitizers

Rosiglitazone and pioglitazone are thiazolidinedione insulin sensitizers with effects on lipid metabolism. Originally discovered and developed empirically without regard to biochemical mechanism (Hofmann & Colca, 1992), it was subsequently shown these compounds activate the nuclear receptor PPARγ with rosiglitazone being the most potent of the original analogs in this regard (Lehmann et al., 1995). While there have been many attempts to improve on the response to these agents, no new insulin sensitizers have been approved since the thiazolidinediones were launched in 1999 (Feldman et al., 2008). This may be because almost all drug development activity has focused on finding PPAR activators similar to rosiglitazone rather than trying to understand and exploit their effects on mitochondria (Colca & Kletzien, 2006). Although pioglitazone and rosiglitazone have similar effects on insulin sensitivity, pioglitazone has superior effects on circulating lipids, particularly with respect to lowering circulating triglycerides and raising circulating HDL cholesterol (Berhanu et al., 2006; Goldberg et al., 2005). Moreover, prospective clinical trials reveal that pioglitazone can reduce cardiovascular events (Erdmann et al., 2007; Wilcox et al., 2007), an effect that is not shared by rosiglitazone (Home et al., 2009). Thus, it is likely there will be differences in clinical outcomes with these compounds over time (Winkelmayer, Setoguchi, Levin, & Solomon, 2008). Indeed, when taken together, these findings suggests that in the beneficial effects on lipid metabolism and the reduction of cardiovascular events associated with these agents may be independent of their interaction with PPARγ. Indeed, it appears that activation of PPARγ is a factor in driving fluid retention, a negative side effect that may predispose to congestive heart failure. Efforts continue to identify insulin sensitizers with positive effects on lipid metabolism, with several agents now in clinical development (Colca, McDonald, Malapaka, Xu, & Kletzien, 2008).

III. Conclusion

Statin-induced reductions in circulating cholesterol are of significant clinical benefit for many of those at risk for cardiovascular disease, whether or not the individual has elevated levels of cholesterol. The level of circulating cholesterol considered unacceptably high has progressively decreased over the last 10 years, from <200 mg/dl to <130 mg/dl, and remains a moving target. As statins are now the standard of care for reducing lipid levels, any new therapy developed for the treatment of cardiovascular disease will be administered with them. However, even with the widespread use of statins, the morbidity and mortality associated with cardiovascular disease remains high and continues to be a major factor in rising health-care costs. In the future it is likely that multiple agents will be administered to address as many risk factors as possible, many of which are related to lipid metabolism. Thus, in addition to lowering LDL cholesterol, efforts must be made to reduce triglycerides, increase HDL cholesterol, as well as reduce vascular inflammation, thrombosis, and blood pressure. There are many mechanisms to consider and others that remain to be discovered. An ideal treatment is one that directly addresses the underlying mechanisms involved in the pathophysiology of cardiovascular disease, and which synergizes with statins.

Conflict of Interest: The authors are cofounders and stockholders in a drug development company that is developing treatments for diabetes. These agents might also be used to treat dyslipidemia and macrovascular disease.

References

Aldridge, M. A., & Ito, M. K. (2001). Colesevelam hydrochloride: A novel bile acid-binding resin. *The Annals of Pharmacotherapy*, 35, 898–907.

Altmann, S. W., Davis, Jr., H. R., Zhu, L.-J., Yao, X., Hoos, L. M., Tetzloff, G., et al. (2004). Niemann-Pick C1 Like 1 protein is critical for intestinal cholesterol absorption. *Science*, 303, 1201–1204.

Barbier, O., Torra, I. P., Duguay, Y., Blanquart, C., Fruchart, J.-C., Glineur, C., et al. (2002). Pleiotropic actions of peroxisome proliferator-activated receptors in lipid metabolism and atherosclerosis arterioscler. *Arteriosclerosis, Thrombosis, and Vascular Biology*, 22, 717–726.

Barter, P. J., & Kastelein, J. J. P. (2006). Targeting cholesterol ester transfer protein for the prevention and management of cardiovascular disease. *Journal of the American College of Cardiology*, 47, 492–497.

Bays, H. E., Weiss, R. J., Rhyne, J. M., Chen, Y., Lopez, C., & Spezzi, A. H. (2007). Abstract 682: Lapaqistat acetate monotherapy: Effects of a novel squalene synthase inhibitor on LDL-C levels and other lipid parameters in patients with primary hypercholesterolemia. *Circulation*, 116, II_127.

Berhanu, P., Kipnes, M. S., Khan, M. A., Perez, A. T., Kupfer, S. F., Spanheimer, R. G., et al. (2006). Effects of pioglitazone on lipid and lipoprotein profiles in patients with type 2 diabetes and dyslipidaemia after treatment conversion from rosiglitazone while continuing stable statin therapy. *Diabetes and Vascular Disease Research*, 3, 39–44.

Brousseau, M. E., Schaefer, E. J., Wolfe, M. L., Bloeden, L. T., Digenio, A. G., Clark, R. W., et al. (2004). Effects of an inhibitor of cholesterol ester transfer protein on HDL cholesterol. *New England Journal of Medicine*, 350, 1505–1515.

Charlton-Menys, V., & Durrington, P. N. (2008). Human cholesterol metabolism and therapeutic molecules. *Experimental Physiology*, 93, 27–42.

Colca, J. R., & Kletzien, R. F. (2006). What has prevented the expansion of insulin sensitisers? *Expert Opinion on Investigational Drugs*, 15(3), 205–210.

Colca, J. R., McDonald, W. G., Malapaka, R., Xu, H. E., & Kletzien, R. F. (2008). PPAR-sparing insulin sensitizers; path for development and clinical evaluation. *Diabetologia*, *51*(Suppl. 1), S21.

Davidson M. H., Maki, K. C., Zavoral, J. H., Yu, S., Popovici, C., & Price, G. D. (2007). Abstract 193: Lapaquistat acetate, a novel squalene synthase inhibitor, co-administered with atorvastatin reduces plasma lipids and C-reactive protein levels in subjects with primary hypercholesterolemia. *Circulation*, *116*, II_17.

de Grooth, G. J., Klerkx, A. H. E. M., Stroes, E. S. G., Stalenhoef, A. F. H.,. Kastelein, J. J. P., & Kuivenhoven, J. A. (2004). A review of CETP and its relation to atherosclerosis. *Journal of Lipid Research*, *45*, 1967–1974.

Endo, A., Tsujita, Y., Kuroda, M., & Tanzawa, K. (1977). Inhibition of cholesterol synthesis in vitro and in vivo by ML-236A and ML-236B, competitive inhibitors of 3-hydroxy-3-methylglutaryl-coenzyme A reductase. *European Journal of Biochemistry*, *77*(1), 31–36.

Erdmann, E., Dormandy, J. A., Charbonnel, B., Massi-Benedetti, M., Moules, I. K., & Skene, A. M., on behalf of the PROactive Investigators. (2007). The effect of pioglitazone on recurrent myocardial infarction in 2,445 patients with type 2 diabetes and previous myocardial infarction: Results from the PROactive (PROactive 05) Study. *Journal of the American College of Cardiology*, *49*, 1772–1780.

Feldman, P. L., Lambert, M. H., & Henke, B. R. (2008). PPAR modulators and PPAR pan agonists for metabolic diseases: The next generation of drugs targeting peroxisome proliferator-activated receptors? *Current Topics in Medicinal Chemistry*, *8*(9), 728–749.

Garcia-Calvo M., Lisnock, J., Bull, H. G., Hawes, B. E., Burnett, D. A., Braun, M. P., et al. (2005). The target of ezetimibe is Niemann-Pick C1-Like 1 (NPC1L1). *Proceedings of the National Academy of Sciences, USA*, *102*, 8132–8137.

Goldberg, R. B., Kendall, D. M., Deeg, M. A., Buse, J. B., Zagar, A. J., Pinaire, J. A., et al., for the GLAI Study Investigators. (2005). A comparison of lipid and glycemic effects of pioglitazone and rosiglitazone in patients with type 2 diabetes and dyslipidemia. *Diabetes Care*, *28*, 1547–1554.

Hebert, P. R., Gaziano, J. M., Chan, K. S., & Hennekens, C. H. (1997). Cholesterol lowering with statin drugs, risk of stroke, and total mortality: An overview of randomized trials. *JAMA*, *278*, 313–321.

Hiyoshi, H., Yanagimachi,M., Ito, M., Ohtsuka, I., Yoshida, I., Saeki, T., et al. (2000). Effect of ER-27856, a novel squalene synthase inhibitor, on plasma cholesterol in rhesus monkeys: Comparison with 3-hydroxy-3-methylglutaryl-CoA reductase inhibitors. *Journal of Lipid Research*, *41*, 1136–1144.

Hiyoshi, H., Yanagimachi, M., Ito, M., Yasuda, N., Okada, T., Ikuta, H., et al. (2003). Squalene synthase inhibitors suppress triglyceride biosynthesis through the farnesol pathway in rat hepatocytes. *Journal of Lipid Research*, *44*, 128–135.

Hofmann, C. A., & Colca, J. R. (1992). New oral thiazolidinedione antidiabetic agents act as insulin sensitizers. *Diabetes Care*, *15*, 1075–1078.

Home, P. D., Pocock, S. J., Beck-Nielsen, H., Curtis, P. S., Gomis, R., Hanefeld, M., et al., for the RECORD Study Team. (2009). Rosiglitazone evaluated for cardiovascular outcomes in oral agent combination therapy for type 2 diabetes (RECORD): A multicentre, rando-mised, open-label trial. *The Lancet*, *373*(9681), 2125–2135.

Huff, M. W., Pollex, R. L., & Hegele, R. A. (2006). NPC1L1: Evolution from pharmacological target to physiological sterol transporter. *Arteriosclerosis, Thrombosis, and Vascular Biology*, *26*, 2433–2438.

Iqbal, J., & Hussain, M. M. (2009). Intestinal lipid absorption. *American Journal of Physiology, Endocrinology and Metabolism*, *296*(6), E1183–E1194.

Issemann, I., Prince, R. A., Tugwood, J. D., & Green, S. (1993). The peroxisome proliferator-activated receptor: Retinoid X receptor heterodimer is activated by fatty acids and fibrate hypolipidaemic drugs. *Journal of Molecular Endocrinology*, *11*, 37–47.

Joseph, S. B., & Tontonoz, P. (2003). LXRs: New therapeutic targets in atherosclerosis? *Current Opinion in Pharmacology, 3*(2), 192–197.

Joy, T. J., & Hegele, R. A. (2009). Narrative review: Statin-related myopathy. *Annals of Internal Medicine, 150,* 858–868.

Kastelein, J. J. P., van Leuven, S. I., Burgess, L., Evans, G. W., Kuivenhoven, J. A., Barter, P. J., et al. (2007). Effect of torceptrapib on carotid atherosclerosis in familial hypercholesterolemia. *New England Journal of Medicine, 356,* 1620–1630.

Kastelein, J. J. P., Wedel, M. K., Baker, B. F., Su, J., Bradley, J. D., Yu, R. Z., et al. (2006). Potent reduction of apolipoprotein B and low-density lipoprotein cholesterol by short-term administration of an antisense inhibitor of apolipoprotein B. *Circulation, 114,* 1729–1735.

Kitayama, K., Koga, T., Inaba, T., & Fujioka, T. (2006). Multiple mechanisms of hypocholesterolemic action of pactimibe, a novel acyl-coenzyme A: Cholesterol acyltransferase inhibitor. *European Journal of Pharmacology, 543*(1–3), 123–132.

Kuivenhoven, J. A., de Grooth, G. J., Kawamura, H., Klerkx, A. H., Wilhelm, F., Trip, M. D., et al. (2005). Effectiveness of inhibition of cholesterol ester transfer protein by JTT-705 in combination with pravastatin in type 2 dyslipidemia. *American Journal of Cardiology, 95,* 1085–1088.

Lada, A. T., Davis, M., Kent, C., Chapman, J., Tomoda, H., Omura, S., et al. (2004). Identification of ACAT1- and ACAT2-specific inhibitors using a novel, cell-based fluorescence assay: Individual ACAT uniqueness. *Journal of Lipid Research, 45,* 378–386.

Lehmann, J. M., Moore, L. B., Smith-Oliver, T. A., Wilkison, W. O., Willson, T. M., & Kliewer, S. A. (1995). An antidiabetic thiazolidinedione is a high affinity ligand for peroxisome proliferator-activated receptor [gamma] (PPAR [gamma]). *Journal of Biological Chemistry, 270,* 12953–12956.

Lewis, G. F., & Rader, D. L. (2005). New insights into the regulation of HDL metabolism and reverse cholesterol transport. *Circulation Research, 96,* 1221–1232.

Li, A. C., & Glass, C. K. (2004). PPAR- and LXR-dependent pathways controlling lipid metabolism and the development of atherosclerosis. *Journal of Lipid Research, 45,* 2161–2173.

Lloyd-Jones, D., Adams, R., Carnethon, M., De Simone, G., Ferguson, T. B., Flegal, K., et al., for the American Heart Association Statistics Committee and Stroke Statistics Subcommittee. (2009). Heart Disease and Stroke Statistics—2009 Update: A report from the American Heart Association Statistics Committee and Stroke Statistics Subcommittee. *Circulation, 119,* e21–e181.

McTaggart, F., Brown, G. R., Davidson, R. G., Freeman, S., Holdgate, G. A., Mallion, K. B., et al. (1996). Inhibition of squalene synthase of rat liver by novel 3' substituted quinuclidines. *Biochemical Pharmacology, 51*(11), 1477–1487.

Meuwese, M. C., de Groot, E., Duivenvoorden, R., Trip, M. D., Ose, L., Maritz, F. J., et al., for the CAPTIVATE Investigators. (2009). ACAT inhibition and progression of carotid atherosclerosis in patients with familial hypercholesterolemia the CAPTIVATE randomized trial. *JAMA, 301*(11), 1131–1139.

Quinet, E. M., Basso, M. D., Halpern, A. R., Yates, D. W., Sheffan, R. J., Clerin, V., et al. (2009). LXR ligand lowers LDL cholesterol in primates, is lipid neutral in hamster, and reduces atherosclerosis in mouse. *Journal of Lipid Research,* 10.1194/jlr.M900037-JLR200.

Ridker, P. M., Danielson, E., Fonseca, F. A. H., Genest, J., Gotto, Jr., A. M., Kastelein, J. J. P., et al., for the JUPITER Study Group. (2008). Rosuvastatin to prevent vascular events in men and women with elevated C-reactive protein. *New England Journal of Medicine, 359,* 2195–2207.

Rigamonti, E., Chinetti-Gbaguidi, G., & Staels, B. (2008). Regulation of macrophage functions by PPAR-{alpha}, PPAR-{gamma}, and LXRs in mice and men. *Arteriosclerosis, Thrombosis, and Vascular Biology, 28,* 1050–1059.

Rosenblum, S. B., Huynh, T., Afonso, A., Davis, Jr, H. R., Yumibe, N., Clader, J. W., et al. (1998). Discovery of 1-(4-fluorophenyl)-(3R)-[3-(4-fluorophenyl)-(3S)-hydroxypropyl]-

(4S)-(4 -hydroxyphenyl)-2-azetidinone (SCH 58235): A designed, potent, orally active inhibitor of cholesterol absorption. *Journal of Medicinal Chemistry, 41*(6), 973–980.

Rudel, L. L., Lee, R. G., & Parini, P. (2005). ACAT2 is a target for treatment of coronary heart disease associated with hypercholesterolemia. *Arteriosclerosis, Thrombosis, and Vascular Biology, 25*, 1112–1118.

Simes, R. S., Marschner, I. C., Hunt, D., Colquhoun, D., Sullivan, D., Stewart, R. A. H., et al. (2002). Relationship between lipid levels and clinical outcomes in the long-term intervention with pravastatin in ischemic disease (LIPID) trial: To what extent is the reduction in coronary events with pravastatin explained by on-study lipid levels? *Circulation, 105*, 1162–1169.

Steinberg, D. (2006). Thematic review series: The pathogenesis of atherosclerosis. An interpretive history of the cholesterol controversy, part V: The discovery of the statins and the end of the controversy. *Journal of Lipid Research, 47*, 1339–1351.

Steiner, G., Kastelein, J. J. P., Kallend, D., & Stroes, E. S. G. (2008). *Cardiovascular safety of the cholesterol ester transfer protein inhibitor R1658/JTT-705: Results from phase 2 trials* Presented on March 31, 2008 at the 57th Annual Scientific Session of the American Congress of Cardiology (ACC), Chicago, USA, Abstract #1028–166.

Tall, A. R., Yvan-Charvet, L., & Wang, N. (2007). The failure of torceptrapib: Was it the molecule or the mechanism? *Arteriosclerosis, Thrombosis, and Vascular Biology, 27*, 257–260.

van Heek, M., & Davis, H. (2002). Pharmacology of ezetimibe. *European Heart Journal,* Suppl. 4: J5–J8.

Weingartner, O., Bohm, M., & Laufs, U. (2009). Controversial role of plant sterol esters in the management of hypercholesterolaemia. *European Heart Journal, 30*(4), 404–409.

Wilcox, R., Bousser, M.-G., Betteridge, D. J., Schernthaner, G., Pirags, V., Kupfer, S., et al., for the PROactive Investigators. (2007). Effects of pioglitazone in patients with type 2 diabetes with or without previous stroke: Results from PROactive (PROspective pioglitAzone Clinical Trial In macroVascular Events 04). *Stroke, 38*, 865–873.

Winkelmayer, W. C., Setoguchi, S., Levin, R., & Solomon, D. K. (2008). Comparison of cardiovascular outcomes in elderly patients with diabetes who initiated rosiglitazone vs pioglitazone therapy. *Archives of Internal Medicine, 168*, 2368–2375.

Gianluigi Tanda, Amy H. Newman, and Jonathan L. Katz

Psychobiology (GT, JLK), and Medicinal Chemistry (AHN) Sections, Medications
Discovery Research Branch, Intramural Research Program, Department of Health and
Human Services, National Institute on Drug Abuse, National Institutes of Health,
Baltimore, Maryland 21224

Discovery of Drugs to Treat Cocaine Dependence: Behavioral and Neurochemical Effects of Atypical Dopamine Transport Inhibitors

Abstract

Stimulant drugs acting at the dopamine transporter (DAT), like
cocaine, are widely abused, yet effective medical treatments for this
abuse have not been found. Analogs of benztropine (BZT) that, like
cocaine, act at the DAT have effects that differ from cocaine and in

Advances in Pharmacology, Volume 57

1054-3589/08 $35.00
10.1016/S1054-3589(08)57007-4

some situations block the behavioral, neurochemical, and reinforcing actions of cocaine. Neurochemical studies of dopamine levels in brain and behavioral studies have demonstrated that BZT analogs have a relatively slow onset and reduced maximal effects compared to cocaine. Pharmacokinetic studies, however, indicated that the BZT analogs rapidly access the brain at concentrations above their *in vitro* binding affinities, while binding *in vivo* demonstrates apparent association rates for BZT analogs lower than that for cocaine. Additionally, the off-target effects of these compounds do not fully explain their differences from cocaine. Initial structure–activity studies indicated that BZT analogs bind to DAT differently from cocaine and these differences have been supported by site-directed mutagenesis studies of the DAT. In addition, BZT analog-mediated inhibition of uptake was more resistant to mutations producing inward conformational DAT changes than cocaine analogs. The BZT analogs have provided new insights into the relation between the molecular and behavioral actions of cocaine and the diversity of effects produced by dopamine transport inhibitors. Novel interactions of BZT analogs with the DAT suggest that these drugs may have a pharmacology that would be useful in their development as treatments for cocaine abuse.

I. Introduction

A. The Dopamine Transporter, a Biological Target for Human Diseases, and Psychostimulant Abuse

Dopamine (DA) neurotransmission subserves a multitude of normal physiological functions in the central nervous system (CNS), with many factors affecting DA homeostasis. DA neurotransmission is regulated dynamically at the synaptic level by several mechanisms including negative feedback circuits induced by DA receptor occupancy that modulate neuronal activity, as well as DA synthesis. However, termination of the actions of DA by rapidly reducing its synaptic concentrations is critical. This occurs via metabolic degradation pathways, including monoamine oxidase and catechol-oxy-methyl-transferase enzymes, and by DA uptake (Iversen, Iversen, Bloom, & Roth, 2008). DA uptake sites or DA transporters (DATs) are membrane-bound proteins that efficiently transport DA from the extra- to the intra-cellular space and represent the major mechanism for the rapid termination of DA neurotransmission.

One of the most prominent of the diseases that involve dysfunctional DA neurotransmission is Parkinson's disease (PD) in which degeneration of the DA system leads to a reduction in neurotransmission in dopaminergic terminal areas that are important not only for somatic–motor functions but also for emotional–affective functions (Lees, Hardy, & Revesz, 2009).

Indeed some of the typical symptoms of PD involve a difficulty to initiate movements, as well as depression and apathy (Chaudhuri & Schapira, 2009). Drugs that target the DAT, methylphenidate and d-amphetamine, are clinically effective treatments, and genetic variants in the DAT have been implicated in the etiology of attention deficit hyperactivity disorder (ADHD) (e.g., Hahn & Blakely, 2007). A DA component is also involved in other diseases involving emotional and affective functions, including schizophrenia, autism, Tourette's syndrome, and depression (Meisenzahl, Schmitt, Scheuerecker, & Moller, 2007; Steeves & Fox, 2008; Stein, 2008).

The DAT is also the main target for stimulant drugs of abuse, such as cocaine, amphetamine, methamphetamine, and methylenedioxymethamphetamine (Zhu & Reith, 2008). Stimulant abuse and addiction are recognized to be major public health and socioeconomical issues (see, e.g., Substance Abuse and Mental Health Services Administration, 2007, http://www.oas.samhsa.gov), and research efforts over the last two decades have shed light on the neurobiological basis of cocaine dependence (Kalivas, 2007; Nestler, 2005). And while promising new strategies for the development of medical treatments have been reported (e.g., Kharkar, Dutta, & Reith, 2008; Newman & Katz, 2009; Runyon & Carroll, 2008), cocaine addiction remains a condition for which effective medical treatments have not yet been identified.

Cocaine acts in the CNS at several pharmacological targets. For example, its local anesthetic effects have been well documented together with its effects on Na^+ channels (Catterall & Mackie, 2006). However, the main activity contributing to the reinforcing effects of cocaine and its consequent abuse liability involves the blockade of plasma membrane monoamine transporters (see review by Carroll, Howell, & Kuhar, 1999). Although cocaine inhibits the transport of dopamine, serotonin, and norepinephrine from the synapse into nerve terminals, blockade of the DAT is considered the main effect through which the pharmacology of cocaine contributes to its behavioral and reinforcing actions (Kuhar, Ritz, & Boja, 1991; Ritz, Boja, George, & Kuhar, 1989).

B. The DAT as a Pharmacological Target for Candidate Drugs as Psychostimulant Abuse Medications, the Atypical DAT Inhibitors Benztropine Analogs

It has been hypothesized that drugs blocking the DAT will have reinforcing effects similar to those of cocaine (Kuhar et al., 1991). However, of the several chemical classes of DAT inhibitors synthesized in the past 15–20 years, some have behavioral effects that differ from those of cocaine (Newman & Kulkarni, 2002). Because of these variations in behavioral effects, these "atypical" DAT inhibitors are being actively investigated to find clues that may help in the search for psychostimulant abuse medications.

Agonist or substitution therapies have been successful in the treatment of opioid (Mattick, Breen, Kimber, & Davoli, 2009) and nicotine abuse (Stead, Perera, Bullen, Mant, & Lancaster, 2008). As such, drugs that block the DAT, but with lower abuse potential compared to cocaine, have been the focus of many of the drug discovery programs directed at cocaine-abuse treatments. One of the most studied compounds, GBR 12909 (Fig. 1), which shares some basic pharmacological features with addictive psychostimulants, has preclinical effects suggestive of a clinically effective treatment. Specifically, treatment with GBR 12909 decreases cocaine self-administration in animals, at doses that do not affect the behaviors reinforced with food presentation (see review by Rothman, Baumann, Prisinzano, & Newman, 2008). However, the appearance of cardiovascular effects in clinical trials prevented its further development (Vocci, Acri, & Elkashef, 2005).

Several classes of DAT inhibitors that were tested preclinically for their potential as treatments for stimulant abuse have been reviewed elsewhere (e.g., Kharkar et al., 2008; Meltzer, 2008; Prisinzano & Rice, 2008; Runyon & Carroll, 2008). The present review focuses on analogs of benztropine (3α-diphenylmethoxytropane, BZT, Fig. 1). This parent compound was initially of interest because it shares structural features with both cocaine and GBR 12909 (Fig. 1). Therefore, solely from a structural perspective, BZT and its analogs were of interest. Moreover, though BZT is in clinical use for treatment of early-stage PD for many years, there are only a few case reports of its abuse, mainly related to its anticholinergic effects (see, e.g., Grace, 1997). Finally, Colpaert, Niemegeers, and Janssen (1979) showed that BZT did not fully substitute in rats trained to discriminate cocaine from saline injections. These considerations suggested that BZT analogs could be of interest for cocaine-abuse treatment and may have advantages over DAT inhibitors that share cocaine-like preclinical indications of abuse liability. To pursue this possibility, we initiated a program of synthesis and evaluation of BZT analogs. A comprehensive review of the chemistry of these compounds has been recently published (Newman & Katz, 2008). In this chapter we review preclinical and clinical research that has been conducted on BZT analogs as it relates to the potential of these compounds as medications for cocaine abuse.

C. Definitions

JJC 1-059: *N*-(3-((3*S*,5*R*)-3,5-dimethyl-4-(3-phenylpropyl)piperazin-1-yl) propyl)-4-fluoro-*N*-(4-fluorophenyl)aniline

JJC 2-010: 3-(4-(3-(bis(4-fluorophenyl)amino)propyl)piperazin-1-yl)-1-phenylpropan-1-ol

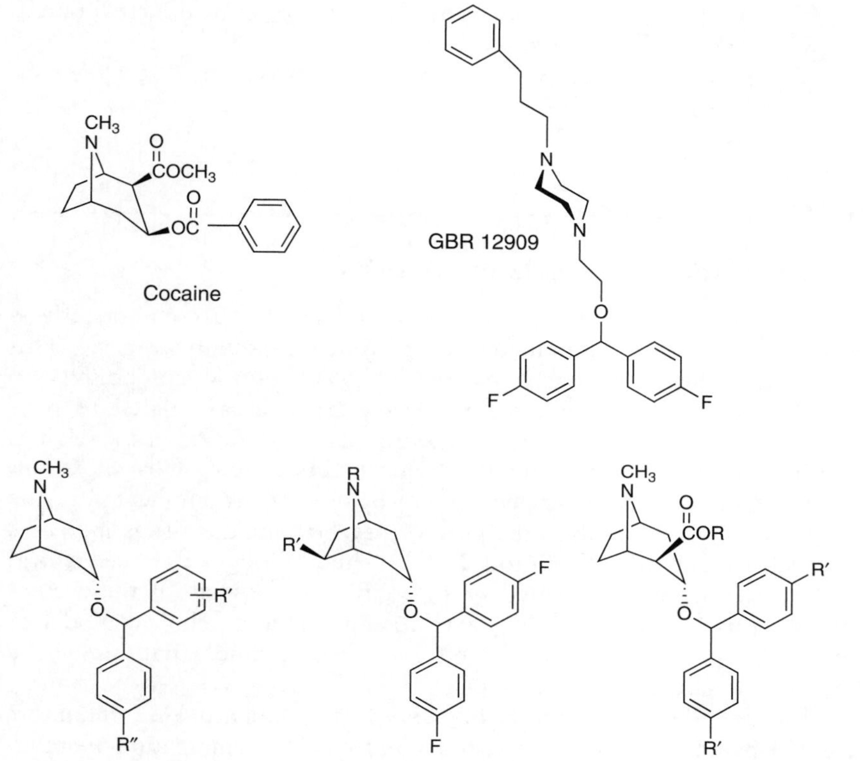

Cocaine

GBR 12909

Benztropine; R′=R″=H
4′-F-BZT; R′=4-F R″=H
4′-Cl-BZT; R′=4-Cl, R″=H
3′-Cl-BZT; R′=3-Cl, R″=H
3′,4′-diCl-BZT; R′=3,4-diCl, R″=H
3′,4′-diCl, 4″-F-BZT; R′=3,4-diCl, R″=F
3′,4′-diF-BZT; R′=3,4-diF, R″=H
3′,4″-diF-BZT; R′=3-F, R″=F
4′,4″-diCl-BZT; R′=4-Cl, R″=Cl
4′-Br,4″-F-BZT; R′=4-Br, R″=F

AHN 2-003; R=R′=H
AHN 1-055; R=CH₃, R′=H
AHN 2-005; R=CH₂CH=CH₂, R′=H
JHW 007; R=CH₂CH₂CH₂CH₃, R′=H
GA 2-99; R=CH₂CH₂NH₂, R′=H
GA 103; R=CH₂CH₂CH₂CH₂Ph, R′=H
PG01053; R=CH₃, R′=OH

MFZ 2-71; R=CH₂CH₃, R′=F
MFZ 4-86; R=CH₂CH₃, R′=Cl
MFZ 4-87; R=CH₃, R′=Cl

FIGURE 1   Chemical structures of cocaine, GBR 12909 and the BZT analogs referred to in the present manuscript. For a more complete description of the chemistry of the BZT analogs see Newman and Katz (2009).

GBR 12909: 1-[2-[bis(4-fluorophenyl)methoxy]ethyl]-4-(3-phenylpropyl) piperazine
WIN 35,428: (−)-2β-carbomethoxy-3β-(4-fluorophenyl)tropane
RTI-371: 3β-(4-methylphenyl)-2β-[3-(4-chlorophenyl)isoxazol-5-yl]tropane
RTI-121: (−)-2β-carboisopropoxy-3β-(4-iodophenyl)tropane

RTI-55: 3β-(4-iodophenyl)tropan-2 beta-carboxylic acid methyl ester
RTI-31: (−)-2β-carbomethoxy-3β-(4′-chlorophenyl)tropane
CP 55940: 2-[(1S,2R,5S)-5-hydroxy-2-(3-hydroxypropyl) cyclohexyl]-
5-(2-methyloctan-2-yl)phenol

II. Behavioral Studies

A. Stimulation of Ambulatory Activity

Stimulation of ambulatory activity is one of the common effects produced by psychostimulants after systemic administration. This behavior is likely mediated by the ability of these compounds to interact with DA transmission in specific brain areas related to physiological functions other than control of motor activities (Zahm, 1999). It is interesting to note that local application of psychostimulants in specific dopaminergic terminal fields that are implicated in the subjective effects and abuse liability of psychostimulant drugs increases ambulatory activity (Ikemoto, 2002). Thus, though this behavioral activity is not directly related to the reinforcing effects of these compounds, this behavior provides a relatively simple preclinical model to investigate psychostimulant-like effects of compounds that may have liability for abuse.

The dose-dependent effects of cocaine and standard DAT inhibitors (e.g., methylphenidate, mazindol, and nomifensine) on stimulation of ambulatory activity can be graphically represented as a bell-shaped, inverted-U curve, with increased stimulation of activity at low to intermediate doses and a decrease of effects at the larger doses (filled symbols in Fig. 2 show cocaine effects). The latter may be the result of the appearance of behaviors other than ambulation, that is, stereotypies, proconvulsive effects, seizures, or convulsions, that are likely incompatible with locomotion. BZT analogs can produce different levels of ambulatory activity, but they most often do not stimulate activity to the same level as that produced by cocaine or cocaine-like drugs (Katz, Izenwasser, Kline, Allen, & Newman, 1999; Katz, Kopajtic, Agoston, & Newman, 2004; Katz et al., 2001; Newman, Allen, Izenwasser, & Katz, 1994; Newman et al., 1995; Tanda, Ebbs, Newman, & Katz, 2005; Tolliver et al., 1999) (Fig. 2, for chemical structures see Fig. 1). In contrast, standard DA uptake inhibitors, such as cocaine and methylphenidate, have maximal effects that are generally comparable, if relatively restricted time points for measurement are selected, eliminating duration of action as an influence on the measurement of maximal effects (Izenwasser, Terry, Heller, Witkin, & Katz, 1994). Thus, the effects of BZT analogs on this behavioral activity were atypically blunted as compared to those of cocaine.

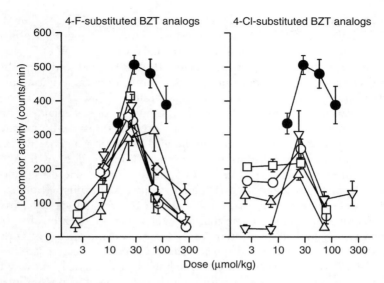

FIGURE 2   Dose-dependent effects of 4-F- and 4-Cl-substituted BZT analogs on locomotor activity in mice. Ordinates: horizontal activity counts after drug administration. Abscissae: dose of drug in μmol/kg, log scale. Each point represents the average effect determined in eight mice. The data are from the 30-min period during the first 60 min after drug administration, in which the greatest stimulant effects were obtained. Note that the 4-F-substituted compounds (left panel) were generally more efficacious than the 4-Cl-substituted compounds, and no members of either group had efficacy comparable to that of cocaine. Left panel symbols: filled circles: cocaine; open circles: 4′-F-BZT; squares: 4′,4″-diF-BZT; triangles: 3′,4′-diCl,4″-F-BZT; downward triangles: 3′,4′-diF-BZT; diamonds: 3′,4″-diF-BZT; hexagons: 4′-Br,4″-F-BZT. Right panel symbols: filled circles: cocaine; open circles: 4′-Cl-BZT; squares: 4′-Cl-BZT (with the diphenylether system at the asymmetric C3 of the tropane ring, in the equatorial, β, configuration); triangles: 4′,4″-diCl-BZT; downward triangles: 3′,4′-diCl-BZT. See Fig. 1 for compound structures. Modified from Katz et al. (1999).

Binding of BZT analogs indicated that they have high affinity for the DAT and are selective for that target over the other monoamine transporters (Katz et al., 1999), suggesting that the reduced effectiveness of these compounds was not due to a low affinity for the DAT protein. Structure–activity studies indicated that the BZT analogs with a fluoro-substitution in the para-position on either of the phenyl rings were less effective than cocaine, but were the most effective among the BZT analogs. Those with chloro-substitutions had affinities comparable to those of the fluoro-substituted analogs, but were even less effective in stimulating locomotor activity than cocaine (Fig. 2).

BZT analogs, when administered before cocaine, can modify cocaine-induced stimulation of ambulatory activity. For example, in rats injected i.p. with 40 mg/kg of 4′-Cl-BZT, cocaine (10 mg/kg, i.p.) administered 2 h later stimulated ambulatory behavior to a greater extent than after saline injection (Tolliver et al., 1999). In contrast, Desai, Kopajtic, Koffarnus, Newman, and Katz (2005) showed that the BZT analog, JHW 007, blocked the locomotor-stimulant effects of cocaine. JHW 007 produced a significant DAT occupancy that was not followed by significant cocaine-like stimulant effects. However, the apparent association rate of JHW 007 *in vivo* was slow. Control mice pretreated with saline showed a dose-dependent stimulation of ambulatory counts by increasing doses of cocaine, with maximum activity shown at 40 mg/kg. Cocaine-induced locomotor activity was completely antagonized in mice pretreated with a 10 mg/kg dose of JHW 007, while another BZT analog, AHN-2005, only reduced the effects of the highest doses of cocaine tested (Desai, Kopajtic, Koffarnus, et al., 2005). Similarly, a combination of AHN 1-055 with cocaine attenuated the cocaine-induced locomotor stimulation (Velazquez-Sanchez et al., 2009). In contrast, *d*-amphetamine pretreatment increased the effects of cocaine, suggesting that the absence of an increase in cocaine effects produced by AHN 1-055 was not the result of a "ceiling" being reached, above which further increases could not be obtained. In addition, the possibility that ambulatory activity was reduced through competition with other behaviors, such as focused stereotypes, was ruled out. Combined *d*-amphetamine and cocaine treatments produced both robust locomotion and stereotyped behavior. In contrast, AHN 1-055 did not enhance the stereotyped behavior produced by cocaine alone. These data suggest that the attenuation of the effects of cocaine by AHN 1-055 was not due to the induction of competing behaviors, and that its effects in combination with cocaine are distinctly different from those produced by classic psychostimulants (Velazquez-Sanchez et al., 2009).

B. Cocaine Discrimination

Drug discrimination is a behavioral procedure in which the subjective effects produced by the administration of a drug can be studied in human or animal subjects (Holtzman, 1990). The more minute details of the procedures differ from one experiment to another, but subjects are always trained to emit one response after injection of the training drug and a different response after injection of its vehicle. These responses are only intermittently reinforced, so the only stimulus for the subject regarding which of the two responses will be reinforced is the injection (drug or vehicle) administered before testing (for further details see Holtzman, 1990). The subjective effects of cocaine using this procedure have been extensively studied (Woods, Winger, & France, 1987), and only drugs that act through brain mechanisms similar to those of cocaine produce cocaine-like responding. Drugs like WIN 35,428, methylphenidate, or *d*-amphetamine will generalize to (or substitute for) the cocaine discriminative stimulus. There is also a correlation between the potencies of various DAT inhibitors in substituting for cocaine and their affinity for the DAT, though the relationship is complicated by the modeling of the binding data for one or two DAT sites (Katz, Izenwasser, & Terry, 2000). Further, monoamine uptake inhibitors with affinity, primarily for either SERT or NET, generally do not fully substitute for the cocaine discriminative stimulus (Baker, Riddle, Saunders, & Appel, 1993; Kleven, Anthony, & Woolverton, 1990).

BZT analogs have demonstrated different degrees of effectiveness in substituting for cocaine, and most do not fully substitute for the cocaine discriminative stimulus (see, e.g., Katz et al., 1999) (Fig. 3). BZT analogs with para-fluoro substituents of the diphenylether system are among the more effective, while BZT analogs with other para-substitutions, despite

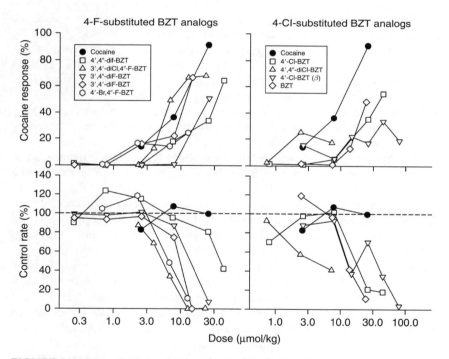

FIGURE 3 Effects of BZT analogs in rats trained to discriminate injections of cocaine from saline. Ordinates for top panels: percentage of responses on the cocaine-appropriate key. Ordinates for bottom panels: rates at which responses were emitted (as a percentage of response rate after saline administration). Abscissae: drug dose in μmol/kg (log scale). Each point represents the effect in four to six rats. The percentage of responses emitted on the cocaine-appropriate key was considered unreliable and not plotted if fewer than half of the subjects responded at that dose. Note that the fluoro-substituted compounds (left panels) were generally more effective in substituting for cocaine than the Cl-substituted compounds. See Fig. 1 for compound structures. Modified from Katz et al. (1999).

binding affinities comparable to those of the fluoro-substituted compounds (Newman & Katz, 2009), are clearly less effective (Fig. 3). It is important to note that the lower efficacy of these compounds in drug-discrimination studies has been suggested as reflecting a slow onset of central effects compared to cocaine or other cocaine-like DAT inhibitors. Thus in some experiments, BZT analogs were administered at different times before testing. However, with the exception of AHN 1-055, none of the BZT analogs studied produced a larger cocaine-like discriminative effect when tested at times from 5 to 120 min before the session (Katz et al., 1999, 2004). AHN 1-055 fully substituted for cocaine when administered 90 min before testing, but not at other times.

Due to their reduced effectiveness, BZT analogs have also been tested for their ability to interfere with the discriminative stimulus effects of cocaine. Combinations of standard DAT inhibitors with cocaine typically resulted in a leftward shift in the cocaine dose–effect curve. In a series of experiments with analogs of BZT substituted with Cl-groups in the 3'-, 4'-, 3',4'-, and 4',4'-positions of the diphenylether system, it was shown that despite of their reduced efficacy in substituting for cocaine, these analogs shifted the cocaine discriminative-stimulus dose–effect curve leftward (Katz et al., 2001). In contrast, N-substituted analogs of BZT (e.g., AHN 2-005, JHW 007) did not appreciably shift the cocaine dose–effect curve (Katz et al., 2004). Thus, there are differences among the BZT analogs with regard to their interactions with cocaine.

Studies have implicated nucleus accumbens (NAc) DA transmission in the discriminative stimulus effects of stimulants (e.g., Callahan, De La Garza, & Cunningham, 1997; Dworkin & Smith, 1988). Tanda, Ebbs, Newman, & Katz (2006) examined the subjective effects of cocaine and N-substituted BZT analogs in rats discriminating cocaine from saline and their effects on extracellular DA in the NAc shell. All of the compounds tested dose-dependently (1, 3, and 10 mg/kg i.p.) increased NAc DA levels, however, their maximum effects were different and were obtained at different times after injection. Although cocaine and AHN 1-055 dose-dependently generalized with the cocaine discriminative stimulus, AHN 1-055 only did so 90 min after injection. Both AHN 2-005 and JHW 007 produced a substitution greater than vehicle, though neither drug fully substituted for cocaine at any dose or time after administration. The subjective effects or cocaine were linearly related to the extracellular levels of DA, and independent of time after injection. However, the BZT analogs were less effective in producing a cocaine-like discriminative stimulus effect even at times and doses that produced a stimulation of DA levels that was equal to or greater than that shown with cocaine to be effective in producing exclusive cocaine-like responding. Other studies have also documented differences in behavioral response to similar concentrations of DA produced by psychostimulants (Zolkowska et al., 2009). Thus, comparable levels of DA stimulated by the BZT analogs produced less substitution than did cocaine, and the behavioral effects obtained at a given level of DA elevation for BZT analogs depended on the time after injection, suggesting a rapid desensitization to the effects of DA accompanying the administration of BZT analogs.

C. Self-Administration

Drug self-administration is a behavioral procedure in which responses of a subject directly produce drug injections. The consistent features of the many variants of the procedure involve training a subject to emit a simple response that produces an intravenous injection of the compound. Often subjects are trained with one known compound, such as cocaine, and tested with various doses of unknown compounds, as well as vehicle. When rates of response are greater than those maintained with vehicle injection, the compound is said to have reinforcing effects (see Katz, 1989, for further details). Behavior maintained by drug self-injection is often considered the gold standard for the study of the reinforcing effects, and thus the abuse liability, of drugs.

The reinforcing effects of cocaine have been extensively documented (Woods et al., 1987). The reinforcing effects of BZT analogs were initially compared to those of cocaine in two studies. In the first, rhesus monkeys were trained to self-administer cocaine, and BZT and its 3'-Cl- and 4'-Cl-analogs were subsequently tested. Rates of responding maintained by BZT and its analogs were relatively low compared to those maintained by cocaine (Woolverton et al., 2000). In this study drugs were delivered after each 10th lever press (fixed-ratio 10-response or FR 10 schedule).

The reinforcing effects of 3'-Cl-, 4'-Cl-, and 3',4'-diCl-BZT were further tested in a second study and compared to those of cocaine and GBR 12909 under the FR 10 schedule (Woolverton, Hecht, Agoston, Katz, & Newman, 2001). The rate of self-administration obtained under the FR schedule with 3'-Cl- and 4'-Cl-BZT, but not with 3',4'-diCl-BZT, was greater than vehicle, but much lower than that maintained by cocaine or by GBR 12909 in the same monkeys. The rate of self-administration of 3',4'-diCl-BZT was not greater than that maintained by vehicle. In a second part of the study, rhesus monkeys were trained to respond under a progressive-ratio schedule, in which the number of responses required for self-administration increases progressively until the subject stops responding. The number of responses completed before the subject stops responding is often considered a measure of the effectiveness of a compound as a reinforcing stimulus (Hodos, 1961). Cocaine and GBR 12909 were the most effective reinforcers, and the BZT analogs were the least efficacious, with the rank order as follows: cocaine> GBR 12909 > 3'-Cl-BZT = 4'-Cl-BZT > 3',4'-diCl-BZT. In a more recent study using rats, progressive-ratio performance maintained by cocaine was

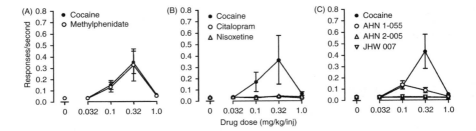

FIGURE 4 Substitution of different doses of cocaine or other monoamine uptake inhibitors and BZT analogs in rats trained to self-administer cocaine (0.32 mg/kg/injection). Ordinates: responses per second. Abscissae: injection dose (mg/kg/injection). Each point represents the mean (vertical bars represent SEM) of 6 to 11 subjects. Panel A: cocaine (filled circles) and methylphenidate (open circles). Panel B: cocaine (filled circles) and citalopram (open circles) or nisoxetine (triangles). Panel C: cocaine (filled circles) and AHN 1-055 (open circles), AHN 2-055 (triangles up), or JHW 007 (triangles down). Modified from Hiranita et al. (2009).

greater than that maintained by AHN 1-055, which was only marginally greater than that maintained by vehicle (Ferragud et al., 2009).

Recently, the reinforcing effects of N-substituted BZT analogs were assessed in rats responding under an FR 5 schedule and compared to those of standard DAT inhibitors (Hiranita, Soto, Newman, & Katz, 2009). The DAT inhibitor, methylphenidate, maintained responding like cocaine (Fig. 4A), whereas the SERT and NET inhibitors, citalopram and nisoxetine, respectively, did not (Fig. 4B). Under the same experimental conditions, neither AHN 2-005 nor JHW 007 maintained rates of responding above those maintained by vehicle (Fig. 4C). AHN 1-055 maintained i.v. self-administration behavior, though maximal rates of responding were at a low level as compared to cocaine or methylphenidate (Fig. 4C). Reinforcing effects of AHN 1-055 were also demonstrated by Ferragud et al. (2009) using an FR 1-response injection schedule. In addition, after a 2-week period in which subjects did not have the opportunity to respond, the responding previously maintained by AHN 1-055 was reduced to the rates previously obtained with vehicle whereas responding previously maintained by cocaine persisted.

Pre-session treatments with methylphenidate (p.o.) shifted the dose–response curve for cocaine self-administration leftward (Fig. 5A), suggesting that methylphenidate did not antagonize the reinforcing effects of cocaine, but rather added to them (Hiranita et al., 2009). At variance with methylphenidate, AHN 2-005 and JHW 007 (p.o.) shifted the cocaine dose–response curve downward (Fig. 5C and D), suggesting an antagonistic effect of these compounds on cocaine self-administration (Hiranita et al., 2009).

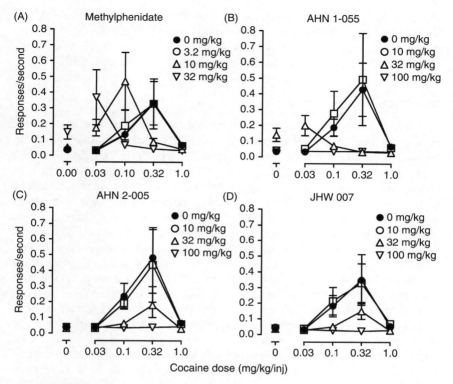

FIGURE 5 Effects of pre-session treatment with methylphenidate and N-substituted BZT analogs on cocaine self-administration. Ordinates: responses per second. Abscissae: injection dose (mg/kg/injection). Each point represents the mean with SEM ($n = 6$ to 10). Methylphenidate, AHN 1-055, AHN 2-005, or JHW 007 were administered orally at 60, 180, 240, or 300 min before sessions, respectively. Modified from Hiranita et al. (2009).

The effects of AHN 1-055 were more complex, with intermediate doses of the compound increasing responding at lower doses of cocaine, but decreasing responding for the higher cocaine doses. Also, higher doses of AHN 1-055 shifted the cocaine dose–response curve downward, thus significantly decreasing and antagonizing cocaine-maintained self-administration behavior (Fig. 5B). Importantly, the BZT analog-induced changes in cocaine self-administration were obtained at p.o. doses that had no effects on responding maintained by food reinforcement under conditions similar to those used for the studies of cocaine-maintained responding (Ferragud et al., 2009; Hiranita et al., 2009).

A slower onset of action as compared to cocaine and other psychostimulants may explain the lower efficacy of BZT analogs as reinforcers. Because of the importance of contingency between the response and the effect of the compound, slow onset of action results in delays in reinforcement. A substantial literature in behavioral science confirms delay in reinforcement as a factor that decreases the effectiveness of all reinforcers (Skinner, 1938), as well as cocaine (e.g., Beardsley & Balster, 1993).

D. Place Conditioning

Place conditioning is a behavioral procedure used to indirectly assess the reinforcing or aversive effects of compounds. As with drug discrimination, the actual details of the procedure can differ from one experiment to the next, but all consist of placing the subject on one side of an enclosure after compound administration and on the other side after vehicle injection. The texture of floors, illumination, and other features of the two sides differ substantially. The majority of published studies proceed in three different phases, starting with a "pre-conditioning" test of how the subject distributes its time on the two sides of the chamber. The second "conditioning" phase involves confining the subject to one of the two sides by closing a door between them. When the subject is confined on one side it is pretreated with a compound, and when confined to the other side it is injected with vehicle. A final "testing" phase follows in which subjects have free access to both sides of the chamber (door open) in a compound-free condition, and the time spent in each side is recorded. It has been repeatedly found that appropriate doses of psychostimulants administered during the conditioning phase increase the time spent by animals in the compound-paired compartment during the testing phase, that is, place conditioning.

As noted above, one hypothesis for the lower reinforcing efficacy of BZT analogs in self-administration studies as compared to cocaine might result from the delayed onset of their effects. For example, Tanda et al. (2005, 2009) have shown that BZT analogs increase extracellular levels of DA in dialysates from the NAc at a lower rate as compared to cocaine (see Section E). In self-administration studies, a slow onset of effect would produce a delay of reinforcement that might decrease the rate or amount of behavior maintained. Even a fully effective drug such as cocaine maintains less behavior when its presentation is delayed in a self-administration study (e.g., Balster & Schuster, 1973). In a place conditioning study, the time between compound treatment and placement of the subject in the chamber can be varied to accommodate a delay in onset of effect and thus not alter the effectiveness of the compound.

Place conditioning with BZT analogs administered from immediately to 90 min before conditioning trials was investigated by Li, Newman, and Katz (2005), and results were compared to those obtained with cocaine administration. The effects of cocaine were robust and replicated the type of dose-dependent effects previously reported (see review by Tzschentke, 1998). The N-substituted BZT analogs, AHN 2-005, AHN 1-055, and JHW 007, were less effective and only occasionally produced an increase in time spent in the compound-paired compartment. For example, AHN 2-005 (0.1–10.0 mg/kg) produced a significant place conditioning only at the dose of 3 mg/kg when administered 45 min before the conditioning session. At all other times and doses, the effects of AHN 2-005 were not different from vehicle. Administration of JHW 007 (1.0–10.0 mg/kg) significantly increased time spent in the compound-paired compartment only when the dose of 10 mg/kg i.p. was administered 45 min before the subject was placed in the conditioning chamber, but not when placed in the chamber immediately or 90 min before trials, or at any of the other doses or times. The N-methyl-substituted BZT analog, AHN 1-055, had effects no different from those of saline across a range of doses from 0.3 to 3.0 mg/kg even when administered i.p. up to 90 min before conditioning sessions (Li et al., 2005).

In agreement with Li et al. (2005), in a recent report (Velazquez-Sanchez et al., 2009), AHN 1-055 did not produce place conditioning in mice when administered 1 h before the conditioning sessions using a higher range of doses compared to those used by Li et al. (2005). Velazquez-Sanchez et al. (2009) also showed that AHN 1-055 blocked the conditioning and reinforcing effects of cocaine measured in the place conditioning paradigm. These effects of AHN 1-055 paralleled its effects on preventing cocaine-induced early-gene activation (Velazquez-Sanchez et al., 2009) in the NAc and dorsomedial striatum, providing a neurobiological correlate to the antagonism of cocaine conditioning by the BZT analog.

Thus, place conditioning experiments with BZT analogs consistently indicate decreased effectiveness compared with cocaine. Further, when the delayed onset of effects of BZT analogs was taken into account, these experiments further suggest that the reduced cocaine-like behavioral effects of BZT analogs could not be entirely accounted for by a slower onset of action.

E. Neurochemistry

Most of the behavioral and reinforcing effects of cocaine have been related to its ability to block the DAT, which consequently leads to increased DA neurotransmission. The effects of cocaine on extracellular DA levels in different dopaminergic terminal areas in brain have been extensively studied using microdialysis (Kuczenski & Segal, 1992; Pontieri, Tanda, & Di Chiara, 1995; Tanda, Pontieri, Frau, & Di Chiara, 1997) and voltammetry techniques (Greco & Garris, 2003).

The effects of 4'-Cl-BZT were compared with those of cocaine on stimulation of DA levels in microdialysis studies in rats. One study was performed with probes implanted only in the NAc (Tolliver et al., 1999), and a second study was performed with microdialysis probes implanted in specific DA terminal areas, including the shell and core of the NAc, the medial prefrontal cortex, and the dorsal striatum (Tanda et al., 2005). Results from each study show that both cocaine and 4'-Cl-BZT dose-dependently stimulated DA levels in all brain regions tested. Across the range of doses studied, cocaine was twofold to threefold more potent than 4'-Cl-BZT in stimulating DA levels in the brain regions studied (Tanda et al., 2005). The differences were most pronounced in the shell of the NAc where cocaine was not only slightly more potent but also more effective than 4'-Cl-BZT (Fig. 6). A different pattern was observed in the prefrontal cortex where 4'-Cl-BZT was more effective than cocaine. Whereas the effects of cocaine were rapid and transient, the effects of 4'-Cl-BZT lasted longer with DA levels still significantly elevated more than 5 h after administration of the higher doses. The long-lasting effects of 4'-Cl-BZT are likely the result of the slow elimination rate of BZT analogs (see later). It should also be noted that although 4'-Cl-BZT effects were longer lasting compared to cocaine, its rate of increase in DA levels was much slower than that for cocaine (Fig. 6). A recent study using mice confirms a lower rate of increase in DA levels and a longer duration of action compared to cocaine for the BZT analog, JHW 007 (Tanda et al., 2009). The duration of the effects of JHW 007 on extracellular DA levels was longer than 24 h at i.p. doses of 10 and

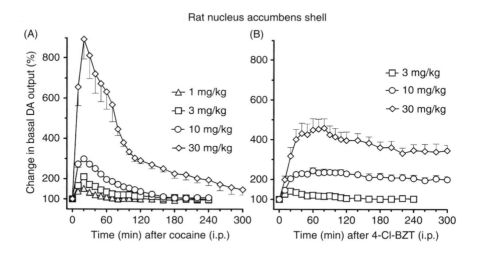

FIGURE 6   Time course of effects of systemic administration of cocaine (Panel A) or 4-Cl-BZT (Panel B) on extracellular levels of DA in dialysates from the NAC shell. Results are means (with vertical bars representing SEM) of the amount of DA in 10-min dialysate samples, expressed as percentage of basal values, uncorrected for probe recovery. Modified from Tanda et al. (2005).

17 mg/kg. The same pattern of activation of DA transmission, lower rate of increase and longer duration of action compared to cocaine, has been also confirmed for 4'-4''-Cl-BZT, MFZ-4-86, and MFZ-4-87 (G. Tanda, unpublished observations).

The antagonist effects of JHW 007 on cocaine-induced stimulation of ambulatory activity and on cocaine-maintained self-administration suggest the interaction between JHW 007 and cocaine might involve alteration of cocaine-induced stimulation of extracellular DA levels. For this reason, the effects of combinations of different doses of JHW 007 and cocaine on stimulation of DA levels in the NAc shell were examined in mice and compared with combinations of cocaine and the DAT blocker, WIN 35,428 (Tanda et al., 2009). Isobolographic analysis (Tallarida, 2000, 2007) showed that combinations of cocaine and WIN 35,428 produced an increase in extracellular DA levels that was greater than a simple additive effect. In contrast, the effects of JHW 007 in combination with cocaine were consistently less than additive. At times after injection and at several doses, JHW 007 decreased the effects of cocaine on extracellular DA levels in the NAc shell (Fig. 7). These results, showing a less than predicted level of DA stimulated by cocaine, are in agreement with the behavioral effects of combinations of JHW 007 with cocaine (Desai, Kopajtic, Koffarnus, et al., 2005; Hiranita et al., 2009) and suggest that JHW 007 may reduce the effectiveness of cocaine in increasing DA levels in brain areas related to its reinforcing actions.

F. Human Studies

BZT is the only drug in its class approved for human use, due to its efficacy in early stages of PD, an effect thought to be due to its antimuscarinic effects. There is only one report in which BZT has been evaluated as a potential cocaine-abuse medication in humans (Penetar et al., 2006) in which 16 healthy recreational cocaine users were administered BZT (1, 2 or 4 mg) or placebo 2 h before the subjects were allowed to self-administer cocaine intranasally (0.9 mg/kg). Physiological and subjective measures of cocaine effects were monitored in the ensuing 2 h. BZT alone did not change cardiovascular parameters or subjective effects evaluated by visual analog scales. In contrast, cocaine produced several subjective responses, most notably an increase in the visual analog scale ratings of "high" and "stimulated" and an increase in heart rate. Pretreatment with BZT did not modify any effect produced by cocaine. The absence of adverse subjective and physiological effects suggests that higher doses of BZT could be tested in human subjects to better evaluate its therapeutic potential as a medication for cocaine abuse.

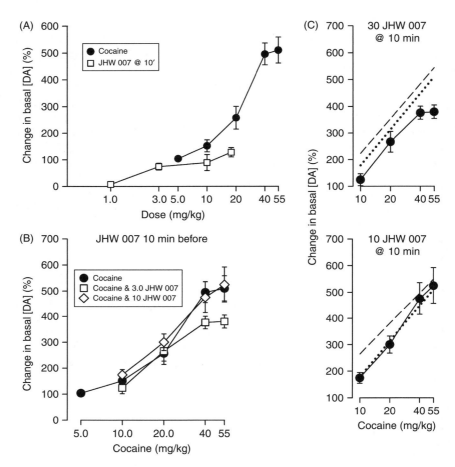

FIGURE 7 Effects of combinations of cocaine and JHW 007 at 10 min after injection on extracellular levels of DA. Panel A: dose-dependent maximal effects of JHW 007 administered 10 min before compared with those of cocaine administered immediately before assessments. Ordinates: change in extracellular DA levels as a percentage of basal values before injection. Abscissae: dose of drug in mg/kg (log scale). Panel B: observed effects of the combinations. Ordinates: change in extracellular DA levels as a percentage of basal values during the 30-min period after cocaine administration. Abscissae: dose of cocaine in mg/kg (log scale). Panel C: Observed effects compared with the predicted effects of the combinations. Ordinates and abscissae are as in Panel B. The calculated (predicted) additive dose–effect curve for cocaine in the presence of 3.0 (top) or 10.0 (bottom) mg/kg of JHW 007 is shown by the dashed straight line and the effects of cocaine alone are shown by the dotted line. The experimental (obtained) values are shown by the connected circles. Modified from Tanda et al. (2009).

III. Pharmacokinetic Studies _____

As noted before, one of the initial hypotheses to explain the lower effectiveness of BZT analogs as compared to cocaine, and the relatively slower onset of effect for behavioral and neurochemical measures, was a slower CNS penetration of BZT analogs. The pharmacokinetic parameters of selected BZT analogs have been studied and compared to those of cocaine (Othman, Newman, & Eddington, 2007; Othman, Syed, Newman, & Eddington, 2007; Raje, Cao, Newman, Gao, & Eddington, 2003; Raje et al., 2006). In these studies, performed in rats, compounds were administered i.v. to eliminate differences in rate of absorption from the injection site. The most prominent difference between the BZT analogs and cocaine was the substantially slower disappearance of the BZT analogs from plasma and brain. The longer duration of action described for several BZT analogs with regard to elevation of NAc DA levels can be explained by their lower plasma and brain elimination rates compared to cocaine.

Interestingly, all the BZT analogs studied were found at high concentrations in brain within minutes after injection with initial levels from 4 to 15 µg/g of tissue (Othman, Newman, et al., 2007; Othman, Syed, et al., 2007; Raje et al., 2003, 2006). The initial compound levels equate to 3–27 µM, depending on the particular compound and exceed the K_i values of 11–30 nM (Newman & Katz, 2009). The relatively fast appearance of the BZT analogs in brain contrasts with the slow onset of their neurochemical and behavioral effects.

IV. Studies of *In Vivo* Binding of BZT Analogs at the DAT and Relationship with Behavioral and Neurochemical Effects _____

Studies of *in vivo* displacement of [^{125}I]RTI-121 by cocaine was dose and time dependent with a maximum effect 30 min after injection (Desai, Kopajtic, Koffarnus, et al., 2005). The BZT analogs, AHN 1-055, AHN 2-005, and JHW 007, also displaced [^{125}I]RTI-121 binding in a dose- and time-related manner (Desai, Kopajtic, French, Newman, & Katz, 2005; Desai, Kopajtic, Koffarnus, et al., 2005). However, AHN 1-055 and AHN 2-005 showed a maximum displacement of [^{125}I]RTI-121 at approximately 150 min after injection, and displacement by JHW 007 did not show a plateau up to 4.5 h after its administration (Fig. 8). Further, there was no evidence of any decrease in the displacement of [^{125}I]RTI-121 by the BZT analogs over the times studied, which follows from the slow elimination rate of BZT analogs described in the pharmacokinetic studies. When the apparent association rate of JHW 007 for the

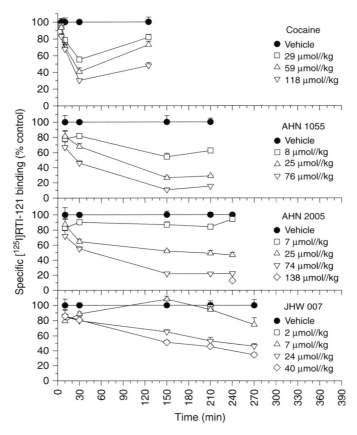

FIGURE 8   Time course of displacement of specific [^{125}I]RTI-121 accumulation in striatum of mice following IP injection of cocaine, AHN 1-055, AHN 2-005, or JHW 007. Ordinates: specific [^{125}I]RTI-121 binding as a percentage of that obtained after vehicle injection. Abscissae: time. For each point the number of replicates was from 5 to 10 or 13. Note that maximal displacement of [^{125}I]RTI-121 was obtained with cocaine at 30 min after injection and at later times with the other compounds. Modified from Desai, Kopajtic, French, et al. (2005) and Desai, Kopajtic, Koffarnus, et al. (2005).

DAT was calculated as a function of the displacement of RTI-121 (as a percentage of specific RTI-121 binding) per minute over the linear portions of the curves, the apparent association of JHW 007 was more than 10-fold lower than that for cocaine (Desai, Kopajtic, Koffarnus, et al., 2005). A lower association rate for BZT analogs might fully account for the pharmacokinetic findings that they penetrate the CNS relatively rapidly and the *in vivo* pharmacology showing a slow onset of effects relative to other stimulant drugs such as cocaine.

The relationship between DAT occupancy and behavioral effects was assessed by examining the relationship between displacement of RTI-121 and the stimulation of locomotor activity (Desai, Kopajtic, French, et al., 2005; Desai, Kopajtic, Koffarnus, et al., 2005) (Fig. 9). There was a significant relationship between DAT occupancy by cocaine and its stimulation of locomotor activity at the various doses and time points. However, one

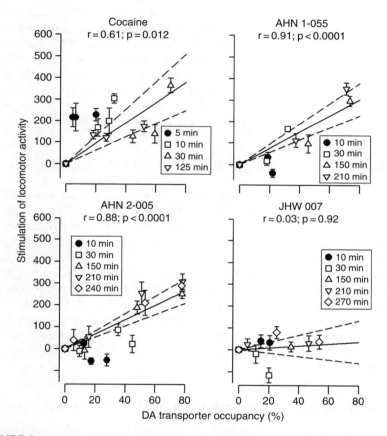

FIGURE 9 Relationship between dopamine transporter occupancy, determined in studies of displacement of [125I]RTI-121 in striatum, and locomotor stimulant effects of cocaine, AHN 1-055, AHN 2-005, or JHW 007. Ordinates: difference between mean horizontal activity counts after drug and after saline. Abscissae: percent displacement of [125I]RTI-121. For each drug, the solid line represents the linear regression of percent occupancy of the DA transporter and horizontal locomotor activity when the line is forced to intersect the origin, the point representing no occupancy and no effect. Dashed lines represent 95% confidence limits for the regression lines. Note that the locomotor stimulant effects of cocaine are less strongly related to DA transporter occupancy than are the effects of AHN 1-055, AHN 2-005, or JHW 007. Modified from Desai, Kopajtic, French, et al. (2005) and Desai, Kopajtic, Koffarnus, et al., (2005).

interesting aspect of this correlation is that a disproportionately greater effect on locomotor activity than could be predicted by DAT occupancy was obtained during the first 5 min after cocaine injection. This effect of cocaine makes the association of the two variables unexpectedly poor as compared to previous comparisons of affinity and potency in self-administration among various DAT inhibitors (Bergman, Madras, Johnson, & Spealman, 1989; Ritz, Lamb, Goldberg, & Kuhar, 1987).

Differences from these previous outcomes are likely related to the manner in which the binding studies were conducted (e.g., *in vivo* vs. *in vitro* binding methods; equilibrium vs. dynamic aspects of binding; single compound vs. comparisons of various compounds) or the behavioral endpoint (locomotor activity vs. self administration). Nonetheless, as the divergence from the regression was observed with data obtained soon after injection, association rate was suggested to play an important role in the stimulant effects of cocaine (e.g., Volkow, Fowler, & Wang, 2002).

V. Influence of Off-Target Actions of BZT Analogs

The parent compound, BZT, has affinity for M_1 muscarinic and H_1 histamine receptors. Binding studies performed on BZT analogs have shown that most of them are selective DAT inhibitors as compared to other monoamine transporters, however, many have affinity for M_1 and H_1 receptors (Katz, Libby, Kopajtic, Husbands, & Newman, 2003; Katz et al., 2001, 2004). Thus it is possible that sites other than DAT may contribute to the differences between the behavioral effects of BZT analogs as compared to cocaine. Several studies were initiated to examine these possibilities. If the off-target effects of the BZT analogs (those not mediated by the DAT) attenuate their cocaine-like activity, then the effects of cocaine should be antagonized, at least partially, by the administration of a compound selective for the off-target site.

A. Antagonist Activities at Muscarinic M_1 Receptors

The non-selective anticholinergics, atropine and scopolamine, potentiate several behavioral effects of CNS stimulants (e.g., Carlton & Didamo, 1961; Scheckel & Boff, 1964). This type of interaction was also found for cocaine and either atropine or scopolamine in drug-discrimination procedures (Katz et al., 1999). Atropine and scopolamine also potentiated the locomotor stimulant effects of cocaine (Katz et al., 1999). Thus a potentiation rather than antagonism of cocaine effects occurs with muscarinic antagonists. From these experiments it appears that the muscarinic antagonism produced by some of the BZT analogs does not account for the attenuation of their cocaine-like behavioral effects. BZT analogs have a preferential affinity for muscarinic M_1 receptors (Tanda et al., 2007) as compared to the M_2–M_5 receptors, a pattern different from of the nonselective muscarinic antagonists, atropine and scopolamine (see, e.g., Buckley, Bonner, Buckley, & Brann, 1989). The muscarinic antagonists trihexyphenidyl and telenzepine that have preferential affinity for muscarinic M_1 receptors were studied in combination with cocaine (Tanda et al., 2007). Both of these antagonists dose-dependently and selectively potentiated the effects of cocaine on DA levels in the shell as compared to the core of the NAc and the medial prefrontal cortex (the effects of telenzepine in the NAc are shown in Fig. 10). As increases in DA in the shell of the NAc have been

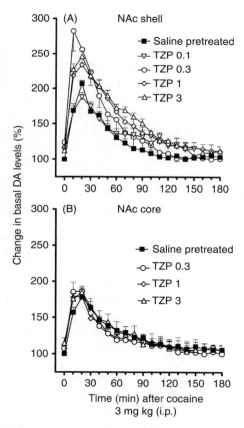

FIGURE 10 Time courses for the effects of pretreatments with increasing doses of telenzepine (TZP) on cocaine-stimulated DA extracellular levels in dialysates from the NAc shell (Panel A) and NAc core (Panel B). Cocaine (3.0 mg/kg i.p.) was administered at time=0. Each point represents means (with vertical bars representing SEM) of the amount of DA in 10-min dialysate samples, expressed as percentage of basal values, uncorrected for probe recovery. Modified from Tanda et al. (2007).

related the acute reinforcing effects of cocaine (Pontieri et al., 1995) and other drugs abused by humans (Pontieri, Tanda, Orzi, & Di Chiara, 1996; Tanda, Kopajtic, & Katz, 2008; Tanda, Pontieri, & Di Chiara, 1997), the potentiation of the effects of cocaine on DA levels selectively in the NAc shell is in disagreement with the hypothesis that M_1 antagonist effects might be responsible for attenuating the reinforcing effects of BZT analogs.

It should also be noted that the rate of increase in extracellular DA levels obtained with the combination of M_1 receptor antagonists and cocaine is higher than that obtained with cocaine alone (Fig. 10). This faster rate of increase is also at variance with that observed for BZT analogs, which is lower as compared to cocaine, indicating that the muscarinic effects of BZT analogs do not account for the different effects on dopaminergic effects. Moreover, in agreement with their ability to potentiate cocaine-induced DA levels telenzepine and trihexyphenidyl can potentiate cocaine-induced subjective effects, producing small leftward shifts in the discriminative stimulus dose effects of cocaine (Tanda & Katz, 2007). However, these M_1 antagonists differed in their ability to interact with cocaine-induced stimulation of locomotor activity, with trihexyphenidyl potentiating the stimulatory effects of cocaine and telenzepine attenuating the effects of cocaine (Tanda et al., 2007). Thus, these experiments suggest that affinity of BZT analogs for, and their actions at, muscarinic M_1 receptors are unlikely to be the cause of their reduced cocaine-like behavioral and reinforcing effects.

In agreement with these studies, BZT analogs with reduced affinity at muscarinic M_1 receptors that retain high affinity and selectivity for the DAT (Agoston, Wu, et al., 1997; Kulkarni, Grundt, Kopajtic, Katz, & Newman, 2004; Robarge et al., 2000; Zou, Kopajtic, Katz, & Newman, 2003) have been evaluated (Katz et al., 2004). Of the BZT analogs tested, AHN 1-055 had the highest affinity for the DAT and M_1 receptors, 11.8 and 11.6 nM, respectively, and it was also among the more effective of the BZT analogs in stimulating ambulatory activity to levels that approached those seen with cocaine. AHN 2-005 and JHW 007 had 29.9 and 24.6 nM affinity for DAT and 177 and 399 nM for M_1 receptors, respectively, but had substantially lower efficacy than cocaine in stimulating locomotor activity or substituting for cocaine as a discriminative stimulus (Katz et al., 2004).

A few studies have also investigated more directly the influence of antagonism at muscarinic receptors on cocaine-induced reinforcing effects. In one study (Ranaldi & Woolverton, 2002), rhesus monkeys were trained to self-administer cocaine under fixed- and progressive-ratio schedules. In most cases, combinations of cocaine and scopolamine maintained less self-administration than did cocaine alone. The authors concluded that anticholinergic actions contribute to the diminished self-administration of BZT analogs relative to cocaine and suggested that the mechanism involves either antagonism of the reinforcing effect of cocaine or punishment of the cocaine self-administration behavior by the anticholinergic activity.

Wilson and Schuster (1973) found atropine to *increase* rates of responding maintained by cocaine, a result that is not consistent with punishment by the anticholinergic agent, as punishment would involve a *decrease* in response rate. Further the atropine-induced increases in response rates were similar to the effect of lowering the cocaine dose. As atropine was administered before the experimental session and independently of responding, it was not functioning as a punishing stimulus. All of these considerations imply a pharmacologically noncompetitive antagonism (if any) of the reinforcing effects of cocaine by anticholinergic effects. Li et al. (2005) evaluated the effects of atropine in a place conditioning procedure. Atropine alone produced a trend toward conditioned place avoidance, and in combination with cocaine there was also a trend toward decreases in effectiveness of cocaine. In contrast to the implications of the Wilson and Schuster (1973) results described earlier, these trends suggest a behavioral rather than pharmacological basis to the interaction of anticholinergics with the reinforcing effects of cocaine and further suggest a punishing effect of anticholinergic agents. However, due to the inconsistencies between the Li et al. and Wilson and Schuster findings, definitive conclusions regarding the basis for the interaction of anticholinergics with cocaine for reinforcement are not possible at this time.

The hypothesis that the anticholinergic effects of the BZT analogs punish behavior relates specifically to self-administration procedures using the BZT analogs. In contrast, non-competitive pharmacological interactions between cocaine-like and antimuscarinic effects could operate more broadly across the range of behavioral end points. As noted earlier, there is a range of pharmacological effects that differ between the BZT analogs and cocaine-like DAT inhibitors, including drug discrimination, locomotor activity (Katz et al., 1999), and c-Fos expression (Velazquez-Sanchez et al., 2009). The preponderance of data suggests that antimuscarinic effects enhance rather than antagonize many of the behavioral effects of cocaine-like stimulants. However, whether antimuscarinic actions enhance or attenuate any cocaine-like effects of individual BZT analogs will need to be empirically determined and may depend on the behavioral end point and the spectrum of effects of the doses used of the particular BZT analog.

B. Antagonist Activities at Histamine Receptors

Antagonists of histamine receptors have been tested in drug-discrimination studies alone and in combination with various behaviorally effective doses of cocaine in rats trained to discriminate cocaine from saline injections (Campbell, Kopajtic, Newman, & Katz, 2005). Results from these experiments show that promethazine and triprolidine, selective H_1 antagonists, did not modify the subjective effects of cocaine at any dose tested, while other H_1 antagonists (e.g., chlorpheniramine and mepyramine) potentiated the subjective effects of cocaine, producing a leftward shift of the cocaine dose–effect curve. The effects of these latter two agents were likely mediated by their activity as DAT inhibitors (Bergman & Spealman, 1986; Tanda et al., 2008; Tuomisto & Tuomisto, 1980). Similarly, the ratios of H_1 to DAT affinities for BZT analogs were not significantly related to and did not predict outcome for their locomotor stimulant effects (Campbell et al., 2005).

As noted, certain histamine receptor antagonists also have actions that are mediated by the DAT, and some of these drugs have psychostimulant-like reinforcing effects in animal models of abuse (Bergman, 1990; Bergman & Spealman, 1986; Wang & Woolverton, 2007, 2009). In microdialysis studies, i.v. administration of diphenhydramine, and the enantiomers of chlorpheniramine, dose-dependently and selectively elevated DA levels in the shell as compared to the core of the NAc (Tanda et al., 2008), as it has been shown for virtually all drugs abused by humans (Pontieri et al., 1995, 1996; Tanda, Pontieri, et al., 1997). However, triprolidine, a selective H_1 antagonist, did not modify extracellular DA levels of dopamine. Together these results show that affinity for both H_1 and DAT in diphenhydramine and chlorpheniramine does not prevent certain cocaine-like behavioral effects. As this applies to BZT analogs, it suggests that their H_1 antagonist actions are probably not responsible for their reduced cocaine-like behavioral effects in animal models of drug abuse.

C. Involvement of Other Receptors/Sites

Most BZT analogs have a high degree of selectivity for the DAT versus SERT and NET while cocaine has similar affinity for DAT and SERT with lower affinity for the NET (Katz et al., 1999, 2004). Thus, the lack of activity of BZT analogs on other monoamine transporters would suggest that agents lacking activity at these sites will be less effective than cocaine in producing effects related to drug abuse. However, several studies have indicated that the self-administration of a variety of monoamine transport inhibitors is related to the affinity of compounds for the DAT and not affinity at NET or SERT (Bergman et al., 1989; Ritz et al., 1987). In addition, compounds relatively selective for the DAT retain reinforcing effects (e.g., Howell, Czoty, Kuhar, & Carrol, 2000; Roberts et al., 1999) while selective SERT or NET inhibitors do not show a cocaine-like behavioral profile (e.g., Hiranita et al., 2009; Howell & Byrd, 1995; Woolverton, 1987). Collectively these studies indicate that lack of effects at the SERT and NET does explain the reduced cocaine-like behavioral effects of BZT analogs.

Among other targets that might be involved in the reduced cocaine-like behavioral effects are the sigma receptors. Antagonists of sigma receptors may modulate various effects of cocaine, including stimulation of locomotor activity and reinforcing effects in place of conditioning procedures (see Matsumoto, Liu, Lerner, Howard, & Brackett, 2003, for a review). However, sigma antagonists failed to reduce the self-administration of cocaine (Martin-Fardon, Maurice, Aujla, Bowen, & Weiss, 2007).

Cannabinoid CB_1 receptors have also been implicated in the neurobiology of cocaine addiction (Arnold, 2005; Tanda, 2007) and Navarro, Howard, Pollard, & Carroll (2009) have suggested that positive allosteric modulators of the cannabinoid CB_1 receptor can contribute to cocaine-antagonist effects of atypical DAT inhibitors. One compound, RTI-371, is a cocaine analog that binds to the DAT but blocks the locomotor stimulation produced by cocaine (Navarro et al., 2009). Screening of RTI-371 at various sites found it to be a positive allosteric modulator of CB_1 receptors. RTI-371 and several other DAT-selective inhibitors with atypical actions on locomotor activity, including the BZT analog JHW 007, increased the efficacy of the CB_1 agonist, CP 55940 in a calcium mobilization assay. From those results, Navarro et al. suggested that enhanced endocannabinoid neurotransmission may contribute to the cocaine-antagonist effects observed with these atypical DAT inhibitors. Consistent with this hypothesis are findings that cannabinoid agonists, including endogenous cannabinoids, reduce spontaneous ambulatory activity through their actions at central cannabinoid CB_1 receptors (Ameri, 1999). Activation of D_2 receptors by increased DA levels stimulated by atypical blockers could enhance endogenous cannabinoid levels (Giuffrida et al., 1999), and the positive allosteric modulation of CB_1 receptors by atypical DAT inhibitors might potentiate cannabinoid neurotransmission, that might in turn counteract the stimulatory effects of these atypical DAT blockers, a hypothesis that clearly warrants further study.

VI. Studies of DAT Structure as Related to Its Function ———

Initial structure–activity studies suggested that BZT and its BZT analogs bind to the DAT differently from cocaine and it congeners (Newman et al., 1995) and subsequent site-directed mutagenesis studies of the DAT supported those conclusions. Several studies have demonstrated differences in the effects of mutating the DAT on the binding of BZT or its analogs compared to analogs of cocaine (Chen, Zhen, & Reith, 2004). For example, mutating aspartate to glutamate at position 79 in the DAT increased the potency of BZT and its analogs in inhibiting DA uptake, whereas cocaine and various classical DAT were unaffected by the mutation (Ukairo et al., 2005). Additionally, the affinity of BZT and GBR 12909 was affected by the concentration of sodium differently from cocaine in several DAT mutants (Chen & Reith, 2004), again suggesting differences from cocaine in how the BZT analogs bind to the DAT. Photoaffinity labeling studies also support the concept of different binding domains for cocaine and its analogs compared to the BZT analogs

(Agoston et al., 1997; Parnas et al., 2008; Vaughan, Agoston, Lever, & Newman, 1999; Vaughan et al., 2007; Zou et al., 2001).

Other evidence supports the notion that the interaction of BZT with the DAT is different from that of other DAT inhibitors, exemplified by cocaine. Reith, Berfield, Wang, Ferrer, and Javitch (2001) compared, among other drugs, the abilities of cocaine and BZT to affect the reaction of a methanethiosulfonate (MTS) reagent to various cysteine residues within the human DAT. A previous study (Ferrer & Javitch, 1998) showed that reaction of MTS reagents with Cys-90 (located within an extracellular loop) increased [^{3}H]WIN 35,428 binding, and cocaine enhanced the reaction of Cys-90 with MTS reagents, resulting in even greater augmentation of [^{3}H] WIN 35,428 binding. In contrast, cocaine decreased the reaction of MTS reagents with Cys-135 and Cys-342 (located within cytoplasmic loops). In contrast to cocaine, BZT had no effect on the reaction of Cys-90 with an MTS reagent, and the decrease in the reaction of Cys-135 with an MTS reagent produced by cocaine was not obtained with BZT (Reith et al., 2001). These results support the idea that different DATs bind to the DAT in different ways and suggest that there may be differences in the conformational changes in the transporter produced by this binding.

Loland et al. (2008) compared the effects of DAT inhibitors on the accessibility of [2-(trimethylammonium)ethyl]-methanethiosulfonate (MTSET) to a cysteine residue inserted into the human DAT (I159C) expressed in COS-7 cells. This cysteine is thought to be inaccessible when the DAT assumes an inwardly facing conformation, but accessible when the DAT assumes an outward conformation. Cocaine potentiated the DAT inhibition produced by MTSET alone, consistent with the induction of a DAT conformation open to the extracellular environment, and thus MTSET. In contrast, BZT analogs protected against the DAT inhibition produced by MTSET, suggesting that these compounds stabilize the DAT in a closed conformation to which the MTSET had limited access.

A previous study suggested that Tyr335 in the DAT is critical for regulating the open/closed conformational equilibrium of the DAT (Loland, Norregaard, Litman, & Gether, 2002). A Y335A DAT mutation impaired DA transport and decreased the potency of cocaine as an inhibitor of DA uptake. Cocaine and several cocaine analogs were approximately 100-fold less potent as DAT inhibitors in Y335A mutants compared to WT DAT (Loland et al., 2008). In contrast, BZT analogs were only 7-fold to 58-fold less potent against the Y335A mutant (Loland et al., 2008). Further, there was a good relationship between the decrease in potencies of the BZT analogs due to the DAT mutation and their effectiveness in stimulating locomotor activity and in substituting for cocaine in rats trained to discriminate cocaine injections from those of saline (Fig. 11). One BZT analog, MFZ 2-71, was of particular interest because it showed a Y335A mutation-dependent loss in DAT inhibitory potency that approached that seen with

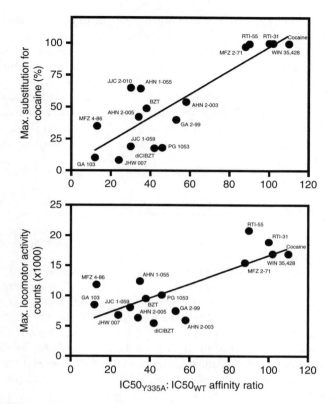

FIGURE 11   The relationship between dopamine uptake potency ratios of various dopamine transporter ligands in COS-7 cells transfected with the Y335A mutant and WT DAT (affinity ratio) and behavioral activity. Top panel: correlation of affinity ratio and the degree to which the drugs substituted for cocaine in rats trained to discriminate cocaine from vehicle injections. The correlation coefficient (r^2) was 0.74 ($p<0.0001$). Bottom panel: correlation of affinity ratio and the maximal locomotor activity stimulation in mice. The correlation coefficient (r^2) was 0.59 ($p<0.0005$). The affinity ratio was calculated from the IC_{50} values for inhibition of [^{3}H] dopamine uptake by the compound in COS-7 cells transiently expressing either DAT WT or Y335A. Modified from Loland et al. (2008).

cocaine. In addition, MFZ 2-71 had behavioral effects like those of cocaine; it not only produced a cocaine-like stimulation of locomotor activity, but it also substituted fully in subjects trained to discriminate cocaine from saline injections. Thus the BZT analog MFZ 2-71 shows promise for differentiating structural features of the BZT structure that promote conformational changes of the DAT which may lead to effects unlike those of cocaine and may indeed contribute to cocaine-antagonist actions.

Modeling of the DAT complexed with DA and DAT inhibitors, using as a basis the structure of the bacterial leucine transporter, showed that the binding of DAT inhibitors and substrates (including DA and amphe-tamine derivatives) overlapped, indicative of a competitive inhibition (Beuming et al., 2008). In contrast to the binding of cocaine, the binding of BZT analogs preserved the hydrogen bond between Asp79 and Tyr156; that bond has been proposed to function as a gate regulating translocation of substrate (Loland, Granas, Javitch, & Gether, 2004). The preservation of the Asp79-Tyr156 bond with the binding of a BZT analog is consistent with the findings of Loland et al. (2008) suggesting different conformational changes induced in the DAT by the binding of cocaine and BZT analogs.

VII. Conclusion

During the past two decades many advances have been made in the understanding of the behavioral and reinforcing effects of cocaine, as well as the neurobiology underlying the effects that lead to its abuse and to addic-tion. Though a long road remains before a medical treatment against cocaine abuse is available, many new pharmacological tools have been discovered, and among them are the BZT analogs. These compounds have provided new insights into the molecular and behavioral actions of cocaine and the diversity of effects produced by DAT inhibitors. Several BZT analogs have been used in studies of the molecular structure of the DAT to elucidate the binding domains of DAT inhibitors, and how differences in the interaction of these compounds with DAT contribute to their pharmacolo-gical differences. In preclinical studies, different BZT analogs can attenuate or block the behavioral, neurochemical, and/or reinforcing actions of cocaine, and may represent the starting point to develop new medications for the treatment of cocaine addiction.

Acknowledgements

This work was supported by the Intramural Research Program of the Department of Health and Human Services, National Institute on Drug Abuse, National Institutes of Health. We would like to thank the many post-doctoral fellows that helped with the work described from our laboratories, and especially: T. Kopajtic, J. Cao, B. Campbell, D. French-Evans, and P. Ballerstadt.

Conflict of Interest: J.L.K. and A.H.N. are inventors, and the NIH the owner of patents on some of the compounds described in this chapter. The rights to commercial development of the compounds in two of these patents have been licensed to Phase 2 Discovery, Inc. of Cincinnati, Ohio a biotech focused on developing compounds for the treatment of brain disorders and Shire, a global specialty biopharmaceutical company that develops and markets drugs in the CNS area.

References

Agoston, G. E., Vaughan, R., Lever, J. R., Izenwasser, S., Terry, P. D., & Newman, A. H. (1997). A novel photoaffinity label for the dopamine transporter based on substituted 3 alpha-[bis(4′-fluorophenyl)methoxy]tropane. *Bioorganic & Medicinal Chemistry Letters, 7*(23), 3027–3032.

Agoston, G. E., Wu, J. H., Izenwasser, S., George, C., Katz, J., Kline, R. H., et al. (1997). Novel N-substituted 3 alpha-[bis(4′-fluorophenyl)methoxy]tropane analogues: Selective ligands for the dopamine transporter. *Journal of Medicinal Chemistry, 40*(26), 4329–4339.

Ameri, A. (1999). The effects of cannabinoids on the brain. *Progress in Neurobiology, 58*(4), 315–348.

Arnold, J. C. (2005). The role of endocannabinoid transmission in cocaine addiction. *Pharmacology, Biochemistry and Behavior, 81*(2), 396–406.

Baker, L. E., Riddle, E. E., Saunders, R. B., & Appel, J. B. (1993). The role of monoamine uptake in the discriminative stimulus effects of cocaine and related compounds. *Behavioural Pharmacology, 4*(1), 69–79.

Balster, R. L., & Schuster, C. R. (1973). Fixed-interval schedule of cocaine reinforcement: Effect of dose and infusion duration. *Journal of the Experimental Analysis of Behavior, 20*(1), 119–129.

Beardsley, P. M., & Balster, R. L. (1993). The effects of delay of reinforcement and dose on the self-administration of cocaine and procaine in rhesus monkeys. *Drug and Alcohol Dependence, 34*(1), 37–43.

Bergman, J. (1990). Psychomotor stimulant effects of the stereoisomers of chlorpheniramine. *Psychopharmacology (Berl), 100*(1), 132–134.

Bergman, J., Madras, B. K., Johnson, S. E., & Spealman, R. D. (1989). Effects of cocaine and related drugs in nonhuman primates. III. Self-administration by squirrel monkeys. *Journal of Pharmacology and Experimental Therapeutics, 251*(1), 150–155.

Bergman, J., & Spealman, R. D. (1986). Some behavioral effects of histamine H1 antagonists in squirrel monkeys. *Journal of Pharmacology and Experimental Therapeutics, 239*(1), 104–110.

Beuming, T., Kniazeff, J., Bergmann, M. L., Shi, L., Gracia, L., Raniszewska, K., et al. (2008). The binding sites for cocaine and dopamine in the dopamine transporter overlap. *Nature Neuroscience, 11*(7), 780–789.

Buckley, N. J., Bonner, T. I., Buckley, C. M., & Brann, M. R. (1989). Antagonist binding properties of five cloned muscarinic receptors expressed in CHO-K1 cells. *Molecular Pharmacology, 35*(4), 469–476.

Callahan, P. M., De La Garza, R., 2nd, & Cunningham, K. A. (1997). Mediation of the discriminative stimulus properties of cocaine by mesocorticolimbic dopamine systems. *Pharmacology, Biochemistry and Behavior, 57*(3), 601–607.

Campbell, V. C., Kopajtic, T. A., Newman, A. H., & Katz, J. L. (2005). Assessment of the influence of histaminergic actions on cocaine-like effects of 3alpha-diphenylmethoxytropane analogs. *Journal of Pharmacology and Experimental Therapeutics, 315*(2), 631–640.

Carlton, P. L., & Didamo, P. (1961). Augmentation of the behavioral effects of amphetamine by atropine. *Journal of Pharmacology and Experimental Therapeutics, 132*, 91–96.

Carroll, F. I., Howell, L. L., & Kuhar, M. J. (1999). Pharmacotherapies for treatment of cocaine abuse: Preclinical aspects. *Journal of Medicinal Chemistry, 42*(15), 2721–2736.

Catterall, W. A., & Mackie, K. (2006). Local anesthetics. In L. Brunton (Ed.), *Goodman & Gilman's 11th edition, The pharmacological basis of therapeutics* (pp. 369–386). New York: McGraw Hill Medical Publishing Edition Division.

Chaudhuri, K. R., & Schapira, A. H. (2009). Non-motor symptoms of Parkinson's disease: Dopaminergic pathophysiology and treatment. *Lancet Neurology, 8*(5), 464–474.

Chen, N., & Reith, M. E. (2004). Interaction between dopamine and its transporter: Role of intracellular sodium ions and membrane potential. *Journal of Neurochemistry, 89*(3), 750–765.

Chen, N., Zhen, J., & Reith, M. E. (2004). Mutation of Trp84 and Asp313 of the dopamine transporter reveals similar mode of binding interaction for GBR12909 and benztropine as opposed to cocaine. *Journal of Neurochemistry, 89*(4), 853–864.

Colpaert, F. C., Niemegeers, C. J., & Janssen, P. A. (1979). Discriminative stimulus properties of cocaine: Neuropharmacological characteristics as derived from stimulus generalization experiments. *Pharmacology, Biochemistry and Behavior, 10*(4), 535–546.

Desai, R. I., Kopajtic, T. A., French, D., Newman, A. H., & Katz, J. L. (2005). Relationship between in vivo occupancy at the dopamine transporter and behavioral effects of cocaine, GBR 12909 [1-{2-[bis-(4-fluorophenyl)methoxy]ethyl}-4-(3-phenylpropyl)piperazine], and benztropine analogs. *Journal of Pharmacology and Experimental Therapeutics, 315*(1), 397–404.

Desai, R. I., Kopajtic, T. A., Koffarnus, M., Newman, A. H., & Katz, J. L. (2005). Identification of a dopamine transporter ligand that blocks the stimulant effects of cocaine. *Journal of Neuroscience, 25*(8), 1889–1893.

Dworkin, S. I., & Smith, J. E. (1988). Neurobehavioral pharmacology of cocaine. *NIDA Research Monograph, 88*, 185–198.

Ferragud, A., Velázquez-Sánchez, C., Hernández-Rabaza, V., Nácher, A., Merino, V., Cardá, M., et al. (2009). A dopamine transport inhibitor with markedly low abuse liability suppresses cocaine self-administration in the rat. *Psychopharmacology*, DOI 10.1007/s00213-009-1653-x.

Ferrer, J. V., & Javitch, J. A. (1998). Cocaine alters the accessibility of endogenous cysteines in putative extracellular and intracellular loops of the human dopamine transporter. *Proceedings of the National Academy of Sciences of the United States of America, 95*(16), 9238–9243.

Giuffrida, A., Parsons, L. H., Kerr, T. M., Rodriguez de Fonseca, F., Navarro, M., & Piomelli, D. (1999). Dopamine activation of endogenous cannabinoid signaling in dorsal striatum. *Nature Neuroscience, 2*(4), 358–363.

Grace, R. F. (1997). Benztropine abuse and overdose—case report and review. *Adverse Drug Reactions and Toxicological Reviews, 16*(2), 103–112.

Greco, P. G., & Garris, P. A. (2003). In vivo interaction of cocaine with the dopamine transporter as measured by voltammetry. *European Journal of Pharmacology, 479*(1–3), 117–125.

Hahn, M. K., & Blakely, R. D. (2007). The functional impact of SLC6 transporter genetic variation. *Annual Review of Pharmacology and Toxicology, 47*, 401–441.

Hiranita, T., Soto, P. L., Newman, A. H., & Katz, J. L. (2009). Assessment of reinforcing effects of benztropine analogs and their effects on cocaine self-administration in rats: Comparisons with monoamine uptake inhibitors. *Journal of Pharmacology and Experimental Therapeutics, 329*(2), 677–686.

Hodos, W. (1961). Progressive ratio as a measure of reward strength. *Science, 134*, 943–944.

Holtzman, S. G. (1990). Discriminative stimulus effects of drugs: Relationship to potential for abuse. *Modern methods in pharmacology, testing and evaluation of drugs of abuse (Vol. 6, pp. 193–210). Wilmington, DE: Wiley Liss Inc.

Howell, L. L., & Byrd, L. D. (1995). Serotonergic modulation of the behavioral effects of cocaine in the squirrel monkey. *Journal of Pharmacology and Experimental Therapeutics, 275*(3), 1551–1559.

Howell, L. L., Czoty, P. W., Kuhar, M. J., & Carrol, F. I. (2000). Comparative behavioral pharmacology of cocaine and the selective dopamine uptake inhibitor RTI-113 in the squirrel monkey. *Journal of Pharmacology and Experimental Therapeutics, 292*(2), 521–529.

Ikemoto, S. (2002). Ventral striatal anatomy of locomotor activity induced by cocaine, D-amphetamine, dopamine and D1/D2 agonists. *Neuroscience, 113*(4), 939–955.

Iversen, L. L., Iversen, S. D., Bloom, F. E., & Roth, R. H. (2008). Catecholamines. In *Introduction to neuropsychopharmacology* (pp. 150–213). New York: Oxford University Press.

Izenwasser, S., Terry, P., Heller, B., Witkin, J. M., & Katz, J. L. (1994). Differential relationships among dopamine transporter affinities and stimulant potencies of various uptake inhibitors. *European Journal of Pharmacology, 263*(3), 277–283.

Kalivas, P. W. (2007). Neurobiology of cocaine addiction: Implications for new pharmacotherapy. *American Journal on Addictions, 16*(2), 71–78.

Katz, J. L. (1989). Drugs as reinforcers: Pharmacological and behavioral factors. In J. M. Liebman & S. J. Cooper (Eds.), *The neurobiological basis of reward* (pp. 164–213). Oxford: Clarendon Press.

Katz, J. L., Agoston, G. E., Alling, K. L., Kline, R. H., Forster, M. J., Woolverton, W. L., et al. (2001). Dopamine transporter binding without cocaine-like behavioral effects: Synthesis and evaluation of benztropine analogs alone and in combination with cocaine in rodents. *Psychopharmacology (Berl), 154*(4), 362–374.

Katz, J. L., Izenwasser, S., Kline, R. H., Allen, A. C., & Newman, A. H. (1999). Novel 3alpha-diphenylmethoxytropane analogs: Selective dopamine uptake inhibitors with behavioral effects distinct from those of cocaine. *Journal of Pharmacology and Experimental Therapeutics, 288*(1), 302–315.

Katz, J. L., Izenwasser, S., & Terry, P. (2000). Relationships among dopamine transporter affinities and cocaine-like discriminative-stimulus effects. *Psychopharmacology (Berl), 148* (1), 90–98.

Katz, J. L., Kopajtic, T. A., Agoston, G. E., & Newman, A. H. (2004). Effects of N-substituted analogs of benztropine: Diminished cocaine-like effects in dopamine transporter ligands. *Journal of Pharmacology and Experimental Therapeutics, 309*(2), 650–660.

Katz, J. L., Libby, T. A., Kopajtic, T., Husbands, S. M., & Newman, A. H. (2003). Behavioral effects of rimcazole analogues alone and in combination with cocaine. *European Journal of Pharmacology, 468*(2), 109–119.

Kharkar, P. S., Dutta, A. K., & Reith, M. E. A. (2008). Structure-activity relationship study of piperidine derivatives for dopamine transporters. In M. L. Trudell & S. Izenwasser (Eds.), *Dopamine transporters, chemistry, biology, and pharmacology* (pp. 233–264). New York: John Wiley & Sons.

Kleven, M. S., Anthony, E. W., & Woolverton, W. L. (1990). Pharmacological characterization of the discriminative stimulus effects of cocaine in rhesus monkeys. *Journal of Pharmacology and Experimental Therapeutics, 254*(1), 312–317.

Kuczenski, R., & Segal, D. S. (1992). Differential effects of amphetamine and dopamine uptake blockers (cocaine, nomifensine) on caudate and accumbens dialysate dopamine and 3-methoxytyramine. *Journal of Pharmacology and Experimental Therapeutics, 262*(3), 1085–1094.

Kuhar, M. J., Ritz, M. C., & Boja, J. W. (1991). The dopamine hypothesis of the reinforcing properties of cocaine. *Trends in Neurosciences, 14*(7), 299–302.

Kulkarni, S. S., Grundt, P., Kopajtic, T., Katz, J. L., & Newman, A. H. (2004). Structure-activity relationships at monoamine transporters for a series of N-substituted 3alpha-(bis [4-fluorophenyl]methoxy)tropanes: Comparative molecular field analysis, synthesis, and pharmacological evaluation. *Journal of Medicinal Chemistry, 47*(13), 3388–3398.

Lees, A. J., Hardy, J., & Revesz, T. (2009). Parkinson's disease. *Lancet, 373*(9680), 2055–2066.

Li, S. M., Newman, A. H., & Katz, J. L. (2005). Place conditioning and locomotor effects of N-substituted, 4′,4″-difluorobenztropine analogs in rats. *Journal of Pharmacology and Experimental Therapeutics, 313*(3), 1223–1230.

Loland, C. J., Desai, R. I., Zou, M. F., Cao, J., Grundt, P., Gerstbrein, K., et al. (2008). Relationship between conformational changes in the dopamine transporter and cocaine-like subjective effects of uptake inhibitors. *Molecular Pharmacology, 73*(3), 813–823.

Loland, C. J., Granas, C., Javitch, J. A., & Gether, U. (2004). Identification of intracellular residues in the dopamine transporter critical for regulation of transporter conformation and cocaine binding. *Journal of Biological Chemistry, 279*(5), 3228–3238.

Loland, C. J., Norregaard, L., Litman, T., & Gether, U. (2002). Generation of an activating Zn(2+) switch in the dopamine transporter: Mutation of an intracellular tyrosine constitutively alters the conformational equilibrium of the transport cycle. *Proceedings of the National Academy of Sciences of the United States of America, 99*(3), 1683–1688.

Martin-Fardon, R., Maurice, T., Aujla, H., Bowen, W. D., & Weiss, F. (2007). Differential effects of signa1 receptor blockade on self-administration and conditioned reinstatement motivated by cocaine vs natural reward. *Neuropsychopharmacology, 32*(9), 1967–1973.

Matsumoto, R. R., Liu, Y., Lerner, M., Howard, E. W., & Brackett, D. J. (2003). Sigma receptors: Potential medications development target for anti-cocaine agents. *European Journal of Pharmacology, 469*(1–3), 1–12.

Mattick, R. P., Breen, C., Kimber, J., & Davoli, M. (2009). Methadone maintenance therapy versus no opioid replacement therapy for opioid dependence. *Cochrane Database of Systematic Reviews*, (3), CD002209.

Meisenzahl, E. M., Schmitt, G. J., Scheuerecker, J., & Moller, H. J. (2007). The role of dopamine for the pathophysiology of schizophrenia. *International Review of Psychiatry, 19*(4), 337–345.

Meltzer, P. C. (2008). Non-nitrogen containing dopamine transporter-uptake inhibitors. In M. L. Trudell & S. Izenwasser (Eds.), *Dopamine transporters, chemistry, biology, and pharmacology* (pp. 265–304). New York: John Wiley & Sons.

Navarro, H. A., Howard, J. L., Pollard, G. T., & Carroll, F. I. (2009). Positive allosteric modulation of the human cannabinoid (CB) receptor by RTI-371, a selective inhibitor of the dopamine transporter. *British Journal of Pharmacology, 156*(7), 1178–1184.

Nestler, E. J. (2005). The neurobiology of cocaine addiction. *Science & Practice Perspectives, 3*(1), 4–10.

Newman, A. H., Allen, A. C., Izenwasser, S., & Katz, J. L. (1994). Novel 3 alpha-(diphenyl-methoxy)tropane analogs: Potent dopamine uptake inhibitors without cocaine-like behavioral profiles. *Journal of Medicinal Chemistry, 37*(15), 2258–2261.

Newman, A. H., & Katz, J. L. (2008). The benztropines: Atypical dopamine-uptake inhibitors that provide clues about cocaine's mechanism at the dopamine transporter. In M. L. Trudell & S. Izenwasser (Eds.), *Dopamine transporters, chemistry, biology, and pharmacology* (pp. 171–210). New York: John Wiley & Sons.

Newman, A. H., & Katz, J. L. (2009). Atypical dopamine uptake inhibitors that provide clues about cocaine's mechanism at the dopamine transporter. *Topics in Medicinal Chemistry, 4*, 95–129.

Newman, A. H., Kline, R. H., Allen, A. C., Izenwasser, S., George, C., & Katz, J. L. (1995). Novel 4′-substituted and 4′,4″-disubstituted 3 alpha-(diphenylmethoxy)tropane analogs as potent and selective dopamine uptake inhibitors. *Journal of Medicinal Chemistry, 38*(20), 3933–3940.

Newman, A. H., & Kulkarni, S. (2002). Probes for the dopamine transporter: New leads toward a cocaine-abuse therapeutic—a focus on analogues of benztropine and rimcazole. *Medicinal Research Reviews, 22*(5), 429–464.

Othman, A. A., Newman, A. H., & Eddington, N. D. (2007). Applicability of the dopamine and rate hypotheses in explaining the differences in behavioral pharmacology of the chloro-benztropine analogs: Studies conducted using intracerebral microdialysis and population pharmacodynamic modeling. *Journal of Pharmacology and Experimental Therapeutics, 322*(2), 760–769.

Othman, A. A., Syed, S. A., Newman, A. H., & Eddington, N. D. (2007). Transport, metabolism, and in vivo population pharmacokinetics of the chloro benztropine analogs, a class of compounds extensively evaluated in animal models of drug abuse. *Journal of Pharmacology and Experimental Therapeutics, 320*(1), 344–353.

Parnas, M. L., Gaffaney, J. D., Zou, M. F., Lever, J. R., Newman, A. H., & Vaughan, R. A. (2008). Labeling of dopamine transporter transmembrane domain 1 with the tropane ligand N-[4-(4-azido-3-[125I]iodophenyl)butyl]-2beta-carbomethoxy-3beta-(4-chloro phenyl)tropane implicates proximity of cocaine and substrate active sites. *Molecular Pharmacology, 73*(4), 1141–1150.

Penetar, D. M., Looby, A. R., Su, Z., Lundahl, L. H., Eros-Sarnyai, M., McNeil, J. F., et al. (2006). Benztropine pretreatment does not affect responses to acute cocaine administration in human volunteers. *Human Psychopharmacology, 21*(8), 549–559.

Pontieri, F. E., Tanda, G., & Di Chiara, G. (1995). Intravenous cocaine, morphine, and amphetamine preferentially increase extracellular dopamine in the "shell" as compared with the "core" of the rat nucleus accumbens. *Proceedings of the National Academy of Sciences of the United States of America*, 92(26), 12304–12308.

Pontieri, F. E., Tanda, G., Orzi, F., & Di Chiara, G. (1996). Effects of nicotine on the nucleus accumbens and similarity to those of addictive drugs. *Nature*, 382(6588), 255–257.

Prisinzano, T. E., & Rice, K. C. (2008). Structure-activity relationshipof GBR 12909 ligands. In M. L. Trudell & S. Izenwasser (Eds.), *Dopamine transporters, chemistry, biology, and pharmacology* (pp. 211–232). New York: John Wiley & Sons.

Raje, S., Cao, J., Newman, A. H., Gao, H., & Eddington, N. D. (2003). Evaluation of the blood-brain barrier transport, population pharmacokinetics, and brain distribution of benztropine analogs and cocaine using in vitro and in vivo techniques. *Journal of Pharmacology and Experimental Therapeutics*, 307(2), 801–808.

Raje, S., Cornish, J., Newman, A. H., Cao, J., Katz, J. L., & Eddington, N. D. (2006). Investigation of the potential pharmacokinetic and pharmaco-dynamic drug interaction between AHN 1–055, a potent benztropine analog used for cocaine abuse, and cocaine after dosing in rats using intracerebral microdialysis. *Biopharmaceutics & Drug Disposition*, 27(5), 229–240.

Ranaldi, R., & Woolverton, W. L. (2002). Self-administration of cocaine: Scopolamine combinations by rhesus monkeys. *Psychopharmacology (Berl)*, 161(4), 442–448.

Reith, M. E., Berfield, J. L., Wang, L. C., Ferrer, J. V., & Javitch, J. A. (2001). The uptake inhibitors cocaine and benztropine differentially alter the conformation of the human dopamine transporter. *Journal of Biological Chemistry*, 276(31), 29012–29018.

Ritz, M. C., Boja, J. W., George, F. R., & Kuhar, M. J. (1989). Cocaine binding sites related to drug self-administration. *NIDA Research Monograph*, 95, 239–246.

Ritz, M. C., Lamb, R. J., Goldberg, S. R., & Kuhar, M. J. (1987). Cocaine receptors on dopamine transporters are related to self-administration of cocaine. *Science*, 237(4819), 1219–1223.

Robarge, M. J., Agoston, G. E., Izenwasser, S., Kopajtic, T., George, C., Katz, J. L., et al. (2000). Highly selective chiral N-substituted 3alpha-[bis(4'-fluorophenyl)methoxy]tropane analogues for the dopamine transporter: Synthesis and comparative molecular field analysis. *Journal of Medicinal Chemistry*, 43(6), 1085–1093.

Roberts, D. C., Phelan, R., Hodges, L. M., Hodges, M. M., Bennett, B., Childers, S., et al. (1999). Self-administration of cocaine analogs by rats. *Psychopharmacology (Berl)*, 144 (4), 389–397.

Rothman, R. B., Baumann, M. H., Prisinzano, T. E., & Newman, A. H. (2008). Dopamine transport inhibitors based on GBR12909 and benztropine as potential medications to treat cocaine addiction. *Biochemical Pharmacology*, 75(1), 2–16.

Runyon, S. P., & Carroll, F. I. (2008). Tropane-based dopamine transporter-uptake inhibitors. In M. L. Trudell & S. Izenwasser (Eds.), *Dopamine transporters, chemistry, biology, and pharmacology* (pp. 125–170). New York: John Wiley & Sons.

Scheckel, C. L., & Boff, E. (1964). Behavioral effects of interacting imipramine and other drugs with *d*-amphetamine, cocaine, and tetrabenazine. *Psychopharmacologia*, 5, 198–208.

Skinner, B. F. (1938). *The behavior of organisms: An experimental analysis*. New York, London: D. Appleton-Century Company, Incorporated.

Stead, L. F., Perera, R., Bullen, C., Mant, D., & Lancaster, T. (2008). Nicotine replacement therapy for smoking cessation. *Cochrane Database of Systematic Reviews* (1), CD000146.

Steeves, T. D., & Fox, S. H. (2008). Neurobiological basis of serotonin-dopamine antagonists in the treatment of Gilles de la Tourette syndrome. *Progress in Brain Research*, 172, 495–513.

Stein, D. J. (2008). Depression, anhedonia, and psychomotor symptoms: The role of dopaminergic neurocircuitry. *CNS Spectrums*, 13(7), 561–565.

Substance Abuse and Mental Health Services Administration, Office of Applied Studies, DEPARTMENT OF HEALTH AND HUMAN SERVICES (2007). Results from the

2007 National Survey on Drug Use and Health: National Findings. Retrieved from http://www.oas.samhsa.gov/nsduh/2k7nsduh/2k7Results.pdf.

Tallarida, R. J. (2000).*Drug synergism and dose-effect data analysis*. Boca Raton, FL: CRC/Chapman-Hall.

Tallarida, R. J. (2007). Interactions between drugs and occupied receptors. *Pharmacology and Therapeutics*, *113*(1), 197–209.

Tanda, G. (2007). Modulation of the endocannabinoid system: Therapeutic potential against cocaine dependence. *Pharmacological Research*, *56*(5), 406–417.

Tanda, G., Ebbs, A., Newman, A. H., & Katz, J. L. (2005). Effects of 4′-chloro-3 alpha-(diphenylmethoxy)-tropane on mesostriatal, mesocortical, and mesolimbic dopamine transmission: Comparison with effects of cocaine. *Journal of Pharmacology and Experimental Therapeutics*, *313*(2), 613–620.

Tanda, G., Ebbs, A., Newman, A. H., & Katz, J. L. (2006). Analogs of benztropine as cocaine-abuse medications: Drug discrimination and microdialysis studies in rats. In *Abstracts, 37th Annual Meeting of the Society for Neuroscience, Atlanta, GA*.

Tanda, G., Ebbs, A. L., Kopajtic, T. A., Elias, L. M., Campbell, B. L., Newman, A. H., et al. (2007). Effects of muscarinic M1 receptor blockade on cocaine-induced elevations of brain dopamine levels and locomotor behavior in rats. *Journal of Pharmacology and Experimental Therapeutics*, *321*(1), 334–344.

Tanda, G., & Katz, J. L. (2007). Muscarinic preferential M(1) receptor antagonists enhance the discriminative-stimulus effects of cocaine in rats. *Pharmacology, Biochemistry and Behavior*, *87*(4), 400–404.

Tanda, G., Kopajtic, T. A., & Katz, J. L. (2008). Cocaine-like neurochemical effects of antihistaminic medications. *Journal of Neurochemistry*, *106*(1), 147–157.

Tanda, G., Newman, A., Ebbs, A. L., Tronci, V., Green, R. J., Tallarida, R. J., et al. (2009). Combinations of cocaine with other dopamine uptake inhibitors: Assessment of additivity. *Journal of Pharmacology and Experimental Therapeutics*, *330*(3), 802–809.

Tanda, G., Pontieri, F. E., & Di Chiara, G. (1997). Cannabinoid and heroin activation of mesolimbic dopamine transmission by a common mu1 opioid receptor mechanism. *Science*, *276*(5321), 2048–2050.

Tanda, G., Pontieri, F. E., Frau, R., & Di Chiara, G. (1997). Contribution of blockade of the noradrenaline carrier to the increase of extracellular dopamine in the rat prefrontal cortex by amphetamine and cocaine. *European Journal of Neuroscience*, *9*(10), 2077–2085.

Tolliver, B. K., Newman, A. H., Katz, J. L., Ho, L. B., Fox, L. M., Hsu, K., Jr., et al. (1999). Behavioral and neurochemical effects of the dopamine transporter ligand 4-chlorobenztropine alone and in combination with cocaine in vivo. *Journal of Pharmacology and Experimental Therapeutics*, *289*(1), 110–122.

Tuomisto, J., & Tuomisto, L. (1980). Effects of histamine and histamine antagonists on the uptake and release of catecholamines and 5-HT in brain synaptosomes. *Medical Biology*, *58*(1), 33–37.

Tzschentke, T. M. (1998). Measuring reward with the conditioned place preference paradigm: A comprehensive review of drug effects, recent progress and new issues. *Progress in Neurobiology*, *56*(6), 613–672.

Ukairo, O. T., Bondi, C. D., Newman, A. H., Kulkarni, S. S., Kozikowski, A. P., Pan, S., et al. (2005). Recognition of benztropine by the dopamine transporter (DAT) differs from that of the classical dopamine uptake inhibitors cocaine, methylphenidate, and mazindol as a function of a DAT transmembrane 1 aspartic acid residue. *Journal of Pharmacology and Experimental Therapeutics*, *314*(2), 575–583.

Vaughan, R. A., Agoston, G. E., Lever, J. R., & Newman, A. H. (1999). Differential binding of tropane-based photoaffinity ligands on the dopamine transporter. *Journal of Neuroscience*, *19*(2), 630–636.

Vaughan, R. A., Sakrikar, D. S., Parnas, M. L., Adkins, S., Foster, J. D., Duval, R. A., et al. (2007). Localization of cocaine analog [125I]RTI 82 irreversible binding to transmembrane domain 6 of the dopamine transporter. *Journal of Biological Chemistry, 282*(12), 8915–8925.

Velazquez-Sanchez, C., Ferragud, A., Hernandez-Rabaza, V., Nacher, A., Merino, V., Carda, M., et al. (2009). The dopamine uptake inhibitor 3-[bis(4'-fluorophenyl) metoxy]-tropane reduces cocaine-induced early-gene expression, locomotor activity, and conditioned reward. *Neuropsychopharmacology, 34,* 2497–2507.

Vocci, F. J., Acri, J., & Elkashef, A. (2005). Medication development for addictive disorders: The state of the science. *American Journal of Psychiatry, 162*(8), 1432–1440.

Volkow, N. D., Fowler, J. S., & Wang, G. J. (2002). Role of dopamine in drug reinforcement and addiction in humans: Results from imaging studies. *Behavioural Pharmacology, 13*(5–6), 355–366.

Wang, Z., & Woolverton, W. L. (2007). Self-administration of cocaine-antihistamine combinations: Super-additive reinforcing effects. *European Journal of Pharmacology, 557*(2–3), 159–160.

Wang, Z., & Woolverton, W. L. (2009). Super-additive interaction of the reinforcing effects of cocaine and H1-antihistamines in rhesus monkeys. *Pharmacology, Biochemistry and Behavior, 91*(4), 590–595.

Wilson, M. C., & Schuster, C. R. (1973). The effects of stimulants and depressants on cocaine self-administration behavior in the rhesus monkey. *Psychopharmacologia, 31*(4), 291–304.

Woods, J. H., Winger, G. D., & France, C. P. (1987). Reinforcing and discriminative stimulus effects of cocaine: Analysis of pharmacological mechanisms. In S. Fisher, A. Raskin, &d E. H. Uhlenhuth (Eds.), *Cocaine, clinical and biobehavioral aspects* (pp. 21–65). New York & Oxford: Oxford University Press.

Woolverton, W. L. (1987). Evaluation of the role of norepinephrine in the reinforcing effects of psychomotor stimulants in rhesus monkeys. *Pharmacology, Biochemistry and Behavior, 26*(4), 835–839.

Woolverton, W. L., Hecht, G. S., Agoston, G. E., Katz, J. L., & Newman, A. H. (2001). Further studies of the reinforcing effects of benztropine analogs in rhesus monkeys. *Psychopharmacology (Berl), 154*(4), 375–382.

Woolverton, W. L., Rowlett, J. K., Wilcox, K. M., Paul, I. A., Kline, R. H., Newman, A. H., et al. (2000). 3'- and 4'-chloro-substituted analogs of benztropine: Intravenous self-administration and in vitro radioligand binding studies in rhesus monkeys. *Psychopharmacology (Berl), 147*(4), 426–435.

Zahm, D. S. (1999). Functional-anatomical implications of the nucleus accumbens core and shell subterritories. *Annals of the New York Academy of Sciences, 877,* 113–128.

Zhu, J., & Reith, M. E. (2008) Role of the dopamine transporter in the action of psychostimulants, nicotine, and other drugs of abuse. *CNS & neurological disorders drug targets, 7,* 393–409.

Zolkowska, D., Jain, R., Rothman, R. B., Partilla, J. S., Roth, B. L., Setola, V., et al. (2009). Evidence for the involvement of dopamine transporters in behavioral stimulant effects of modafinil. *Journal of Pharmacology and Experimental Therapeutics, 329*(2), 738–746.

Zou, M. F., Kopajtic, T., Katz, J. L., & Newman, A. H. (2003). Structure-activity relationship comparison of (S)-2beta-substituted 3alpha-(bis[4-fluorophenyl]methoxy)tropanes and (R)-2beta-substituted 3beta-(3,4-dichlorophenyl)tropanes at the dopamine transporter. *Journal of Medicinal Chemistry, 46*(14), 2908–2916.

Zou, M. F., Kopajtic, T., Katz, J. L., Wirtz, S., Justice, J. B., Jr., & Newman, A. H. (2001). Novel tropane-based irreversible ligands for the dopamine transporter. *Journal of Medicinal Chemistry, 44*(25), 4453–4461.

David A. Taylor and Abdel A. Abdel-Rahman

Department of Pharmacology and Toxicology, Brody School of Medicine at East Carolina University, Greenville, North Carolina 27834

Novel Strategies and Targets for the Management of Hypertension

Abstract

Hypertension, as the sole or comorbid component of a constellation of disorders of the cardiovascular (CV) system, is present in over 90% of all patients with CV disease and affects nearly 74 million individuals in the United States. The number of medications available to treat hypertension has dramatically increased during the past 3 decades to some 50 medications as new targets involved in the normal regulation of blood pressure have been identified, resulting in the development of new agents in those classes with improved therapeutic profiles (e.g., renin–angiotensin–aldosterone system; RAAS). Despite these new agents, hypertension is not adequately managed

Advances in Pharmacology, Volume 57
© 2009 Elsevier Inc. All rights reserved.

1054-3589/08 $35.00
10.1016/S1054-3589(08)57008-6

in approximately 30% of patients, who are compliant with prescriptive therapeutics, suggesting that new agents and/or strategies to manage hypertension are still needed. Some of the newest classes of agents have targeted other components of the RAS, for example, the selective renin inhibitors, but recent advances in vascular biology have provided novel potential targets that may provide avenues for new agent development. These newer targets include downstream signaling participants in pathways involved in contraction, growth, hypertrophy, and relaxation. However, perhaps the most unique approach to the management of hypertension is a shift in strategy of using existing agents with respect to the time of day at which the agent is taken. This new strategy, termed "chronotherapy," has shown considerable promise in effectively managing hypertensive patients. Therefore, there remains great potential for future development of safe and effective agents and strategies to manage a disorder of the CV system of epidemic proportion.

I. Introduction

A. Definition and Characteristics of Hypertension

The cardiovascular (CV) system is comprised of the heart and blood vessels and functions to deliver oxygenated blood to tissues and organs throughout the body and return deoxygenated blood to the pulmonary circulation to remove carbon dioxide and replenish the oxygen supply. Many factors regulate the efficiency with which this process occurs, with a major component being the arterial pressure under which the system operates (Fig. 1; also see Section II). When any one or a combination of these factors fails to adequately regulate the defined set point for blood pressure maintenance in an individual, the blood pressure will either drop below normal levels or be raised to exceed the normal operating range. The failure to homeostatically maintain pressure within normal ranges initiates a series of intrinsic regulatory pathways that attempt to reconcile pressure as illustrated in Fig. 2. Hypertension is characterized by abnormally high blood pressure as evidenced by a diastolic (resting) blood pressure ≥ 90 mm Hg, a systolic blood pressure ≥ 140 mm Hg, or a combination of both.

Hypertension presents as one of two major classifications defined as "essential hypertension" (a disorder in which no definitive cause of the disease can be identified) or "secondary hypertension" (a disorder in which high blood pressure is due to a specific organic basis). The most common form of hypertension is "essential hypertension" which accounts for nearly 90% of all cases, suggesting that defined and readily demonstrable causes underlying the disease can be identified in only a few individuals. This also

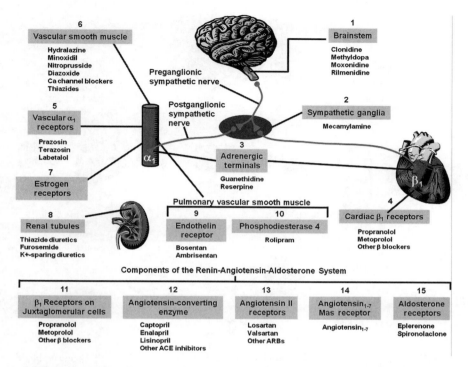

FIGURE 1   Schematic representation of anatomical and cellular sites of action of agents that are currently used in the treatment of high blood pressure or that could serve as potential future targets. A more complete listing of currently available classes and agents is provided in Table II.

suggests that the management of the disorder may require many different approaches as the basis for the elevated pressure may differ among individuals. In part due to the varying basis of the disorder, a large number of agents have been employed that are directed toward different components of the regulatory control process in efforts to manage the condition (Fig. 1). Furthermore, a number of risk factors have been identified as contributors to the development of "essential hypertension" that are associated with the development of other CV diseases as well. This places hypertension in the unenviable position of not only being a significant CV disorder in its own right but also being an independent major risk factor in many other CV diseases.

However, the definition of and management of high blood pressure have been the subject of constant debate and discussion. The Joint National Committee on Prevention, Detection, Evaluation and Treatment of High Blood Pressure (JNC) is a panel of experts that are

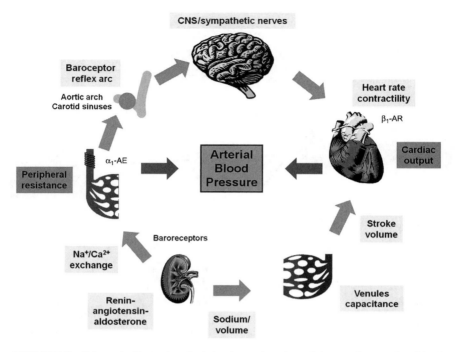

FIGURE 2 Schematic illustration depicting how physiological factors that regulate blood pressure interrelate and impact on either peripheral resistance, cardiac output, or both. The regulatory control of blood pressure occurs through a complex dynamic interplay between the intrinsic and extrinsic factors. New agents that will be effective in the treatment of hypertension must be able to interact in a positive manner with this regulatory cycle of factors.

regularly convened to develop the guidelines for defining high blood pressure as well as the recommendations for appropriate management. The seventh report of the JNC (JNC-7) published in 2003 (Chobanian et al., 2003; Fields et al., 2004) replaced the previous report (JNC-VI) and established new categories of "hypertension" based on systolic and diastolic pressure (Table I). Based upon the debate and changing recommendations regarding management, the National Institutes of Health and the National Heart, Lung, and Blood Institute are planning to present an updated new set of guidelines (JNC-8) in the spring of 2010. The latest guidelines from the JNC established a new category called "prehypertension" defined by a systolic pressure of 120–139 mm Hg or a diastolic pressure of 80–89 mm Hg. The three stages of hypertension described by JNC-VI were replaced by two stages in which Stage 1 was defined as a systolic pressure of 140–159 mm Hg and/or a diastolic pressure of 90–99 mm Hg and Stage 2 was defined by pressures of ≥ 160 and/or ≥ 100 mm Hg. The panel provided

TABLE I Comparisons of Classifications of Blood Pressure and Severity of Hypertension

Classification	American Society of Hypertension				JNC-7			
	Normal	Stage 1	Stage 2	Stage 3	Normal	Prehypertensive	Stage 1	Stage 2
Descriptive terms: (systolic/diastolic pressures)	Normal BP (≤120 mm Hg/≤80 mm Hg) and no CVD signs	Occasional BP elevations (140–160 mm Hg/80–100 mm Hg) or early CVD signs	Sustained BP elevation (140–160 mm Hg/80–100 mm Hg) or progressive CVD signs	Marked and sustained BP elevations (≥160 mm Hg/≥100 mm Hg) or advanced CVD	(≤120 mm Hg systolic/≤80 mm Hg diastolic)	(120–139 mm Hg systolic/80–89 mm Hg diastolic)	(140–159 mm Hg systolic/90-99 diastolic)	(≥160 mm Hg systolic/≥100 mm Hg diastolic)
Cardiovascular risk factors	None or few	Several	Many	Many	Not included	Not included	Not included	Not included
Early disease markers (e.g., C-reactive protein, microalbuminuria, von Willebrand factor)	None	Usually present	Clearly present	Clearly present with progression	Not included	Not included	Not included	Not included
Target-organ damage (e.g., kidneys, eyes, heart, blood vessels)	None	None	Early signs present	Clearly present with or without CVD events	Not included	Not included	Not included	Not included

Abbreviation: JNC, Joint National Committee on Prevention, Detection, Evaluation and Treatment of High Blood Pressure; CVD, cardiovascular disease.

recommendations and specific treatment guidelines for each of the stages that were based upon the urgency for treatment. In addition, the American Society of Hypertension has developed a new definition/classification of hypertension based on both systolic and diastolic blood pressure values and the absence or presence of risk factors for other CV diseases. This system defines normal blood pressure as less than 120/80 mm Hg with no risk factors or early markers (e.g., C-reactive protein (CRP) von Willebrand factor, and other markers of inflammation) for CV disease. According to the new classification, the three stages of hypertension correspond to the JNC-7 stages as follows (Table I): Stage 1— blood pressure is 120/80–139/89 mm Hg, several CV risk factors and early disease markers and signs of functional or structural changes in the heart and small arteries but no end-organ damage; Stage 2—blood pressure is ≥140/90 mm Hg with widespread disease markers and early evidence of end-organ damage as well as risk factors; Stage 3—blood pressure is sustained at ≥140/90 mm Hg even when treated with the presence of end-organ damage and an increased potential for existing CV events (Brookes, 2008). Since the management of hypertension has been subject to a number of modifications since JNC 7, the National Heart, Lung, and Blood Institute has indicated that it will distribute an update to the report (JNC 8) in the spring of 2010 (Brookes, 2008).

Hypertension is a condition of elevated blood pressure that affects a larger portion of the population (see Section I.B) so that it is important to begin preventive measures as early as possible. The changing definitions and classifications of hypertension have contributed substantially to the confusion regarding the appropriate management of the disorder. One early approach, called "stepped care," always initiated therapy with diuretics and "stepped" through other available agents such α- or β-receptor blockers as the need arose. However, several factors contributed to the decline of this approach including the development of new agents, the need for individualization of therapy, and the recognition that many other factors that could be controlled including environment contributed to the disorder. Clearly lifestyle modifications which include alterations in diet and nutrition to reduce sodium intake and increased consumption of fruits, vegetables, and fat-free products combined with reduced alcohol consumption and increased physical activity are among the most important methods currently recommended for preventive and early management of the disorder and should be encouraged even in patients with normal blood pressure. As hypertension progresses and becomes sustained, medications from selective classes are added to reduce the high level of blood pressure. As illustrated in Fig. 1 and Table II, these agents differentially target factors that may contribute to the development of hypertension or that are involved in the normal physiological regulation of blood pressure. These agents are among the first drugs employed when lifestyle modifications fail and are considered the "first line of therapy" or "first-line agents." The structures of some members of this group of agents and some of the other agents

TABLE II Drug Classes and Agents Currently Used in the Therapeutic Management of Hypertension

A. Diuretics			
Thiazides	Loop diuretics	Potassium sparing diuretics	Aldosterone antagonists
Hydrochlorothiazide, chlorothiazide	Furosemide, ethacrynic acid, bumetanide, torsemide	Amiloride, spironolactone, triamterene, eplerenone	Spironolactone, eplerenone

B. Agents acting in the autonomic nervous system
B1. Autonomic ganglia
Mecamylamine, trimethaphan
B2. Sympathetic nervous system inhibitors (sympatholytics)
B2a. Nerve terminal blockers
Reserpine, guanethidine, guanadrel
B2b. α-blockers

Nonselective irreversible	Nonselective reversible	α_1-selective
Phenoxybenzamine	Phentolamine	Prazosin, terazosin, doxazosin

B2c. β-blockers

Nonselective	β_1-selective
Propranolol, timolol, nadolol, pindolol, acebutolol, carteolol, penbutolol	Atenolol, betaxolol, esmolol, metoprolol, nebivolol

B2d. Mixed blockers
Carvedilol, labetalol

(Continued)

TABLE II (*Continued*)

B2e. Centrally acting sympatholytics

α_2-receptor agonists	Imidazoline receptor agonists
Clonidine, guanabenz, guanfacine, methyldopa (via metabolite, α-methyl-norepinephrine)	Clonidine, moxonidine, rilmenidine

C. Renin–Angiotensin–Aldosterone System

β-blockers	Renin inhibitors	Angiotensin-converting enzyme inhibitors	Angiotensin II receptor (type I) blockers	Aldosterone receptor blockers
Propranolol, metoprolol and others (see above)	Aliskiren	Benazepril, captopril, enalapril, fosinopril, lisinopril, moexipril, perindopril, quinapril, ramipril, trandolapril	Candesartan, eprosartan, irbesartan, losartan, olmesartan, telmisartan, valsartan	Spironolactone, eplerenone

D. Agents acting directly on vascular smooth muscle

D1. Calcium channel blockers (calcium entry blockers)

Dihydropyridines	Miscellaneous
Amlodipine, clevidipine, felodipine, isradipine, nicardipine, nifedipine, nisoldipine	Diltiazem, verapamil

D2. Direct acting vasodilators

Diazoxide, hydralazine, minoxidil, nitroprusside

D3. Dopamine receptor agonists

Fenoldopam

E. Agents used for hypertensive emergency and urgency

Fenoldopam, nitroprusside, trimethaphan, nicardipine, esmolol employed are illustrated in Table III. The "first-line agents" include diuretics (especially the thiazides), angiotensin-converting enzyme inhibitors (ACEIs like captopril and enalapril), angiotensin receptor blocking agents (ARBs like losartan), calcium channel blockers (e.g., nifedipine), and β-blockers (e.g., propranolol). Under conditions of greater severity of the elevated pressure in spite of adequate compliance, there may be a need to combine these "first-line" agents with other agents that inhibit sympathetic nerve activity either peripherally or from the central nervous system (CNS). In cases of hypertensive emergency or urgency (e.g., hypertensive crisis), vasodilator agents that act directly on the smooth muscle of the arteries and veins are employed (Table II). The large number of agents currently available to manage hypertension reflects the challenge that this disorder presents to health-care providers.

B. Epidemiology of CV Disease

The constellation of CV disorders and diseases identified in Table IV is interrelated in a very complex manner and in 2005–2006 represented approximately 80 million individuals or over 30% of the US population of indicating that this family of disorders and diseases is approaching epidemic proportions (American Heart Association, 2009). The diseases involved include coronary heart disease (CHD); acute coronary syndrome (ACS which includes myocardial infarction (STEMI and non-STEMI), angina pectoris (coronary artery disease), or unstable angina); stroke; hypertension; congestive heart failure (CHF); arrhythmias; peripheral artery disease; rheumatic heart disease; valvular heart disease; and venous thromboembolism (Ramachandran, Benjamin, Sullivan, & D'Agostino, 2009; Taylor, 2007). Based upon the National Health and Nutrition Examination Survey, CV diseases and disorders were responsible for more than one-third of the global mortality burden and the American Heart Association estimated that the annual direct and indirect economic impact of CV diseases and stroke for 2009 exceeds $475 billion in the United States (American Heart Association, 2009). CV diseases target men, women, and children of all ethnic groups but prevalence and rates of mortality appear to be greater in African-Americans as well as in individuals older than 70 (CDC, 2005). Of particular concern is the fact that the prevalence of CV disease and disorders is expected to continue to rise in the population over the next two decades and will remain the leading cause of both death and disability in the world for decades to come. This is especially disconcerting when considering the fact that most CV diseases and disorders are preventable through lifestyle modification and, when severe enough, can be effectively managed using drugs. Of even greater concern is the alarming worldwide increase in specific major risk factors for CV diseases and hypertension that include tobacco use; physical inactivity; poor nutrition; dyslipidemia; obesity and overweight; and diabetes.

TABLE III Structures of Some Primary First-Line Antihypertensive Drugs and Selected Other Structures

Diuretics

Thiazide	Loop	K⁺-sparing	Aldosterone antagonists
Hydrochlorothiazide	Furosemide	Amiloride	Spironolactone

Angiotensin-converting enzyme inhibitors

Sulfhydryl-containing
captopril

Dicarboxylate-containing
enalaprilat

Phosphonate-containing fosinoprilat

Angiotensin receptor blocking agents
Losartan

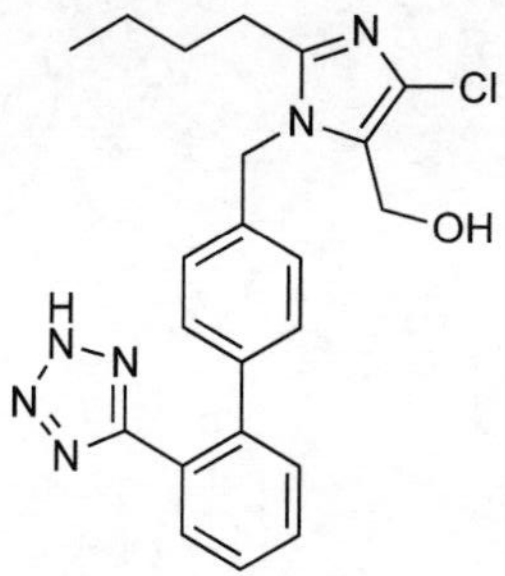

Eprosartan

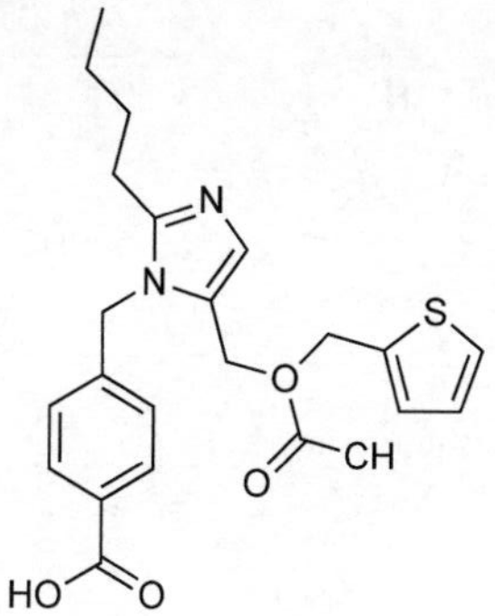

Calcium channel blockers
Dihydropyridines
Nifedipine

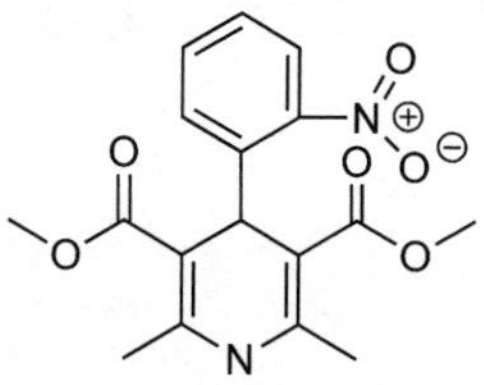

Others
Diltiazem

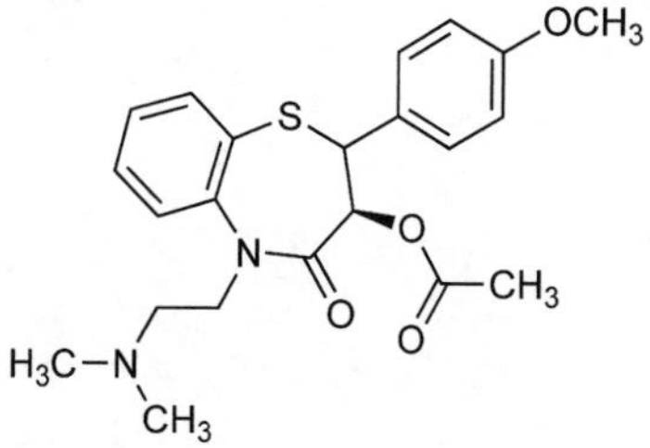

(Continued)

TABLE III (*Continued*)

Sympatholytic agents
α-Adrenoceptor
  blockers
  Nonselective
  Phentolamine

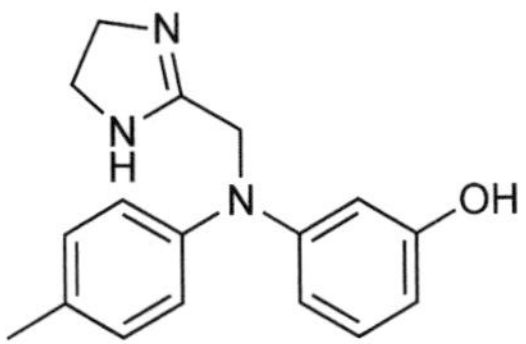

α₁-Selective
Prazosin

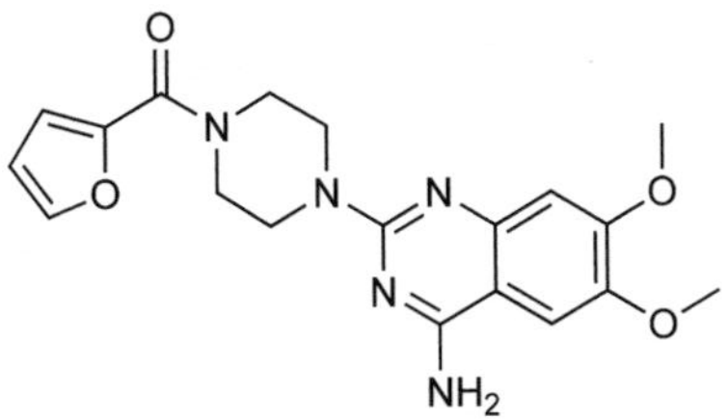

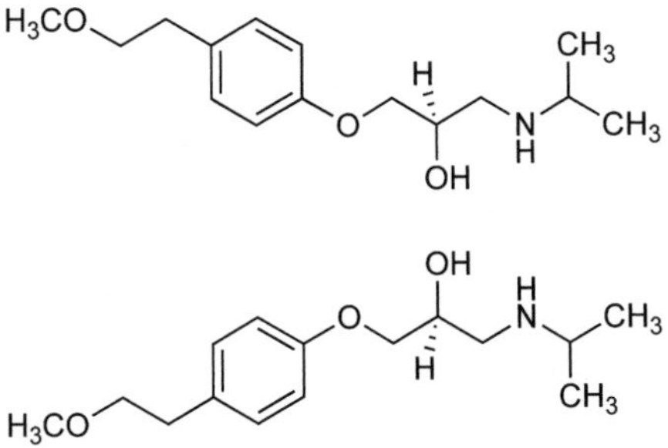

Mixed receptor blockers
Carvedilol

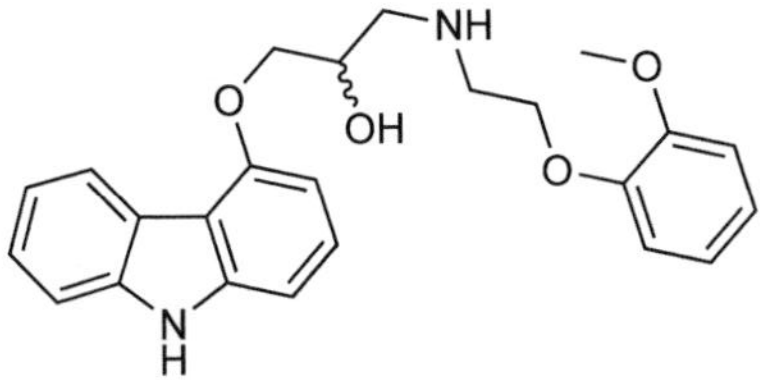

β-Adrenoceptor blockers
  Nonselective
  Propranolol

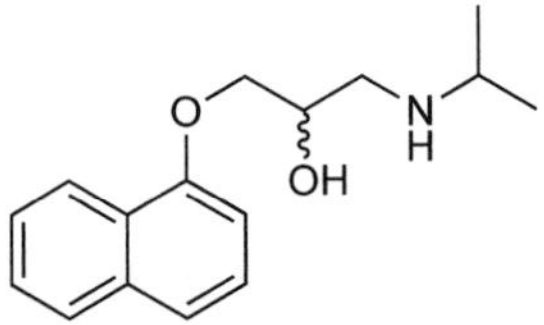

β₁-Selective
Metoprolol (racemic)

Other agents

Clonidine

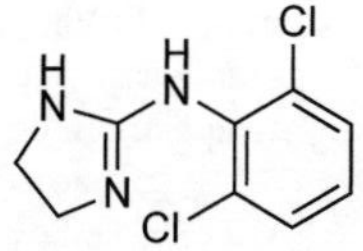

α-methyldopa

Nebivolol (β₁-selective)

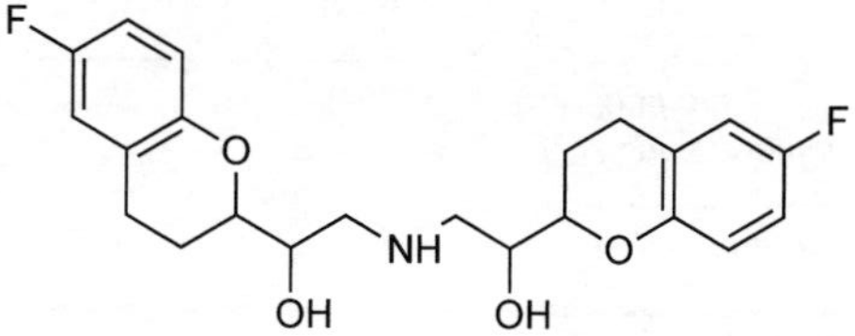

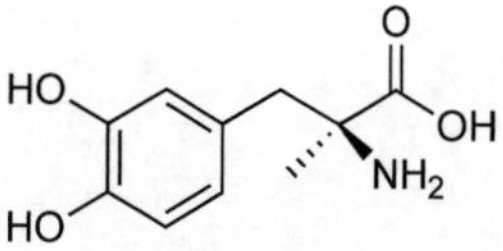

ICI 118551 (β₂-selective)

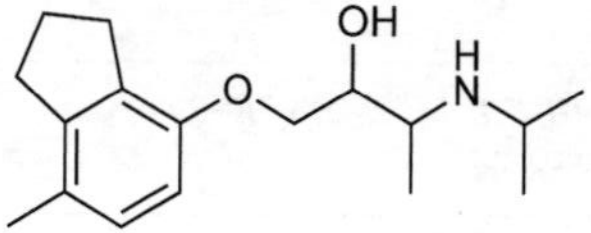

TABLE IV Prevalence Disease Comprising Cardiovascular Disorders in the United States of America

CVD	Population prevalence[a]		Males (millions)	Percentage of disease	Females (millions)	Percentage of disease
	Actual population (millions)	Percentage of total CVD burden				
Coronary heart disease	16.8	21	8.7	51.8	8.1	48.2
Acute myocardial infarction	7.9	9.9	4.7	59.5	3.2	40.5
Angina pectoris	9.8	12.2	4.3	43.9	5.5	56.1
Stroke	6.5	8.1	2.6	40	3.9	60
Congestive heart failure	5.7	7.1	2.4	56.2	2.5	43.8
Hypertension	73.6	92	35.3	48	38.3	52
Congenital cardiovascular defects	0.65-1.3	1.4	–	–	–	–

Abbreviations: CVD, cardiovascular disease.
[a]Total population exhibiting one or more CVDs = 80 million (36% of US population).

Hypertension impacts the largest number of individuals (Table IV) and is present in 92% of all patients that evidence any CV disease. The second largest disease in the constellation is CHD which is only present in about 21% of the patients with CV disease. The American Heart Association estimates that nearly 80 million individuals in the United States have high blood pressure (defined as a systolic blood pressure greater than 140 mm Hg, diastolic blood pressure greater than 90 mm Hg, currently taking antihypertensive medication or having been told twice by a physician or other health professional that high blood pressure is present) and that high blood pressure contributes to nearly 50% of all CV diseases either independently or as a comorbid factor.

In the United States, the prevalence of hypertension has remained relatively constant since 1999 with established high blood pressure being diagnosed in nearly 30% of the population. There was an age-related increase in hypertension that ranged from 7% in individuals 18–39 years of age to 67% in patients 60 years old or older. There also appeared to be clear ethnic orientation for the disease with non-Hispanic African-Americans exhibiting a significantly higher incidence (41%) compared to non-Hispanic whites (28%) and Mexican Americans (22%). In addition, it appears that the disease develops at an earlier age in African-Americans. Furthermore, an additional 25% of Americans over age 18 falls into the JNC-7 category of "prehypertension" which suggests that early prevention could be an important component in the treatment regimen. Even more significant is the fact that among those patients diagnosed with hypertension, 78% were aware of the presence of the disease but only 68% were taking antihypertensive medications. Even more surprising was the fact that in individuals taking medications to control the disease, only 36% were adequately controlled.

CV diseases are the leading cause of mortality irrespective of gender or ethnicity and account for nearly 1 million deaths per year of the 80 million individuals affected by the diseases (American Heart Association, 2009). CV diseases are the leading cause of death in both females and males with no apparent differences between white and non-Hispanic African-Americans. The mortality associated with hypertension was significantly greater in females compared to males (59% versus 41%, respectively) and African-American women appear to exhibit a much greater prevalence of the disease than white females (45% versus 31%, respectively). CV diseases appeared less significant contributors to the mortality of Hispanic and Latino men and women. However, there is a much larger prevalence of diabetes mellitus in this population which has been associated as a comorbid risk factor with many other CV diseases including hypertension. As better epidemiological studies are conducted this idea that the Hispanic population may have lesser risk of mortality due to hypertension or other CV diseases is being challenged (Pickering & Ogedegbe, 2009). The impact of CV diseases and disorders on the health of the population is substantial and the difficulty associated with appropriate management of the disease suggests that newer modalities will likely be developed to improve therapeutic outcomes.

C. Role of Hypertension in Other Pathologies

Hypertension plays an integral role in many CV diseases as well as other diseases and pathologies (e.g., end stage kidney disease and diabetes). As summarized in Fig. 2 major contributors to the development of hypertension can also be adversely affected by the developing hypertension as the normal physiological regulatory pathways begin to fail to perform adequately leading to a feed-forward loop that exacerbates the disorder. As indicated in Table III, the fact that hypertension is a comorbid factor in many other CV diseases is clearly apparent by the fact that the disease appears in 92% of all patients with CV disease. Hypertension that remains untreated is considered to be a major risk factor for sudden death due to myocardial infarction as well as a risk factor for cerebral vascular disease, CHD, CHF, and renal failure. Furthermore, the end-organ damage associated with untreated hypertension is a major consideration when deciding the appropriate management plan (see Fig. 2). The development of CHF due to longstanding not well-controlled hypertension is well documented. Chronic kidney disease that is produced by high blood pressure-induced decreases in renal perfusion has also been clearly established (USRDS, 2007). In addition, nearly 73% of all diabetics are hypertensive so the relationship between these two disorders as comorbid risk factors while well established is not well understood with respect to cause and effect. There is accumulating evidence that the two diseases may be interrelated. A similar relationship exists between obesity and hypertension as well as other comorbid risk factors that may be related to the presence of hypertension. The clear relationship between hypertension and other CV diseases such as stroke and ACS is also well recognized by the health-care community (see Taylor, 2007).

In contrast to the CV diseases that may be a function of the development or presence of hypertension, there are other diseases and pathologies that have been associated with hypertension. Some of the disorders include visual problems and blindness that develop, as the eye becomes the target end organ for reduced blood flow. Similarly, the relationship between hypertension and other comorbid factors like diabetes and erectile dysfunction is well documented in both the lay and the scientific media. It is interesting to note that erectile dysfunction may not only be produced by these diseases but also be a side effect of the drugs that are used to manage the diseases. One of the major target end organs that are especially vulnerable to sustained elevated pressure is the kidney. This organ is essential for regulating fluid volume and eliminating toxic material so that any reduction in function could rapidly escalate into serious health problems. The reduction in glomerular blood flow due to high pressure in the afferent arteriole renders the kidney ineffective in removing fluid and toxic material. Similarly, as blood flow to the liver begins to decline, the capacity of the liver to provide the necessary metabolic functions begins to decline. Finally, reduced blood flow to the CNS due to high blood pressure can increase the risk for stroke and other centrally mediated disorders such as seizures and dementia that can be precipitated by the anoxia associated with low blood flow.

D. Pharmacogenomics of Hypertension

The contribution of genetics to CV disease can be viewed on two different levels. The first is related to defining the genetics of the pathophysiology of the disease and the genetics of the molecular targets for drug development, while the second is related to understanding the basis for individual variation in the response to currently employed agents as well as those under development.

Identifying the genetic determinants that contribute to the development of hypertension would provide enormous assistance not only with the understanding of the pathophysiology of the disease but also with determining the molecular and cellular targets appropriate for therapeutic management of the disorder. However, progress in understanding the genetic aspects of CV disease and hypertension, in particular, have been slowed by the fact that the diseases have multifactorial pathologies and are very closely interrelated (Lee, 2007). Furthermore, the genetic traits that lead to the disease in one animal model or in any given individual may differ from the traits that are important in others (Cowley, Liang, Roman, Greene, & Jacob, 2004; Malek et al., 2006). Additional complexity in defining the pharmacogenomics of hypertension is derived from the fact that phenotypic characteristics impact both the development of the disease and the ability of individual patients to respond to therapeutic agents. For example, recent advances in the treatment of CHF (Taylor et al., 2004) have identified a differential responsiveness to drugs based upon ethnicity with the successful management of heart failure in African-Americans using the fixed combination of hydralazine and isosorbide dinitrate (BiDil®). These observations have markedly increased interest in the possibility of developing new therapies based upon the genetics and ethnicity of the individual patient (Taylor et al., 2004). It should be emphasized that the primary focus of this discussion is "essential hypertension" which is a comorbid component of many of the spectrum of CV diseases which are frequently not associated with known genetic predispositions. It is clear that essential hypertension develops as the result of a polygenic modification in which the contribution may differ among individuals. Estimates of the relative contribution of genetic components to the development of hypertension have ranged from 30 to 50% penetration probabilities.

The fact that multiple genes are involved suggests that an effective approach to understanding the foundation of the disease may rely on identification of quantitative trait loci (QTLs). Based upon the rat genome, nearly 200 QTLs have been identified as associated with blood pressure in the spontaneously hypertensive rat, which is a standard model employed by many investigators to evaluate the basis of the disease and the potential therapeutic utility of drugs (Pravenec & Kren, 2005). The identification of QTLs involved in the regulation of blood pressure is complicated by the fact that blood pressure is a systemic phenotype that displays the highest level of complexity within the genome. The fact that the genes that regulate cardiac development and function, vascular smooth muscle development and function, kidney function, and nervous system function all can contribute to the status of blood pressure increases the number of analyses and linkages that need to be developed. In addition, there is evidence that many of these genes can be influenced environmentally adding even greater variation (Takahashi and Smithies, 2004). Furthermore, there are accumulating data that suggest that in certain individuals the specific phenotype they express contains genetic variability in the specific cellular and molecular entities (e.g., angiotensin-converting enzyme (ACE), α- and β-adrenoceptors, angiotensin II (Ang II) receptors) targeted by agents utilized in the management of the disease. Animal studies employing antisense technology have demonstrated the feasibility of this approach using retroviral delivery of antisense cDNA to elements of the RAAS (Pachori et al., 2000, 2002; Wang et al., 1999, 2004). While these genes do offer primary targets for gene therapy, this type of approach will face many challenges if it is to be successful.

A second level of pharmacogenomic contribution to hypertension is related to the genetic contributions responsible for patient susceptibility. Nearly one-third of patients receiving antihypertensive medication are not adequately controlled and there is a great inter-patient variability in response to the first-line pharmacological agents that are employed. Furthermore, a similar degree of inter-patient variability exists for the development of adverse effects including serious, life-threatening responses. One of the benefits of the post-genomic era has been the ability to characterize genetic polymorphisms that impact on patient responses to pharmacological agents. Much of the emphasis has been focused on characterizing the drug-metabolizing enzyme profile of individual patients that permits appropriate drug selection prior to administration. While a number of these polymorphisms exist that impact upon CV drug metabolism, there are only a small number in which the impact of the genetic polymorphism is of significant clinical importance (Johnson & Cavallari, 2005). One of these relates to the genetic polymorphism of the cytochrome p450 enzyme isoform, CYP2C9, where there are a number of single nucleotide polymorphisms that modify the functional capacity of the enzyme that is responsible for the metabolism of warfarin. The presence of one or more variant allele in an individual (nearly 40% of all Caucasians carry at least one variant allele) substantially alters the dose of warfarin required to produce a reduction in clotting. There are other polymorphisms that regulate β-blocker metabolism by CYP2D6 that seem to exert lesser impact on pharmacological efficacy.

In contrast to the effect of phenotypic differences in drug metabolism, there are emerging studies that suggest that genetic modifications in the target of many different drugs may impact on drug efficacy or toxicity. For example, there are genetic alterations in α-adducin, a protein responsible for renal tubular reabsorption that is a target for diuretics in which the modification alters the response to diuretics (Cusi et al., 1997). There are also genetic modifications in the alpha subunits of the G-proteins that couple to β-receptors that modify the responsiveness to this class of agents. Finally, polymorphisms have been associated with the Ang II receptor subtype 1 (AT_1R) gene (Baudin, 2002) and ACE (Saeed, Saboohi, Osman, Bokhari, & Frossard, 2003) that may be involved with altered efficacy of ARBs and ACEIs. Polymorphisms have also been identified that are responsible for adverse effects of drugs in some patients. Much of the emphasis in this area has focused on the genetic predisposition of individuals to the development of prolonged QT interval of the ECG and the production of Torsades de Pointe (Johnson & Cavallari, 2005). Several mutations in both sodium channel genes and potassium channel genes have been identified that increase the susceptibility of patients to the development of this life-threatening arrhythmia (Roden, 2009). Thus, the need to profile an individual's genetic composition of drug-metabolizing enzymes and other factors of importance that may be identified in the future may increase as the population becomes more resistant to the therapeutic effects of drugs and there is greater emphasis on managing each patient individually.

II. Physiological Regulation of Blood Pressure

Blood pressure is the product of total peripheral resistance (TPR) times the cardiac output (CO). Therefore, to maintain blood pressure at physiological level, many factors that influence vascular resistance and cardiac function need to be tightly controlled. The homeostatic regulation of arterial pressure is multifaceted and includes neural, hormonal, and local control of the vasculature (Figs. 1 and 2). In addition to the ability of these factors to directly modulate vascular resistance, the neural, humoral, and local modulators that affect two other organs, the heart and kidney, indirectly influence blood pressure and, therefore, contribute to the overall control of arterial pressure (Fig. 2). We will present a brief overview of the major physiological systems that influence arterial pressure in order to develop the basis by which targets for drugs that have been identified in the past as well as to present some potential new areas of exploration that may come in the future as a result of increased knowledge concerning vascular biology. The fact that hypertension is not well controlled in a significant number of hypertensive individuals supports that concept that there is a continuing need to develop new agents and that these newer targets may provide a better ability to match the agent to the specific individual being treated.

A. Primary Factors Controlling Vascular Tone

In recent years, advances made in the field of vascular biology have significantly enhanced knowledge of the molecular and cellular mechanisms involved in the regulation of vascular tone. While this section will focus mainly on the control of arterial vasculature, it is imperative to note that changes in venous vascular tone can have clear implications on venous return, which impacts CO and ultimately blood pressure (Fig. 2). To fully appreciate the interplay between different factors that influence vascular tone, we will first discuss the independent contribution of each of the major factors that influence the vascular tone. It must, however, be realized that the interplay between the different factors is dynamic and none of the known systems that influence vascular biology operates in isolation.

B. Role of the CNS in Regulating Blood Pressure

Early studies have clearly demonstrated the importance of the CNS in short- as well as long-term maintenance of blood pressure (Figs. 1 and 2). Well-defined localized neuroanatomical lesions and localized microinjection of highly selective neurotoxins have mapped brain areas that control blood pressure as well as their function. Furthermore, the importance of the spinal cord in modulating the neural output to the vasculature was established by demonstrating the drastic reduction in arterial pressure following destruction of the spinal cord, particularly the thoracolumbar segments. Hemodynamic complications and CV collapse are known consequences of irreversible spinal cord injury that results in interruption of autonomic nervous system (ANS) control of the vasculature. Interestingly, if adequate ventilation is maintained following spinal cord injury, the body seems to have the capacity to regenerate and consequently regain some of the lost sympathetic tone. Although this process takes a relatively long time to occur, there is experimental and limited clinical evidence that demonstrated steady increases in blood pressure from its lowest point achieved following accidental or experimental spinal cord injury. While these paradigms cause physical changes in neural outflow, the most compelling evidence that demonstrated the importance of a fully functioning neural outflow was obtained following the discovery of the impact of pharmacological interventions capable of interrupting neural transmission at the level of the autonomic ganglia (Fig. 1). Depending on their potency, some of these drugs caused "reversible" reductions in blood pressure to a nadir only achieved following cervical spinal cord transection. Indeed, the use of agonists and antagonists as research tools has enhanced understanding of the role of the CNS in controlling blood pressure.

C. Role of the ANS

The two subdivisions of the ANS, the *sympathetic nervous system* (SNS) *and parasympathetic nervous systems* (PNS), play major physiological roles in controlling CV function. While both nervous systems reciprocally control heart rate, the dominance of one over the other is influenced by many factors that include physical activity, the sleep/awake phase, and the emotional state of the individual (Hermida, Calvo, Ayala, Mojon, & Lopez, 2002; Zaros, Pires, Bacci, Moraes, & Zanesco, 2009). At rest, the PNS plays only a minor role in controlling vascular resistance. Anatomically, there is no parasympathetic innervation to the vascular smooth muscle. However, sympathetic vasodilating innervation to the skeletal muscle vasculature in certain vascular beds is mediated via the release of acetylcholine (ACh) from these sympathetic nerve terminals. Circulating ACh can indirectly contribute to vascular resistance via two mechanisms. First, ACh activation of presynaptic cholinergic nicotinic receptors on noradrenergic nerve terminals can result in increased norepinephrine release. Conversely, ACh activation of presynaptic muscarinic receptors can cause inhibition of norepinephrine release from noradrenergic nerve terminals. Second, activation of muscarinic cholinergic receptors on endothelial cells enhances nitric oxide (NO) release (Furchgott & Zawadski, 1980; Palmer, Ferrige, & Moncada, 1987). These contrasting effects of cholinergic modulation of norepinephrine and NO release are anticipated to contribute differentially to vascular tone control depending upon the circumstances present at that time.

The contribution of the other ANS subdivision, the SNS, has been well recognized for many decades. Starting within the CNS, noradrenergic neurotransmission plays pivotal role in determining the level of activity of presympathetic neurons in the brainstem (Fig. 1). Depending on the neuroanatomical site, the adrenergic receptor, and neuronal signaling implicated, the activation of adrenergic receptors located in the brainstem can lead to either activation or inhibition of SNS. Therefore, neuronal signaling triggered by the activation of adrenergic receptors in the CNS, and particularly in the brainstem, has physiological and pathophysiological implications. Indeed, enhanced central sympathetic activity is a well-recognized hallmark of most forms of experimental as well as clinical hypertension. It must be emphasized that central and/or peripheral sympathetic overactivity can also result in vasoconstriction and elevation of blood pressure independent of other contributing modulators of vascular tone. However, as discussed above, at the integrative level, the SNS is engaged in feed-forward interplay with other important regulators of vascular tone. For example, there is ample experimental evidence that supports the presence of positive feedback interplay between the SNS and the RAAS. The latter plays an important role in the normal physiological control of blood pressure as well as in the pathophysiology of hypertension (Table II). Given the importance of the SNS overactivity in hypertension, it was logical to develop medications that could selectively inhibit SNS activity by developing drugs able to interrupt generation of sympathetic activity within the CNS, neural transmission at the autonomic ganglion level, release of norepinephrine from adrenergic nerve terminals or by blocking vascular adrenergic receptor(s) (see Table II, Fig. 1). Sympathetic innervation of other organ systems (e.g., heart and kidney) can indirectly influence blood pressure and appears to serve as an important target for at least some of the currently available antihypertensive medications that do not directly impact vascular tone.

D. Role of the Kidney

The importance of the kidney in blood pressure control and the pathophysiology of hypertension has long been recognized as demonstrated in at least two of the early models of hypertension that are classical models of hypertension (see Section III.B). The original concept that the kidney contributes to blood pressure homeostasis by controlling total fluid volume and electrolyte balance has been extended to include the ability of the kidney to be more directly involved in blood pressure control at the level of the vascular smooth muscle cells (VSMCs) via the RAAS as illustrated in Fig. 2. The kidney is a unique organ because its sympathetic innervation is involved in feed-forward regulation of the RAAS. As shown in Figs. 1 and 2, norepinephrine released from the renal sympathetic nerve activates β_1-adrenergic receptors to cause release of renin, which eventually leads to generation of Ang II and other angiotensin fragments (see Tables II and III).

E. Role of the RAAS

The importance of the RAAS in blood pressure control as well as in the pathophysiology of hypertension is well known (Katovich, Grobe & Raizada 2008; Laragh, 1993). Until the discovery of endothelin (ET), Ang II was considered the most potent vasoconstrictor peptide. It is approximately 40 times more potent than norepinephrine as a vasoconstrictor. In addition to its direct vasoconstrictor function, Ang II exhibits many additional direct and indirect effects that ultimately result in increased vascular resistance and cell hypertrophy that contribute to characteristics of hypertension (see Section II.G). Most notable is the ability of neuronally synthesized Ang II within the brainstem to increase SNS activity and its contribution to neurogenic hypertension (Phillips & de Oliveira, 2008); this effect is further intensified by the ability of Ang II to enhance the release of NE from noradrenergic nerve terminals as well as by its capacity to sensitize the vascular smooth muscle to the vasoconstrictor effect of NE. There are also well-recognized direct and indirect (via aldosterone) renal effects of Ang II that result in sodium and water retention along with hypokalemia. Finally, Ang II and aldosterone enhance central sympathetic activity (Kumar, Goodchild, Li, & Pilowsky, 2006) and vascular smooth muscle growth, which eventually contributes to increased vascular resistance as well as to the remodeling that occurs in the vasculature, myocardium, and kidney as the disease progresses (Iwanami, Mogi, Iwai, & Horiuchi, 2009). The effects triggered by Ang II, including the release of aldosterone from the adrenal cortex, are mediated by the activation of AT_1R. Conversely, in recent years, the roles of other angiotensin fragments (e.g., Ang_{1-7}) and receptors (e.g., AT_2R) in blood pressure control and in the pathophysiology of hypertension have become recognized (Lazartigues, Feng, & Lavoie, 2007; Rodrigues et al., 2007; Trask & Ferrario, 2007; Katovich, Grobe & Raizada, 2008). Signaling triggered by the activation of AT_2R or Mas receptor by their natural ligands, Ang II and Ang_{1-7}, respectively, results in vasodilation and reduction in vascular resistance. Activation of the Mas receptor by Ang_{1-7} leads to vasodilatation, natriuresis, anti-proliferation, and an increase in the bradykinin–NO signaling. Akt phosphorylation, protein kinase C (PKC) activation, and mitogen-activated protein (MAP) kinase inhibition have also been implicated in Ang_{1-7}–Mas receptor signaling pathway (Iwai & Horiuchi, 2009). Ang_{1-7} lowers blood pressure via peripheral as well as central mechanisms of action that might involve bradykinin and NO in addition to producing direct antihypertrophic and antifibrotic effects (Iusuf, Henning, van Gilst, & Roks, 2008; Katovich, Grobe, & Raizada, 2008). A third peptide, Ang III, produced from its precursor Ang II has been implicated in central control of blood pressure. Within the brain, conversion of Ang II to Ang III by aminopeptidase A (APA) accounts, at least partly, for the centrally mediated pressor and sympathoexcitatory effects caused by Ang II. This view is supported by (i) the ability of intracerebroventricular Ang II and Ang III to produce similar increases in blood pressure and both Ang II and Ang III exhibit similar agonist activity at central AT_1R (Reaux-Le Goazigo et al., 2005); and (ii) pharmacologic inhibition of central APA lowers blood pressure (Bodineau, Frugière, Marc, Claperon, & Llorens-Cortes, 2008; Reaux-Le Goazigo et al., 2005). Therefore, the ability of the RAAS to exhibit counterbalancing effects on vascular resistance will impact blood pressure homeostasis. Obviously an imbalance that results in exacerbated AT_1R signaling may be expected to lead to hypertension that is referred to as high-renin hypertension.

F. Role of the Endothelium

The conceptual role of the endothelium has changed from that of just the lining layer of the interior of the arterial wall to being a major contributor to vascular tone control. The discovery that damaged (dysfunctional) endothelium in isolated artery preparations abrogated the vasodilatory effect of ACh led to the discovery of endothelium-derived relaxing factor which was later identified to be NO (Furchgott & Zawadski, 1980; Palmer et al., 1987). Many studies have been conducted to elucidate the synthetic pathway and importance of NO in vascular biology and the pathophysiology of hypertension. This gaseous molecule with very short half-life is synthesized from L-arginine via the action of the enzyme NO synthase. This enzyme exists is three different isoforms (i.e., endothelial (eNOS), neuronal (nNOS), and inducible (iNOS) isoforms) that are differentially distributed among tissues and, with the exception of iNOS, are constitutive enzymes. Regulation of the activity and expression of these enzymes determines the level of NO generation and hence its contribution to vascular tone. NO produces vasodilation by enhancing the generation of intracellular cyclic GMP (cGMP; see Section II.G). In recent years, an important discovery has been made with regard to the significance of the "coupled" versus "uncoupled" state of eNOS and nNOS in CV biology. The coupling of eNOS or nNOS to caveolin and tetrahydrobiopterin (BH4) maintains the activity of the enzyme within physiological limits. By contrast, uncoupling of either form of the enzyme, which eventually shifts the balance to greater association of the enzyme with the facilitatory allosteric protein calmodulin, results in the generation of superoxide and other reactive oxygen species (ROS) that can negatively impact smooth and cardiac muscle cell structure and function (see Section II.G). The latter is implicated in cardiac injury following eNOS uncoupling and in coronary vasoconstriction following nNOS uncoupling. The endothelium also releases potent vasoconstrictors with the most notable being the peptide, ET, that is considered the most potent vasoconstrictor known to date and plays an important role in maintaining vascular tone by activating the endothelin-A (ET_A) receptor . Therefore, pathophysiological overactivity of ET receptor signaling is expected to increase total vascular resistance. However, perhaps due to differential distribution of the ET receptors in different vascular beds, overactivity of ET receptor signaling has also been implicated in pathological pulmonary vasoconstriction and pulmonary hypertension (Aubert & Juillerat-Jeanneret, 2009; Channick, Sitbon, Barst, Manes, & Rubin, 2004; Kabunga & Coghlan, 2008).

G. Cell Signaling Systems Regulating Vascular Tone

The final common element in determining vascular tone is the contractile state of VSMCs. The contractile state of any vascular smooth muscle at any point in time is related to the combined activity of the extrinsic and intrinsic factors that are impacting upon the cell and, specifically, the free intracellular calcium concentration. As illustrated in Fig. 1 and Tables II and III, therapeutic agents target many of the extrinsic factors described above that include the activity of the ANS, the RAAS, and the endothelial release of substances that either produce vasoconstriction (e.g., ET) or vasodilation (e.g., NO, endothelium-derived hyperpolarizing factors, adenosine, prostacyclin, and others). With improved knowledge of vascular biology, many of the components of these signaling pathways have been identified and characterized and now serve as potential elements for new agent development.

The endothelium is also responsive to changes in the turbulence of flow through a process identified as shear stress that is an important factor in understanding the pathophysiology of cell function and structure changes that occur during and after the development of hypertension. Shear stress causes multiple alterations in endothelial function with respect to the release of signaling factors as well as the physical structure of the endothelium and VSMCs. Both in *in vitro,* endothelial cell monolayers and in the arterial endothelium, shear stress causes endothelial cells to align in the direction of flow and to alter the cytoskeleton (Griendling, Harrison, & Alexander, 2009). In addition to the physical changes, shear stress causes endothelial cell function to change due to activation of K^+ channels, increased secretion of both vasoconstrictor and vasodilating factors, increased uptake of low-density lipoproteins, increased expression of growth factors (Davies, 1995), and elevated influx of Ca^{++} due to increased release of ATP-activated $P2X_4$ receptors (Yamamoto et al., 2003). These actions may play an important role in the remodeling of the vasculature that occurs as a chronic response to elevated mean arterial pressure (i.e., hypertension). The endothelial cell signaling pathways by which the mechanical signals are converted to functional responses have been intensively investigated and have resulted in the identification of multiple pathways that ultimately impact upon the extracellular matrix and cell–cell adhesion molecules (Shyy & Chien, 2002; Li, Huang, & Hsu, 2005). These pathways involve extracellular glycosaminoglycans and adhesion molecules such as the selectin, platelet endothelial cell adhesion molecule-1 (PECAM-1). These molecules have been proposed to play a role in endothelial cell migration by activating integrins that engage members of the Rho GTPases (e.g., Rac) to promote actin polymerization. Alternatively, shear stress may activate different Rho GTPases (e.g., p160ROCK) that leads to disassembly of focal adhesions. Thus, the downstream signaling modulates a number of cell functions that lead to structural modification (Li, Huang, & Hsu, 2005; Shyy & Chien, 2002).

VSMCs respond to external stimulation by producing contraction or relaxation depending on the cell signaling pathway that is engaged. In addition, many external signals can evoke both acute responses and long-term changes in cell function that impact cell growth and/or hypertrophy leading to physical changes in cell structure. These latter changes often appear associated with specific pathologies including hypertension. Interestingly, either contraction or dilation can be initiated by the same hormonal stimulus that may also evoke some of the nuclear signaling events so the final response observed is determined by the ability of the cell to innately regulate both acute and long-term signaling and the phenotype and environment in which the cell exists. The mechanism(s) by which VSMCs contract and relax have been studied and presented in great detail (Griendling et al., 2009; Rang, Dale, Ritter, & Moore, 2003; Watts, 2010; Webb, 2003) and are only described briefly. Ultimately, contraction is created by altering free intracellular calcium concentrations binding to calmodulin, which converts the myosin light-chain kinase to its activated form. Contraction occurs when the activated kinase phosphorylates the myosin light chain causing it to detach from actin filaments. The free actin filaments activate the myosin Mg^{++}-ATPase, which forms actin–myosin cross-bridges with thick filaments in smooth muscle and thin filaments in striated muscle. The process is reversed by another enzyme, myosin phosphatase, which is responsible for removing the phosphate from the myosin light chain. Another family of proteins activated through G-protein-coupled receptors (GPCR) stimulation that impact on this process is the guanine nucleotide exchange factors whose activation phosphorylates the small molecular weight G-protein, Rho. Rho phosphorylation stimulates the activity of Rho kinase, which inhibits myosin phosphatase leading to an increased level of myosin light-chain phosphorylation (Griendling et al., 2009; Webb, 2003). The Rho kinase inhibitor, Y-27632, alters the formation of actin stress fibers, focal adhesion, and cellular contraction suggesting that it was a potential target for the development of agents that could treat glaucoma (Rao, Deng, Kumar, & Epstein, 2001). The ability of different agonists to activate these components of the cycle varies such that the contraction develops in two different phases. The two phases include an acute rapid component that is sometimes following by a prolonged phase of contraction. Of particular importance is the fact that endogenous hormones as well as receptor selective agonists differ in the capacity to produce these various stages. For example, contraction associated with norepinephrine tends to be prolonged while that observed with Ang II presents as a transient contraction (Rang et al., 2003).

In most vascular smooth muscle, depolarization is associated with calcium influx generated by opening L-type voltage-dependent calcium channels unlike skeletal and most cardiac muscle where depolarization is associated with sodium influx (Harder & Sperelakis, 1979; Rang et al., 2003; Watts, 2010). Contraction of all muscle types is dependent upon the concentration of free calcium in the cytoplasm which in smooth muscle can be modulated by influx as well as triggered release. Therefore, vascular smooth muscle is particularly sensitive to agents that modulate the membrane potential and those that block voltage-dependent calcium channels. The primary extrinsic regulators of free intracellular calcium include a number of circulating or autocrine hormones that activate one member of the super family of GPCR. These receptors and hormones include α_1-adrenoceptors (norepinephrine and epinephrine), AT_1 receptor (Ang II), H_1 receptor (histamine), and ET_A receptor (ET) among others (Watts, 2010; Webb, 2003). The process is the well-documented classic signaling cascade initiated by the interaction of a serpentine receptor and a heterotrimeric G-protein. For the receptors identified above, the G_q α subunit dissociates from the βγ subunits and activates either phospholipase Cβ to generate inositol trisphosphate (IP3) and diacylglycerol (DAG) or phospholipase D (PLD) to produce DAG (Watts, 2010; Webb, 2003). Some IP3 releases calcium from intracellular stores by activating IP3 receptors on the endoplasmic reticulum, while some IP3 is phosphorylated to inositol tetraphosphate which may promote additional calcium influx (Rang et al., 2003). The βγ subunits activate ion channels (e.g., L-type voltage-gated calcium channels or others) to increase extracellular calcium influx. DAG stimulates PKC, an enzyme that phosphorylates many substrates that act in the contractile process and as transcription factors (Griendling et al., 2009; Watts, 2010). Thus, contraction of vascular smooth muscle through GPCR-mediated mechanisms has the potential to induce two different types of contraction (i.e., transient and rapid or sustained and slow) as well as activate intracellular transcription processes that may be important for long-term events like muscle remodeling.

The long-term consequences following activation of a GPCR are thought to be due to the elevation of free intracellular calcium and the activation of PKC. PKC activates downstream partners in the mitogen-activated pathway kinase cascade including extracellular signal-regulated kinases (ERKs) and Jun kinase, both of which activate transcription factors (Griendling et al., 2009; Watts, 2010). In addition to the effects on contractile proteins, elevated intracellular calcium also activates the MAP kinase pathway through receptor-tyrosine kinases via the Ras/Raf cascade as well as factors in signaling pathways that promote cell growth (Griendling et al., 2009; Rang et al., 2003). In particular, the suggestion was made that one member of the family of proteins known as regulators of G-protein signaling, might be an important target for drug development (Tang et al., 2003) though drugs with this specific mechanism of action would also be expected to negatively impact upon the immune system (Doggrell, 2004) and none have been introduced into clinical practice at this time. The biochemical signaling pathways involved in regulating smooth muscle growth and hypertrophy have attracted considerable attention with the identification of several growth factors and regulators of transcription that may play significant roles (Griendling et al., 2009; Newby, Southgate, & Assender, 1992; Ueba, Kawakami, & Yaginuma, 1997). Many of these factors activate tyrosine kinase receptors, which may provide another protein family target for new drug development. A number of growth factors that have been proposed to regulate the extracellular matrix that permits hypertrophy and hyperplasia may also offer novel targets for drug development. Relaxation of vascular smooth muscle uses several intracellular signaling pathways including guanylyl and adenylyl cyclases (Rang et al., 2003; Watts, 2010; Webb, 2003). Activation of guanylyl cyclase stimulates production of cGMP that activates protein kinase G and promotes dephosphorylation of the myosin light chain. Similarly, cyclic AMP (cAMP) produced by activation of adenylyl cyclase stimulates protein kinase A and modifies the phosphorylation state of the myosin light chain (Rang et al., 2003; Watts, 2010). The intracellular levels of both cAMP and cGMP are controlled through the activity of a large number of phosphodiesterase (PDE) enzyme isoforms that vary in cyclic nucleotide specificity and tissue distribution and function that make them attractive targets for drug development. While initially employed in acute heart failure (inamrinone-like agents), other inhibitors of select PDE isoforms have been developed that are therapeutically targeted to the management of erectile dysfunction and asthma. Though these agents have been successful in the treatment of erectile dysfunction, the success of agents in the management of asthma has been disappointing but there has been some limited success with their use for the treatment of pulmonary hypertension (see Section IV.C.2).

III. Experimental Models of Hypertension

A. Introduction

A number of animal models for hypertension exist (see Badyal, Lata, & Dadhich, 2003; Scriabine, 2007; Herrera & Ruiz-Opazo, 2009). Based upon the polygenic nature of the disease and the multiple complicating factors, it is not surprising that many models of hypertension would be available. Our understanding of the pathogenesis and utility of drugs used to manage hypertension has been greatly expanded over the past many decades by employing such animal models. These models have also been used to develop new agents to manage hypertension (Badyal et al., 2003; Scriabine, 2007). A variety of different animal models can be useful since essential hypertension (the primary focus for drug development) is a multifactorial condition. Animal models of hypertension and antihypertensive drugs have proven to be very predictive and reliable with respect to compound efficacy even for such a complex disease.

Animal models of hypertension range from those that are genetic and spontaneous to ones that are produced experimentally either by surgical manipulation or by dietary influences or chemical administration. Equally important is the fact that the animal models are created using different phenotypic bases, which provides even greater predictability about the effectiveness of drugs in various forms of essential hypertension. The early animal models relied on larger animals and, in particular, dogs. However, the increasing cost of purchase and maintenance and regulatory control of these animals have shifted greater attention to smaller animals including rats and mice. For an animal model to be effective in the drug development process, it should be able to accurately predict the potential utility of agents, not be difficult or costly to run in large numbers and be comparable to some form of human hypertension. This last characteristic is important and could be partly responsible for the fact that the number of animal models is large. Therefore, models will be discussed using major representatives of a model system rather than an exhaustive discussion of each model system.

B. Surgically Induced Hypertension (Renovascular Hypertension)

The development of hypertension following surgical intervention by occluding the main renal artery is one of the more commonly employed animal models for studying hypertension. Partial constriction of the renal artery of a dog elevated mean arterial pressure to the level of hypertension over a period of 3–4 days, which then remained constant (Goldblatt, Lynch, Hanzel, & Summerville, 1934). Similar effects were observed in a number of other species and the Goldblatt model has been used to induce hypertension in rabbits and monkeys as well as rats and mice. The model leads to the establishment of hypertension resulting from the permanent or transient occlusion of the renal artery with or without unilateral nephrectomy. This has led to the development of three different "Goldblatt" models based upon the nature of the surgical intervention. These are referred to as the two kidney/one clip (2K1C) model, the one kidney/one clip (1K1C) model, and the two kidney/two clip (2K2C) model.

Each surgery employs different levels of involvement with the 2K1C being the simplest with banding or clipping only occurring on one renal artery while leaving both kidneys intact. This intervention causes elevations in plasma renin activity leading to renin-dependent hypertension early that is supplanted by a volume-dependent hypertension after about 6 weeks. In contrast, the 1K1C model employs a unilateral nephrectomy of the kidney opposite to the one in which the renal artery is clipped. This intervention leaves plasma renin levels relatively normal with very rapid salt and water accumulation leading primarily to a volume-dependent hypertension. Finally, in the 2K2C model, the clipping leads to ischemia of both kidneys, which elevates plasma renin levels and also permits salt and water retention thereby emulating the complicated forms of human hypertension that possess both renin-dependent and renin-independent but volume-dependent hypertension. The development of these models in small animals (i.e., rats and mice) has increased their utility in compound assessment by saving compound when dosed on a weight basis, reducing cost and providing the ability to use an appropriate sample size for better statistical analysis.

A number of other renovascular or surgically induced forms of hypertension have been employed in dogs, rabbits, and rats. These models include (1) compression of the renal parenchyma by either "wrapping" one or both of the kidneys in cellophane (Page, 1939) or surgically compressing the kidney with ligatures (Grollman, 1955); (2) compression of the aorta (coarctation) above or near the renal arteries (Brilla, Pick, Tan, Janicki, & Weber, 1990; Thiedemann, Holubarsch, Medugarac, & Jacob, 1983); or (3) actual reduction in renal mass (Anderson, Meyer, Rennke, & Brenner, 1985). The models using compression of the renal parenchyma can be performed using a protocol that "wraps" or ligates both kidneys or wraps or ligates a single kidney and removes the contralateral kidney (Badyal et al., 2003). Another form of surgically induced hypertension is accomplished by denervation of the sinoaortic baroreceptor afferents (Krieger, 1964; Reis, Doba, & Nathan, 1976). This form of surgical manipulation has been employed in dogs, rabbits, and rats (Cowley, Liard, & Guyton, 1973; Krieger, 1964). In dogs, the elevation in blood pressure resolves after only a few days, making this procedure appropriate for evaluating acute hypertension (Badyal et al., 2003). In contrast, aortic baroreceptor denervation or lesioning of the nucleus tractus solitarius in rats produces a sustained elevation in pressure (Krieger, 1964; Reis et al., 1976) that is similar in nature to that produced by surgical manipulation of the kidneys (i.e., renovascular hypertension) and desoxycorticosterone acetate (DOCA)-induced hypertension (see below). Thus, renovascular and surgically induced models of hypertension have considerable utility in evaluating potential antihypertensive agents as these models emulate very common forms of human hypertension.

C. Dietary-Induced Hypertension

The importance of diet in the treatment of hypertension has long been recognized and, most recently, an important component of any treatment regimen. Some animal models have utilized diet as a method of inducing hypertension to develop a model that emulates some aspects of the human disorder. The role of enhanced sodium intake coupled to normal or reduced sodium elimination is a significant contribution to the development of hypertension. Chronic exposure to excess salt via the diet produces hypertension in rats, rabbits, and chicks, and in dogs with one kidney removed. In rats, excess sodium intake produces morphological changes that mimic those observed in human hypertension (Dahl, 1960). Dahl and his associates developed genetic strains of rats that exhibit altered sensitivity and resistance to the effects of chronic dietary salt exposure providing better insights into the cellular and molecular mechanisms that may underlie the development of hypertension in response to excessive salt intake. Of particular interest is that these strains of rats have led to the identification of three distinct genes that are involved in the regulation of salt sensitivity (Lighthall, Hamilton, & Hamlyn, 2004). Other models have employed the use of the NO synthase inhibitor, L-NNA, the glucocorticoid, dexamethasone, or the tetrahydrobiopterin (BH4) inhibitor, 2,4-diamino-6-hydroxypyrimidine, delivered chronically in the drinking water to induce hypertension (Mitchell, Wallerath, & Förstermann, 2007).

D. Endocrine and Drug-Induced Hypertension

Mineralocorticoids are physiologically important for the regulation of sodium and water in humans and other species. Selye was the first to describe the hypertension produced by DOCA and salt administration (Selye & Bois, 1957). This form of production of hypertension has been employed in primates, pigs, dogs, and rodents with much success. A variation of this protocol has been employed with rats in which a unilateral nephrectomy was performed followed by DOCA administration that led to the development of sustained hypertension (Katholi & Naftilon, 1980). With additional salt administration that is absolutely required for development, this form of hypertension has been associated with increased release of vasopressin leading to water retention and vasoconstriction and elevated activity of the RAAS leading to elevated SNS activity. The sustained form of hypertension appears to be low-renin salt dependent and has been used to evaluate the ability of ET antagonists to reduce blood pressure as the ET system is involved in the production of low-renin hypertension (van den Meiracker, 2002). Another intriguing observation obtained from this particular model of hypertension is the potential involvement of the peroxisome proliferator-activated receptor γ (PPARγ) in the development of hypertension. Rosiglitazone, an activator of PPARγ, prevented the development of hypertension in this animal model (Iglarz et al., 2003) thus identifying a new target for drug discovery.

While the DOCA–salt model is one of the more routinely used forms of endocrine-induced hypertension, recent advances in knowledge regarding the regulation of blood pressure have suggested other interventions that may be important, leading to the development of other models that include chronic administration of AT II using osmotic mini-pumps and the cholinergic agonists, physostigmine, or oxotremorine. The cholinergic agonists appear to produce hypertension caused by activation of the CNS cholinergic systems that regulate the peripheral SNS (Buccafusco, 1996). Hypertension has also been developed following chronic inhibition of NO generation (Mitchell et al., 2007) using chronic exposure to the nonselective NO synthase inhibitor, Nω-nitro-L-arginine methyl ester (L-NAME), or other NO synthase inhibitors delivered through the drinking water. The role of vascular endothelium-mediated production of NO in the regulation of TPR has become the focus of considerable interest as a potential new target for drug discovery.

Another component of an endocrine role in hypertension is the involvement of estrogens in the development of hypertension. Estrogens administered to estrogen-deficient rats and humans can produce hypotension (see Section IV.F), while postmenopausal women develop blunted blood pressure responses during the normal day–night cycle when compared to premenopausal women of the same age (Mercuro et al., 2004; Owens, Stoney, & Matthews, 1993). In addition, transgenic mice deficient in the estrogen receptor β (ERβ) develop sustained hypertension and an exaggerated vasoconstrictor response to α-adrenoceptor agonists (Zhu et al., 2002). Polymorphisms of the ERβ genes (*ESR1* and *ESR2*) are also associated with elevated blood pressure (Ogawa, Emi, & Shiraki, 2000; Peter et al., 2005). Interestingly, in both these genetic abnormalities the sustained elevations in blood pressure do not appear to be gender related since comparable changes in blood pressure are observed in both males and females.

E. Genetic and Transgenic Models of Hypertension

There are currently well over 200 inbred strains of rats used to study human disease with a number of these models having been employed to investigate the pathogenesis and management of CV diseases (see Cowley et al., 2004; Kwitek et al., 2006). In fact, there is increasing attention to describing the genomics associated with the development of these inbred strains to better understand the epigenetics surrounding the development of the disorder of hypertension (Cowley et al., 2004; Lee, 2007; Malek, et al., 2006). In the post-genomic era, the groundwork laid by defining the genetics of these various animal models will be important as investigators attempt to define appropriate QTLs that may associate with one or more phenotypic characteristic intrinsic to the animal model. Since hypertension is a multifactorial, polygenic disorder, the inability to define a single gene as being causative is not surprising. However, as attempts continue to develop gene therapy it will be critical to be certain that any approach targets the appropriate genes. However, since success with gene therapy has been rare, it is unlikely to provide a satisfactory management scheme for a disease like hypertension that is subject to multiple interventions including environmental.

Though the first strain of rats with inheritable hypertension was the genetically hypertensive (GH) rat, the most common genetic model of hypertension is the spontaneously hypertensive rat (SHR) (Okamoto & Aoki, 1963). The GH rat develops hypertension through a progressive increase in systemic vascular resistance making it a useful model for one component of human hypertension. A number of substrains of the SHR, developed by selective inbreeding, have generated animals that are stroke prone (SHRsp) or express other inheritable abnormalities such as hyperlipidemia and obesity (the Lyon rat) in addition to hypertension (Rapp, 2000). The mechanisms underlying the pathogenesis of hypertension in the SHR have historically been tested by comparison to the genetic control strain, the Wistar Kyoto (WKY) rat that was developed from the same population base. However, many investigators suggest that these animals may not represent an appropriate control (Festing & Bender, 1984; Johnson, Ely, & Turner, 1992; Kurtz, Montano, Chan, & Kabra, 1989; Rapp, 2000) since there are considerable genetic differences from the SHR. Nonetheless, this model has been successfully used to investigate the genetic mechanisms underlying the pathogenesis of hypertension and to evaluate potential antihypertensive drugs and mechanism of action of existing agents. The predictive nature of this is very high due to the very low number of false positives that are produced through initially screening.

Another animal strain of interest is the Dahl salt sensitive (SS/Jr) strain (Dahl, Heine, & Tassinari, 1962a, 1962b; Rapp, 1982). This strain has become popular because hypertension develops spontaneously in response to exposure to dietary salt and the availability of another strain that is resistant to development of hypertension when exposed to the same dietary salt level (the DH/Jr) may be an even more intriguing genetic model to use to distinguish why these animals do not respond to salt (Dahl et al., 1962a, 1962b; Rapp, 1982). Another model, the Sabra model of hypertension (Ben-Ishay, Saliternik, & Welner, 1972), responds to salt but is phenotypically distinct from the Dahl model (Ben-Ishay & Yagil, 1994). This model develops hypertension in response to dietary salt but does not develop spontaneous hypertension and may provide a model system that is specifically able to identify the genetic basis for salt selectivity (Yagil et al., 1996). The value of these animal models is based upon the fact that among humans, between 15 and 29% of normotensive or borderline hypertensive Caucasians, respectively, and 27 and 50% of normotensive and borderline hypertensive African-American subjects, respectively, are believed to be salt sensitive (Sullivan, 1991). Thus, the models may represent a significant component of the human hypertensive population and provide valuable predictive tools for therapeutic agents that possess efficacy against the disease.

Other animal models of spontaneous hypertension include the Milan strain (Bianchi, Ferrari, & Barber, 1984) that develops hypertension apparently due to alterations in cytoskeletal membrane protein genes that encode proteins such as the Na^+–K^+ ATPase. The Lyon strain (Vincent & Sassard, 1994), developed in 1969 from outbred Sprague–Dawley animals, is characterized by mild-to-moderate hypertension that is also associated with increased weight, hyperlipidemia, and increased sensitivity to salt (Vincent et al., 1993). This model is useful in the context of the high prevalence of hyperlipidemia and obesity in the population at large. The Wistar fatty rat (Kava, Peterson, West, & Greenwood, 1990) from a cross between the Zucker and WKY rats displays hypertension associated with hyperinsulinemia representing the first rat model of obese type 2 diabetes (Sone, Suzuki, Takahashi, & Yamada, 2001). Only males develop hypertension concomitant with hyperinsulinemia, hyperlipidemia, hyperglycemia, glucose intolerance, and reduced insulin sensitivity, making it a useful animal model predictive of agents that may be effective in managing type 2 diabetics where hypertension is a comorbid component. The Fawn-Hooded Hypertensive rat originated as a cross between German-Brown and Lashley white rats that developed hypertension associated with abnormal platelet function and renal abnormalities caused by hyperalbuminemia (Kuijpers & Gruys, 1984; Kuijpers, Provoost, & De Jong, 1986; Kuijpers, Van Zutphen, & De Jong, 1987). This strain was further extended by inbreeding programs to develop a normotensive control strain (Provoost & De Keijzer, 1993; Verseput, Provoost, Van Tol, Koomans, & Joles, 1997). Considerable efforts have been focused on developing transgenic models of hypertension in both rat and mouse. In the rat, this effort has focused on transgenic manipulation of the RAAS system. The TGR (mREN2) 27 transgenic rat is hypertensive apparently due to overexpression of renin that was produced by the introduction of the murine *Ren-2* gene into the rat germ line (Mullins, Peters, & Ganten, 1990; Paul, Wagner, Hoffmann, Urata, & Ganten, 1994). However, attempts to manipulate the genes encoding other components of the RAAS have not yielded useful models. Nonetheless, efforts continue to assess the potential for transgenic mutation of other targets, including atrial natriuretic peptide and arginine vasopressin. Transgenic mice that lack the estrogen receptor (ER) (see above) display hypertension and offer a useful model system for studying the impact of menopause on CV function. Considerable efforts have been made to develop transgenic models but the fact that candidate QTLs for various components of essential hypertension occur in all rat genes except 6, 11, 12, and 15 (Scriabine, 2007) suggests that this may be a challenging task.

IV. Novel Targets/Agents for Therapeutic Management of Hypertension

At least 970 million individuals are affected by hypertension worldwide and by 2025, it is predicted that approximately 1.6 billion people will be diagnosed as hypertensive (World Heart Federation, 2009). Approximately 30% of these individuals will not be adequately controlled despite the current therapeutics available (Fig. 1, Table IV) reinforcing the need for new drug classes. Additionally, newer generations from existing drug classes (Tables II and III) with better efficacy and reduced side effects may lead to improved drug therapy for hypertension.

A. Novel Targets for Regulating the ANS

The ANS, particularly the SNS, is a logical therapeutic target for the management of hypertension with some of the older antihypertensives being introduced on the premise that interrupting SNS activity would attenuate the excessive vasoconstriction modulated by the SNS. For example, when introduced nearly 50 years ago, α-methyldopa was thought to lower blood pressure in hypertensive individuals by functioning as a "false neurotransmitter" in the peripheral SNS by interfering with norepinephrine synthesis (Cannon, Whitlock, Morris, Angers, & Laragh, 1962), a premise that was later deemed incorrect. The actual mechanism was due to activation of α_{2A}-adrenoceptors in the brainstem by α-methyl-norepinephrine (a metabolite of α-methyldopa) resulting in an inhibition of central sympathetic tone that ultimately resulted in a reduction in arterial pressure. Similar effects occurred with clonidine. Extensive studies on the neural control of blood pressure using agents like clonidine led to a novel class of centrally acting drugs that targeted a non-adrenergic receptor in the brainstem (Garty, Deka-Starosta, Chang, Kopin, & Goldstein, 1990; Koss, 1983; Tibirica, Mermet, Feldman, Gonon, & Bousquet, 1989). This class of drugs that includes rilmenidine and moxonidine targets the imidazoline receptor in the rostral ventrolateral medulla (RVLM) to reduce sympathetic tone in the periphery (Bousquet, Dontenwill, Greney, & Feldman, 1998; El-Mas & Abdel-Rahman, 2000; Feldman et al., 1998; Li, Wang & Abdel-Rahman, 2005; Mao & Abdel-Rahman, 1998; Wang, Li, & Abdel-Rahman, 2005). Research on the I_1-imidazoline receptor (I_1R) has been hampered by the lack of pure I_1R agonists, as rilmenidine and moxonidine also exhibit weak α_{2A}-adrenoceptor (α_{2A} AR) agonist activity (Bousquet et al., 1998; Feldman et al., 1998; Szabo, 2002). Mouse nischarin, a homolog of the human imidazoline receptor antisera-selective (IRAS; Alahari, 2003; Alahari, Lee, & Juliano, 2000) discovered when transfection of IRAS cDNA into the CHO cells led to the expression of high-affinity I_1R binding sites for moxonidine and rilmenidine (Piletz, Wang, & Zhu, 2003), made it possible to delineate the signaling and function of these proteins *in vitro* (Lim & Hong, 2004; Reddig, Xu, & Juliano, 2005; Sun, Chang, & Ernsberger, 2007; Zhang & Abdel-Rahman, 2006) that was common with that of I_1R. In addition, CHO cells stably expressing IRAS exhibit enhanced phosphatidylcholine-specific phospholipase C and ERK signaling (Li et al., 2006); the latter signaling pathway is triggered by rilmenidine or moxonidine in PC12 cells (Zhang, El-Mas, & Abdel-Rahman, 2001) that lack the α_{2A}-AR (Ernsberger et al., 1995; Separovic, Kester, & Ernsberger, 1996). It is noteworthy that phosphorylated extracellular regulated kinase (pERK1/2) generation in the RVLM has been implicated in the hypotension caused by I_1R activation (Zhang & Abdel-Rahman, 2005) and that nischarin homology exists among different species (Piletz et al., 2003; Sun et al., 2007). Despite differences in the methodologies used for the development of polyclonal nischarin antibodies and anti-nischarin antisense oligodeoxynucleotides (ODNs), these molecular probes have facilitated the identification of nischarin expression and the impact of its knockdown on I_1R-mediated signaling in PC12 cells (Sun et al., 2007; Zhang & Abdel-Rahman, 2006). The use of these molecular probes was crucial for elucidating the biological function of the nischarin/I_1R at the integrative level. Reported findings present the first evidence that knocking down nischarin expression in the brainstem using antisense ODN virtually abolishes the neurochemical (enhanced pERK1/2 production in the RVLM) and hypotensive responses elicited by central I_1 receptor activation. These findings support the hypothesis that brainstem (i.e., RVLM) nischarin serves as, or at least shares, a common signaling pathway with the I_1 receptor (Zhang & Abdel-Rahman, 2008). Further studies are needed to elucidate the mechanisms implicated in nischarin signaling *in vivo* and its role in central regulation of blood pressure as well as its potential as a molecular target for new antihypertensive medications. Interestingly, recent studies have established the dependence of clonidine-evoked hypotension on central adenosine A_{2A} receptor signaling, which involves downstream activation of brainstem ERK1/2–NOS pathway (Nassar & Abdel-Rahman, 2006, 2008, 2009). These findings have identified central adenosine receptors as potential novel targets for new antihypertensive drugs. On the other hand, the sympathoinhibitory and hypotensive action of clonidine could be counteracted by concurrent administration of ethanol (Mao & Abdel-Rahman, 1998; Mao, Li, & Abdel-Rahman, 2003). This hemodynamic interaction is clinically serious because ethanol also exacerbates the α_{2A}-AR-mediated sedative effects of clonidine (Bender & Abdel-Rahman, 2009; Mao & Abdel-Rahman, 1996).

Nebivolol, a third-generation β_1-adrenoceptor selective blocker that lacks intrinsic sympathomimetic activity (Table III), exhibits pharmacological and pharmacodynamic properties that are distinct compared with other β-blockers. In addition to selectively blocking the β_1-adrenoceptor, nebivolol promotes endothelium-dependent vasodilation through the NOS–NO pathway in different regional vascular beds (Weiss, 2006). Recent studies have shown that nebivolol increases renal tissue levels of bioavailable NO and reduces renal fibrosis in an animal model of high-renin hypertension (Whaley-Connell et al., 2009). In addition, nebivolol has been proposed to offer some advantage in the management of obese and moderately obese patients due to the fact that the combination of actions apparently has no effect on lipid and carbohydrate metabolism in obese patients (Manrique, Whaley-Connell, & Sowers, 2009).

B. Novel Targets Engaged with the Renin–Angiotensin–Aldosterone System

The RAAS plays important role in blood pressure control as well as in the pathophysiology of hypertension. As mentioned above (Section II.E), hypertension that is caused by or associated with hyperactivity in the RAAS is classified as high-renin hypertension. Such a classification has clinical ramifications because individuals with high-renin hypertension are usually treated with drug(s) that inhibit RAAS activity unless such drugs are contraindicated. It is important to note, however, that it is rather difficult to categorize an individual as high-renin hypertensive based merely on plasma renin level and/or activity. Even with the advent of more reliable biochemical tests (e.g., aldosterone:renin ratio), there is some skepticism toward utilizing the high- versus low-renin hypertension classification as a basis for prescribing medications for the treatment of hypertension for at least two reasons. First, the notion that hypertension in African-Americans is of the *low-renin type* has become well accepted despite the lack of unequivocal evidence to support this notion. Unfortunately, general acceptance of this notion has resulted in denying many African-American hypertensive patients appropriate treatment with RAAS-inhibiting drugs (ACEIs and ARBs). The recent use of BiDil® (Taylor et al., 2004) has also opened opportunities to investigate other forms of management based upon ethnicity. Second, there are additional benefits conferred by these drugs that go beyond the reduction in blood pressure given a well-established contribution of Ang II, acting via activation of AT_1R, to increased cellular production of ROS a proinflammatory molecule that is a major contributor to kidney and endothelial dysfunction as well as cardiac myocyte injury that occurs in hypertensive individuals (Lu et al., 2009; Ren et al., 2008). ACEIs and ARBs are expected to confer renal and CV protective effects independent of their blood pressure lowering effects.

The additional benefits of ACEIs are not limited to the heart, kidney, and vasculature, but also extend to the brain. Although mechanistic studies are needed to elucidate the mechanism of action, evidence-based medicine highlights the findings of the observational Cardiovascular Health Study that demonstrated the ability of ACEIs to reduce cognitive decline in individuals by 65% per year of exposure (World Heart Federation, 2009). This effect is *centrally* mediated because the benefit conferred was associated only with therapy with ACEIs that cross the blood–brain barrier (captopril, lisinopril, perindopril, ramipril, and trandolapril) and was independent of the antihypertensive effect of the drug; this notion is supported by the inability of *non-centrally active ACEIs* (benazepril, enalapril, moexipril, and quinapril) to confer this benefit despite the reduction in blood pressure (Sink et al., 2009). On the other hand, ACEIs and ARBs are contraindicated in patients with renal artery stenosis because these agents will compromise the ability of the kidney to autoregulate glomerular filtration via enhanced Ang II–AT_1R signaling in the efferent arteriole. It must be emphasized that the newest antihypertensive medication (the only antihypertensive drug approved over the past decade) targets the RAAS at it origin. Aliskiren, a direct renin inhibitor (DRI) (Riccioni, Vitulano, D'Orazio, & Bellocci, 2009), lowers blood pressure by acting as direct inhibitor of renin catalytic activity that has prompted interest in pursuing other agents with this primary site and mechanism of action. Combination therapy with aliskiren and an ACEI or ARB resulted in significant additional blood pressure reductions over monotherapy in patients with mild-to-moderate hypertension. The antihypertensive effect conferred by the combination was also associated with a reduction in surrogate markers of end-organ damage in patients with heart failure or diabetic nephropathy, with generally similar safety and tolerability to the component monotherapies (Düsing & Sellers, 2009). These recent findings with the combination therapy with aliskiren/ACEI or aliskiren/ARB are clinically significant given the superior clinical outcomes with these combinations over ACEI/ARB combination. However, whether these benefits conferred by combining aliskiren and ACEI or ARB will have favorable long-term outcomes remain to be determined (Düsing & Sellers, 2009).

I. Development of Domain-Selective ACEIs

Advances in molecular biology, combinatorial chemistry, high-throughput screening, protein structure analysis, and bioinformatics have led to the development of the concept of "structure-based drug development." The development of first-generation ACEIs succeeded through a combination of hard work and serendipity since the agents were developed without the availability of purified enzyme and without knowledge of the protein sequence or three-dimensional structure. The determination of the three-dimensional crystal structure (Natesh, Schwager, Sturrock, & Acharya, 2003) has now provided scientists with the tools required to begin to explore novel approaches to inhibition of the enzyme that may lead to better therapeutic agents with greater selectivity and fewer adverse effects. Through these efforts, a number of potential novel agents have been developed that include the vasopeptidase inhibitors such as omapatrilat (Acharya, Sturrock, Riordan, & Ehlers, 2003) as well as agents that target selective domains identified in the ACE tertiary structure by X-ray crystallography (Redelinghuys, Nchinda, & Sturrock, 2005). The vasopeptidase inhibitors were highly regarded early in their development as they targeted both the ACE and the neutral endopeptidase enzyme (another metallopeptidase-like ACE) that is responsible for degradation of the natriuretic peptides that are diuretic and vasodilatory and appear to be elevated in conditions such hypertension and CHF (Weber, 2001). Unfortunately, the first generation of these agents has not fulfilled the promise that they possessed due to the fact that the incidence of side effects (i.e., angioedema and cough) did not appear to be reduced compared to the ACEIs. In contrast, the identification of two distinct domains of ACE that each has an active site that appears to possess selective substrate and inhibitor selectivity (Redelinghuys et al., 2005) has provided another opportunity for the development of novel therapeutic agents focused upon the RAAS. The two domains have begun to be characterized functionally with both the C and the N domain apparently responsible for the hydrolysis of bradykinin and the N domain also responsible for hydrolysis of Ang I and Ang_{1-7} (see below) as well as amyloid β-peptide that is elevated in Alzheimer's disease (Redelinghuys et al., 2005). The development of novel agents that possess domain selectivity is an attractive target that will require substantial effort as the domains display nearly 90% homology. However, the diligent effort and serendipity that permitted the development of selective ACEIs may also provide the health-care community with new agents to manage hypertension.

2. Ang_{1-7}–Mas Receptor Agonists

Novel targets for new RAAS-related drugs have also been identified from studies on RAAS signaling. One target of interest is the newly identified Ang II fragment, Ang_{1-7}, which is formed from its precursor Ang II by the catalytic activity of ACE2 (Iwai & Horiuchi, 2009). Although the signaling pathway of the ACE2–Ang_{1-7} axis has not yet been fully elucidated, the Mas oncogene has been suggested as a receptor for Ang_{1-7} and activation of the Mas receptor by Ang_{1-7} leads to vasodilatation, natriuresis, anti-proliferation, and an increase in the bradykinin–NO signaling. Akt phosphorylation, PKC activation, and MAP kinase inhibition have also been implicated in Ang_{1-7}–Mas receptor signaling pathway. Although Ang_{1-7} is derived from Ang I and Ang II, the catalytic efficiency of ACE2 is approximately 400-fold higher with Ang II as a substrate than with Ang I (see Iwai & Horiuchi, 2009). Therefore, the ACE2–Ang_{1-7}–Mas receptor axis in the RAAS can be an important target for the therapy of CV and metabolic disorders. Overall, this axis appears to act as a counter-regulatory system against the ACE–Ang II–AT_1R axis (Iwai & Horiuchi, 2009). Importantly, such an axis might contribute to the antihypertensive and other beneficial CV effects conferred by ARBs by shifting accumulated Ang II to be converted into Ang_{1-7}. Currently, there are no available Ang_{1-7} agonists for the treatment of hypertension. The use of Ang_{1-7} is not clinically feasible because of the pharmacokinetic limitations of the peptide (Iusuf et al., 2008). Nonetheless, the development of nonpeptide analogs of Ang_{1-7} constitutes a novel target for the management of hypertension. If successful, this new strategy will be the first to directly activate the vasodilating side of the RAAS.

3. Inhibitors of CNS APA and Phosphatidylinositol 3-Kinase (PI3-K)

As discussed above, the brain has its own synthetic pathway(s) for generating Ang II and other related peptides (Bodineau et al., 2008; Reaux-Le Goazigo et al., 2005). Despite this knowledge, little attention has been directed towards developing medications that target the RAAS in the brain. Genetic and pharmacological interventions that specifically targeted the brain RAS have clearly identified a role for brain Ang II, acting directly on its receptors, and Ang III (derived from Ang II via APA) in hypertension. Elegant genetic studies have shown that inhibition of brain RAS decreased blood pressure in hypertensive rats (Baltatu, Campos, & Bader, 2004; Davisson, 2003; Kagiyama, Varela, Phillips, & Galli, 2001). Realizing that APA catalytic degradation of Ang II resulted in the formation of the potent pressor peptide Ang III in the brain constituted a basis for considering APA a novel target for the treatment of hypertension (see Reaux-Le Goazigo et al., 2005). Experimental findings with a potent systemically active APA inhibitor, RB150, has furnished a foundation for developing a new class of centrally acting drugs that specifically inhibit Ang III formation in the brain (Bodineau et al., 2008; Fournie-Zaluski et al., 2004; Reaux-Le Goazigo et al., 2005). There is also evidence that suggests the involvement of heightened neuronal phosphatidylinositol 3-kinase (PI3-K) signaling in the central sympathoexcitatory action of Ang II in the SHR (Sun, Du, Sumners, & Raizada, 2003; Yang & Raizada, 1999). These findings highlight another potential therapeutic target within the brain for the treatment of hypertension via inhibiting the central RAS.

C. Novel Strategies for the Management of Pulmonary Hypertension

Pulmonary arterial hypertension might develop independent of systemic hypertension and can result in life-threatening right heart failure (see Kabunga & Coghlan, 2008; McLaughlin et al., 2004). Therefore, highly selective and fast-acting pulmonary artery vasodilators will have clinical utility. The urgency with which pulmonary hypertension requires attention makes this disorder one of particular interest in order to prevent the relatively high rate of mortality that is caused by this type of hypertension. The following are proposed novel strategies for the treatment of elevated pulmonary arterial pressure.

1. ET_A Receptor Antagonists

Currently, two ET receptor antagonists are available for the treatment of pulmonary hypertension, bosentan and ambrisentan. The development of the ET receptor antagonists for treatment of pulmonary hypertension was based on the findings that the endothelium releases potent vasoconstrictors with the most notable being the peptide, ET. This peptide is considered the most potent vasoconstrictor known to date and plays an important role in maintaining vascular tone by activating the ET_A receptor. Therefore, pathophysiological overactivity of ET_A receptor signaling is expected to increase total vascular resistance. However, perhaps due to differential distribution of the ET receptors in different vascular beds, overactivity of ET receptor signaling has been implicated in pathological pulmonary vasoconstriction and pulmonary hypertension (Aubert & Juillerat-Jeanneret, 2009; Channick et al., 2004; Kabunga & Coghlan, 2008). Other ET_A receptor antagonists include sitaxsentan. However, because ET_A receptor antagonists may cause hepatotoxicity that could be fatal, liver function must be routinely monitored in patients receiving these drugs (Humbert, Sitbon, & Simonneau, 2004).

2. Phosphodiesterase-4 Inhibitors

Phosphodiesterase-4 (PDE-4) inhibitors have been promoted for the management of asthma based on the findings that PDE-4 overexpression or overactivity is associated with cellular inflammation and reduction in the dilation ability of bronchial smooth muscle. These cellular changes seem to extend to other types of smooth muscles as well. However, upregulation of PDE-4 expression/activity seems to be tissue specific. For example, in a mouse model of pulmonary hypertension, the early phase of pulmonary arterial hypertension was associated with the upregulation of PDE-4 isoform as well as cellular inflammation. PDE-4 activation elicits remodeling of pulmonary circulation at least in part by enhancing the expression of ET and other mediators of inflammatory response. In support of these findings are the recent observations with the PDE-4 inhibitor rolipram, which interfered with the development of pulmonary hypertension by modulating vascular tone (De Franceschi et al., 2008). Two mechanisms were suggested: (i) directly, via inhibition of cAMP cellular degradation, and/or (ii) indirectly, by reducing the magnitude of vasoconstriction secondary to a reduction in the inflammatory response (De Franceschi et al., 2008). The ET receptor antagonists, bosentan and ambrisentan, are recommended for the treatment of pulmonary hypertension (Fig. 1). However, if PDE-4 inhibitors could be developed as novel therapeutic agents for the treatment of pulmonary hypertension, they would produce their effect, at least partly, by acting upstream to inhibit ET expression and signaling which have a theoretical advantage. Further, such new drugs will be needed to treat pulmonary hypertension, which has been difficult to manage due to the availability of a limited number of drugs to treat this condition. Interestingly, as discussed earlier, enhanced expression/activity of PDE-4 seems to occur in some specific vascular beds rather than being a generalized phenomenon. In support of this notion is the ability of selective (rolipram) as well as nonselective (theophylline) PDE-4 inhibitors to elicit retinal blood vessel vasodilation in the absence of significant changes in systemic blood pressure (Miwa, Mori, Nakahara, & Ishii, 2009). Therefore, although at present PDE-4 inhibitors might not be used for management of systemic hypertension, they seem to hold promise for their use for the treatment of pulmonary hypertension as well as for the treatment of retinal vascular disorders. Major limitations that hindered the clinical use of rolipram and similar drugs are the side effects (mainly nausea and vomiting); however, a novel PDE-4 inhibitor, NIS-62949, with a wider therapeutic window as compared to older-generation PDE-4 inhibitors might bring this class of drugs closer to clinical use (Dastidar et al., 2009).

Another class of PDE inhibitors (PDE-5) has been used for the treatment of pulmonary hypertension (Humbert et al., 2004). This class of drugs is most noteworthy for use in the management of erectile dysfunction. Recently, sildenafil was used in a multicenter clinical trial sponsored by the NIH to test its efficacy and safety for the treatment of pulmonary hypertension in sickle-cell anemia patients. The clinical trial has been stopped nearly 1 year early due to safety concerns. Compared with placebo, participants taking sildenafil were significantly more likely to have serious medical problems with most common being episodes of severe pain called sickle-cell crises, which resulted in hospitalization. No deaths have been associated with the drug in the clinical trial (NIH News, 2009).

3. β_2-Adrenoceptor Selective Blockers with Partial Agonist Activity

Like PDE-4 inhibitors, discussed above, a β_2-adrenergic receptor antagonist/partial agonist has been shown to cause selective vasodilation of the pulmonary arteries. ICI 118,551 is a β_2-adrenoceptor blocker with partial agonist activity that exhibits 500-fold selectivity toward β_2-AR over β_1-AR. ICI 118,551 decreases pulmonary vascular tone via a G-protein/NO-coupled pathway (Wenzel et al., 2009). This drug shares with the third-generation β-blockers, for example, nebivolol, the ability to directly induce vasodilation via NO release from the endothelium. The exact mechanism that underlies the selectivity of this drug for the pulmonary vascular bed is not fully understood and was not due to its β-adrenoceptor blockade as other β-blockers failed to produce similar effects. The most likely mechanism of action is the ability of the drug to act as β_2-agonist as well as triggering pulmonary vasorelaxation via a G-protein/NO-coupled pathway. ICI 118,551 can also attenuate the vasoconstriction elicited by norepinephrine and 5-hydroxytryptamine (5-HT) more selectively in pulmonary vascular beds compared with the aorta (Wenzel et al., 2009).

D. Chronotherapy as Novel Strategy for Management of Hypertension

The goal of therapeutic intervention in hypertension is to adequately control BP to reduce CV morbidity and mortality. Common therapeutic strategies used to improve blood pressure control in a hypertensive patient are (i) increasing the dose of the medication, (ii) change of antihypertensive drug(s), and (iii) prescribe drug combinations that have synergistic effects. Regardless of the strategy adopted, in most cases the drug or drug combination is administered as a once daily medication in the morning to increase patient compliance. Indeed, up to 89% of treated hypertensive patients take their antihypertensive medication in a single morning dose (Hermida et al., 2002). This therapeutic approach would be theoretically valid only if all patients had similar circadian blood pressure pattern and/or all antihypertensive medications have long half-lives. However, based on blood pressure chronobiology, there are differences between individuals with regard to night dipping and morning surges of blood pressure and many of the currently available drugs have relatively short half-lives (Hermida & Ayala, 2009). Blood pressure circadian rhythm shows a decrease (dipper) during sleep and a surge during the morning hours. The findings show that a "non-dipper" circadian blood pressure pattern represents a risk factor for left ventricular hypertrophy, cerebrovascular disease, CHF, vascular dementia, and myocardial infarction (Hermida, Ayala, Mojón, Alonso, & Fernández, 2009). On the other hand, recent evidence suggests that "dippers" and patients who receive antihypertensive medications to enhance blood pressure dipping during sleep are better protected against the adverse CV events associated with hypertension (Morgan, 2009). The normalization of the circadian blood pressure pattern to a dipper profile is a novel therapeutic approach (Hermida, Ayala, & Portaluppi, 2007). Based on this approach, a number of clinical studies have been undertaken with different antihypertensive medications to determine the benefit of taking such medications at bedtime (Morgan, 2009). The bedtime antihypertensive drug administration strategy has been attempted with a number of drugs including nifedipine (Hermida, Ayala, Mojón, et al., 2009), ACEIs (Hermida & Ayala, 2009) and ARBs (Hermida, Ayala, Chayan, Mojon, & Fernandez, 2009) and the findings of these studies showed better management of hypertension as well as reduced risk of adverse CV outcomes.

E. Estrogen and ER Agonists as Viable Antihypertensive Medications for the Treatment of Hypertension in Postmenopausal Women

It is now clear that CV disease has become an important risk for all individuals including women with increasing numbers of women exhibiting all forms of CV disease in greater prevalence than previously (Peter et al., 2005). Hypertension in women is often underdiagnosed or inadequately treated, especially after menopause when CV risk increases. Endogenous estrogens maintain vasodilation and contribute to blood pressure control in premenopausal women (Meyer, Hass, & Barton, 2006). The loss of endogenous estrogen production and aging after menopause are accompanied by an elevation in blood pressure and are likely contributing factors to hypertension, which occurs in 75% of postmenopausal women in the United States (Amigoni, Morelli, Parazzinin, & Chateneoud, 2000; Ong, Cheung, Man, Lau, & Lam, 2007). The effects of endogenous estrogen are mediated via ERs, which include the "classic" receptor $ER\alpha$ and $ER\beta$. These receptors are implicated in the genomic effects of estrogen but are also associated with the plasma membrane and mediate rapid activation of intracellular signaling cascades. The latter signaling pathways have been linked to increases in NO bioavailability and inhibition of (i) VSMC and myocardial growth (Kuroski de Bold, 1999; Sangaralingham, Tse, & Pang, 2007), (ii) AT_1R expression and function (Dean, Tan, O'Brien, & Leenen, 2005; Krishnamurthi et al., 1999), (iii) SNS and enhancement of baroreflex function (El-Mas & Abdel-Rahman, 2009). Experimental studies have demonstrated the contribution of ERs to the regulation of blood pressure but these findings were not readily extrapolated to human physiology due to the complex

CV effects of estrogen in women. Contributing factors to the inconsistent CV effects of estrogen in women include the form, dose, and route of administration (patch vs. oral) of estrogen as well as the age of women at the start of estrogen therapy (Barton & Meyer, 2009). For example, the elevated blood pressure associated with premature ovarian failure is reduced by 17β-estradiol and not by ethinylestradiol therapy (Langrish et al., 2009). Furthermore, transdermal estrogen causes more consistent reduction in blood pressure than oral estrogen (Mueck & Seeger, 2004) and acute sublingual estrogen lowers blood pressure in hypertensive but not in normotensive postmenopausal women (Fisman, Tenenbaum, Shapira, Motro, & Pines, 1999). In addition to ER-dependent signaling it is also important to consider the contribution of ER-independent effects (e.g., antioxidant mechanisms of estrogens to the overall effects of estrogens on blood pressure). Further, activation of the G-protein-coupled estrogen receptor (formerly known as GPR30), which is highly expressed in human VSMCs and arteries, causes (i) acute vasodilation in arteries from rodents and humans, (ii) reduces blood pressure *in vivo* even under normotensive conditions, and (iii) inhibits human VSMC proliferation, similar to that observed with 17β-estradiol (Prossnitz & Barton, 2009; Prossnitz & Maggiolini, 2009). Future studies are warranted to help delineate the role of individual pathways contributing to the function of each of the currently known three ERs to blood pressure control and the vasoprotective effects of estrogens so that novel selective ER modulators can be developed as antihypertensive therapeutics for the management of hypertension in postmenopausal women. Finally, research is needed to determine the impact of lifestyle on the CV effects of estrogen. For example, estrogen activation of NOS–NO signaling is exacerbated in the presence of moderate amounts of alcohol (El-Mas & Abdel-Rahman, 2001). This hemodynamic interaction occurs between ethanol and endogenous as well as exogenous estrogen and leads to hypotension secondary to a reduction in cardiac function (El-Mas, Fan, & Abdel-Rahman, 2008; El-Mas, Zhang, & Abdel-Rahman, 2006). Recent evidence implicates non-genomic ER signaling in the enhanced NO generation elicited by estrogen–ethanol combination via the PI3-K–AKt–NOS pathway (El-Mas, Fan, & Abdel-Rahman, 2009; Li & Abdel-Rahman, 2009).

V. Conclusion

CV diseases constitute a major cause of morbidity and mortality in the United States and across the world. One of the primary contributors to CV diseases is hypertension. The most common form of hypertension is a polygenic, multifactorial disease. Furthermore, individuals vary considerably in the factors that are responsible for the expression of the disease. In addition, nearly one-third of the patients that are diagnosed with hypertension are not adequately controlled in spite of excellent compliance with medications. For that reason, there are ever-increasing numbers of therapeutic agents that have been developed to treat the disease. These agents have progressively targeted factors that are involved in the regulation of blood pressure from a systems approach (e.g., ganglionic blocking agents) to a more focused approach on the molecules that are involved in the signaling (e.g., receptors and post-receptor signaling components). The fact that patients differ in their responsiveness to antihypertensive agents on the basis of pharmacogenetically determined pharmacokinetic and pharmacodynamic differences suggests that novel agents will continue to be developed. There have been a number of significant advances in the development of new agents that have been focused on two major components: (1) improving response level and rate; and (2) decreasing adverse effect production. There has also been a new approach to the management of hypertension that has utilized existing agents but modified the timing of administration to become effective therapeutics when considering the natural circadian rhythms. It is clear that novel agents will continue to develop that target more selective components of the signaling pathways that may be altered as part of the pathophysiology that underlies hypertension. The fact that predictions indicate that hypertension as well as CV diseases in general will continue to rise at epidemic proportions suggests that considerable attention needs to be devoted to developing new agents with better therapeutic profiles in the future.

Conflict of Interest Disclosure: Neither Dr. Abdel Abdel-Rahman nor Dr. David Taylor has any financial holdings or involvement in any industrial or other entity that would appear as a conflict of interest in the information provided.

References

Acharya, K.R., Sturrock, E.D., Riordan, J.F., & Ehlers, M. R. W. (2003). ACE revisited: A new target for structure-based drug design. *Nature Reviews Drug Discovery, 2,* 891–902.

Alahari, S. K. (2003). Nischarin inhibits RAC induced migration and invasion of epithelial cells by affecting signaling cascades involving PAK. *Experimental Cell Research, 288,* 415–424.

Alahari, S. K., Lee, J. W., & Juliano, R. L. (2000). Nischarin, a novel protein that interacts with the integrin alpha5 subunit and inhibits cell migration. *Journal of Cell Biology, 151,* 1141–1154.

American Heart Association. (2009). *Heart Disease and Stroke Statistics, 2009-Update.* Retrieved July 2009, from http://www.americanheart.org/

Amigoni, S., Morelli, P., Parazzinin, F., & Chateneoud, L. (2000). Determinants of elevated blood pressure in women around menopause: results from cross-sectional study in Italy. *Maturitas, 34,* 25–32.

Anderson, S., Meyer, T. W., Rennke, H. G., & Brenner, B. M. (1985). Control of glomerular hypertension limits glomerular injury in rats with reduced renal mass. *Journal of Clinical Investigation, 76,* 612–619.

Aubert, J. D., & Juillerat-Jeanneret, L. (2009). Therapeutic potential of endothelin receptor modulators: Lessons from human clinical trials. *Expert Opinion on Therapeutic Targets,* *13*(9), 1069–1084.

Badyal, D. K., Lata, H., & Dadhich, A. P. (2003). Animal models of hypertension and effect of drugs. *Indian Journal of Pharmacology, 35,* 349–362.

Baltatu, O., Campos, L. A., & Bader, M. (2004). Genetic targeting of the brain renin-angiotensin system in transgenic rats: impact on stress-induced renin release. *ACTA Physiologica Scandinavica, 181*(4), 579–584.

Barton, M., & Meyer, M. R. (2009). Postmenopausal hypertension mechanisms and therapy. *Hypertension, 54,* 11–18.

Baudin, B. (2002). Angiotensin II receptor polymorphisms in hypertension. Pharmacogenomic considerations. *Pharmacogenomics, 3,* 1–9.

Bender, T. S., & Abdel-Rahman, A. A. (2009). Alpha 2A-adrenergic receptor signaling under-lies synergistic enhancement of ethanol-induced behavioral impairment by clonidine. *Alcoholism, Clinical and Experimental Research, 33*(3), 408–418.

Ben-Ishay, D., & Yagil, Y. (1994). The Sabra hypertension-prone and -resistant strains. In W. H. Birkenhager & J. L. Reid (Series Eds.) & D. Ganten & W. de Jong (Vol. Eds.), *Handbook of hypertension: Vol. 4. Experimental and genetic models of hypertension,* (p. 272). Amsterdam: Elsevier Science B. V.

Ben-Ishay, D., Saliternik, R., & Welner, A. (1972). Separation of two strains of rats with inbred dissimilar sensitivity to DOCA-salt hypertension. *Experientia, 28,* 1321–1322.

Bianchi, G., Ferrari, P., & Barber, B. R. (1984). The Milan hypertensive strain. In W. H. Birkenhager & J. L. Reid (Series Eds.) & D. Ganten & W. de Jong (Vol. Eds.), *Handbook of hypertension: Vol. 4. Experimental and genetic models of hypertension,* (pp. 328–349). Amsterdam: Elsevier Science B. V.

Bodineau, L., Frugière, A., Marc, Y., Claperon, C., & Llorens-Cortes, C. (2008). Aminopepti-dase A inhibitors as centrally acting antihypertensive agents. *Heart Failure Reviews, 13*(3), 311–319.

Bousquet, P., Dontenwill, M., Greney, H., & Feldman, J. (1998) I1-imidazoline receptors: an update. *Journal of Hypertension (Supplement), 16*(3), S1–5.

Brilla, C. G., Pick, P., Tan, L. B., Janicki, J. S., & Weber, K. T. (1990). Remodelling of rat right and left ventricle in experimental hypertension. *Circulation Research, 67,* 1355–1364.

Brookes, L. (2008). New US National Hypertension Guidelines—JNC 8—To Be Announced? Retrieved July 2009, from, http://www.medscape.com/

Buccafusco, J. J. (1996). The role of central cholinergic neurons in the regulation of blood pressure and in experimental hypertension. *Pharmacological Reviews, 48,* 179–211.

Cannon, P. J., Whitlock, R. T., Morris, R. C., Angers, M., & Laragh, J. H. (1962). Alpha methyl dopa in malignant hypertension. *JAMA, 179,* 673–681.

Centers for Disease Control and Prevention (CDC). (2005). Racial/ethnic disparities in pre-valence, treatment, and control of hypertension—United States, 1999–2002. *MMWR. Morbidity and Mortality Weekly Report, 54,* 7–9.

Channick, R. N., Sitbon, O., Barst, R. J., Manes, A., & Rubin, L. J. (2004). Endothelin receptor antagonists in pulmonary arterial hypertension. *Journal of the American College of Cardiology, 43*(12 Suppl S), 62S–67S.

Chobanian, A. V., Bakris, G. L., Black, H. R., Cushman, W. C., Green, L. A., Izzo, J. L., Jr., et al. and the National High Blood Pressure Educational Program Coordinating Commit-tee (2003). Seventh report of the Joint Committee on Prevention, Detection, Evaluation and Treatment of High Blood Pressure. *Hypertension, 42,* 1206–1252.

Cowley, A. W., Liard, J. F., & Guyton, A. C. (1973). Role of baroreceptor reflexes in daily control of arterial pressure and other variables in dog. *Circulation Research, 32,* 564–578.

Cowley, A. W., Jr., Liang, M., Roman, R. J., Greene, A. S., & Jacob, H. J. (2004). Consomic rat model systems for physiological genomics. *ACTA Physiologica Scandinavica, 181,* 585–592.

Cusi, D., Barlassina, C., Azzani, T., Casari, G., Citterio, L., Devoto, M. et al., (1997). Polymorphisms of alpha-adducin and salt sensitivity in patients with essential hypertension. *Lancet, 349,* 1353–1357.

Dahl, L. K. (1960). Possible role of salt intake in the development of essential hypertension. In K. D. Pork & P. T. Cottier (Eds.), *Essential hypertension-an international symposium,* (pp. 53–65). Berlin: Springer-Verlag.

Dahl, L. K., Heine, M., & Tassinari, L. (1962a). Role of genetic factors in susceptibility to experimental hypertension due to chronic excess salt ingestion. *Nature, 194,* 480–482.

Dahl, L. K., Heine, M., & Tassinari, L. (1962b). Effects of chronic excess slat ingestion. *Journal of Experimental Medicine, 115,* 1173–1190.

Dastidar, S. G., Ray, A., Shirumalla, R., Rajagopal, D., Chaudhary, S., Nanda, K., et al. (2009). Pharmacology of a novel, orally active PDE4 inhibitor. *Pharmacology, 83*(5), 275–286.

Davies, P. F. (1995). Flow-mediated endothelial mechanotransduction. *Physiological Reviews, 75,* 519–560.

Davisson, R. L. (2003). Physiological genomic analysis of the brain renin-angiotensin system. *American Journal of Physiology. Regulatory, Integrative and Comparative Physiology, 285*(3), R498–R511.

Dean, S. A., Tan, J., O'Brien, E. R., & Leenen, F. H. (2005). 17beta-estradiol downregulates tissue angiotensin-converting enzyme and ANG II type 1 receptor in female rats. *American Journal of Physiology. Regulatory, Integrative and Comparative Physiology, 288*(3), R759–766.

De Franceschi, L., Platt, O. S., Leboeuf, C., Beuzard, Y., Malpeli, G., Payen, E., et al. (2008). Protective effects of phosphodiesterase-4 (PDE-4) inhibition in the early phase of pulmonary arterial hypertension in transgenic sickle cell mice. *FASEB Journal, 22,* 1849–1860.

Doggrell, S. A. (2004). Is RGS-2 a new drug development target in cardiovascular disease? *Expert Opinion on Therapeutic Targets, 8*(4), 355–358.

Düsing, R., & Sellers, F. (2009). ACE inhibitors, angiotensin receptor blockers and direct renin inhibitors in combination: a review of their role after the ONTARGET trial. *Current Medical Research and Opinion, 25*(9), 2287–2301.

El-Mas, M. M., & Abdel-Rahman, A. A. (2000). Clonidine diminishes c-jun gene expression in the cardiovascular sensitive areas of the rat brainstem. *Brain Research, 856*(1–2), 245–249.

El-Mas, M. M., & Abdel-Rahman, A. A. (2001). An association between the estrogen-dependent hypotensive effect of ethanol and an elevated brainstem c-jun mRNA in female rats. *Brain Research, 912*(1), 79–88.

El-Mas, M. M., & Abdel-Rahman, A. A. (2009, April 27). Longitudinal assessment of estrogen effects on blood pressure and cardiovascular autonomic activity in female rats. *Clinical and Experimental Pharmacology and Physiology,* [Epub ahead of print].

El-Mas, M. M., Fan, M., & Abdel-Rahman, A. A. (2008). Endotoxemia-mediated induction of cardiac inducible nitric-oxide synthase expression accounts for the hypotensive effect of ethanol in female rats. *Journal of Pharmacology and Experimental Therapeutics, 324*(1), 368–375.

El-Mas, M. M., Fan, M., & Abdel-Rahman, A. A. (2009). Facilitation of myocardial PI3K/Akt/nNOS signaling contributes to ethanol-evoked hypotension in female rats. *Alcoholism, Clinical and Experimental Research, 33*(7), 1158–1168.

El-Mas, M. M., Zhang, J., & Abdel-Rahman, A. A. (2006). Upregulation of vascular inducible nitric oxide synthase mediates the hypotensive effect of ethanol in conscious female rats. *Journal of Applied Physiology, 100*(3), 1011–1018.

Ernsberger, P., Graves, M. E., Graff, L. M., Zakieh, N., Nguyen, P., Collins, L. A., et al. (1995). I1-imidazoline receptors. Definition, characterization, distribution, and transmembrane signaling. *Annals of the New York Academy of Sciences, 763,* 22–42.

Feldman, J., Greney, H., Monassier, L., Vonthron, C., Bruban, V., Dontenwill, M., et al. (1998). Does a second generation of centrally acting antihypertensive drugs really exist? *Journal of the Autonomic Nervous System, 72*(2–3), 94–97.

Festing, M. F., & Bender, K. (1984). Genetic relationships between inbred strains of rats: An analysis based on genetic markers at 28 biochemical loci. *Genetical Research, 44*, 271–281.

Fields, L. E., Burt, V. L., Cutler, J. A., Hughes, J., Roccella, E. J., & Sorlie, P. (2004). *Hypertension, 44*, 398–404.

Fisman, E. Z., Tenenbaum, A., Shapira, I., Motro, M., & Pines, A. (1999). The acute effects of sublingual estradiol on left ventricular diastolic function in normotensive and hypertensive postmenopausal women. *Maturitas, 33*, 145–152.

Fournie-Zaluski, M. C., Fassot, C., Valentin, B., Djordjijevic, D., Reaux-Le Goazigo, A., Corvol, P., et al. (2004). Brain renin-angiotensin system blockade by systemically active aminopeptidase A inhibitors: a potential treatment of salt-dependent hypertension. *Proceedings of the National Academy of Sciences of the United States of America, 101*(20), 7775–7780.

Furchgott, R. F., & Zawadski, J. V. (1980). The obligatory role of endothelial cells in the relaxation of arterial smooth muscle by acetylcholine. *Nature, 228*, 373–376.

Garty, M., Deka-Starosta, A., Chang, P., Kopin, I. J., & Goldstein, D. S. (1990). Effects of clonidine on renal sympathetic nerve activity and norepinephrine spillover. *Journal of Pharmacology and Experimental Therapeutics, 254*(3), 1068–1075.

Goldblatt, H., Lynch, J., Hanzel, R. F., & Summerville, W. W. (1934). Studies on experimental hypertension-II: The production of persistent elevation of systolic blood pressure by means of renal ischaemia. *Journal of Experimental Medicine, 59*, 347–379.

Griendling, K. K., Harrison, D. G., & Alexander, R. W. (2009). Biology of the vessel wall. In V. Fuster, R. A. O'Rourke, R. A. Walsh, & P. Poole-Wilson (Eds.), *Hurst's the heart* (12th ed., chap. 7, King, S. B., Roberts, R., Nash, I. S., & Prystowsky, E. N., Assoc. Eds.). Retrieved July 2009, from http://www.accessmedicine.com/content.aspx?aID=3062385

Grollman, A. (1955). The effect of various hypotensive agents on the arterial blood pressure of hypertensive rats and dogs. *Journal of Pharmacology and Experimental Therapeutics, 174*, 263–270.

Harder, D. R., & Sperelakis, N. (1979). Action potentials induced in guinea pig arterial smooth muscle by tetraethylammonium. *American Journal of Physiology, 237*, C75–C80.

Hermida, R. C., & Ayala, D. E. (2009). Chronotherapy with the angiotensin-converting enzyme inhibitor ramipril in essential hypertension: improved blood pressure control with bedtime dosing. *Hypertension, 54*, 40–46.

Hermida, R. C., Ayala, D. E., & Portaluppi, F. (2007). Circadian variation of blood pressure: The basis for the chronotherapy of hypertension. *Advanced Drug Delivery Reviews, 59*, 904–922.

Hermida, R. C., Ayala, D. E., Mojón, A., Alonso, I., & Fernández, J. R. (2009). Reduction of morning blood pressure surge after treatment with nifedipine GITS at bedtime, but not upon awakening, in essential hypertension. *Blood Pressure Monitoring, 14*(4), 152–159.

Hermida, R. C., Ayala, D. E., Chayan, L., Mojon, A., & Fernandez, J. R. (2009). Administration-time-dependent effects of olmesartan on the ambulatory blood pressure of essential hypertension patients. *Chronobiology International, 26*, 61–79.

Hermida, R. C., Calvo, C., Ayala, D. E., Mojon, A., & Lopez, J. E. (2002). Relationship between physical activity and blood pressure in dipper and non-dipper hypertensive patients. *Journal of Hypertension, 20*, 1097–1104.

Herrera, V. L. M., & Ruiz-Opazo, N. (2009). Rat as a model system for hypertension drug discovery. *Drug Discovery Today: Disease Models*, doi:10.1016/j.ddmod.2009.03.003.

Humbert, M., Sitbon, O., & Simonneau, G. (2004). Treatment of pulmonary arterial hypertension. *New England Journal of Medicine, 351*, 1425–1436.

Iglarz, M., Touyz, R. M., Viel, E. C., Paradis, P., Amiri, F., Diep, Q. N., et al. (2003). Peroxisome proliferator-activated receptor-alpha and receptor-gamma activators prevent cardiac fibrosis in mineralocorticoid-dependent hypertension. *Hypertension, 20*, 737–743.

Iusuf, D., Henning, R. H., van Gilst, W. H., & Roks, A. J. (2008). Angiotensin-(1–7): Pharmacological properties and pharmacotherapeutic perspectives. *European Journal of Pharmacology, 585*, 303–312.

Iwai, M., & Horiuchi, M. (2009). Devil and angel in the renin-angiotensin system: ACE-angiotensin II-AT(1) receptor axis vs. ACE2-angiotensin-(1–7)-Mas receptor axis. *Hypertension Research, 32*, 533–536.

Iwanami, J., Mogi, M., Iwai, M., & Horiuchi, M. (2009). Inhibition of the renin-angiotensin system and target organ protection. *Hypertension Research, 32*(4), 229–237.

Johnson, J. A., & Cavallari, L. H. (2005). Cardiovascular pharmacogenomics. *Experimental Physiology, 90*(3), 283–289.

Johnson, M. L., Ely, D. L., & Turner, M. E. (1992). Genetic divergence between the Wistar-Kyoto rat and the spontaneously hypertensive rat. *Hypertension, 19*, 425–427.

Kabunga, P., & Coghlan, G. (2008). Endothelin receptor antagonism: role in the treatment of pulmonary arterial hypertension related to scleroderma. *Drugs, 68*(12), 1635–1645.

Kagiyama, S., Varela, A., Phillips, M. I., & Galli, S. M. (2001). Antisense inhibition of brain renin-angiotensin system decreased blood pressure in chronic 2-kidney, 1 clip hypertensive rats. *Hypertension, 37*(2 Part 2), 371–375.

Katholi, R. E., & Naftilon, A. J. (1980). Importance of renal sympathetic tone in development of DOCA-Salt hypertension in rat. *Hypertension, 2*, 266–272.

Katovich, M. J., Grobe, J. L., &Raizada, M. K. (2008). Angiotensin-(1-7) as an antihypertensive, antifibrotic target. *Current Hypertension Reports, 10*(3), 227–232.

Kava, R., Peterson, R. G., West, D. B., & Greenwood, M. R. C. (1990). Wistar diabetic fatty rat. *ILAR News, 32*, 9–13.

Koss, M. C. (1983). Analysis of CNS sympatho-inhibition produced by guanabenz. *European Journal of Pharmacology, 90*(1), 19–27.

Krieger, E. M. (1964). Neurogenic hypertension in the rat. *Circulation Research, 15*, 511–521.

Krishnamurthi, K., Verbalis, J. G., Zheng, W., Wu, Z., Clerch, L. B., & Sandberg, K. (1999). Estrogen regulates angiotensin AT1 receptor expression via cytosolic proteins that bind to the 5′ leader sequence of the receptor mRNA. *Endocrinology, 140*(11), 5435–5438.

Kuijpers, M. H. M., & Gruys, E. (1984). Spontaneous hypertension and hypertensive renal disease in the fawn-hooded rat. *British Journal of Experimental Pathology, 65*, 181–190.

Kuijpers, M. H. M., Provoost, A. P., & De Jong, W. (1986). Development of hypertension and proteinuria with age in fawn-hooded rats. *Clinical and Experimental Pharmacology and Physiology, 13*, 201–209.

Kuijpers, M. H. M., Van Zutphen, B. F. M., & De Jong, W. (1987). The fawn-hooded rat. *Hypertension, 9* Suppl I, I-34–I-36.

Kumar, N. N., Goodchild, A. K., Li, Q., & Pilowsky, P. M. (2006). An aldosterone-related system in the ventrolateral medulla oblongata of spontaneously hypertensive and Wistar-Kyoto rats. *Clinical and Experimental Pharmacology and Physiology, 33*(1–2), 71–75.

Kuroski de Bold, M. L. (1999). Estrogen, natriuretic peptides and the renin-angiotensin system. *Cardiovascular Research, 41*(3), 524–531.

Kurtz, T. W., Montano, M., Chan, L., & Kabra, P. (1989). Molecular evidence of genetic heterogeneity in Wistar-Kyoto rats: Implications for research with the spontaneously hypertensive rat. *Hypertension, 13*, 188–192.

Kwitek, A. E., Jacob, J. G., Baker, J. E., Dwinell, M. R., Forster, H. V., Greene, A. S., et al. (2006). BN phenome: Detailed characterization of the cardiovascular, renal, and pulmonary systems of the sequenced rat. *Physiological Genomics, 25*, 303–313.

Langrish, J. P., Mills, N. L., Bath, L. E., Warner, P. E., Webb, D. J., Kelnar, C. J., et al. (2009). Cardiovascular effects of physiological and standard sex hormone replacement regimen in premature ovarian failure. *Hypertension, 53*, 805–811.

Laragh, J. H. (1993). The renin system and new understanding of the complications of hypertension and their treatment. *Arzneimittelforschung, 43*, 247–254.

Lazartigues, E., Feng, Y., & Lavoie, J. L. (2007). The two fACEs of the tissue renin-angiotensin systems: implication in cardiovascular diseases. *Current Pharmaceutical Design, 13*(12), 1231–1245.

Lee, N. H. (2007). Physiogenomic strategies and resources to associate genes with rat models of heart, lung and blood disorders. *Experimental Physiology, 92*(6), 992–1002.

Li, F., Wu, N., Su, R. B., Zheng, J. Q., Xu, B., Lu, X. Q., et al. (2006). Involvement of phosphatidylcholine-selective phospholipase C in activation of mitogen-activated protein kinase pathways in imidazoline receptor antisera-selected protein. *Journal of Cellular Biochemistry, 98*, 1615–1628.

Li, G., & Abdel-Rahman, A. A. (2009). Estrogen-dependent enhancement of NO production in the nucleus tractus solitarius contributes to ethanol-induced hypotension in conscious female rats. *Alcoholism, Clinical and Experimental Research, 33*(2), 366–374

Li, G., Wang, X., & Abdel-Rahman, A. A. (2005). Neuronal norepinephrine responses of the rostral ventrolateral medulla and nucleus tractus solitarius neurons distinguish the I_1-from the alpha2-receptor-mediated hypotension in conscious SHRs. *Journal of Cardiovascular Pharmacology, 46*(1), 52–62.

Li, S., Huang, N. F., & Hsu, S. (2005). Mechanotransduction in endothelial cell migration. *Journal of Cellular Biochemistry, 96*, 1110–1126.

Lighthall, G. K., Hamilton, B. P., & Hamlyn, J. M. (2004). Identification of salt-sensitive genes in the kidneys of Dahl rats. *Journal of Hypertension, 22*, 1487–1494.

Lim, K. P., & Hong, W. (2004). Human nischarin/imidazoline receptor antisera-selected protein is targeted to the endosomes by a combined action of a PX domain and a coiled-coil region. *Journal of Biological Chemistry, 279*, 54770–54782.

Lu, Y.-M., Han, F., Shioda, N., Moriguchi, S., Shirasaki, Y., Qin, Z.-H., et al. (2009). Phenylephrine-induced cardiomyocyte injury is triggered by superoxide generation through uncoupled endothelial nitric-oxide synthase and ameliorated by 3-[2-[4-(3-chloro-2-methylphenyl)-1-piperazinyl]ethyl]-5,6-dimethoxyindazole (DY-9836), a novel calmodulin antagonist. *Molecular Pharmacology, 75*(1), 101–112.

Malek, R. L., Wang, H.-Y., Kwitek, A. E., Greene, A. S., Bhagabati, N., Borchardt, G., et al. (2006). Physiogenomic resources for rat models of heart, lung and blood disorders. *Nature Genetics, 38*(2), 234–239.

Manrique, C., Whaley-Connell, A., & Sowers, J. R. (2009). Nebivolol in obese and non-obese hypertensive patients. *Journal of Clinical Hypertension, 11*, 309–315.

Mao, L., & Abdel-Rahman, A. A. (1996). Synergistic behavioral interaction between ethanol and clonidine in rats: role of alpha-2 adrenoceptors. *Journal of Pharmacology and Experimental Ttherapeutics, 279*(2), 443–449.

Mao, L., & Abdel-Rahman, A. A. (1998). Ethanol counteraction of clonidine-evoked inhibition of norepinephrine release in rostral ventrolateral medulla of rats. *Alcoholism, Clinical and Experimental Research, 22*(6), 1285–1291.

Mao, L., Li, G., & Abdel-Rahman, A. A. (2003). Effect of ethanol on reductions in norepinephrine electrochemical signal in the rostral ventrolateral medulla and hypotension elicited by I_1-receptor activation in spontaneously hypertensive rats. *Alcoholism, Clinical and Experimental Research, 27*(9), 1471–1480.

McLaughlin, V. V., Presberg, K. W., Doyle, R. L., Abman, S. H., McCrory, D. C., Fortin, T., et al. (2004). Prognosis of pulmonary arterial hypertension: ACCP evidence-based clinical practice guidelines. *Chest, 126*(Suppl 1), 78S–92S.

Mercuro, G., Zoncu, S., Saiu, F., Mascia, M., Melis, G. B., & Rosano, G. M. (2004). Menopause induced by oophorectomy reveals a role of ovarian estrogen on the maintenance of pressure homeostasis. *Maturitas, 47*, 131–138.

Meyer, M. R., Hass, E., & Barton, M. (2006). Gender differences of cardiovascular disease: New perspectives for estrogen receptor signaling. *Hypertension, 47*, 1019–1026.

Mitchell, L. B. M., Wallerath, T., & Förstermann, U. (2007). Animal models of hypertension. In J. M. Walker (Series Ed.) & N. Sreejayan & J. Ren (Vol. Eds.), *Methods in molecular medicine. Vascular biology protocols* (chap. 6, pp. 105–111). Totowa, NJ: Humana Press.

Miwa, T., Mori, A., Nakahara, T., & Ishii, K. (2009). Intravenously administered phosphodiesterase 4 inhibitors dilate retinal blood vessels in rats. *European Journal of Pharmacology, 602*, 112–116.

Morgan, T. O. (2009). Does it matter when drugs are taken? *Hypertension, 54*, 23–24.

Mueck, A. O., & Seeger, H. (2004). Effect of hormone therapy on blood pressure in normotensive and hypertensive postmenopausal women. *Maturitas, 49*, 189–203.

Mullins, J. J., Peters, J., & Ganten, D. (1990). Fulminant hypertension in transgenic rats harbouring the mouse Ren-2 gen. *Nature, 344*, 541–544.

Nassar, N., & Abdel-Rahman, A. A. (2006). Central adenosine signaling plays a key role in centrally mediated hypotension in conscious aortic barodenervated rats. *Journal of Pharmacology and Experimental Therapeutics, 318*(1), 255–261.

Nassar, N., & Abdel-Rahman, A. A. (2008). Brainstem phosphorylated extracellular signal-regulated kinase 1/2-nitric-oxide synthase signaling mediates the adenosine A2A-dependent hypotensive action of clonidine in conscious aortic barodenervated rats. *Journal of Pharmacology and Experimental Therapeutics, 324*(1), 79–85.

Nassar, N., & Abdel-Rahman, A. A. (2009). Brainstem adenosine A1 receptor signaling masks phosphorylated extracellular signal-regulated kinase 1/2-dependent hypotensive action of clonidine in conscious normotensive rats. *Journal of Pharmacology and Experimental Therapeutics, 328*(1), 83–89.

Natesh, R., Schwager, S. L. U., Sturrock, E. D., & Acharya, K. R. (2003). Crystal structure of the human angiotensin-converting enzyme-lisinopril complex. *Nature, 421*, 551–554.

Newby, A. C., Southgate, K. M., & Assender, J. W. (1992). Inhibition of vascular smooth muscle cell proliferation by endothelium-dependent vasodilators. *Herz, 17*(5), 291–299.

NIH News. (2009). Retrieved from http://www.nih.gov/news/health/jul2009/nhlbi-28.htm

Ogawa, S., Emi, M., & Shiraki, M. (2000). Association of estrogen receptor beta (ESR2) gene polymorphism with blood pressure. *European Journal of Human Genetics, 45*, 327–330.

Okamoto, K., & Aoki, K. (1963). Development of a strain of spontaneously hypertensive rats. *Japanese Circulation Journal, 27*, 282–293.

Ong, K. L., Cheung, B. M., Man, Y. B., Lau, C. P., & Lam, K. S. (2007). Prevalence, awareness, treatment, and control of hypertension among United States adults 1999–2004. *Hypertension, 49*, 69–75.

Owens, J., Stoney, C., & Matthews, K. (1993). Menopausal status influences ambulatory blood pressure levels and blood pressure levels and blood pressure changes during mental stress. *Circulation, 88*, 2794–2802.

Pachori, A. S., Numan, M. T., Ferrario, C. M., Diz, D. M., Raizada, M. K., & Katovich, M. J. (2002). Blood pressure-independent attenuation of cardiac hypertrophy by AT(1) R-AS gene therapy. *Hypertension, 39*, 969–975.

Pachori, A. S., Wang, H., Gelband, C. H., Ferrario, C. M., Katovich, M. J., & Raizada, M. K. (2000). Inability to induce hypertension in normotensive rat expressing AT(1) receptor antisense. *Circulation Research, 86*, 1167–1172.

Page, I. H. (1939). The production of persistent arterial hypertension by cellophane perinephritis. *JAMA, 113*, 2046.

Palmer, R. M. J., Ferrige, A. G., & Moncada, S. (1987). Nitric oxide release accounts for the biological activity of endothelium-derived relaxing factor. *Nature, 327*, 524–526.

Paul, M., Wagner, J., Hoffmann, S., Urata, H., & Ganten, D. (1994). Transgenic rats: New experimental models for the study of candidate genes in hypertension research. *Annual Review of Physiology, 56*, 811–829.

Peter, I., Shearman, A. M., Zucker, D. R., Schmid, C. H., Demissie, S., Cupples, L. A., et al. (2005). Variation in estrogen related genes and cross-sectional and longitudinal blood pressure in the Framingham Heart Study. *Journal of Hypertension, 23,* 2193–2200.

Phillips, M. I., & de Oliveira, E. M. (2008). Brain renin angiotensin in disease. *Journal of Molecular Medicine, 86*(6), 715–722.

Pickering, T. G., & Ogedegbe, G. (2009). Epidemiology of hypertension. In V. Fuster, R. A. O'Rourke, R. A. Walsh, & P. Poole-Wilson (Eds.), *Hurst's the heart* (12th ed., chap. 68, S. B. King, R. Roberts, I. S. Nash, & E. N. Prystowsky, Assoc. Eds.). Retrieved July 2009, from http://www.accessmedicine.com/content.aspx?aID=3055828

Piletz, J. E., Wang, G., & Zhu, H. (2003). Cell signaling by imidazoline-1 receptor candidate, IRAS, and the nischarin homologue. *Annals of the New York Academy of Sciences, 1009,* 392–399.

Pravenec, M., & Kren, V. (2005). Genetic analysis of complex cardiovascular traits in the spontaneously hypertensive rat. *Experimental Physiology, 90,* 273–276.

Prossnitz, E. R., & Barton, M. (2009). Signaling, physiological functions and clinical relevance of the G protein-coupled estrogen receptor GPER. *Prostaglandins & Other Lipid Mediators, 89*(3–4), 89–97.

Prossnitz, E. R., & Maggiolini, M. (2009). Mechanisms of estrogen signaling and gene expression via GPR30. *Molecular and Cellular Endocrinology, 308*(1–2), 32–38.

Provoost, A. P., & De Keijzer, M. H. (1993). The fawn-hooded rat: a model for chronic renal failure. In N. Gretz & M. Strauch (Eds.), *Experimental and genetic rat models of chronic renal failure* (pp. 100–114). Basel, Switzerland: Karger.

Ramachandran, S. V., Benjamin, E. J., Sullivan, L. M., & D'Agostino, R. B., (2009). The burden of increasing worldwide cardiovascular disease. In V. Fuster, R. A. O'Rourke, R. A. Walsh, & P. Poole-Wilson (Eds.), *Hurst's the heart* (12th ed., chap. 2, S. B. King, R. Roberts, I. Nash, & E. N. Prystowsky, Assoc. Eds.). Retrieved from http://www.accessmedicine.com/content.aspx?aID=3059745

Rang, H. P., Dale, M. M., Ritter, J. M., & Moore, P. K. (2003). Cellular mechanisms: Excitation, contraction and secretion. In H. P. Rang, M. M. Dale, J. M. Ritter, & P. K. Moore (Eds.), *Pharmacology fifth edition* (pp. 51–68). London: Elsevier Science.

Rao, P. V., Deng, P.-F., Kumar, J., & Epstein, D. L. (2001). Modulation of aqueous humor outflow facility by the Rho kinase-specific inhibitor Y-27632. *Investigative Ophthalmology & Visual Science, 42,* 1029–1037.

Rapp, J. P. (1982). Dahl salt-susceptible and salt-resistant rats. *Hypertension, 4,* 753–763.

Rapp, J. P. (2000). Genetic analysis of inherited hypertension. *Physiological Reviews, 80,* 135–172.

Reaux-Le Goazigo, A., Iturrioz, X., Fassot, C., Claperon, C., Roques, B. P., & Llorens-Cortes, C. (2005). Role of angiotensin III in hypertension. *Current Hypertension Reports, 7*(2), 128–134.

Reddig, P. J., Xu, D., & Juliano, R. L. (2005). Regulation of p21-activated kinase-independent Rac1 signal transduction by nischarin. *Journal of Biological Chemistry, 280,* 30994–31002.

Redelinghuys, P., Nchinda, A. T., & Sturrock, E. D. (2005). Development of domain-selective angiotensin I-converting enzyme inhibitors. *Annals of the New York Academy of Sciences, 1056,* 160–175.

Reis, D. J., Doba, N., & Nathan, M. A. (1976). Neurogenic arterial hypertension produced by brainstem lesion. In Onesti, G., Fernanades, M., & Kim, K. E. (Eds.), *Regulation of blood pressure by the central nervous system* (pp. 35–51). New York: Grune and Stratton.

Ren, J., Duan, J., Thomas, D. P., Yang, X., Sreejayan, N., Sowers, J. R., et al. (2008). IGF-I alleviates diabetes-induced RhoA activation, eNOS uncoupling, and myocardial dysfunction. *American Journal of Physiology. Regulatory, Integrative and Comparative Physiology, 294*(3), R793–R802.

Riccioni, G., Vitulano, N., D'Orazio, N., & Bellocci, F. (2009). Aliskiren, the first approved renin inhibitor: Clinical application and safety in the treatment of hypertension. *Advances in Therapy, 26*(7), 700–710.

Roden, D. M. (2009). Antiarrhythmic drugs. In L. L. Brunton, J. S. Lazo, & K. L. Parker (Eds.), *Goodman & Gilman's the pharmacological basis of therapeutics,* (11th ed., chap. 34). Retrieved July, 2009, from http://www.accessmedicine.com/content

Rodrigues, M. C., Campagnole-Santos, M. J., Machado, R. P., Silva, M. E., Rocha, J. L., Ferreira, P. M., et al. (2007). Evidence for a role of AT(2) receptors at the CVLM in the cardiovascular changes induced by low-intensity physical activity in renovascular hypertensive rats. *Peptides, 28*(7), 1375–1382.

Saeed, M. M., Saboohi, K, Osman, A. S., Bokhari, A. M., & Frossard, P. M. (2003). Association of the angiotensin-converting enzyme (ACE) gene G2350A dimorphism with essential hypertension. *Journal of Human Hypertension, 17,* 719–723.

Sangaralingham, S. J., Tse, M. Y., & Pang, S. C. (2007). Estrogen protects against the development of salt-induced cardiac hypertrophy in heterozygous proANP gene-disrupted mice. *Journal of Endocrinology, 194*(1), 143–152.

Scriabine, A. (2007). 6.32 Hypertension. In M. Williams (Ed.), *Comprehensive medicinal chemistry II. Volume 6* (J. B. Taylor & D. J. Triggle, Editors-in-chief, pp. 705–728). Oxford, UK: Elsevier Ltd.

Selye, H., & Bois, P. (1957). The hormonal production of nephrosclerosis and periarteritis nodosa in the primate. *British Medical Journal, 1,* 183–186.

Separovic, D., Kester, M., & Ernsberger, P. (1996). Coupling of I1-imidazoline receptors to diacylglyceride accumulation in PC12 rat pheochromocytoma cells. *Molecular Pharmacology, 49,* 668–675.

Shyy, J. Y.-J., & Chien, S. (2002). Role of integrins in endothelial mechanosensing of shear stress. *Circulation Research, 91,* 769–775.

Sink, K. M., Leng, X., Williamson. J., Kritchevsky, S. B., Yaffe, K., Kuller, L., et al. (2009). Angiotensin-converting enzyme inhibitors and cognitive decline in older adults with hypertension: results from the Cardiovascular Health Study. *Archives of Internal Medicine, 169,* 1195–1202.

Sone, H., Suzuki, H., Takahashi, A., & Yamada, N. (2001). Disease model: Hyperinsulinemia and insulin resistance. Part A—targeted disruption of insulin signaling or glucose transport. *Trends in Molecular Medicine, 7,* 320–322.

Sullivan, J. M. (1991). Salt sensitivity: definition, conception, methodology, and long-term issues. *Hypertension, 17*(Suppl. I), I-61–I-68.

Sun, C., Du, J., Sumners, C., & Raizada, M. K. (2003). PI3-kinase inhibitors abolish the enhanced chronotropic effects of angiotensin II in spontaneously hypertensive rat brain neurons. *Journal of Neurophysiology, 90*(5), 3155–3160.

Sun, Z., Chang, C. H., & Ernsberger, P. (2007). Identification of IRAS/Nischarin as an I1-imidazoline receptor in PC12 rat pheochromocytoma cells. *Journal of Neurochemistry, 101,* 99–108.

Szabo, B. (2002). Imidazoline antihypertensive drugs: a critical review on their mechanism of action. *Pharmacology and Therapeutics, 93*:1–35.

Takahashi, N., & Smithies, O. (2004). Human genetics, animal models and computer simulations for studying hypertension. *Trends in Genetics, 20,* 136–145.

Tang, M., Wang, G., Lu, P., Karras, R. H., Aronovitz, M., Heximer, S. P., et al. (2003). Regulator of G-protein signaling-2 mediates vascular smooth muscle relaxation and blood pressure. *Nature Medicine, 9,* 1506–1512.

Taylor, A. L., Ziesche, S., Yancy, C., Carson, P., D'Agostino, R., Jr., Ferdinand, K., et al., (2004). Combination of isosorbide dinitrate and hydralazine in blacks with heart failure. *New England Journal of Medicine, 351,* 2049–57.

Taylor, D. A. (2007). 6.31 Cardiovascular overview. In M. Williams (Ed.), *Comprehensive medicinal chemistry II. Volume 6* (J. B. Taylor & D. J. Triggle, Editors-in-chief, pp. 693–704). Oxford, UK: Elsevier Ltd.

Thiedemann, K. U., Holubarsch, C., Medugarac, I., & Jacob, R. (1983). Connective tissue contraction and myocardial stiffness in pressure overload hypertrophy: a combined study of morphologic, morphometric, biochemical and mechanical parameters. *Basic Research in Cardiology, 78,* 140–155.

Tibirica, E., Mermet, C., Feldman, J., Gonon, F., & Bousquet, P. (1989). Correlation between the inhibitory effect on catecholaminergic ventrolateral medullary neurons and the hypotension evoked by clonidine: A voltammetric approach. *Journal of Pharmacology and Experimental Therapeutics, 250*(2), 642–647.

Trask, A. J., & Ferrario, C. M. (2007). Angiotensin-(1-7): pharmacology and new perspectives in cardiovascular treatments. *Cardiovascular Drug Reviews, 25*(2), 162–174.

Ueba, H., Kawakami, M., & Yaginuma, T. (1997). Shear stress as an inhibitor of vascular smooth muscle cell proliferation. Role of transforming growth factor-beta 1 and tissue type plasminogen activator. *Arteriosclerosis, Thrombosis, and Vascular Biology, 17*(8), 1512–1516.

United States Renal Data System. (2007). USRDS 2007 Annual Data Report. Bethesda, MD: National Institute of Diabetes and Digestive and Kidney Diseases, National Institutes of Health, U. S. Department of Health and Human Services. Retrieved August 2009, from http://kidney.niddk.nih.gov/kudiseases/pubs/highblood/

van den Meiracker, A. H. (2002). Endothelins and venous tone in DOCA-salt hypertension. *Journal of Hypertension, 20,* 587–589.

Verseput, G. H., Provoost, A. P., Van Tol, A., Koomans, H. A., & Joles, J. A. (1997). Hyperlipidemia is secondary to proteinuria and is completely normalized by angiotensin-converting enzyme inhibition in hypertensive fawn-hooded rats. *Nephron, 77,* 346–352.

Vincent, M., & Sassard, J. (1994). Lyon strains. In J. Swales (Ed.), *Textbook of hypertension* (pp. 455–457). Oxford, UK: Blackwell Scientific Publications.

Vincent, M., Boussairi, E. H., Cartier, R., Lo, M., Sassolas, A., Cerutti, C., et al. (1993). High blood pressure and metabolic disorders are associated in the Lyon hypertensive rat. *Journal of Hypertension, 11,* 1179–1185.

Wang, H., Katovich, M. J., Gelband, C. H., Reaves, P. Y., Phillips, M. I., & Raizada, M. K. (1999). Sustained inhibition of angiotensin I-converting enzyme (ACE) expression and long-term antihypertensive action by virally mediated delivery of ACE antisense cDNA. *Circulation Research, 85,* 614–622.

Wang, H.-W., Gallinat, S., Li, H.-W., Sumners, C., Raizada, M. K., & Katovich, M. J. (2004). Elevated blood pressure in normotensive rats produced by 'knockdown' of the angiotensin type 2 receptor. *Experimental Physiology, 89,* 313–322.

Wang, X., Li, G., & Abdel-Rahman, A. A. (2005). Site-dependent inhibition of neuronal c-jun in the brainstem elicited by imidazoline I1 receptor activation: role in rilmenidine-evoked hypotension. *European Journal of Pharmacology, 514*(2–3), 191–199.

Watts, S. (2010). Vasodilators and nitric oxide synthase. In L. Wecker, L. M. Crespo, G. Dunaway, C. Faingold, & S. Watts (Eds.), *Brody's human pharmacology molecular to clinical* (5th ed., chap. 24). Philadelphia, PA: Mosby Elsevier.

Webb, R. C. (2003). Smooth muscle contraction and relaxation. *Advances in Physiology Education, 27,* 201–206.

Weber, M. A. (2001). Vasopeptidase inhibitors. *Lancet, 358,* 1525–1532.

Weiss, R. (2006). Nebivolol: A novel beta-blocker with nitric oxide-induced vasodilatation. *Vascular Health and Risk Management, 2,* 303–308.

Wenzel, D., Knies, R., Matthey, M., Klein, A. M., Welschoff, J., Stolle, V., et al. (2009). β_2-Adrenoceptor Antagonist ICI 118,551 decreases pulmonary vascular tone in mice via a G protein/nitric oxide-coupled pathway. *Hypertension, 54,* 157–163.

Whaley-Connell, A., Habibi, J., Johnson, M., Tilmon, R., Rehmer, N., Rehmer, J., et al. (2009). Nebivolol reduces proteinuria and renal NADPH oxidase-generated reactive oxygen species in the transgenic Ren2 rat. *American Journal of Nephrology, 30,* 354–360.

World Heart Federation. (2009). Cardiovascular disease risk factors - Hypertension. Retrieved from http://www.world-heart-federation.org/cardiovascular-health/cardiovascular-disease-risk-factors/hypertension/#c560

Yagil, C., Katni, G., Rubattu, S., Stolpe, C., Kreutz, R., Lindpaintner, K., et al. (1996). Development, genotype and phenotype of a new colony of the Sabra hypertension prone (SBH/y) and resistant (SBN/y) rat model of salt sensitivity and resistance. *Journal of Hypertension, 14*, 1175–1182.

Yamamoto, K., Sokabe, T., Ohura, N., Nakatsuka, H., Kamiya, A., & Ando, J. (2003). Endogenously released ATP mediates shear stress-induced Ca^{2+} influx into pulmonary artery endothelial cells. *American Journal of Physiology. Heart and Circulatory Physiology, 285*, H793–H803.

Yang, H., & Raizada, M. K. (1999). Role of phosphatidylinositol 3-kinase in angiotensin II regulation of norepinephrine neuromodulation in brain neurons of the spontaneously hypertensive rat. *Journal of Neuroscience, 19*(7), 2413–2423.

Zaros, P. R., Pires, C. E., Bacci, M., Jr., Moraes, C., & Zanesco, A. (2009). Effect of 6-months of physical exercise on the nitrate/nitrite levels in hypertensive postmenopausal women. *BMC Women's Health, 19*, 9–17.

Zhang, J., & Abdel-Rahman, A. A. (2005). Mitogen-activated protein kinase phosphorylation in the rostral ventrolateral medulla plays a key role in imidazoline (i1)-receptor-mediated hypotension. *Journal of Pharmacology and Experimental Therapeutics, 314*, 945–952.

Zhang, J., & Abdel-Rahman, A. A. (2006). Nischarin as a functional imidazoline (I1) receptor. *FEBS Letters, 580*, 3070–3074.

Zhang, J., & Abdel-Rahman, A. A. (2008). Inhibition of nischarin expression attenuates rilmenidine-evoked hypotension and phosphorylated extracellular signal-regulated kinase 1/2 production in the rostral ventrolateral medulla of rats. *Journal of Pharmacology and Experimental Therapeutics, 324*, 72–78.

Zhang, J., El-Mas, M. M., & Abdel-Rahman, A. A. (2001). Imidazoline I(1) receptor-induced activation of phosphatidylcholine-specific phospholipase C elicits mitogen-activated protein kinase phosphorylation in PC12 cells. *European Journal of Pharmacology, 415*, 117–125.

Zhu, Y., Bian, Z., Lu, P., Karas, R. H., Bao, L., Cox, D., et al. (2002). Abnormal vascular function and hypertension in mice deficient in estrogen receptor beta. *Science, 295*, 505–508.

Jeffrey M. Witkin and Xia Li

Neuroscience Discovery Research, Lilly Research Laboratories, Eli Lilly and Company,
Indianapolis, Indiana, 46285

New Approaches to the Pharmacological Management of Major Depressive Disorder

Abstract

Despite effective and safe therapies for major depressive disorder (MDD), the current arsenal of antidepressant therapies does not fully satisfy the needs of patients or physicians. Many patients are only partial responders or are treatment resistant and side effects interfere with compliance. The majority of antidepressants directly affect monoamine neurotransmission within the central nervous system. Moving beyond this mechanism has been a challenge because of the lack of knowledge about the underlying etiology and pathophysiology of

Advances in Pharmacology, Volume 57
© 2009 Elsevier Inc. All rights reserved.

1054-3589/08 $35.00
10.1016/S1054-3589(08)57009-8

MDD. Provided in this report is a review of some of the major new advances in MDD research that suggest the possibility of novel and improved future therapeutic options. Emphasis is placed on studies of unipolar, but not bipolar, depression. New therapies include dual and triple monoamine uptake inhibitors, non-conventional antidepressants such as tianeptine, and a number of augmentation strategies. In addition, studies are underway on a number of mechanisms of action that might yield the next therapeutic advance. These include agents that interact with endocannabiniod systems, examination of natural products, and compounds that influence neuropeptide systems such as galanin and melanin-concentrating hormone, and growth and neurotrophic factors. Epigenetic mechanisms involving histone modification are also being explored. An area of intensive investigation is glutamate neurotransmission. Data support the hypothesis that NMDA receptor antagonists are effective in MDD individuals resistant to conventional therapies. The potential of metabotropic glutamate receptors as novel targets is also discussed. Accumulating evidence supports the idea that amplification of AMPA receptor function is a critical link in the transduction processes involved antidepressant effects.

I. Introduction

Disorders of mood including major depressive disorder (MDD) and bipolar depression affect the lives of millions worldwide. Although existing pharmacological treatments are effective and generally well tolerated, there is significant room for improvement, both in terms of efficacy and side effects. Provided in this report is an overview of the major areas of experimental inquiry that address this medical need and thereby pave the way for the next generation of antidepressant drugs. Work in this area is particularly difficult because of the lack of information on disease etiology and pathophysiolgy and the limitations of the preclinical animal models. Nonetheless, a broad range of neurobiological mechanisms are being considered for next-generation antidepressants. In many cases small molecules have already been identified that selectively impact the relevant systems. For some, new chemical entities have been advanced in development to orally active molecules that can be used to address proof of principle in the clinic. As emphasis is placed in the present review on unipolar depression, those wishing to review information on bipolar depression are urged to consult any number of excellent articles (DiazGranados & Zarate, 2008; Kozikowski et al., 2007; Rowe, Wiest, & Chuang, 2007; Zarate, Singh, & Manji, 2006). Besides new pharmacological approaches for treating MDD, other treatment modalities such a deep brain stimulation are under development (Hamani et al., 2009; Rakofsky, Holtzheimer, & Nemeroff, 2009).

II. Mood Disorders

Mood disorders are one of the most prevalent medical conditions in the world. According to the Diagnostic and Statistical Manual of Mental Disorders (DSM IV), mood disorders are characterized by (1) depressed mood; (2) greatly diminished interest and pleasure in life events; (3) weight gain or loss; (4) sleep alterations; (5) agitation; (6) fatigue, loss of energy; (7) thoughts of worthlessness or inappropriate guilt; (8) decreased capacity to concentrate, think and make decisions; and (9) suicidal ideation. A host of conditions are classified under mood disorders including bipolar depression, major depression, masked depression, dysthymic disorder, psychotic depression, and cyclothymic disorder (Dubovsky & Buzan, 1999). The prevalence of these disorders is 9–20% of the population in the Western hemisphere and is expected to increase as the population ages.

III. Antidepressants

A. Conventional Agents

Modern pharmacotherapy has been employed for the treatment of depression since the introduction of the monoamine oxidase inhibitors and the tricyclic monoamine uptake inhibitors in the 1950s. Besides being useful for reducing the symptoms associated with depression, these agents have been valuable tools in defining neurochemical systems associated with these disorders. Thus, the observation that a structurally and pharmacologically diverse group of antidepressants share in common the ability to increase the synaptic concentration of norepinephrine, serotonin, and/or dopamine is one of the foundations of the biogenic amine theory of depression (Iversen, 2005).

Although marked enhancements in the safety and side-effect profile of antidepressants have been engineered into modern therapeutics, further improvements are needed. In this regard, treatment response and remission rates are the areas of greatest unmet need. It has been estimated that up to 50% of patients do not respond to antidepressant treatment (Rush et al., 2006). Of those responding to these agents, remission is only partial in up to 70%. Moreover, some 30% of depressed subjects do not respond to antidepressant therapy despite being prescribed multiple pharmacological agents (Rush et al., 2006). These patients, termed treatment resistant, remain without therapeutic relief from their core symptoms. For most depressed subjects, some symptoms of MDD are often not affected by antidepressants. These include cognitive dysfunction and fatigue.

The rate of onset of action is another area of intense interest and study. Although some effects of antidepressants are observed within hours of administration, full-blown improvement can take several weeks of continuous treatment (Katz et al., 2004). As outlined below, a variety of experimental approaches are being taken to address these areas of unmet need.

B. Dual and Triple Reuptake Inhibitors

In recent years, selective dual inhibitors of serotonin and norepinephrine have been introduced as antidepressants. While these compounds affect the same neurotransmitter systems as older agents, such as desipramine or tranylcypromine, they are better tolerated (Millan, 2009). It was hoped that these compounds might provide not only enhanced efficacy over the serotonin selective reuptake inhibitors (SSRIs) but also a more rapid onset of action and be more generally efficacious (Schmitt et al., 2009; Tran, Bymaster, McNamara, & Potter, 2003). Clinical experience indicates the dual uptake inhibitors, such as venlafaxine and duloxetine, are valuable treatment options for MDD (Benedict, Arellano, De Cock, & Baird, 2009).

There is substantial evidence that dopamine plays a significant role in the regulation of mood. Because of this, significant effort has been expended on the discovery and development of new chemical entities that inhibit the uptake of serotonin, norepinephrine, and dopamine in the hope that the dopamine-driven mood enhancement would be beneficial in the treatment of depression (Aluisio et al., 2008; Liang et al., 2008; Millan, 2009; Skolnick & Basile, 2007; Skolnick, Popik, Janowsky, Beer, & Lippa, 2003; Skolnick et al., 2006).

C. Non-conventional Agents

Tianeptine (Brink, Harvey, & Brand, 2006; Wagstaff, Ormrod, & Spencer, 2001), in contrast to the monoamine-based antidepressants discussed above, enhances the synaptic uptake of serotonin with minimal effects on norepinephrine and dopamine uptake. Tianeptine is a generally well-tolerated medication which, like the SSRIs, has both antidepressant and anxiolytic activity. Preclinical work suggests that tianeptine has neuroprotective effects against stress-induced dendritic atrophy in the hippocampus, and has neurogenic actions (Kasper & McEwen, 2008) and might engender these effects via modulation of glutamate neurotransmission (Zoladz, Park, Muñoz, Fleshner, & Diamond, 2008).

Mirtazepine (Croom, Perry, & Plosker, 2009), in addition to facilitating the availability of norepinephrine and serotonin, is an α_2-adrenoceptor and histamine H_1 receptor antagonist. It displays both antidepressant and anxiolytic activity and appears to be especially beneficial in improving sleep in MDD populations. Meta-analysis suggests superior efficacy in acute phases of treatment and in melancholic patients and a faster onset of action for mirtazepine as compared to conventional agents.

Pramipexole is a dopamine $D_{2/3}$ receptor agonist approved for use in the treatment of Parkinson's disease. It has also displayed efficacy as a treatment for unipolar and bipolar depression and possibly of cycling in bipolar disorder (see Aiken, 2007). However, side effects, such as sleep attacks, induction of compulsive behaviors, and psychotic symptoms limit the utility of pramipexole. Whether these side effects are more common in Parkinson's disease than in pure MDD remains to be seen. Preclinical data support the clinical responses observed with pramipexole and confirm its mechanism of action. Thus, this agent has an antidepressant-like profile in the forced-swim test in both normal and adrenocorticotropin hormone-treated rats, and these effects are attenuated by both a selective dopamine D_2 and a selective dopamine D_3 receptor antagonist (Kitagawa et al., 2009). Pramipexole, and the $D_{2/3}$ receptor agonist (+)-7-OH-DPAT, decrease the hyperactivity and brain alterations in rats that result from bilateral lesions of the olfactory bulbs, an animal model used to screen for antidepressant drugs (Breuer et al., 2009). Other structurally distinct dopamine $D_{2/3}$ receptor agonists display antidepressant activity and, in some cases, anxiolytic-like effects (Millan et al., 2004).

D. Augmentation Approaches

One standard approach to treating MDD patients who are unresponsive or only partially responsive to an antidepressant is to coadminister an augmenting agent, such as bupropion. Aripiprazole, an antipsychotic, has received FDA approval as an adjunct treatment of MDD. Aripiprazole increases antidepressant response when added to monotherapy with escitalopram, fluoxetine, paroxetine controlled release, sertraline, or venlafaxine extended release (Berman et al., 2009).

Several clinical studies have also shown that olanzapine, an antipsychotic, augments the antidepressant response to fluoxetine, an SSRI, when the combined product (Symbyax) is administered to treatment-resistant patients (Debattista & Hawkins, 2009; Trivedi et al., 2009).

E. Mechanisms of Action

When considering new approaches for the treatment of depression, selection of a molecular target must take into consideration the known pharmacology of conventional and atypical antidepressants, factors that precipitate or increase MDD symptoms, and the lag time between drug administration and full therapeutic benefit. Because most currently used antidepressants directly influence central monoaminergic transmission, the biogenic amine theory of depression continues to predominate (Iversen, 2005; Millan, 2009). As relapse sometimes involves environmental stressors and neurotoxic responses to glucocorticoids, a hypothesis on the underlying mechanism of action of antidepressants is that antidepressants are neuroprotective. This theory holds that antidepressants enhance the production of neurotrophic factors, such as brain-derived neurotrophic factor (BDNF), that provide cellular protection, growth, and resilience in brain areas involved in affective illness (Duman, 2004). Support for this idea is based on the fact that BDNF has neurotrophic and neuroprotective effects, and that it can promote neurogenesis. Further, the neurogenic effects of antidepressants are thought to be mediated by BDNF (Duman, 2004). Finally, neurogenesis appears necessary for the antidepressant-like effects of drugs (Santarelli et al., 2003). The pathways through which antidepressants influence BDNF production have been described, along with some inconsistencies in the BDNF model of depression (Alt, Nisenbaum, Bleakman & Witkin, 2006).

F. Assessment of Antidepressant Potential

There are no functionally homologous animal models of MDD. However, some aspects of MDD can be modeled in laboratory animals and certain models readily and reliably detect the biological actions of antidepressants *in vivo* (Cryan, Markou, & Lucki, 2002; O'Neill & Moore, 2003; Willner & Mitchell, 2002). A host of animal models are routinely employed to screen for potential antidepressant activity. Two of the most efficient and commonly used assays are the forced-swim test (mouse or rat) and the mouse tail-suspension test. In both cases, antidepressants generally decrease the immobility of rodents placed in an inescapable situation (a swim tank or suspension in space). Other animal models require subchronic antidepressant treatment to observe a behavioral change, more closely mimicking the human temporal situation than the acute tests. Included among the subchronic models are the reduction of submissive behavior paradigm, the novelty-suppressed feeding assay, the chronic unpredictable stress assay, the olfactory bulbectomy model, and learned helplessness (Alt et al., 2006; Cryan et al., 2002; Willner & Mitchell, 2002).

IV. New Targets in Discovery and Development

Because so little is known about the precise abnormalities associated with or the etiology of depression, the number of potential targets for new therapeutics is quite large. Detailed below are many of the mechanistic approaches that have been most popular over the past few years.

A. Endocannabiniod Agents

Cannabis and its major psychoactive component (–)-trans-Δ^9-tetrahydrocannabinol are known to have effects on anxiety and mood. The endocannabinoid system is a highly regulated network. The endocannabinoids, of which arachidonoylethanolamide (anandamide) and 2-arachidonoylglycerol (2-AG) are members of a novel class of regulatory neurolipid molecules located in the central nervous system (CNS). These substances operate as retrograde signaling messengers, modulate neuronal plasticity, as well as adjust the momentary strength of excitatory and inhibitory neurotransmission (Di Marzo, 2009). The synaptic effects (availability) of the endocannabinoids are controlled by specific reuptake processes and/or enzymatic degradation by fatty acid amidohydrolase (FAAH) and monoacylglycerol lipase (Di Marzo, 2009). Although the molecular entity responsible for endocannabinoid reuptake has not been identified, compounds that inhibit uptake and/or FAAH-induced enzymatic degradation have been identified. Among the agents that block anandamide uptake are LY2077885 and OMDM-1 (Felder et al., 2006; Witkin, Tzavara, & Nomikos, 2005). Compounds that inhibit FAAH also increase brain concentrations of anandamide. Of these, URB597 is the most characterized molecule. There are at least two G-protein-coupled cannabinoind receptors (CB_1 and CB_2) that bind endocannabinoids and exogenous cannabinoid ligands (Di Marzo, 2009). Endocannabinoids can also act through the stimulation of the vanilloid type 1 (TRPV1) cation channel-gating receptor (Di Marzo, 2009; Witkin, Tzavara, Davis, Li, & Nomikos, 2005).

Data suggest that amplification of endocannabinoid systems engender anxiolytic, antidepressant, analgesic and other pharmacological actions of potential therapeutic import. There is increasing, although not uniform, agreement that a cannabinoid agonist can, under some conditions, display antidepressant-like behavioral and biochemical effects, including neurogenesis (Table I) (Bambico & Gobbi, 2008; Bambico, Duranti, Tontini, Tarzia, & Gobbi, 2009; Tzavara & Witkin, 2008; Witkin, Tzavara, & Nomikos, 2005). In a number of cases, the agonists appear to act primarily through CB_1 receptors. For example, the CB_1 receptor antagonist, rimonabant, prevents the antidepressant-like effects of endocannabinoid agonists but not of imipramine (Adamczyk, Gołda, McCreary, Filip, & Przegaliński, 2008; Shearman et al., 2003). Further support for antidepressant-like effects of these molecules comes from *in vivo* studies demonstrating their enhancement of the antidepressant-like activity of conventional antidepressants. For example, the indirect endocannabinoid agonist, AM404, enhances the antidepressant-like effects of imipramine or citalopram, whereas the FAAH

TABLE I Effects of Cannabinoid Agonists in Tests Detecting Conventional Antidepressants

Compound	Method—species	Findings[a]	Reference
URB597	TST—mouse	Decreased immobility	Gobbi et al. (2005)
URB597	Modified TST—mouse	Decreased immobility	Naidu et al. (2007)
URB597	TST—mouse	No effect from 1 to 10 mg/kg	Naidu et al. (2007)
None	TST—mouse	Decreased immobility in FAAH(−/−)	Naidu et al. (2007)
Anandamide	TST—mouse	**Increases in immobility**	Naidu et al. (2007)
URB597	CMS—mouse	Decreased weight loss	Bortolato et al. (2007)
		Increased sucrose drinking	
URB597	FST—rat	Decreased immobility	Gobbi et al. (2005)
AM404, HU-210	FST—rat	Decreased immobility as with DMI	Hill and Gorzalka (2005)
AM404, URB597, CP55,940	FST—rat	Decreased immobility	Adamczyk et al. (2008)
URB597	FST—rat	Decreased immobility	Hill et al. (2007)
HU-210	FST—rat	Decreased immobility	Jiang et al. (2005)
HU-210	FST—rat	Hippocampal X-irradiation prevented antidepressant-like effects	Jiang et al. (2005)
ACEA	FST—rat	Decreased immobility	Rutkowska and Jachimczuk (2004)
AM404, URB597, CP55,940	Restraint—rat	Blockade of corticosterone increases	Patel et al. (2004)
URB597, CP55,940	Restraint—rat	Blockade of decreased sucrose intake and preference	Rademacher and Hillard (2007)
URB597	Electrophysiology—rat	Increased firing of dorsal raphe 5-HT and locus coeruleus NE neurons	Gobbi et al. (2005)
CP47,497	Tetrabenazine-induced ptosis—mouse	**No blockade to 10 mg/kg**	Weissman, Milne, and Melvin (1982)

Data from dose–effect studies only. CMS, chronic mild stress; DMI, desipramine; FST, forced-swim test; 5-HT, serotonin; NE, norepinephrine; TST, tail-suspension test.

[a] Negative findings are shown in bold.

inhibitor, URB597, augments the effects of imipramine only (Adamczyk et al., 2008). The CB_1 receptor agonist, ACEA, enhances the ability of fluoxetine to decrease immobility in the mouse forced-swim test to levels much greater than can be attained with either drug alone (Rutkowska & Jachimczuk, 2004). Further evidence linking endocannabinoids and anti-depressants is the finding that 3 weeks of desipramine treatment increases CB_1 receptor density in rat hippocampus and hypothalamus (Hill et al., 2006). These biochemical changes are associated with decreases in forced-swim-induced corticosterone secretion and c-fos induction in the paraventricular nucleus. As both the corticosterone and c-fos effects are prevented by AM251 pretreatment, it appears that the CB_1 receptor is mediating these effects (Hill et al., 2006). Furthermore, as noted above, there are data linking neurogenesis to the behavioral effects of the CB_1 receptor agonist HU-210. As hippocampal neurogenesis appears to be a component of the response to antidepressants (Santarelli et al., 2003), it is notable that HU-210 induces neurogenesis and decreases immobility in the rat forced-swim test (Jiang et al., 2005); X-rays directed at hippocampal structures disrupted both the neurogenesis and antidepressant-like effects of HU-210 (Jiang et al., 2005).

Convergent biological data have also implicated CB_1 receptor antagonism as an inducer of antidepressant-like activity (Tzavara & Witkin, 2008; Witkin, Tzavara, & Davis, et al., 2005). Thus, functional antagonism of CB_1 receptors produces antidepressant-like behavioral and biochemical effects (Table II). A variety of molecules are effective in animal models that detect different behavioral effects of antidepressants and these antagonists affect brain neurochemistry in a manner consistent with antidepressant activity. These effects are observed in different species, are attenuated by CB_1 agonists, and are not observed in CB_1 receptor null mice (Table II).

While endocannabinoid receptor agonists and antagonists have been suggested to play a role in mood, there are side-effect liabilities associated with their use. Thus, endocannabinoid receptor agonists may have abuse and dependence liabilities (Tzavara & Witkin, 2008; Witkin, Tzavara, & Davis, et al., 2005), while inhibitors of FAAH may not (Solinas, Yasar, & Goldberg, 2007). Endocannabinoid antagonists might cause mood disturbances. Indeed, two of these agents, rimonabant and taranabant, were reported to cause anxiety/mood problems when examined clinically as treatments for obesity (Moreira, Grieb, & Lutz, 2009).

There are some, although limited, data suggesting that CB_2 receptors may also be potential targets for novel antidepressants (Onaivi et al., 2008).

B. Natural Products

A variety of natural products and their derivatives have displayed the potential to be therapies for neurological and psychiatric disorders,

TABLE II Effects of Cannabinoid Receptor Antagonist/Inverse-Agonists in Tests Predictive of an Impact in Mood Disorders

Compound	Method—species	Findings[a]	Reference
Rimonabant	FST—mouse	Decreased immobility	Tzavara et al. (2003)
Rimonabant	FST—rat	Decreased immobility as with fluoxetine	Griebel, Stemmelin, and Scatton (2005)
Rimonabant	FST—rat	No effect	Adamczyk et al. (2008)
AM251	FST—mouse	Decreased immobility as with DMI	Shearman et al. (2003)
AM251	FST—mouse	CB$_1$ receptor deletion prevented antidepressant-like effects	Shearman et al. (2003)
AM251	TST—mouse	Decreased immobility as with DMI	Shearman et al. (2003)
Rimonabant	Tonic immobility—gerbil	Decreased immobility as with fluoxetine	Griebel et al. (2005)
Rimonabant	Chronic mild stress—mouse	Decreased fur deterioration. Decreased immobility in FST	Griebel et al. (2005)
Rimonabant	EEG	Antidepressant-like EEG activation	Santucci, Storme, Soubrie, and Le Fur (1996)
AM281	Sexual behavior—male, rough-skinned newts	Blockade of stress and CORT-induced suppression of sexual behavior	Coddington, Lewis, Rose, and Moore (2007)
Rimonabant	Neurochemistry—Rat	Increased efflux of 5-HT, NE, DA, Ach	Tzavara et al. (2003)

Data from dose–effect studies only. Ach, acetylcholine; CORT, corticosterone; DA, dopamine; DMI, desipramine; FST, forced-swim test; 5-HT, serotonin; NE, norepinephrine; TST, tail-suspension test.
[a] Negative findings are shown in bold.

including Alzheimer's disease and MDD. Several have a long history of use as treatments for stress, mood, and anxiety (Kumar, 2006). In addition to the potential that natural product-derived medications might be safer than conventional agents, there is the possibility that such compounds might have novel mechanisms of action and therefore an improved efficacy profile. Indeed, the multiplicity of actions of some of these materials would seem to suggest a high potential for displaying some clinically beneficial effects (Panossian & Wikeman, 2008).

Natural products are grouped into distinct categories based on origin, use, and function. Adaptogens are generally plants or plant extracts that increase the ability of biological substrates to adapt to particular stresses and to balance endocrine changes and alterations in immune function (Brekhman & Dardymov, 1969). These materials reportedly enhance physical and mental capacity, reduce fatigue, improve resistance to disease, and prolong life. Examples of adaptogens include *Rhodiola rosea, Schisandra chinensis, Eleutherococcus senticosus* (Siberian ginseng), and Ginsenosides (*Panax ginseng*). A mixture of such materials was reported to display antidepressant-like effects in rodents and to induce biochemical alterations associated with resilience (Panossian, Wikman, Kaur, & Asea, 2009). Medicinal plants overlap with the adaptogens. These include species such as *Ginkgo biloba*, St. John's wort, Huperzine A, Kaka-kaka, Valeriana, Berberine, *Apocynum venetum*, and Soy isoflavone. Of these, St. John's wort is used for management of mood, although with questionable efficacy (Linde et al., 2005a,b; Linde, Berner, & Kriston, 2008). Berberine is an isoquinoline alkaloid used for many years in some oriental cultures as an antimicrobial and as a treatment for sores. Preclinical studies suggest that berberine has antidepressant-like behavioral and biochemical effects in rodents (Kulkarni & Dhir, 2007, 2008).

Also gaining attention are the omega-3 fatty acids that are present in many natural products. This was stimulated in part by a 1998 report showing a significant negative correlation between fish consumption and the prevalence of MDD (Hibbeln, 1998). The potential value of omega-3 fatty acids as a treatment for a host of neurological and neuropsychiatric disorders is being considered (Freeman et al., 2006). Indeed, the data for MDD has some clinical support in both unipolar and bipolar disorders (Freeman et al., 2006; Montgomery & Richardson, 2008; Ross, Seguin, & Sieswerda, 2007; Turnbull, Cullen-Drill, & Smaldone, 2008).

Herbs represent another category of natural product that could yield antidepressants. Of these, capsaicin, luteolin (Oregano), clove, cinnamon, and curcumin have garnered particular attention. Curcumin (diferuloyl-methane) is the primary constituent of the spice turmeric used in curries (*Curcuma longa*). A host of biological effects and potential therapeutic uses have been attributed to this agent. For example, it is reported to display antimicrobial, anticarcinogenic, and antioxidant properties among others

(Goel, Kunnumakkara, & Aggarwal, 2008; Kulkarni & Dhir, 2009). Curcumin enhances neural cell adhesion molecule (NCAM) polysialylation, a process intimately associated with hippocampal neural processing. Subchronic administration of curcumin to rats increases polysialyated cells in the dentate infragranular zone of the hippocampus and increases water maze learning and consolidation. This effect is related to the inhibition of protein kinase A delta (Conboy et al., 2009). This finding, besides strengthening the molecular basis of spatial learning in hippocampus, suggests that curcumin could enhance cognition. Moreover, given the putative role of hippocampal modulation in mood disorders (see Sections III. E and V. B), such a mechanism might also underlie the antidepressant potential of curcumin.

Curcumin tea has been used for the treatment of stress and mood disorders for over a century, and preclinical studies support the antidepressant potential of this substance. Thus, Xu et al. (2005b) reported that curcumin displays oral antidepressant-like activity in the mouse tail-suspension and forced-swim tests. Curcumin is also active in a chronic unpredictable stress assay for both behavioral and biochemical endpoints (Bhutani, Bishnoi, & Kulkarni, 2009). Curcumin is also active against other behavioral and biochemical changes brought on by chronic unpredictable stress (Li et al., 2009). At a dose shown to display antidepressant-like activity in animal models (10 mg/kg), curcumin increases the brain levels of dopamine, serotonin, and norepinephrine. Since curcumin also inhibits monoamine oxidase A and B (Xu et al., 2005b; Kulkarni, Bhutani, & Bishnoi, 2008), its ability to increase monoamines and induce antidepressant-like behavioral changes could be related to this enzyme inhibition. Rats administered curcumin for 14 consecutive days also display antidepressant-like effects in the forced-swim test and in the olfactory bulbectomy model (Xu et al., 2005a). In the olfactory bulbectomy model, curcumin attenuates the hyperactivity and passive avoidance deficits seen in these animals and reverses the decrease in monoamine levels induced by the lesion (Xu et al., 2005a). Curcumin is also effective against behavioral and neurochemical changes engendered by chronic stress, including effects on neurogenesis pathways (Xu et al., 2006, 2007, 2009). While curcumin augments the antidepressant-like effects of fluoxetine, venlafaxine, and bupropion, it is ineffective in this regard when administered with tricyclic antidepressants; the reason for this differential interaction is not known (Kulkarni et al., 2008).

Antidepressant-like effects of curcumin might involve actions upon serotonin $5\text{-}HT_1$ and $5\text{-}HT_2$ receptors (Wang et al., 2008b). Curcumin also increases brain levels of BDNF, thereby activating trkB receptors. It is speculated these effects are involved in the neuroprotective and antidepressant-like effects of curcumin (Wang et al., 2008a). An interaction of curcumin with the adenylyl cyclase and cAMP processing pathways through serotonin receptors has also been identified. Curcumin also has nanomolar affinity inverse agonist activity at CB_1 receptors. (Seely, Levi, &

Prather, 2009). Thus, the biochemical pharmacology of curcumin is consistent with a possible antidepressant action.

C. Other Potential Mechanisms of Action

1. Galanin 3

Galanin is a 29-amino acid neuropeptide with a C-terminal amide. In humans it has 30 amino acids and is non-amidated. Three G-protein-coupled galanin receptor subtypes, Gal_1, Gal_2, and Gal_3, have been cloned from both human and rat (Branchek, Smith, Gerald, & Walker, 2000). In rat brain, galanin is present in 80–90% of noradrenaline-producing neurons of the locus coeruleus and 30% of serotonin-producing neurons of the dorsal raphe nucleus (Holets, Hokfelt, Rokaeus, Terenius, & Goldstein, 1988). Galanin is also found in corticolimbic regions of the brain, including the amygdala, hippocampus, septum, and hypothalamus (Melander, Hokfelt, & Rokaeus, 1986; O'Donnell, Ahmad, Wahlestedt, & Walker, 1999). Galanin can modulate serotonergic neurotransmission (Razani, Diaz-Cabialem, Fuxe, & Ogren, 2000) and attenuate imipramine- or citalopram-induced extracellular 5-HT release in rats (Yoshitake et al., 2003).

The evidence that Gal_3 might be involved in the control of anxiety and mood comes from studies in which galanin peptides are administered to laboratory animals. However, these data do not generate a fully consistent picture. The most direct evidence for the involvement of Gal_3 receptors in mood and anxiety is derived from investigations with systemically active galanin receptor antagonists. The Gal_3 receptor antagonists SNAP 37889 and SNAP 398299 display anxiolytic- and antidepressant-like effects including reducing vocalizations after maternal separation in guinea pig, attenuating stress-induced hyperthermia in mice, increasing punished drinking in rats, and decreasing immobility in the rat forced-swim test. Increased social interaction and antidepressant-like effect in the forced-swim test are maintained over 21-day treatment (Swanson et al., 2005).

2. Melanin-Concentrating Hormone

There is a body of evidence suggesting that blockade of melanin-concentrating hormone (MCH_1) receptors might be of value in the treatment of MDD and anxiety (Chaki et al., 2005; Shimazaki, Yoshimizu, & Chaki, 2006). In addition to the lateral hypothalamus, MCH-containing fibers project to the isocortex, olfactory regions, hippocampus, amygdala, septum, basal ganglia, thalamus, brainstem, cerebellum, and spinal cord (Bittencourt et al., 1992). Reports from several laboratories indicate a range of antidepressant-like, anxiolytic-like, and antistress endocrine effects of MCH_1 receptor antagonists (Chaki et al., 2005; Gehlert et al., 2009; Shimazaki et al., 2006; Smith et al., 2006). Study of MCH_1 receptor knockout mice confirms that reduction in receptor availability or function yields anxiolytic-like and antidepressant-like effects (Gehlert et al., 2009; Smith et al., 2006). There are also data indicating MCH_1 receptor involvement in the regulation of limbic dopaminergic activity (Smith et al., 2005).

Gehlert et al. (2009) correlated *in vivo* behavioral doses in rodents with the autoradiographically identified interaction of GW803430 with MCH_1 receptors. They found antidepressant-like efficacy of this MCH_1 antagonist in the mouse forced-swim and tail-suspension tests, with the activity in the forced-swim test absent in MCH_1 –/– mice. In a test of the reduction of submissive behavior, subchronic administration of GW803430 is efficacious in rats. A more rapid onset of action of MCH_1 antagonism as compared to conventional antidepressants might be deduced from the finding that SNAP94847 is effective in the novelty-suppressed feeding assay after acute administration, while this effect is generally only observed with antidepressants after subacute treatment (David et al., 2007). Evidence that the MCH_1 antagonist mechanism might be independent of neurogenesis was reported by David et al. (2007), which would also be consistent with the possibility of a rapid onset of action.

Contrary to these findings, an MCH_1 antagonist (SNAP 94847) is inactive in the mouse forced-swim test (David et al., 2007). Further, Basso et al. (2006) were unable to detect antidepressant-like activity in the rat forced-swim, mouse tail-suspension, and Vogel conflict tests with four structurally distinct MCH_1 antagonists, SNAP7941, T226296, A665798, and A777903.

It appears that MCH_1-containing neural pathways can affect the behavioral response to drugs of abuse (DiLeone, Georgescu, & Nestler, 2003), a common comorbidity with mood and anxiety disorders. Blockade of MCH_1 receptors is also associated with a reduction in body weight. In addition, the fact that the MCH_1 antagonist GW803430 augments the antidepressant-like effects of imipramine (Gehlert et al., 2009) suggests that MCH_1 antagonists might be useful as adjuncts for the treatment of MDD. Moreover, like fluoxetine and desmethylimipramine, an MCH_1 receptor antagonist peptide increases phosphorylation of GluR1 at Ser845 (Georgescu et al., 2005) (see Sections III. E and V. B for a discussion of these mechanisms).

3. VGF and FGF

Both nerve growth factor inducible (VGF) and fibroblast growth factor (FGF) are implicated in the symptoms of MDD (Thakker-Varia & Alder, 2009; Turner, Akil, Watson, & Evans, 2006). VGF is a neuropeptide induced by nerve growth factor, CREB, and BDNF under the regulation of neurotrophin-3. Several pieces of evidence suggest VGF and its associated biochemical machinery as potential targets for the treatment of MDD. There is up-regulation of VGF by antidepressant treatments (Alder et al., 2003; Thakker-Varia & Alder, 2009) and VGF increases the expression of several gene products (associated with cell proliferation) that are induced by electroconvulsive therapy or exercise (Hunsberger et al., 2007; Newton et al., 2003). Administration of the VGF peptide, TLQP62, enhances hippocampal neuron proliferation both *in vivo* and *in vitro* (Thakker-Varia et al., 2007), and VGF displays neuroprotective effects against cerebellar granule cell death (Severini et al., 2008). Stress, such as that associated with learned helplessness, immobilization, and forced swimming, down-regulates VGF protein in the hippocampus (Hunsberger et al., 2007; Thakker-Varia & Alder, 2007). All of these findings are consistent with the idea that VGF may play a role in controlling affect.

VGF is influenced by the neurotrophic growth factor mitogen-activated protein (MAP) kinase signaling pathway, with the regulation of VGF by BDNF requiring trkB and MAP kinases. MEK inhibitors block the BDNF-induced VGF production in neuronal cell culture (Alder et al., 2003), and both 5-HT and BDNF stimulate VGF expression independently. Up-regulation of VGF by 5-HT is not blocked by the trk receptor antagonist K252a, but is blocked by a 5-HT_{1A} receptor antagonist (WAY100635) and by a 5-HT_7 receptor antagonist (SB269970). In contrast, these 5-HT receptor antagonists have no effect on BDNF-induced VGF production (Thakker-Varia et al., 2007). The VGF peptide, TLQP-21, induces mobilization of intracellular calcium in cerebellar granule cells (Severini et al., 2008), with the CaMK inhibitor, KN93, blocking the induction of VGF by BDNF (Newton et al., 2003). Moreover, C-terminal cleaved VGF peptides influence synaptic plasticity and display neuroprotective and neurogenesis activities. Thus, the C-terminal VGF peptides, TLQP-62 and AQEE30, enhance synaptic activity in rat hippocampal neurons (Alder et al., 2003), induce synaptic plasticity genes (*Nrn1* and *Syn1*) in PC-12 cells and after *in vivo* hippocampal infusion of VGF (Hunsberger et al., 2007). These peptides also produce antidepressant-like effects in animal behavioral models that are not observed with VGF knockout mice (Hunsberger et al., 2007; Thakker-Varia et al., 2007).

The linkage of FGF and MDD might help explain the high correlation between depression and vascular disorders (Kahl et al., 2009; Newton & Duman, 2004). A relationship between FGF and MDD is suggested by the fact that this peptide, like antidepressants, displays neuroprotective effects and induces neurogenesis in hippocampus. It has also been shown that antidepressants increase activation of FGF2 (Czeh et al., 2001; Mallei, Shi, & Mocchetti, 2002; Maragnoli, Fumagalli, Gennarelli, Racagni, & Riva, 2004) and the FGF2-associated extracellular chaperone, FGF-binding protein (Bachis, Mallei, Cruz, Wellstein, & Mocchetti, 2008). Although up-regulation of FGF2 is sometimes observed after stress (Molten et al., 2001), some stressors, such as defeat stress, down-regulate FGF transcripts, including FGF2, in rat brain (Turner, Calve, Frost, Akil, & Watson, 2008), an effect consistent with post-mortem findings in MDD patients (Evans et al.,

2004). FGF2 (i.c.v.) in rats induces antidepressant-like behavior in both the forced-swim test and the novelty-suppressed feeding assay (Turner Gula, Taylor, Watson, & Akil, 2008).

While an association of adenosine A_{2a} receptors with FGF has recently been reported (Flajolet et al., 2008), the implications of this finding with regard to mood disorders is not fully understood. A relationship of the FGF system with the cell adhesion processing involved in neural plasticity has also been identified (Aonurm-Helm et al., 2008). In this case, mice deficient in NCAM display a depression-like phenotype in the tail-suspension and sucrose-preference tests. Likewise, these mice have reduced adult neurogenesis and reduced levels of phospho-CREB in the hippocampus. FGL, a peptide associated with the NCAM binding site for FGF receptors, attenuates the depression-like phenotype in NCAM −/− mice and increases phospho-CREB. These data not only reinforce the potential role of FGF in mood disorders but also further substantiate the importance of neurogenesis and neural plasticity in the development and treatment of mood disorders.

4. Histone Deacetylase 5

Epigenetic phenomena are likely to affect mood and to influence the pathogenesis and therapeutic relief from MDD. Histone modification is known to be influenced by, and to be involved in, pathways regulating mood and responses to antidepressants (Beglopoulos & Shen, 2006). Thus, intracellular targets influencing histone rearrangement, such as methylation and acetylation, are being carefully scrutinized, with recent data possibly opening a new broad area of investigation. Particular emphasis is being placed on the hypothesis that histone deacetylase (HDAC) inhibitors might facilitate histone remodeling in a way that may underlie depression and antidepressant activity.

Evidence supporting this hypothesis includes the finding that HDAC5 and CREB mRNA are altered in peripheral leukocytes of patients with MDD (Iga et al., 2007). Indirect support also comes from the observation that some non-selective HDAC inhibitors, such as valproate, are used for the treatment of bipolar disorder (Beutler, Li, Nicol, & Walsh, 2005). In addition, like known antidepressants, some HDAC inhibitors are neuroprotective (Gardian et al., 2005).

The tricyclic antidepressant imipramine regulates histone acetylation in rodents (Tsankova et al., 2006). Moreover, defeat stress is reported to downregulate Bdnf II and IV and to increase repressive histone methylation. Chronic administration of imipramine reverses the stress-induced down-regulation of BDNF and increases histone acetylation. These changes are associated with the down-regulation of HDAC5. The overexpression of HDAC5 in hippocampus which nullifies the effects of imipramine further support the involvement of this deacetylase in the action of this antidepressant.

While the data in hippocampus are consistent with the idea that HDAC5 inhibition might be antidepressant, results from the nucleus accumbens present the opposite picture (Renthal et al., 2007). In this case, chronic stress or cocaine selectively down-regulate HDAC5 in this brain structure. Conversely, HDAC5 overexpression decreases the reinforcing effects of cocaine, an effect reversed by HDAC inhibition. Further, HDAC5 deletion in nucleus accumbens sensitized mice to the reinforcing effects of cocaine, an effect attenuated with restoration of HDAC5. HDAC5 deletion in nucleus accumbens also sensitizes mice to the effects of chronic stress and long-term administration of imipramine selectively increases HDAC5 mRNA expression. The balance and integration of HDAC5 inhibition across the CNS must be better defined to fully appreciate its potential as a target for new drugs to treat MDD.

V. Glutamate Modulation

Another major departure from monoaminergic synapses as a focus of mood disorder therapeutics is the effort aimed at discerning the role of glutamatergic neurotransmission in this condition (Hashimoto, 2009; Mathew, Keegan, & Smith, 2005). Research on this topic has concentrated on NMDA receptors (Machado-Vieira, Salvadore, Diazgranados, & Zarate, 2009; Paul & Skolnick, 2003; Skolnick, Popik, & Trullas, 2009), AMPA receptors (Alt et al., 2006; Machado-Vieira, Salvadore, Ibrahim, Diaz-Granados, & Zarate, 2009; Skolnick, 2008), metabotropic receptors (Pilc, Chaki, Nowak, & Witkin, 2008; Witkin, Marek, Johnson, & Schoepp, 2007), downstream signaling pathways (Pilc et al., 2008; Szabo et al., 2009), excitatory amino acid transporters (EAATs), glia, and glutamate cycling (Valentine & Sanacora, 2009). This research has demonstrated that monoamine neurotransmission affects downstream glutamate targets and that AMPA receptor potentiation might be a core mechanism for the control of mood (Alt et al., 2006; Bleakman, Alt, & Witkin, 2007).

A. NMDA Receptors

Based on the finding that NMDA receptor antagonists alter long-term potentiation, Trullas and Skolnick (1990) proposed that NMDA receptor antagonist might have antidepressant properties. This launched a series of investigations demonstrating that blockade of the NMDA receptor ion–channel complex at multiple sites results in antidepressant-like activity in animal models used to identify potential antidepressants and anxiolytics (Paul & Skolnick, 2003; Skolnick et al., 2009). In addition to competitive antagonists acting at the glutamate recognition site, and uncompetitive antagonists acting at the ion channel, negative modulators of the glycine and the polyamine sites have also demonstrated efficacy in these assays. Moreover, zinc, an NMDA receptor ion channel blocker, has been reported to display antidepressant activity in the clinic (Pilc et al., 2008).

In addition to the clinical proof-of-principle studies from Nowak's group, the Trullas–Skolnick hypothesis has received additional substantiation in the clinical findings demonstrating that ketamine, a noncompetitive NMDA receptor antagonist, is efficacious in treatment-resistant MDD patients (Berman et al., 2000; Machado-Vieira, Salvadore, Diazgranados et al., 2009; Skolnick et al., 2009; Zarate et al., 2006). The findings with ketamine are particularly noteworthy in that its intravenous infusion provided almost immediate relief, in contrast to the days or weeks of continuous treatment that is required with conventional therapies (Katz et al., 2004). Moreover, relief from MDD symptoms following a single dose of ketamine lasted for up to 1 week. Extensions of this finding were reported with the disclosure that CP 101,606, an NMDA antagonist with selectivity for the NR2B receptor isoform, is also effective in reducing the symptoms of MDD in treatment-resistant patients on SSRI therapy (Preskorn et al., 2008). While the reported results with ketamine and CP 101,606 are remarkable, other mechanisms have shown related effects. For example, a double-blind, placebo-controlled study demonstrated a rapid and significant effect for i.v. scopolamine in the treatment of MDD (Furey & Drevets, 2006). More work is needed to fully appreciate the kinetic (i.v.) and pharmacological conditions (mechanisms) that are necessary and sufficient to drive these antidepressant responses.

The clinical findings with ketamine and CP 101,606 raise the question of how one might achieve remission with NMDA receptor blockade without the side effects, such as dissociative reactions, associated with this mechanism of action. In this regard, it is notable that the dose of CP 101,606, the receptor subtype-selective antagonist, found to be effective in treating depression did not cause any dissociative reactions (Preskorn et al., 2008). Another way of blocking the NMDA receptor without engendering phencyclidine-like side effects might be through functional blockade of the NMDA receptor-associated glycine site (Witkin, Steele, & Sharpe, 1997).

B. AMPA Receptors

As AMPA receptors have been implicated in mood disorders, they have been considered for some time as potential targets for the design of small molecule therapies (Alt et al., 2006; Bleakman et al., 2007; Machado-Vieira, Salvadore, Ibrahim, et al., 2009; Skolnick, 2008). Evidence that AMPA receptors are involved in MDD comes from a host of sources. For example, administration of known antidepressants generally increases AMPA receptor densities and/or enhances functional phosphorylation of this receptor (Alt et al., 2006). Thus, subchronic administration of an SSRI, such as fluoxetine, or a tricyclic antidepressant, such as desipramine, increases the expression and phosphorylation of AMPA GluR1 (Martinez-Turrillas, Frechilla, & Del Río, 2002; Svenningsson et al., 2002). Similar findings have been reported for other antidepressants, such as tianeptine (Svenningsson et al., 2007) and possible antidepressants, such as MCH_1 receptor antagonists (Georgescu et al., 2005). It has been suggested that increases in AMPA/NMDA currents might be responsible for antidepressant efficacy (Maeng & Zarate, 2007). However, electrophysiological data are not entirely consistent with the idea that antidepressant activity is due to an increase in AMPA current (c.f., Bobula & Hess, 2008; Marek, 2008). Indeed, drugs used to treat bipolar disorder generally have the opposite effect (Alt et al., 2006). The subunit composition of AMPA receptors and their localization are important considerations when attempting to link AMPA receptors and mood (Black, 2005; Todtenkopf et al., 2006). Additionally, AMPA receptor current and membrane localization are controlled by transmembrane AMPA receptor regulatory proteins that have unique, subtype-dependent, central localizations (Bredt & Nicoll, 2003).

Evidence supporting the hypothesis that amplification of signaling through AMPA receptors is related to antidepressant efficacy comes also from preclinical studies using conventional animal models employed for detecting antidepressants (Table III). Positive allosteric modulators of AMPA receptors, sometimes referred to as ampakines or AMPA receptor potentiators, produce antidepressant-like behavioral and biochemical effects. These effects have been reported in mice and rats with molecules from different structural classes. Antidepressant-like behavioral effects following acute dosing have been reported in the mouse forced-swim test, the mouse tail-suspension test, and in the rat forced-swim test. Moreover, AMPA receptor potentiators appear to display a faster onset of action than conventional agents in the dominance/submissive assay that requires subchronic administration to detect efficacy.

Evidence that these antidepressant-like effects of AMPA potentiators are due to AMPA receptor facilitation comes from the finding that AMPA receptor antagonists prevent this effect without altering the antidepressant-like action of imipramine (Li et al., 2001). An AMPA receptor blocker also prevented the antidepressant-like effects of ketamine and other NMDA antagonists, showing again that AMPA potentiation might be a core biochemical antidepressant process (Alt et al., 2006; Dybała, Siwek, Poleszak, Pilc, & Nowak, 2008; Maeng et al., 2008). Biochemical and morphological effects are observed after administration of AMPA receptor potentiators that are consistent with predictions from the neurogenesis hypothesis of depression (see Section III.E). Thus, AMPA potentiators increase BDNF levels and increase neurogenesis *in vitro* and *in vivo* (Table III).

TABLE III Effects of AMPA Receptor Potentiators on Antidepressant-Related Biochemistry and Behavior

Compound	Method—species	Findings	Reference
CX546, CX614	Entorhinal/hippocampal slices—rat	Increased BDNF and trkB mRNA	Lauterborn, Lynch, Vanderklish, and Arai (2000)
CX546	Hippocampus—rat	Increased BDNF mRNA	Lauterborn et al. (2000)
LY392098	Cortical neurons—rat	Increased BDNF	Legutko, Li, and Skolnick (2001)
LY451646	Hippocampus—rat	Increased BDNF	Mackowiak, O'Neill, Hicks, Bleakman, and Skolnick (2002)
LY451646	Hippocampus—rat	Increased cell proliferation	Bai, Bergeron, and Nelson (2003)
Org 26576	Hippocampus—rat	Increased cell proliferation and survival	Su et al. (2009)
LY392098	Forced-swim—mouse	Decreased immobility	Li et al. (2001), Witkin, Need, and Skolnick (2003)
LY392098	Forced-swim—rat	Decreased immobility	Li et al. (2001)
LY392098	Tail-suspension—mouse	Decreased immobility	Li et al. (2001)
LY392098	Forced-swim—mouse	Synergy with conventional antidepressants	Li et al. (2003)
LY404817, LY451646	Tail-suspension—mouse	Decreased immobility	Bai et al. (2001)
LY404817, LY451646	Forced-swim—mouse	Decreased immobility	Bai et al. (2001)
CX516, CX691, CX731	Submissive behavior—rat	Decreased submissive behavior	Knapp et al. (2002)

C. Metabotropic Glutamate Receptors

Metabotropic glutamate (mGlu) receptors regulate glutamate neuronal transmission by modulating the release of neurotransmitters and the post-synaptic responses to glutamate. Biochemical, pharmacological, and behavioral data suggest that mGlu receptor-mediated control of monoa-minergic and ionotropic glutamatergic transmission is intimately linked to mood disorders (Pilc et al., 2008; Witkin & Eiler, 2006; Witkin et al., 2007). Thus, pharmacological modulation of some mGlu receptors can facilitate neuronal stem cell proliferation (neurogenesis) and the release of neurotransmitters associated with antidepressant responses. Other data supporting the idea that mGlu receptors might be targets for novel anti-depressants include the discovery that these sites are localized in mood-disorder-related neural circuits and that these receptors are altered by antidepressant treatments. Moreover, pharmacological manipulation of some mGlu receptors causes behavioral and neurochemical changes in laboratory animals similar to those obtained with conventional antidepres-sants. Research suggests that the mGlu2, mGlu3, and/or mGlu5 receptors are the most appropriate targets for drugs intended to treat affective illness (Witkin et al., 2007).

Antagonists of the mGlu1 and mGlu5 members of the Group I mGlu receptor family display biochemical and behavioral effects consistent with an antidepressant profile (Pilc et al., 2008; Witkin et al., 2007). For exam-ple, chronic mild stress up-regulates mGlu5 receptors in the hippocampal CA1 region of rat brain (Wieronska et al., 2001). In addition, these receptor antagonists display antidepressant-like behavioral effects, with the bulk of the reports focused on mGlu5 because of the availability of selective com-pounds for this site. For example, the structurally related mGlu5 antago-nists, MPEP and MTEP, produce antidepressant-like behavioral effects in both mice and rats in the forced-swim and tail-suspension tests and in olfactory bulbectomized rats (Pilc et al., 2008; Witkin et al., 2007). The target specificity of the effects of these compounds was verified in mGlu5 receptor-deficient mice (Li, Need, Baez, & Witkin, 2006). Belozertseva, Kos, Popik, Danysz, and Bespalov (2007) showed that the mGlu1 receptor antagonist, EMQMCM, is active in both the mouse tail-suspension test and in a modified rat forced-swim test.

Both mGlu2 and mGlu3, Group II mGlu receptors, have also received a great deal of attention as targets for treating mood disorders given the prominent antidepressant-like biochemical and behavioral effects observed when these sites are pharmacologically manipulated (Pilc et al., 2008; Witkin & Eiler, 2006; Witkin et al., 2007). Although there have been reports from one group suggesting the possibility that mGlu2/3 receptor agonists might augment and shorten the time to response of conventional antidepressants (Matrisciano et al., 2002, 2008), most work on these sites has focused on an examination of the effects of receptor antagonists. Two orthosteric antagonists of mGlu2/3 receptors, LY341495 and MGS0039, induce biochemical and behavioral effects consistent with antidepressant activity. These actions include enhancement of monoamine release and antidepressant-like responses in the tail-suspension, forced-swim, and in the learned assay. A relationship between these behavioral and biochemical changes and AMPA receptors has been shown by the fact that both the neurochemical and behavioral effects are prevented by AMPA receptor antagonists (Karasawa, Shimazaki, Kawashima, & Chaki, 2005; Witkin et al., 2007).

While information on Group III mGlu receptors (mGlu4, 6, 7, and 8) is generally lacking, there are suggestions that manipulation of mGlu7 and mGlu8 receptors can induce an antidepressant-like response (Pilc et al., 2008; Witkin et al., 2007).

D. Glial and Transport Modulation

Recent work has focused on the role of glia in mood disorders and the impact of glutamate–glutamine cycling (Valentine & Sanacora, 2009). Particular interest is directed toward studying the glial EAATs which regulate glutamate availability. Evidence of a possible involvement of EAATs in affective illness includes the finding of reduced glial number in MDD patients and reduced amino acid metabolism under conditions of stress. Moreover, riluzole, an agent known to facilitate EAAT-mediated glutamate uptake, displays antidepressant activity in humans and, in preclinical animal models, has been shown to modify stress-induced modifications in glutamate metabolism (Valentine & Sanacora, 2009).

While the glial hypotheses of mood disorders and many electrophysiological findings with antidepressants emphasize a dampening of excitatory neurotransmission by antidepressants, the AMPA/NMDA hypotheses posits an enhancement as the underlying mechanism of the antidepressant response. Thus, the almost immediate onset of antidepressant effects of NMDA antagonists like ketamine might be due to the pulsatile drive at excitatory synapses with AMPA receptors being a pivot point. The ultimate biochemical consequences of the enhancement of excitatory tone in different regions of the CNS, and the ramifications of such changes for MDD, require further intensive experimental analyses. In this regard, attempts should be made to determine whether the lasting changes, such as the relatively long-lived effects of a single dose of ketamine or conventional antidepressants, reflect a reduction in the activity of particular neuronal circuits and neurogenesis. In this regard, it is notable that drugs used to treat monopolar depression have the opposite effect on AMPA receptor activity as those employed for the treatment of bipolar illness (Alt et al., 2006). Perhaps this is related to a switch from excitatory to inhibitory functionality and vice versa, depending on the preexisting state of the system.

VI. Conclusion

There exist a number of treatment options for MDD that include SSRIs, serotonin/norepinephrine reuptake inhibitors, and some novel agents such as tianeptine and mirtazepine. The current investigational thrust toward the discovery of future MDD medicines is directed toward improved efficacy for treatment-resistant patients, reduction in the onset of action of full therapeutic benefit, additional impact upon specific symptoms such as fatigue, as well as a reduction in side-effect impact. Research is currently engaging a diversity of mechanisms as potential future treatment options. This diversity reflects in part a lack of full understanding of the etiology and pathophysiology of MDD. Drug discovery efforts are ongoing in the area of augmenting agents for existing medicines, exploitation of natural product chemistry and biology, a host of neuropeptide targets, mechanisms that facilitate neurogenesis, novel neurotransmitter regulator systems such as the endocannabinoid system, and epigenetic mechanisms. An additional major area of current focus is on modulators of glutamate neurotransmission that include a wide range of potential targets such as NMDA, AMPA, and mGlu proteins. Recent verification of the NMDA hypothesis of depression with the clinical work on ketamine and an NR2B-selective NMDA antagonist along with the data supporting an AMPA-driven mediation of these effects has given additional impetus for focus in these areas.

Acknowledgments

We thank the following colleagues for previous discussions that have helped shape some of the thoughts expressed in this review: Andrew J. Alt, David Bleakman, Holly L. Cates, Shigeyuki Chaki, Christian C. Felder, Donald R. Gehlert, John D. Hixon, Lauren Marangell, Gerard J. Marek, George G. Nomikos, Andrzej Pilc, Gabriel Nowak, Darryle D. Schoepp, Glenn A. Phillips, Phil Skolnick, and Eleni T. Tzavara.

Conflict of Interest: The authors declare no conflicts of interest. Both authors are employees of Eli Lilly and Company. All data reported in the present review are from the public scientific literature.

References

Adamczyk, P., Gołda, A., McCreary, A. C., Filip, M., & Przegaliński, E. (2008). Activation of endocannabinoid transmission induces antidepressant-like effects in rats. *Journal of Physiology and Pharmacology*, *59*, 217–228.

Aiken, C. B. (2007). Pramipexole in psychiatry: A systematic review of the literature. *Journal of Clinical Psychiatry*, *68*, 1230–1236.

Alder, J., Thakker-Varia, S., Bangasser, D. A., Kuroiwa, M., Plummer, M. R., Shors, T. J., et al. (2003). Brain-derived neurotrophic factor-induced gene expression reveals novel actions of VGF in hippocampal synaptic plasticity. *Journal of Neuroscience*, *23*, 10800–10808.

Alt, A., Nisenbaum, E. S., Bleakman, D., & Witkin, J. M. (2006). A role for AMPA receptors in mood disorders. *Biochemical Pharmacology*, *71*, 1273–1288.

Aluisio, L., Lord, B., Barbier, A. J., Fraser, I. C., Wilson, S. J., Boggs, J., et al. (2008). In-vitro and in-vivo characterization of JNJ-7925476, a novel triple monoamine uptake inhibitor. *European Journal of Pharmacology*, *587*, 141–146.

Aonurm-Helm, A., Jurgenson, M., Zharkovsky, T., Sonn, K., Berezin, V., Bock, E., et al. (2008). Depression-like behaviour in neural cell adhesion molecule (NCAM)-deficient mice and its reversal by an NCAM-derived peptide, FGL. *European Journal of Neuroscience*, *28*, 1618–1628.

Bachis, A., Mallei, A., Cruz, M. I., Wellstein, A., & Mocchetti, I. (2008). Chronic antidepressant treatments increase basic fibroblast growth factor and fibroblast growth factor-binding protein in neurons. *Neuropharmacology*, *55*, 1114–1120.

Bai, F., Bergeron, M., & Nelson, D. L. (2003). Chronic AMPA receptor potentiator (LY451646) treatment increases cell proliferation in adult rat hippocampus. *Neuropharmacology*, *44*, 1013–1021.

Bambico, F. R., Duranti, A., Tontini, A., Tarzia, G., & Gobbi, G. (2009). Endocannabinoids in the treatment of mood disorders: Evidence from animal models. *Current Pharmaceutical Design*, *15*, 1623–1646.

Bambico, F. R., & Gobbi, G. (2008). The cannabinoid CB1 receptor and the endocannabinoid anandamide: Possible antidepressant targets. *Expert Opinion on Therapeutic Targets*, *12*, 1347–1366.

Basso, A. M., Bratcher, N. A., Gallagher, K. B., Cowart, M. D., Zhao, C., Sun, M., et al. (2006). Lack of efficacy of melanin-concentrating hormone-1 receptor antagonists in models of depression and anxiety. *European Journal of Pharmacology*, *540*, 115–120.

Beglopoulos, V., & Shen, J. (2006). Regulation of CRE-dependent transcription by presenilins: Prospects for therapy of Alzheimer's disease. *Trends in Pharmacological Sciences*, *27*, 33–40.

Belozertseva, I. V., Kos, T., Popik, P., Danysz, W., & Bespalov, A. Y. (2007). Antidepressant-like effects of mGluR1 and mGluR5 antagonists in the rat forced swim and the mouse tail suspension tests. *European Neuropsychopharmacology*, *17*, 172–179.

Benedict, A., Arellano, J., De Cock, E., & Baird, J. (2009). Economic evaluation of duloxetine versus serotonin selective reuptake inhibitors and venlafaxine XR in treating major depressive disorder in Scotland. *Journal of Affective Disorders*, [Epub ahead of print].

Berman, R. M., Cappiello, A., Anand, A., Oren, D. A., Heninger, G. R., Charney, D. S., et al. (2000). Antidepressant effects of ketamine in depressed patients. *Biological Psychiatry*, *47*, 351–354.

Berman, R. M., Fava, M., Thase, M. E., Trivedi, M. H., Swanink, R., McQuade, R. D., et al. (2009). Aripiprazole augmentation in major depressive disorder: A double-blind, placebo-controlled study in patients with inadequate response to antidepressants. *CNS Spectrrums*, *14*, 197–206.

Beutler, A. S., Li, S., Nicol, R., & Walsh, M. J. (2005). Carbamazepine is an inhibitor of histone deacetylases. *Life Sciences*, *76*, 3107–3115.

Black, M. D. (2005). Therapeutic potential of positive AMPA modulators and their relationship to AMPA receptor subunits. A review of preclinical data. *Psychopharmacology*, *179*, 154–63.

Bleakman, D., Alt, A., & Witkin, J. M. (2007). AMPA receptors in the therapeutic management of depression. *CNS & Neurological Disorders Drug Targets*, 6(2), 117–126.

Bhutani, M. K., Bishnoi, M., & Kulkarni, S. K. (2009). Anti-depressant like effect of curcumin and its combination with piperine in unpredictable chronic stress-induced behavioral, biochemical and neurochemical changes. *Pharmacology, Biochemistry and Behavior*, 92, 39–43.

Bittencourt, J. C., Presse, F., Arias, C., Peto, C., Vaughan, J., Nahon, J. L., Vale, W., & Sawchenko, P. E. (1992). The melanin-concentrating hormone system of the rat brain: an immuno- and hybridization histochemical characterization. *Journal of Comparative Neurology* 319, 218–245.

Bobula, B., & Hess, G. (2008). Antidepressant treatments-induced modifications of glutamatergic transmission in rat frontal cortex. *Pharmacological Reports*, 60, 865–871.

Bortolato, M., Mangieri, R. A., Fu, J., Kim, J. H., Arguello, O., Duranti, A., et al. (2007). Antidepressant-like activity of the fatty acid amide hydrolase inhibitor URB597 in a rat model of chronic mild stress. *Biological Psychiatry*, 62, 1103–1110.

Bredt, D. S., & Nicoll, R. A. (2003). AMPA receptor trafficking at excitatory synapses. *Neuron*, 40, 361–379.

Branchek, T. A., Smith, K. E., Gerald, C., & Walker, M. W. (2000). Galanin receptor subtypes. *Trends in Pharmacological Sciencesm*, 21, 109–117.

Brekhman, I. I. and Dardymov, I. V. (1969). New substances of plant origin which increase non-specific resistance. *Annual Review of Pharmacology*, 9, 419–430.

Breuer, M. E., Groenink, L., Oosting, R. S., Buerger, E., Korte, M., Ferger, B., et al. (2009). Antidepressant effects of pramipexole, a dopamine D(3)/D(2) receptor agonist, and 7-OH-DPAT, a dopamine D(3) receptor agonist, in olfactory bulbectomized rats. *European Journal of Pharmacology*, 616, 134–140.

Brink, C. B., Harvey, B. H., & Brand, L. (2006). Tianeptine: A novel atypical antidepressant that may provide new insights into the biomolecular basis of depression. *Recent Patents on CNS Drug Discovery*, 1, 29–41

Chaki, S., Funakoshi, T., Hirota-Okuno, S., Nishiguchi, M., Shimazaki, T., Iijima, M., et al. (2005). Anxiolytic- and antidepressant-like profile of ATC0065 and ATC0175: Nonpeptidic and orally active melanin-concentrating hormone receptor 1 antagonists. *Journal of Pharmacology and Experimental Therapeutics*, 313, 831–839.

Coddington, E., Lewis, C., Rose, J. D., & Moore, F. L. (2007). Endocannabinoids mediate the effects of acute stress and corticosterone on sex behavior. *Endocrinology*, 148, 493–500.

Conboy, L., Foley, A. G., O'Boyle, N. M., Lawlor, M., Gallagher, H., Murphy, K. J., et al. (2009). Curcumin-induced degradation of PKC delta is associated with enhanced dentate NCAM PSA expression and spatial learning in adult and aged Wistar rats. *Biochemical Pharmacology*, 77, 1254–1265.

Croom, K. F., Perry, C. M., & Plosker, G. L. (2009). Mirtazapine: A review of its use in major depression and other psychiatric disorders. *CNS Drugs*, 23, 427–452.

Cryan, J. F., Markou, A., & Lucki, I. (2002). Assessing antidepressant activity in rodents: Recent developments and future needs. *Trends in Pharmacological Sciences*, 23, 238–245.

Czeh, B., Michaelis, T., Watanabe, T., Frahm, J., de Biurrun, G., van Kampen, M., et al. (2001). Stress-induced changes in cerebral metabolites, hippocampal volume, and cell proliferation are prevented by antidepressant treatment with tianeptine. *Proceedings of the National Academy of Sciences of the United States of America*, 98, 12796–13801.

David, D. J., Klemenhagen, K. C., Holick, K. A., Saxe, M. D., Mendez, I., Santarelli, L., et al. (2007). Efficacy of the MCHR1 antagonist N-[3-(1-{[4-(3,4-difluorophenoxy)phenyl]-methyl}(4-piperidyl))-4-methylphenyl]-2-methylpropanamide (SNAP 94847) in mouse models of anxiety and depression following acute and chronic administration is independent of hippocampal neurogenesis. *Journal of Pharmacology and Experimental Therapeutics*, 321, 237–248.

Debattista, C., & Hawkins, J. (2009). Utility of atypical antipsychotics in the treatment of resistant unipolar depression. *CNS Drugs*, *23*, 369–377.

DiazGranados, N., & Zarate, C. A., Jr. (2008). A review of the preclinical and clinical evidence for protein kinase C as a target for drug development for bipolar disorder. *Current Psychiatry Reports*, *10*, 510–519.

DiLeone, R. J., Georgescu, D., & Nestler, E. J. (2003). Lateral hypothalamic neuropeptides in reward and drug addiction. *Life Sciences*, *73*, 759–768.

Di Marzo, V. (2009). The endocannabinoid system: Its general strategy of action, tools for its pharmacological manipulation and potential therapeutic exploitation. *Pharmacological Research*, *60*, 77–84.

Dubovsky, S. L., & Buzan, R. (1999). Mood disorders. In R. E. Hales, S. C. Yudofsky, & J. A. Talbott (Eds.), *Text book of psychiatry* (3rd ed., pp. 479–565). Washington, DC: American Psychiatric Press.

Duman, R. S. (2004). The neurochemistry of depressive disorders: Preclinical studies. In D. S. Charney & E. J. Nestler (Eds.), *Neurobiology of mental illness* (2nd ed., pp. 421–439). Oxford: Oxford University Press.

Dybała, M., Siwek, A., Poleszak, E., Pilc, A., & Nowak, G. (2008). Lack of NMDA-AMPA interaction in antidepressant-like effect of CGP 37849, an antagonist of NMDA receptor, in the forced swim test. *Journal of Neural Transmission*, *115*, 1519–1520.

Evans, S. J., Choudary, P. V., Neal, C. R., Li, J. Z., Vawter, M. P., Tomita, H., et al. (2004). Dysregulation of the fibroblast growth factor system in major depression. *Proceedings of the National Academy of Sciences of the United States of America*, *101*, 15506–15511.

Felder, C. C., Dickason-Chesterfield, A. K., & Moore, S. A. (2006). Cannabinoids biology: The search for new therapeutic targets. *Molecular Interventions*, *6*, 149–161.

Flajolet, M., Wang, Z., Futter, M., Shen, W., Nuangchamnong, N., Bendor, J., et al. (2008). FGF acts as a co-transmitter through adenosine A(2A) receptor to regulate synaptic plasticity. *Nature Neuroscience*, *11*, 1402–1409.

Freeman, M. P., Hibbeln, J. R., Wisner, K. L., Davis, J. M., Mischoulon, D., Peet, M., et al. (2006). Omega-3 fatty acids: Evidence basis for treatment and future research in psychiatry. *Journal of Clinical Psychiatry*, *67*, 1954–1967. Erratum in: *J Clin Psychiatry*. (2007) 68:338.

Furey, M. L., & Drevets, W. C. (2006). Antidepressant efficacy of the antimuscarinic drug scopolamine: A randomized, placebo-controlled clinical trial. *Archives of General Psychiatry*, *63*, 1121–1129.

Gardian, G., Browne, S. E., Choi, D. K., Klivenyi, P., Gregorio, J., Kubilus, J. K., et al. (2005). Neuroprotective effects of phenylbutyrate in the N171–82Q transgenic mouse model of Huntington's disease. *The Journal of Biological Chemistry*, *280*, 556–563.

Gehlert, D. R., Rasmussen, K., Shaw, J., Li, X., Ardayfio, P., Craft, L., et al. (2009). Preclinical evaluation of melanin-concentrating hormone receptor 1 antagonism for the treatment of obesity and depression. *Journal of Pharmacology and Experimental Therapeutics*, *329*, 429–438

Georgescu, D., Sears, R. M., Hommel, J. D., Barrot, M., Bolaños, C. A., Marsh, D. J., et al. (2005). The hypothalamic neuropeptide melanin-concentrating hormone acts in the nucleus accumbens to modulate feeding behavior and forced-swim performance. *Journal of Neuroscience*, *25*, 2933–2940.

Gobbi, G., Bambico, F. R., Mangieri, R., Bortolato, M., Campolongo, P., Solinas, M., et al. (2005). Antidepressant-like activity and modulation of brain monoaminergic transmission by blockade of anandamide hydrolysis. *Proceedings of the National Academy of Sciences of the United States of America*, *102*, 18620–18625.

Goel, A., Kunnumakkara, A. B., & Aggarwal, B. B. (2008). Curcumin as "Curecumin": From kitchen to clinic. *Biochemical Pharmacology*, *75*, 787–809.

Griebel, G., Stemmelin, J., & Scatton, B. (2005). Effects of the cannabinoid CB1 receptor antagonist rimonabant in models of emotional reactivity in rodents. *Biological Psychiatry, 57*, 261–267.

Hamani, C., Mayberg, H., Snyder, B., Giacobbe, P., Kennedy, S., & Lozano, A. M. (2009). Deep brain stimulation of the subcallosal cingulate gyrus for depression: Anatomical location of active contacts in clinical responders and a suggested guideline for targeting. *Journal of Neurosurgery*, [Epub ahead of print].

Hashimoto, K. (2009). Emerging role of glutamate in the pathophysiology of major depressive disorder. *Brain Research Reviews, 61*, 105–123.

Hibbeln, J. R. (1998). Fish consumption and major depression. *Lancet, 351*, 1213.

Hill, M. N., & Gorzalka, B. B. (2005). Pharmacological enhancement of cannabinoid CB1 receptor activity elicits an antidepressant-like response in the rat forced swim test. *European Neuropsychopharmacology, 15*, 593–599.

Hill, M. N., Ho, W. S., Sinopoli, K. J., Viau, V., Hillard, C. J., & Gorzalka, B. B. (2006). Involvement of the endocannabinoid system in the ability of long-term tricyclic antidepressant treatment to suppress stress-induced activation of the hypothalamic-pituitary-adrenal axis. *Neuropsychopharmacology, 31*, 2591–2599.

Hill, M. N., Karacabeyli, E. S., & Gorzalka, B. B. (2007). Estrogen recruits the endocannabinoid system to modulate emotionality. *Psychoneuroendocrinology, 32*, 350–357.

Holets, V. R., Hokfelt, T., Rokaeus, A., Terenius, L., & Goldstein, M. (1988). Locus coeruleus neurons in the rat containing neuropeptide Y, tyrosine hydroxylase or galanin and their efferent projections to the spinal cord, cerebral cortex and hypothalamus. *Neuroscience, 24*, 893–906.

Hunsberger, J. G., Newton, S. S., Bennett, A. H., Duman, C. H., Russell, D. S., Salton, S. R., et al. (2007). Antidepressant actions of the exercise-regulated gene VGF. *Nature Medicine, 13*, 1476–1482.

Iga, J., Ueno, S., Yamauchi, K., Numata, S., Kinouchi, S., Tayoshi-Shibuya, S., et al. (2007). Altered HDAC5 and CREB mRNA expressions in the peripheral leukocytes of major depression. *Progress in Neuro-Psychopharmacology and Biological Psychiatry, 31*, 628–632.

Iversen, L. (2005). The monoamine hypothesis of depression. In J. Licinio & M. L. Wong (Ed.), *Biology of depression* (pp. 71–86). Weinheim: Wiley-VCH.

Jiang, W., Zhang, Y., Xiao, L., Van Cleemput, J., Ji, S. P., Bai, G., et al. (2005). Cannabinoids promote embryonic and adult hippocampus neurogenesis and produce anxiolytic- and antidepressant-like effects. *Journal of Clinical Investigation, 115*, 3104–3116.

Kahl, K. G., Bens, S., Ziegler, K., Rudolf, S., Kordon, A., Dibbelt, L., et al. (2009). Angiogenic factors in patients with current major depressive disorder comorbid with borderline personality disorder. *Psychoneuroendocrinology, 34*, 353–357.

Karasawa, J., Shimazaki, T., Kawashima, N., & Chaki, S. (2005). AMPA receptor stimulation mediates the antidepressant-like effect of a group II metabotropic glutamate receptor antagonist. *Brain Research, 1042*, 92–98.

Kasper, S., & McEwen, B. S. (2008). Neurobiological and clinical effects of the antidepressant tianeptine. *CNS Drugs, 22*, 15–26.

Katz, M. M., Tekell, J. L., Bowden, C. L., Brannan, S., Houston, J. P., & Berman, N. (2004). Onset and early behavioral effects of pharmacologically different antidepressants and placebo in depression. *Neuropsychopharmacology, 29*, 566–579.

Kitagawa, K., Kitamura, Y., Miyazaki, T., Miyaoka, J., Kawasaki, H., Asanuma, M., et al. (2009). Effects of pramipexole on the duration of immobility during the forced swim test in normal and ACTH-treated rats. *Naunyn-Schmiedebergs Archives of Pharmacology, 380*, 59–66.

Knapp, R. J., Goldenberg, R., Shock, C., Cecil, A., Watkins, J., & Miller, C. (2002). Antidepressant activity of memory-enhancing drugs in the reduction of submissive behavior model. *European Journal of Pharmacology, 440*, 27–35.

Kozikowski, A. P., Gaisina, I. N., Yuan, H., Petukhov, P. A., Blond, S. Y., Fedolak, A., et al. (2007). Structure-based design leads to the identification of lithium mimetics that block mania-like effects in rodents: Possible new GSK-3beta therapies for bipolar disorders. *Journal of the American Chemical Society, 129*, 8328–8332.

Kulkarni, S. K., Bhutani, M. K., & Bishnoi, M. (2008). Antidepressant activity of curcumin: Involvement of serotonin and dopamine system. *Psychopharmacology, 201*, 435–442.

Kulkarni, S. K., & Dhir, A. (2007). Possible involvement of L-arginine-nitric oxide (NO)-cyclic guanosine monophosphate (cGMP) signaling pathway in the antidepressant activity of berberine chloride. *European Journal of Pharmacology, 569*, 77–83.

Kulkarni, S. K., & Dhir, A. (2008). On the mechanism of antidepressant-like action of berberine chloride. *European Journal of Pharmacology, 589*, 163–172.

Kulkarni, S. K., & Dhir, A. (2009). Current investigational drugs for major depression. *Expert Opinion on Investigational Drugs, 18*, 767–788.

Kumar, V. (2006). Potential medicinal plants for CNS disorders: An overview. *Phytotherapy Research, 20*, 1023–1035.

Lauterborn, J. C., Lynch, G., Vanderklish, P., & Arai, A. (2000). Gall CM: Positive modulation of AMPA receptors increases neurotrophin expression by hippocampal and cortical neurons. *Journal of Neuroscience, 20*, 8–21.

Legutko, B., Li, X., & Skolnick, P. (2001). Regulation of BDNF expression in primary neuron culture by LY392098, a novel AMPA receptor potentiator. *Neuropharmacology, 40*, 1019–1027.

Li, X., Tizzano, J. P., Griffey, K., Clay, M., Lindstrom, T., & Skolnick, P. (2001). Antidepressant-like actions of an AMPA receptor potentiator (LY392098). *Neuropharmacology, 40*, 1028–1033.

Li, X., Witkin, J. M., Need, A. B., & Skolnick, P. (2003). Enhancement of antidepressant potency by a potentiator of AMPA receptors. *Cellular and Molecular Neurobiology, 23*, 419–430.

Li, X., Need, A. B., Baez, M., & Witkin, J. M. (2006). mGlu5 Receptor Antagonism is Associated with Antidepressant-Like effects in Mice. *Journal of Pharmacology and Experimental Therapeutics, 319*, 254–259.

Li, Y. C., Wang, F. M., Pan, Y., Qiang, L. Q., Cheng, G., Zhang, W. Y., et al. (2009). Antidepressant-like effects of curcumin on serotonergic receptor-coupled AC-cAMP pathway in chronic unpredictable mild stress of rats. *Progress in Neuro-Psychopharmacology and Biological Psychiatry, 33*, 435–449.

Liang, Y., Shaw, A. M., Boules, M., Briody, S., Robinson, J., Oliveros, A., et al. (2008). Antidepressant-like pharmacological profile of a novel triple reuptake inhibitor (1S,2S)-3-(methylamino)-2-(naphthalen-2-yl)-1-phenylpropan-1-ol (PRC200-SS). *Journal of Pharmacology and Experimental Therapeutics, 327*, 573–583.

Linde, K., Berner, M., Egger, M., & Mulrow, C. (2005a). St John's wort for depression: Meta-analysis of randomised controlled trials. *The British Journal of Psychiatry, 186*, 99–107.

Linde, K., Berner, M. M., & Kriston, L. (2005b). St John's wort for major depression. *Cochrane Database of Systematic Reviews 2*, CD000448.

Linde, K., Berner, M. M., & Kriston, L. (2008). St John's wort for major depression. *Cochrane Database of Systematic Reviews 4*, CD000448.

Machado-Vieira, R., Salvadore, G., Diazgranados, N., & Zarate, C. A., Jr. (2009). Ketamine and the next generation of antidepressants with a rapid onset of action. *Pharmacology and Therapeutics, 123*, 143–50.

Machado-Vieira, R., Salvadore, G., Ibrahim, L. A., Diaz-Granados, N., & Zarate, C. A., Jr. (2009). Targeting glutamatergic signaling for the development of novel therapeutics for mood disorders. *Current Pharmaceutical Design, 15*, 1595–1611.

Mackowiak, M., O'Neill, M., Hicks, C., Bleakman, D., & Skolnick, P. (2002). An AMPA receptor potentiator modulates hippocampal expression of BDNF: An in vivo study. *Neuropharmacology, 43*, 1–10.

Maeng, S., & Zarate, C. A., Jr. (2007). The role of glutamate in mood disorders: Results from the ketamine in major depression study and the presumed cellular mechanism underlying its antidepressant effects. *Current Psychiatry Reports*, 9, 467–474.

Maeng, S., Zarate, C. A., Jr., Du, J., Schloesser, R. J., McCammon, J., Chen, G., et al. (2008). Cellular mechanisms underlying the antidepressant effects of ketamine: Role of alpha-amino-3-hydroxy-5-methylisoxazole-4-propionic acid receptors. *Biological Psychiatry*, 63, 349–352.

Martinez-Turrillas, R., Frechilla, D., & Del Río, J. (2002). Chronic antidepressant treatment increases the membrane expression of AMPA receptors in rat hippocampus. *Neuropharmacology*, 43, 1230–1237.

Matrisciano, F., Storto, M., Ngomba, R. T., Cappuccio, I., Caricasole, A., Scaccianoce, S., et al. (2002). Imipramine treatment up-regulates the expression and function of mGlu2/3 metabotropic glutamate receptors in the rat hippocampus. *Neuropharmacology*, 42, 1008–1015.

Matrisciano, F., Zusso, M., Panaccione, I., Turriziani, B., Caruso, A., Iacovelli, L., et al. (2008). Synergism between fluoxetine and the mGlu2/3 receptor agonist, LY379268, in an in vitro model for antidepressant drug-induced neurogenesis. *Neuropharmacology*, 54, 428–437.

Melander, T., Hokfelt, T., & Rokaeus, A. (1986). Distribution of galanin-like immunoreactivity in the rat central nervous system. *Journal of Comparative Neurology*, 248, 475–517.

Mallei, A., Shi, B., & Mocchetti, I. (2002). Antidepressant treatments induce the expression of basic fibroblast growth factor in cortical and hippocampal neurons. *Molecular Pharmacology*, 61, 1017–1024.

Maragnoli, M. E., Fumagalli, F., Gennarelli, M., Racagni, G., & Riva, M. A. (2004). Fluoxetine and olanzapine have synergistic effects in the modulation of fibroblast growth factor 2 expression within the rat brain. *Biological Psychiatry*, 55, 1095–1102.

Marek, G. J. (2008). Regulation of rat cortical 5-hydroxytryptamine2A receptor-mediated electrophysiological responses by repeated daily treatment with electroconvulsive shock or imipramine. *European Neuropsychopharmacology*, 18, 498–507.

Mathew, S. J., Keegan, K., & Smith, L. (2005). Glutamate modulators as novel interventions for mood disorders. *Revista Brasileira de Psiquiatria*, 27, 243–248.

Millan, M. J. (2009). Dual- and triple-acting agents for treating core and co-morbid symptoms of major depression: Novel concepts, new drugs. *Neurotherapeutics*, 6, 53–77.

Millan, M. J., Brocco, M., Papp, M., Serres, F., La Rochelle, C. D., Sharp, T., et al. (2004). S32504, a novel naphtoxazine agonist at dopamine D3/D2 receptors: III. Actions in models of potential antidepressive and anxiolytic activity in comparison with ropinirole. *Journal of Pharmacology and Experimental Therapeutics*, 309, 936–950.

Molteni, R., Fumagalli, F., Magnaghi, V., Roceri, M., Gennarelli, M., Racagni, G., et al. (2001). Modulation of fibroblast growth factor-2 by stress and corticosteroids: From developmental events to adult brain plasticity. *Brain Research. Brain Research Reviews*, 37, 249–258.

Montgomery, P., & Richardson, A. J. (2008). Omega-3 fatty acids for bipolar disorder. *Cochrane Database of Systematic Reviews*, 16, CD005169.

Moreira, F. A., Grieb, M., & Lutz, B. (2009). Central side-effects of therapies based on CB1 cannabinoid receptor agonists and antagonists: Focus on anxiety and depression. *Best Practice & Research. Clinical Endocrinology & Metabolism*, 23, 133–144.

Naidu, P. S., Varvel, S. A., Ahn, K., Cravatt, B. F., Martin, B. R., & Lichtman, A. H. (2007). Evaluation of fatty acid amide hydrolase inhibition in murine models of emotionality. *Psychopharmacology*, 192, 61–70.

Newton, S. S., Collier, E. F., Hunsberger, J., Adams, D., Terwilliger, R., Selvanayagam, E., et al. (2003). Gene profile of electroconvulsive seizures: Induction of neurotrophic and angiogenic factors. *Journal of Neuroscience*, 23, 10841–10851.

Newton, S. S., & Duman, R. S. (2004). Regulation of neurogenesis and angiogenesis in depression. *Current Neurovascular Research*, 1, 261–267.

O'Donnell, D., Ahmad, S., Wahlestedt, C., & Walker, P. (1999). Expression of the novel galanin receptor subtype GALR2 in the adult rat CNS: Distinct distribution from GALR1. *Journal of Comparative Neurology, 409*, 469–481.

Onaivi, E. S., Ishiguro, H., Gong, J. P., Patel, S., Meozzi, P. A., Myers, L., et al. (2008). Functional expression of brain neuronal CB2 cannabinoid receptors are involved in the effects of drugs of abuse and in depression. *Annals of the New York Academy of Sciences, 1139*, 434–449.

O'Neill, M. F., & Moore, N. A. (2003). Animal models of depression: Are there any? *Human Psychopharmacology, 18*, 239–254.

Panossian, A., Wikman, G., Kaur, P., & Asea, A. (2009). Adaptogens exert a stress-protective effect by modulation of expression of molecular chaperones. *Phytomedicine, 16*, 617–622.

Panossian, A., & Wikman, G. (2008). Pharmacology of Schisandra chinensis Bail.: An overview of Russian research and uses in medicine. *Journal of Ethnopharmacology, 118*, 183–212.

Patel, S., Roelke, C. T., Rademacher, D. J., Cullinan, W. E., & Hillard, C. J. (2004). Endocannabinoid signaling negatively modulates stress-induced activation of the hypothalamic- pituitary-adrenal axis. *Endocrinology, 145*, 5431–5438.

Paul, I. A., & Skolnick, P. (2003). Glutamate and depression: Clinical and preclinical studies. *Annals of the New York Academy of Sciences, 1003*, 250–272.

Pilc, A., Chaki, S., Nowak, G., & Witkin, J. M. (2008). Mood disorders: Regulation by metabotropic glutamate receptors. *Biochemical Pharmacology, 75*, 977–1006.

Preskorn, S. H., Baker, B., Kolluri, S., Menniti, F. S., Krams, M., & Landen, J. W. (2008). An innovative design to establish proof of concept of the antidepressant effects of the NR2B subunit selective N-methyl-D-aspartate antagonist, CP-101,606, in patients with treatment-refractory major depressive disorder. *Journal of Clinical Psychopharmacology, 28*, 631–637.

Rademacher, D. J., & Hillard, C. J. (2007). Interactions between endocannabinoids and stress-induced decreased sensitivity to natural reward. *Progress in Neuro-Psychopharmacology and Biological Psychiatry, 31*, 633–641.

Rakofsky, J. J., Holtzheimer, P. E., & Nemeroff, C. B. (2009). Emerging targets for antidepressant therapies. *Current Opinion in Chemical Biology, 13*, 291–302.

Razani, H., Diaz-Cabialem, Z., Fuxe, K., & Ogren, S. O. (2000). Intraventricular galanin produces a time-dependent modulation of 5-HT1A receptors in the dorsal raphe of the rat. *Neuroreport, 11*, 3943–3948.

Renthal, W., Maze, I., Krishnan, V., Covington, H. E., III, Xiao, G., Kumar, A., et al. (2007). Histone deacetylase 5 epigenetically controls behavioral adaptations to chronic emotional stimuli. *Neuron, 56*, 517–529.

Ross, B. M., Seguin, J., & Sieswerda, L. E. (2007). Omega-3 fatty acids as treatments for mental illness: Which disorder and which fatty acid? *Lipids in Health Disease, 6*, 21.

Rowe, M. K., Wiest, C., & Chuang, D. M. (2007). GSK-3 is a viable potential target for therapeutic intervention in bipolar disorder. *Neuroscience and Biobehavioral Reviews, 31*, 920–931.

Rush, A. J., Trivedi, M. H., Wisniewski, S. R., Nierenberg, A. A., Stewart, J. W., Warden, D., et al. (2006). Acute and longer-term outcomes in depressed outpatients requiring one or several treatment steps: A STAR*D report. *American Journal of Psychiatry, 163*, 1905–1917.

Rutkowska, M., & Jachimczuk, O. (2004). Antidepressant—like properties of ACEA (arachidonyl-2-chloroethylamide), the selective agonist of CB1 receptors. *Acta Poloniae Pharmaceutica, 61*(2), 165–167.

Santarelli, L., Saxe, M., Gross, C., Surget, A., Battaglia, F., Dulawa, S., et al. (2003). Requirement of hippocampal neurogenesis for the behavioral effects of antidepressants. *Science, 301*(5634), 805–809.

Santucci, V., Storme, J. J., Soubrie, P., & Le Fur, G. (1996). Arousal-enhancing properties of the CB1 cannabinoid receptor antagonist SR 141716A in rats as assessed by electroencephalographic spectral and sleep-waking cycle analysis. *Life Sciences, 58*, PL103–PL110.

Schmitt, A. B., Bauer, M., Volz, H. P., Moeller, H. J., Jiang, Q., Ninan, P. T., et al. (2009, March 3). Differential effects of venlafaxine in the treatment of major depressive disorder according to baseline severity. *European Archives of Psychiatry and Clinical Neuroscience, 259*, 329–339.

Seely, K. A., Levi, M. S., & Prather, P. L. (2009). The dietary polyphenols trans-resveratrol and curcumin selectively bind human CB1 cannabinoid receptors with nanomolar affinities and function as antagonists/inverse agonists. *Journal of Pharmacology and Experimental Therapeutics, 330*, 31–39.

Severini, C., Ciotti, M. T., Biondini, L., Quaresima, S., Rinaldi, A. M., Levi, A., Frank, C., & Possenti, R. (2008). TLQP-21, a neuroendocrine VGF-derived peptide, prevents cerebellar granule cells death induced by serum and potassium deprivation. *Journal of Neurochemistry 104*, 534–544.

Shearman, L. P., Rosko, K. M., Fleischer, R., Wang, J., Xu, S., Tong, X. S., et al. (2003). Antidepressant-like and anorectic effects of the cannabinoid CB1 receptor inverse agonist AM251 in mice. *Behavioural Pharmacology, 14*, 573–582.

Shimazaki, T., Yoshimizu, T., & Chaki, S. (2006). Melanin-concentrating hormone MCH1 receptor antagonists: A potential new approach to the treatment of depression and anxiety disorders. *CNS Drugs, 20*, 801–811.

Skolnick, P. (2008) AMPA receptors: A target for novel antidepressants? *Biological Psychiatry, 63*, 347–348.

Skolnick, P., & Basile, A. S. (2007). Triple reuptake inhibitors ("broad spectrum" antidepressants). *CNS & Neurological Disorders Drug Targets, 6*, 141–149.

Skolnick, P., Krieter, P., Tizzano, J., Basile, A., Popik, P., Czobor, P., et al. (2006). Preclinical and clinical pharmacology of DOV 216,303, a "triple" reuptake inhibitor. *CNS Drug Reviews, 12*, 123–134.

Skolnick, P., Popik, P., Janowsky, A., Beer, B., & Lippa, A. S. (2003). "Broad spectrum" antidepressants: Is more better for the treatment of depression? *Life Sciences, 73*, 3175–3179.

Skolnick, P., Popik, P., & Trullas, R. (2009). Glutamate Based Antidepressants: 20 Years On. *Trends in Pharmacological Sciences*, [Epub ahead of print].

Smith, D. G., Tzavara, E. T., Shaw, J., Luecke, S., Wade, M., Davis, R., Salhoff, C., Nomikos, G. G., & Gehlert, D. R. (2005). Mesolimbic dopamine super-sensitivity in melanin-concentrating hormone-1 receptor-deficient mice. *Journal of Neuroscience 25*, 914–922.

Smith, D. G., Davis, R. J., Rorick-Kehn, L., Morin, M., Witkin, J. M., McKinzie, D. L., et al. (2006). Melanin-concentrating hormone-1 receptor modulates neuroendocrine, behavioral, and corticolimbic neurochemical stress responses in mice. *Neuropsychopharmacology, 31*, 1135–1145.

Solinas, M., Yasar, S., & Goldberg, S. R. (2007). Endocannabinoid system involvement in brain reward processes related to drug abuse. *Pharmacological Research, 56*, 393–405.

Svenningsson, P., Bateup, H., Qi, H., Takamiya, K., Huganir, R. L., Spedding, M., et al. (2007). Involvement of AMPA receptor phosphorylation in antidepressant actions with special reference to tianeptine. *European Journal of Neuroscience, 26*, 3509–3517.

Svenningsson, P., Tzavara, E. T., Witkin, J., Fienberg, A. A., Nomikos, G. G., & Greengard, P. (2002). Involvement of striatal and extrastriatal DARPP-32 in biochemical and behavioral effects of fluoxetine (Prozac). *Proceedings of the National Academy of Sciences, 99*, 3182–3187.

Swanson, C. J., Blackburn, T. P., Zhang, X., Zheng, K., Xu, Z. Q., Hokfelt, T., et al. (2005). Anxiolytic- and antidepressant-like profiles of the galanin-3 receptor (Gal3) antagonists SNAP 37889 and SNAP 398299. *Proceedings of the National Academy of Sciences of the United States of America, 102*, 17489–17494.

Szabo, S. T., Machado-Vieira, R., Yuan, P., Wang, Y., Wei, Y., Falke, C., et al. (2009). Glutamate receptors as targets of protein kinase C in the pathophysiology and treatment of animal models of mania. *Neuropharmacology, 56*, 47–55.

Su, X. W., Li, X. Y., Banasr, M., Koo, J. W., Shahid, M., Henry, B., et al. (2009). Chronic treatment with AMPA receptor potentiator Org 26576 increases neuronal cell proliferation and survival in adult rodent hippocampus. *Psychopharmacology, 206*, 215–222.

Thakker-Varia, S., & Alder, J. (2009). Neuropeptides in depression: Role of VGF. *Behavioural Brain Research, 197*, 262–278.

Thakker-Varia, S., Krol, J. J., Nettleton, J., Bilimoria, P. M., Bangasser, D. A., Shors, T. J., et al. (2007). The neuropeptide VGF produces antidepressant-like behavioral effects and enhances proliferation in the hippocampus. *Journal of Neuroscience, 27*, 12156–12167.

Todtenkopf, M. S., Parsegian, A., Naydenov, A., Neve, R. L., Konradi, C., & Carlezon, W. A., Jr. (2006). Brain reward regulated by AMPA receptor subunits in nucleus accumbens shell. *Journal of Neuroscience, 26*, 11665–11669.

Tran, P. V., Bymaster, F. P., McNamara, R. K., & Potter, W. Z. (2003). Dual monoamine modulation for improved treatment of major depressive disorder. *Journal of Clinical Psychopharmacology, 23*, 78–86

Trivedi, M. H., Thase, M. E., Osuntokun, O., Henley, D. B., Case, M., Watson, S. B., et al. (2009). An integrated analysis of olanzapine/fluoxetine combination in clinical trials of treatment-resistant depression. *Journal of Clinical Psychiatry, 70*, 387–396.

Trullas, R., & Skolnick, P. (1990). Functional antagonists at the NMDA receptor complex exhibit antidepressant actions. *European Journal of Pharmacology, 185*, 1–10.

Tsankova, N. M., Berton, O., Renthal, W., Kumar, A., Neve, R. L., & Nestler, E. J. (2006). Sustained hippocampal chromatin regulation in a mouse model of depression and antidepressant action. *Nature Neuroscience, 9*, 519–525.

Turnbull, T., Cullen-Drill, M., & Smaldone, A. (2008). Efficacy of omega-3 fatty acid supplementation on improvement of bipolar symptoms: A systematic review. *Archives of Psychiatric Nursing, 22*, 305–311.

Turner, C. A., Akil, H., Watson, S. J., & Evans, S. J. (2006). The fibroblast growth factor system and mood disorders. *Biological Psychiatry, 59*, 1128–1135.

Turner, C. A., Calvo, N., Frost, D. O., Akil, H., & Watson, S. J. (2008). The fibroblast growth factor system is downregulated following social defeat. *Neuroscience Letters, 430*, 147–150.

Turner, C. A., Gula, E. L, Taylor, L. P., Watson, S. J., & Akil, H. (2008). Antidepressant-like effects of intracerebroventricular FGF2 in rats. *Brain Research, 1224*, 63–68.

Tzavara, E. T., Davis, R. J., Perry, K. W., Li, X., Salhoff, C. Bymaster, F. P., et al. (2003). The CB_1 receptor antagonist SR141716A selectively increases monoaminergic neurotransmission in the medial prefrontal cortex: Implications for therapeutic actions. *British Journal of Pharmacology, 138*, 544–553.

Tzavara, E. T., & Witkin, J. M. (2008). Cannabinoid agonists and antagonists: Potential novel therapies for mood disorders. In A. Köfalvi (Ed.), *Cannabinoids and the brain*. New York: Springer.

Valentine, G. W., & Sanacora, G. (2009). Targeting glial physiology and glutamate cycling in the treatment of depression. *Biochemical Pharmacology, 78*, 431–439.

Wagstaff, A. J., Ormrod, D., & Spencer, C. M. (2001). Tianeptine: A review of its use in depressive disorders. *CNS Drugs, 15*, 231–259

Wang, R., Li, Y. B., Li, Y. H., Xu, Y., Wu, H. L., & Li, X. J. (2008a). Curcumin protects against glutamate excitotoxicity in rat cerebral cortical neurons by increasing brain-derived neurotrophic factor level and activating TrkB. *Brain Research, 1210*, 84–91.

Wang, R., Xu, Y., Wu, H. L., Li, Y. B., Li, Y. H., Guo, J. B., et al. (2008b). The antidepressant effects of curcumin in the forced swimming test involve 5-HT1 and 5-HT2 receptors. *European Journal of Pharmacology, 578*, 43–50.

Weissman, A., Milne, G. M., & Melvin, L. S., Jr. (1982). Cannabimimetic activity from CP-47,497, a derivative of 3-phenylcyclohexanol. *Journal of Pharmacology and Experimental Therapeutics*, *223*, 516–523.

Wieronska, J. M., Branski, P., Szewczyk, B., Palucha, A., Papp, M., Gruca, P., et al. (2001). Changes in the expression of metabotropic glutamate receptor 5 (mGluR5) in the rat hippocampus in an animal model of depression. *Polish Journal of Pharmacology*, *53*, 659–662.

Willner, P., & Mitchell. P. J. (2002). The validity of animal models of predisposition to depression. *Behavioural Pharmacology*, *13*, 169–188.

Witkin, J. M., & Eiler, W. J. A., II. (2006). Antagonism of metabotropic glutamate group II receptors in neurological and neuropsychiatric disorders, *Drug Development Research*, *67*, 757–769.

Witkin, J. M., Marek, G. J., Johnson, B. J., & Schoepp, D. D. (2007). Metabotropic glutamate receptors in the control of mood disorders. *CNS Neurological Disorders Drug Targets*, *6*, 87–100.

Witkin, J. M., Steele, T. D., & Sharpe, L. G. (1997). Effects of strychnine-insensitive glycine receptor ligands in rats discriminating either dizocilpine or phencyclidine from saline. *Journal of Pharmacology and Experimental Therapeutics*, *280*, 46–52.

Witkin, J. M., Tzavara, E. T., Davis, R. J., Li, X., & Nomikos, G. G. (2005). A Therapeutic Role for Cannabinoid CB_1 Receptor Antagonists in Major Depressive Disorders. *Trends in Pharmacological Sciences*, *26*, 609–617.

Witkin, J. M., Tzavara, E. T., & Nomikos, G. G. (2005). A Role for Cannabinoid CB_1 Receptors in Mood and Anxiety Disorders. *Behavioural Pharmacology*, *16*, 315–331.

Xu, Y., Ku, B. S., Cui, L., Li, X., Barish, P. A., Foster, T. C., et al. (2007). Curcumin reverses impaired hippocampal neurogenesis and increases serotonin receptor 1A mRNA and brain-derived neurotrophic factor expression in chronically stressed rats. *Brain Research*, *1162*, 9–18.

Xu, Y., Ku, B. S., Tie, L., Yao, H., Jiang, W., Ma, X., et al. (2006). Curcumin reverses the effects of chronic stress on behavior, the HPA axis, BDNF expression and phosphorylation of CREB. *Brain Research*, *1122*, 56–64.

Xu, Y., Ku, B. S., Yao, H. Y., Lin, Y. H., Ma, X., Zhang, Y. H., et al. (2005a). Antidepressant effects of curcumin in the forced swim test and olfactory bulbectomy models of depression in rats. *Pharmacology, Biochemistry and Behavior*, *82*, 200–206.

Xu, Y., Ku, B. S., Yao, H. Y., Lin, Y. H., Ma, X., Zhang, Y. H., et al. (2005b). The effects of curcumin on depressive-like behaviors in mice. *European Journal of Pharmacology*, *518*, 40–46.

Xu, Y., Lin, D., Li, S., Li, G., Shyamala, S. G., Barish, P. A., et al. (2009). Curcumin reverses impaired cognition and neuronal plasticity induced by chronic stress. *Neuropharmacology*, *57*, 463–471.

Yoshitake, T., Reenila, I., Reenila, I., Ogren, S. O., Hokfelt, T., & Kehr, J. (2003). Galanin attenuates basal and antidepressant drug-induced increase of extracellular serotonin and noradrenaline levels in the rat hippocampus. *Neuroscience Letters*, *339*, 239–242.

Zarate, C. A., Jr., Singh, J., & Manji, H. K. (2006). Cellular plasticity cascades: Targets for the development of novel therapeutics for bipolar disorder. *Biological Psychiatry*, *59*, 1006–1020.

Zoladz, P. R., Park, C. R., Muñoz, C., Fleshner, M., & Diamond, D. M. (2008). Tianeptine: An antidepressant with memory-protective properties. *Current Neuropharmacology*, *6*, 311–321.

Vincent Castagné, Paul C. Moser, and Roger D. Porsolt

Porsolt & Partners Pharmacology, 9 bis rue Henri Martin, 92100 Boulogne-Billancourt, France

Preclinical Behavioral Models for Predicting Antipsychotic Activity

Abstract

Schizophrenia is a major psychiatric disease that is characterized by three distinct symptom domains: positive symptoms, negative symptoms, and cognitive impairment. Additionally, treatment with classical antipsychotic medication can be accompanied by important side effects that involve extrapyramidal symptoms (EPS). The discovery of clozapine in the 1970s, which is efficacious in all three symptom domains and has a reduced propensity to induce EPS, has driven research for new antipsychotic agents with a wider spectrum of activity and a lower propensity to induce EPS. The following chapter reviews existing behavioral procedures in animals for their ability to predict compound efficacy against

Advances in Pharmacology, Volume 57
1054-3589/08 $35.00
10.1016/S1054-3589(08)57010-4

schizophrenia symptoms and liability to induce EPS. Rodent models of positive symptoms include procedures related to hyperfunction in central dopamine and serotonin (5-hydroxytryptamine) systems and hypofunction of central glutamatergic (*N*-methyl-D-aspartate) neurotransmission. Procedures for evaluating negative symptoms include rodent models of anhedonia, affective flattening, and diminished social interaction. Cognitive deficits can be assessed in rodent models of attention (prepulse inhibition (PPI), latent inhibition) and of learning and memory (passive avoidance, object and social recognition, Morris water maze, and operant-delayed alternation). The relevance of the conditioned avoidance response (CAR) is also discussed. A final section reviews animal procedures for assessing EPS liability, in particular parkinsonism (catalepsy), acute dystonia (purposeless chewing in rodents, dystonia in monkeys), akathisia (defecation in rodents), and tardive dyskinesia (long-term antipsychotic treatment in rodents and monkeys).

I. Introduction

The major requirements of an animal procedure are reliability and validity (Floresco et al., 2005). Reliability refers to the readiness with which test data can be reproduced, while validity can be divided into predictive, face, and construct entities (Marino, Knutsen, & Williams, 2008; Willner, 1991; Williams et al., 2008). For predictive validity, the animal procedure must be capable of predicting the clinical effects of the drug in humans. For face validity, the animal procedure must mimic symptoms of the disease. For construct validity, the animal procedure must reproduce etiological factors of the disease. Drug development in psychopharmacology relies mainly on predictive validity, and this is particularly true for the development of antipsychotics (Millan, 2008).

Drug discovery research over the last 20 years has largely focused on target-based approaches or "targephilia" (Enna & Williams, 2009). Unfortunately, in the case of schizophrenia, efforts focused on single targets has not enabled the discovery of drugs that are more effective than those in current use which owe their clinical efficacy to actions at multiple targets (Hughes, 2009; Spedding, Jay, Costa e Silva, & Perret, 2005). Despite the general acceptance that schizophrenia has a major genetic component accounting for perhaps 50% of disease risk, and the considerable research that has been undertaken to elucidate the genetics of schizophrenia (Gogos & Gerber, 2006; Owen, Williams, & O'Donovan, 2009; Williams, Owen, & O'Donovan, 2009), no one gene has yet been identified that can be considered a major risk factor for the disease (Crow, 2007; Williams, 2009). Indeed, none of the currently used antipsychotics would have been discovered by gene-based approaches (Marino et al., 2008). For this reason, the reader is referred to Crow (2007); Enna and Williams (2009), Gogos and Gerber (2006), Owen et al. (2009), Williams (2009) and Williams et al. (2009) for additional information on target-based or genetic models of schizophrenia.

Schizophrenia is a devastating disease with major consequences for patients, their families, and society as a whole (McGrath, Saha, Chant, & Welham, 2008). Schizophrenia is characterized by three major symptom domains: positive symptoms (delusions, hallucinations, bizarre speech and thought, paranoia), negative symptoms (emotional blunting, affective flattening, anhedonia, impoverishment of speech and thought, social withdrawal), and cognitive impairment (deficits in attention, learning, and memory) (Galletly, 2009). Symptoms vary between individuals, as a function of sex and age and also during the course of illness (Webber & Marder, 2008).

Despite intensive research, the etiology of schizophrenia remains far from understood (Keshavan, Tandon, Boutros, & Nasrallah, 2008; Ross, Margolis, Reading, Pletnikov, & Coyle, 2006). Most hypotheses have evolved from the actions of drugs in clinical use. The major hypothesis has therefore centered around a supposed hyperfunction in central dopamine (DA) systems, as the principal mechanism of action of the first clinically active antipsychotics (phenothiazines, thioxanthines, butyrophenones) was to block central DA receptors (Coyle, 2006; Stone, Morrison, & Pilowsky, 2007; Hughes, 2009; Toda & Abi-Dargham, 2007). Furthermore, indirect or direct DA agonists (amphetamine, cocaine, apomorphine) can exacerbate psychotic symptoms (Carlsson, 1988).

The introduction of the atypical antipsychotic, clozapine, in the early 1970s stimulated the search for other hypotheses since clozapine was clearly active as an antipsychotic (Hippius, 1989), but was less potent in blocking DA receptors as compared to the first-generation or typical antipsychotics (Creese et al., 1976) and was devoid of extrapyramidal side effects. Later studies have also suggested that clozapine, in addition to treating positive symptoms, is particularly effective in treatment-resistant patients, against negative symptoms and even against the cognitive deficits associated with schizophrenia (Serretti, De Ronchi, Lorenzi, & Berardi, 2004). Clozapine possesses a "rich" neurochemical profile with affinity for a wide range of receptors including D1, D4, 5-hydroxytryptamine (5-HT)$_{2A}$, 5-HT$_6$, α1, H1, and M1 (Jones, Gallagher, Pisa, & McFalls., 2008). Furthermore, in contrast to typical antipsychotics like haloperidol, the action of clozapine in the central nervous system (CNS) is less markedly localized on DA pathways in the striatal system, the putative origin of EPS (Bartholini, 1976).

While the discovery of clozapine led to a differential classification of antipsychotics into "classicals" and "atypicals" (Marino et al., 2008), the "atypicals" clearly do not form a homogeneous category. To be considered as such, in addition to controlling positive symptoms, they should be effective against negative symptoms, improve cognitive deficits, and induce fewer side effects, in particular EPS.

Discovery strategies for novel antipsychotics for the past 30 years have been dominated by attempts to reproduce the advantages of clozapine, while at the same time avoiding the side effects of clozapine including agranulocytosis, QT prolongation, hypotension, weight gain, and diabetes. Although numerous drugs, for example, amisulpride, aripiprazole, olanzapine, quetiapine, risperidone, sertindole, sulpiride, tiapride and ziprasidone, have been classified as "atypicals," none has yet approached clozapine in terms of its clinical properties (Gardner, Baldessarini, & Waraich, 2005).

The clinical effects of clozapine have led to a second major hypothesis for schizophrenia, 5-HT hyperfunction, as clozapine is a potent blocker at 5-HT$_{2A}$ receptors (Meltzer, 1989). Indeed, even before the DA hypothesis, clinicians were struck by the hallucinogenic properties of lysergic acid diethylamide (LSD) and mescaline which were later found to be potent 5-HT$_{2A}$ receptor agonists (Marino et al., 2008). A third major hypothesis for schizophrenia implicates hypofunction in central glutamatergic systems (Bunney, Bunney, & Carlsson, 1995; Coyle, 2006). Clinicians had been intrigued by the psychotomimetic actions of the N-methyl-D-aspartate (NMDA) antagonists in recreational drug abusers and in controlled human studies. NMDA antagonists mimic the positive, negative, and cognitive symptoms of schizophrenia, exacerbate symptoms in schizophrenic patients, and trigger the re-emergence of symptoms in remitted patients (Lahti, Koffel, LaPorte, & Tamminga, 1995; Petersen & Stillman, 1978). Indeed the glutamatergic hypothesis is considered as a link between the DA and 5-HT hypotheses in that the three systems are clearly interdependent (Marino et al., 2008). The present chapter will therefore discuss animal models derived from these three hypotheses.

Other hypotheses involving central GABAergic hypofunction (Wassef, Baker, & Kochan, 2003), muscarinic and nicotinic cholinergic hypofunction (Kelly & McCreadie, 2000), and histaminic H$_3$ hyperfunction (Ito, 2004) have also been proposed, but proof of concept in clinical trials is not yet available (Marino et al., 2008). These additional hypotheses will not be further covered in the present chapter.

In recent years psychopharmacologists have made considerable efforts to develop animal procedures that constitute direct translations of the symptomatology observed under clinical conditions (Markou, Chiamulera, Geyer, Tricklebank, & Steckler, 2009; McArthur & Borsini, 2008). These efforts are aimed at increasing the relevance of animal procedures for predicting the therapeutic efficacy of a novel substance (Day et al., 2008; Markou et al., 2009; Millan, 2008). The need for new animal models to evaluate new compounds for the treatment of schizophrenia has been highlighted by two recent research initiatives: the NIMH-funded

MATRICs (Measurement and Treatment Research to Improve Cognition in Schizophrenia) battery (Geyer, 2008) and the European Commission initiative NEWMEDS (Novel Methods Leading to New Medications in Depression and Schizophrenia) schizophrenia (Hughes, 2009). The latter is targeted to "develop better animal models ... generate translational technology that could help provide early indicators of efficacy ... and ... to develop tools to improve patient stratification to focus on the complexity and heterogeneity of the disease."

In the field of schizophrenia, such translational approaches have largely concentrated on the cognitive aspects of schizophrenia because these can be investigated in an equivalent fashion both in humans and in animals. More florid psychotic manifestations, such as hallucinations, delusions or paranoia, being essentially human, are less readily amenable to such an approach.

Based on the above considerations, the present chapter will attempt to define the animal criteria most likely to predict clinical antipsychotic activity, concentrating on the three primary symptom domains: positive symptoms, negative symptoms, and cognitive deficit, including some data from our own laboratory. No preclinical assay for antipsychotics would, however, be complete without evaluating procedures for predicting side effects, in particular EPS.

II. Procedures for Evaluating Positive Symptoms

Agitation, hallucinations, delusions, and paranoia represent the main positive symptoms described in schizophrenic patients. Although delusions and paranoia are difficult to model in rodents, agitation and hallucinations are more easily amenable to behavioral testing. Indeed the majority of behavioral tests relevant to agitation use reagent substances administered to animals in order to reproduce an abnormality presumed also to be present in psychotic patients (Geyer & Ellenbroek, 2003; Large, 2007; Mouri, Noda, Enomoto, & Nabeshima, 2007). Although caution must be used in drawing parallels between animal and human behavior, stereotyped behavior in animals has been generally accepted as modeling the stereotyped behavior observed in psychotic patients, whereas hyperactivity would appear to parallel more closely psychotic agitation.

A. Hyperactivity and Stereotypies Induced by DA Agonists

Direct and indirect DA agonists, such as apomorphine, cocaine, and amphetamine, induce hyperactivity at moderate doses and stereotypies at higher doses when administered to rodents (Costall, Marsden, Naylor, & Pycock, 1977; Simon & Chermat, 1972; Thiebot et al., 1982). Activation of

DA D2 receptors located in the ventral striatum (mainly the *nucleus accumbens*) induces hyperactivity whereas stereotypies seem to involve striatal D2 receptors (Costall, Domeney, & Naylor, 1982). Although all classical or typical antipsychotics inhibit amphetamine-induced locomotion and stereotypies, atypical antipsychotics are said to be less effective against stereotypies than classical antipsychotics (O'Neill & Shaw, 1999; Palucha-Poniewiera et al., 2008). These findings have been corroborated by data from our own laboratory (Fig. 1), where haloperidol potently antagonized both amphetamine-induced hyperactivity and stereotypies, whereas clozapine had less marked effects on stereotypies. There was no clear differentiation between the two parameters with the other atypicals tested (olanzapine, quetiapine, risperidone).

The relatively lower efficacy of clozapine against stereotypies as compared with the hyperactivity induced by DA agonists is considered as evidence for its preferential action on D2 receptors located in the striatum (Leite, Guimaraes, & Moreira, 2008). Because EPS are thought to result from decreased activity of DA receptors in the striatum (Bartholini, 1976), a preferential action of a novel substance against DA agonist-induced hyperactivity might thus represent a first indicator of a lower potential to induce EPS in patients (see below).

By design and outcome, behavioral tests using DA agonists are exclusively linked to the DA hypothesis of schizophrenia. However, other potential antipsychotics that have minimal affinity for DA receptors, for example, the 5-HT$_2$ antagonists MDL 100-907 (Moser, Moran, Frank, & Kehne, 1996) and WAY 163909 (Marquis et al., 2007), and diverse client substances which have been evaluated at Porsolt and Partners, clearly antagonize DA agonist effects.

B. Behaviors Induced by 5-HT Agonists

Hallucinogens acting on 5-HT receptors, for example, LSD, psilocybin, and mescaline, induce visual hallucinations in humans and cause characteristic behavioral signs in animals. Thus antagonism of the behavioral effects of serotonergic hallucinogens in animals would appear to provide a possible behavioral model for assessing antipsychotic activity. Administration of mescaline to specific strains of mice induces episodes of paroxysmic scratching (Deegan & Cook, 1958). Mescaline-induced scratching is inhibited by classical and atypical antipsychotics, in particular those which directly or indirectly antagonize 5-HT$_2$ receptors (Cook, Tam, & Rohrbach, 1992). These results are corroborated by data from our own laboratory (Fig. 2), where all the substances tested potently antagonized mescaline-induced scratching.

On the other hand, a wide range of indirectly or directly acting 5-HT receptor agonists without known hallucinogenic properties also

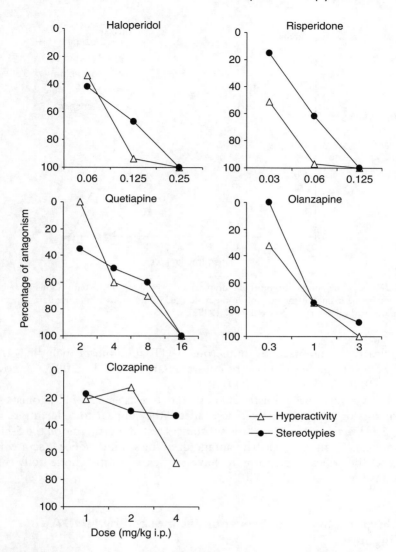

FIGURE 1 The effects of typical and atypical antipsychotics on the hyperactivity and stereotypies induced by D-amphetamine (2 mg/kg i.p.) in the male Rj:NMRI mouse. In-house data generated using the method for hyperactivity of Boissier and Simon (1965) and that for stereotypies as described by Simon and Chermat (1972).

induce clear behavioral effects in rodents; for example, the forepaw treading, head twitches, and lower lip retraction induced by 5-HT_{1A} agonists or the head twitches and wet-dog shakes induced by the 5-HT_2 agonist ($\pm$)-2,5-dimethoxy-4-iodoamphetamine. These effects

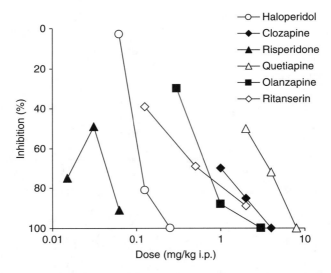

FIGURE 2   The effects of typical and atypical antipsychotics on the paroxysmic scratching induced by mescaline (50 mg/kg p.o.) in the male Rj:C57BL6 mouse. In-house data generated using the method described by Cook et al. (1992).

are clearly antagonized by numerous 5-HT antagonists including antipsychotics targeting 5-HT$_2$ receptors (Gardell et al., 2007; Vanover et al., 2006; Weiner et al., 2001).

It is not therefore robustly established that tests using 5-HT agonists are predictors of antipsychotic activity. Indeed, they appear to reflect more the anti-5-HT activity of some of the substances tested. Furthermore, the 5-HT$_2$ antagonist, ritanserin, clearly antagonized mescaline-induced scratching (Fig. 2), but does not appear to have any clear antipsychotic activity in humans (den Boer et al., 2000)

C. Hyperactivity and Stereotypies Induced by NMDA Antagonists

Antagonists of the NMDA glutamate receptor subtype also induce hyperactivity at moderate doses and ataxia accompanied by stereotypies at higher doses (Carlsson & Carlsson, 1989; Hargreaves & Cain, 1995). The downstream mechanisms leading from NMDA blockade to behavioral effects are still debated and include disinhibition of cortical neurons by inhibitory interneurons, alterations in monoamine systems, and/or increase of glutamate release with subsequent activation of non-NMDA glutamate receptors (Morris, Cochran, & Pratt, 2005). The complexity of the secondary targets of NMDA antagonists is consistent with the concept that schizophrenia involves, but cannot be reduced to, a simple hypoactivity of glutamatergic systems (Coyle, 2006; Stone et al., 2007). Stereotypies and hyperactivity are induced by several psychotomimetic NMDA antagonists such as phencyclidine (PCP), ketamine, and dizocilpine (MK-801) (Morris et al., 2005).

NMDA antagonist-induced hyperactivity and stereotypies in the rat are reversed by both typical and atypical antipsychotics. In general, atypical antipsychotics, for example, clozapine, aripiprazole and olanzapine, are thought to be more effective than typical antipsychotics (Leite et al., 2008; Ninan & Kulkarni, 1999; O'Neill & Shaw, 1999). The situation is thus different from that observed against the effects of DA agonists. Nonetheless, the differential potency against the effects of dopaminergic and glutamatergic substances is not that marked (Natesan, Reckless, Barlow, Nobrega, & Kapur, 2008). Interestingly, the efficacy of antipsychotics (haloperidol, clozapine, olanzapine) against PCP-induced hyperactivity has been reported to become more robust after repeated treatment and testing, whereas their efficacy against amphetamine-induced hyperactivity tends to wane (Sun, Hu, & Li, 2009). Data from our laboratory (Fig. 3) suggest that, even with haloperidol, the acute doses required to antagonize NMDA antagonist-induced stereotypies in the rat are considerably higher than those required to antagonize DA agonist effects. The other substances had little effect on this parameter in our hands.

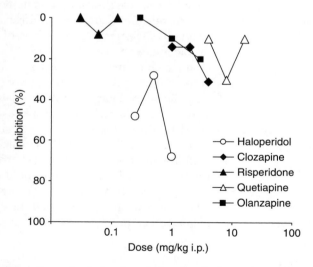

FIGURE 3 The effects of typical and atypical antipsychotics on the stereotypies induced by phencyclidine (4 mg/kg s.c.) in the male Rj:Wistar rat. In-house data generated using the method described by Meltzer et al. (1981).

III. Procedures for Evaluating Negative Symptoms _____

Negative symptoms in schizophrenia include emotional blunting, affective flattening, anhedonia, impoverishment of speech and thought, and social withdrawal. Even in clinical terms these symptoms are more difficult to characterize than the more florid positive symptoms discussed above and, furthermore, are not necessarily specific to schizophrenia. Some of them (impoverished speech and thought) are uniquely human (Crow, 2007) and therefore not amenable to modeling in animals. Other symptoms lend themselves more readily to animal testing and are discussed below.

A. Anhedonia

Anhedonia refers to a decrease in the capacity to feel pleasure and, in addition to representing a negative symptom in schizophrenia, is a core symptom of depression (Anisman & Matheson, 2005). Anhedonia in animals has been assessed through measures of sucrose consumption or intracranial self-stimulation (ICSS) although the two approaches are not interchangeable (Nielsen, Arnt, & Sanchez, 2000).

In normal rats, typical antipsychotics acting preferentially as DA antagonists decrease sucrose consumption and preference although they do not impair sweetness discrimination (Muscat & Willner, 1989; Willner, Papp, Phillips, Maleeh, & Muscat, 1990). In contrast, the atypical antipsychotics olanzapine and quetiapine reverse stress-induced anhedonia (Orsetti et al., 2006, 2007). PCP also decreases sucrose consumption in the rat via an action suggesting impaired reward function (Turgeon & Hoge, 2003). To our knowledge no data are available investigating the effects of typical or atypical antipsychotics on this phenomenon.

ICSS is an operant model in which animals will press a lever to obtain brief electrical stimulations to specific regions of the brain, in particular the medial forebrain bundle (Phillips, Blaha, & Fibiger, 1989). Variations in the level of ICSS current are therefore considered as a measure of reward function, where an increase in the level of ICSS necessary to sustain self-stimulation behavior is taken to indicate a decrease in the rewarding power of the electrical stimulation. Withdrawal from sub-chronic PCP treatment in the rat is associated with an increase in ICSS current threshold suggesting withdrawal-induced anhedonia (Spielewoy & Markou, 2003). Again, to our knowledge, no data are available investigating the effects of classical or atypical antipsychotics on this phenomenon.

B. Affective Flattening

Affective flattening refers to apathy in various situations, including those involving stress. Although there is no animal model for affective flattening, the immobility induced during the forced swim test procedure may reflect a lowered affective state in the rodent (Porsolt, Bertin, & Jalfre, 1977, 1978). PCP increases immobility in the forced swim test in the mouse, particularly after repeated treatment (Corbett, Zhou, Sorensen, & Mondadori, 1999; Noda, Kamei, Mamiya, Furukawa, & Nabeshima, 2000). Furthermore, the effect persists when PCP treatment is discontinued (Noda et al., 2000). More interestingly, PCP-enhanced immobility has been reported to be attenuated by the atypical antipsychotics clozapine, risperidone, olanzapine, and quetiapine, but not by the typical antipsychotics haloperidol, pimozide, or chlorpromazine (Corbett et al., 1999; Nagai et al., 2003; Noda et al., 2000). Antidepressants and anxiolytics devoid of antipsychotic activity did not reverse PCP-induced immobility in the forced swim test (Nabeshima, Mouri, Murai, & Noda, 2006). Taken together, the above data suggest that enhanced immobility in the forced swim test induced by PCP or PCP-discontinuation represents a promising model of affective flattening in schizophrenia.

C. Social Interaction

The social interaction test in the rat has been widely used to evaluate anxiety (File, Ouagazzal, Gonzalez, & Overstreet, 1999), but has also been proposed as a model for antipsychotic activity using acute or repeated administration of NMDA antagonists to decrease social investigation (Becker & Grecksch, 2004; Rung, Carlsson, Ryden, & Carlsson, 2005; Sams-Dodd, 1999).

In the majority of studies, classical antipsychotics such as haloperidol do not reverse acute NMDA antagonist-induced deficits in social investigation (Becker & Grecksch, 2004; Boulay et al., 2004; Rung, Carlsson, Markinhuhta, & Carlsson, 2005). Conflicting data exist for clozapine, which is either inactive (Boulay et al., 2004; Rung, Carlsson, Markinhuhta, et al., 2005) or able to reverse social investigation deficits (Becker & Grecksch, 2004). Comparable effects of acute administration of PCP and MK-801 occur in the mouse (Olszewski et al., 2008; Zou et al., 2008), although this animal is difficult to use because of high general activity, aggressiveness, and sensitivity to stress.

Repeated administration of PCP or MK-801 also decreases social investigation in the rat (Geyer & Ellenbroek, 2003), an effect that persists on discontinuation of PCP (Tanaka et al., 2003). Acute treatment with the atypical agents, ziprasidone and aripiprazole, has been reported to reverse sub-chronic PCP-induced deficits in social investigation in the rat, whereas similar treatment with haloperidol or clozapine was without effect (Snigdha & Neill, 2008a, 2008b). In the mouse, deficits in social investigation induced by sub-chronic PCP treatment have been reversed by clozapine but not haloperidol (Qiao et al., 2001). Similar reversal has been described in the mouse after combined treatment with galantamine and risperidone (Wang et al., 2007).

Taken together, the above data suggest that classical antipsychotics such as haloperidol are not effective in reversing NMDA antagonist-induced deficits in social interaction in the rat or the mouse, whereas more encouraging data have been obtained with various atypical antipsychotics.

IV. Procedures for Evaluating Cognitive Deficits

Cognitive deficits in schizophrenic patients encompass attentional processes, memory, and learning (Galletly, 2009). Although some human cognitive functions do not have equivalents in animals, several tests present interesting translational potential (Castner, Goldman-Rakic, & Williams, 2004; Day et al., 2008; Floresco, Geyer, Gold, & Grace, 2005; Geyer, 2008; Geyer & Ellenbroek, 2003; Markou et al., 2009).

A. Attentional Processes

Cognitive function relies on adequate automatic processes for the treatment of incoming information (Ellenbroek, 2004). The two main behavioral paradigms used in preclinical and in clinical research for attentional processes are pre-pulse inhibition (PPI; Swerdlow, Weber, Qu, Light, & Braff, 2008) and latent inhibition (LI) (Moser, Hitchcock, Lister, & Moran, 2000).

I. Prepulse Inhibition

PPI refers to the decrease in startle reaction to a sudden stimulus by pre-exposure to a weak, non-startling, stimulus. The weak and the strong stimuli are termed prepulse and pulse, respectively (Ellenbroek, 2004; Geyer & Ellenbroek, 2003). PPI is observed in normal subjects and is considered as an index of sensorimotor gating, that is, the capacity to filter incoming information. Schizophrenia and several other brain disorders involve PPI deficits that can be modeled in animals with relatively good translational power. Most preclinical PPI studies have been performed in the rat, where disruption of PPI is induced by pharmacological means (Ellenbroek, 2004; Swerdlow et al., 2008).

The DA agonists, apomorphine and amphetamine, are widely used to disrupt PPI in the rat. Apomorphine-induced PPI deficits can be reversed by haloperidol (Auclair, Kleven, Besnard, Depoortere, & Newman-Tancredi, 2006). Some reports describe reversal of apomorphine-induced PPI deficits by clozapine although its effects are often limited to a narrow dose-range (Martin et al., 2003). Amphetamine effects are reversed by typical and some atypical antipsychotics (Marquis et al., 2007; Martin et al., 2003).

Nonetheless, conflicting data exist regarding clozapine (Martin et al., 2003; Pouzet, Didriksen, & Arnt, 2002).

Antagonists of NMDA glutamate receptors also disrupt PPI in the rat (Martinez, Halim, Oostwegel, Geyer, & Swerdlow, 2000). PCP-induced PPI deficits are resistant to typical and atypical antipsychotics (Pouzet et al., 2002), although one report has described reversal by clozapine (Suemaru et al., 2004). Similarly, deficits in PPI induced by MK-801 have been reported resistant to typical and atypical antipsychotics (Bast, Zhang, Feldon, & White, 2000), although Martin et al. (2003) have described positive effects of clozapine and olanzapine. In the mouse, Adage et al. (2008) report reversal of PCP-induced PPI deficits by clozapine. Interestingly, in data from our laboratory, clear antagonism by clozapine of the deficits in PPI induced in rats by MK-801 was observed (Fig. 4).

Besides pharmacologically induced PPI deficits, spontaneous deficits observed in the DBA/2 strain of mice have been used to detect efficacy of typical and atypical antipsychotics, where acute treatment with risperidone improves PPI in DBA/2 mice (Browman et al., 2004; Fox et al., 2005). Likewise, the Brattleboro rat displays spontaneous deficits in PPI that can be attenuated by typical and atypical antipsychotics (Cilia et al., 2009). Finally, deficits in PPI can also be induced by isolation rearing which,

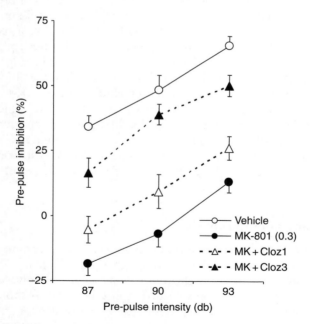

FIGURE 4   The effects of the atypical antipsychotic, clozapine on the deficits in prepulse inhibition induced by MK-801 (0.3 mg/kg s.c.) in the male Rj:Wistar rat. In-house data generated using the method described by Bast et al. (2000).

although time consuming, has been used as a procedure for detecting antipsychotic activity (Southam et al., 2009).

2. Latent Inhibition

LI refers to a cognitive process in which repeated non-rewarded experience of a stimulus retards the ability of that stimulus to subsequently enter into new associations (Lubow & Moore, 1959). It is of particular interest in schizophrenia as it is attenuated during acute phases of the disease (Baruch, Hemsley, & Gray, 1988). A deficit in LI can be induced in animals by acute administration of drugs that increase mesolimbic dopaminergic activity, for example, amphetamine and as a result, LI is a widely used as an animal model with relevance to information processing deficits (Moser et al., 2000; Weiner et al., 2000). There are two ways that LI can be used to study putative antipsychotic agents: reversal of amphetamine disruption or enhancement of low levels of LI (Moser et al., 2000). The latter procedure involves exposing animals to relatively low numbers of stimulus presentations (typically 10 compared to 30–40 for complete LI). Both procedures are sensitive to a wide range of clinically active antipsychotics (Moser et al., 2000). Figure 5 shows the effects of clozapine on LI in the two procedures (Moran, Fischer, Hitchcock, & Moser, 1996).

Although it has been suggested that specific conditions of pre-exposure may allow dissociation of the effects of typical and atypical antipsychotics (Shadach, Gaisler, Schiller, & Weiner, 2000), the majority of reports indicate that neither procedure is able to separate typical and atypical antipsychotics. This, together with theoretical considerations linking LI deficits primarily to positive symptoms, has limited the interest in LI as a novel test for antipsychotics. However, recent studies using MK-801-induced deficits in LI are of interest. In contrast with amphetamine (which disrupts LI), the NMDA receptor antagonist, MK-801, induces abnormally persistent LI (i.e., LI is still observed in conditions where it should not) which may prove to be a useful new model of cognitive deficits with relevance to schizophrenia (Black et al., 2009; Gaisler-Salomon, Diamant, Rubin, & Weiner, 2008).

B. Learning and Memory

There exist a multitude of procedures for evaluating learning and memory in animals, all of possible relevance to schizophrenia. Learning and memory problems present in schizophrenic patients are, however, difficult to differentiate from symptoms occurring in other CNS pathologies. This explains a convergence between preclinical tests performed for antipsychotic development with research for cognitive enhancement (Castner et al., 2004). The present section will focus on procedures which have been used for developing drugs in schizophrenia and will not attempt to cover the whole

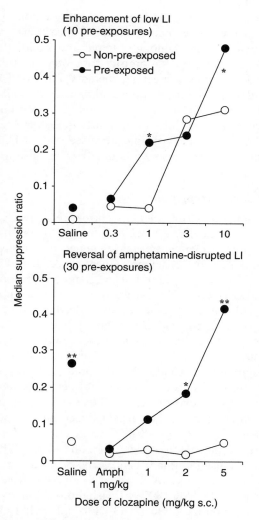

FIGURE 5 The effects of clozapine on latent inhibition in the male Charles River Wistar rat. Figure adapted from Moran et al. (1996).

range of available procedures in the learning and memory domain. The procedures described include passive avoidance, object and social recognition, spatial learning in the Morris water maze (MWM) and operant-delayed alternation in the Skinner box.

1. Passive Avoidance

The one-trial passive avoidance task is one of the oldest procedures for evaluating drug effects on learning and memory (Glick & Zimmerberg,

1972). A rat or a mouse receives an aversive stimulation in a recognizable environment and on a later occasion shows that it has remembered by avoiding the environment. Although simple and rapid, the procedure is notoriously variable from one laboratory to another (Sarter, 2004) and is now rarely used except for screening memory impairing effects. Indeed, most typical and atypical antipsychotics administered alone impair passive avoidance performance (Ishiyama et al., 2007). In contrast, in the same study, the atypical antipsychotics clozapine, quetiapine, and risperidone but not olanzapine or aripiprazole reversed the deficits induced by MK-801. Haloperidol was also without effect against MK-801-induced deficits.

2. Object and Social Recognition

Object recognition is impaired in schizophrenic patients (Gabrovska, Laws, Sinclair, & McKenna, 2003). This has led to the use of the object recognition test for evaluating substances aimed to improve the cognitive deficits in schizophrenia (Castagné, Cuénod, & Do, 2004; Castagné, Rougemont, Cuénod, & Do, 2004). The rat test, based on that described by Ennaceur and Delacour (1988), is a two-session procedure where recognition at the second session is indicated by a decrease in investigation of a familiar object as compared with a new object. The atypical antipsychotics, clozapine and risperidone, but not haloperidol, reverse the deficits in object recognition induced by PCP or MK-801 (Grayson, Idris, & Neill, 2007; Karasawa, Hashimoto, & Chaki, 2008). Other substances with different molecular mechanisms intended for the treatment of cognitive deficits in schizophrenia are also active against NMDA antagonist-induced deficits in object recognition and include the partial α7 nicotinic receptor agonist, SSR 180711, (Pichat et al., 2007), ADX 47273 a positive modulator of metabotropic glutamate receptors (Liu et al., 2008), and GSK 207040, a histamine H_3 receptor antagonist (Southam et al., 2009). Other studies have been performed in mice, where NMDA antagonist-induced deficits in object recognition can be reversed by SSR 180711 (Hashimoto, Ishima, et al., 2008), the glycine transport inhibitors, NFPS (N-[3-([1,1-biphenyl]-4-yloxy)-3-(4-fluorophenyl)propyl]-N-methylglycine), and D-serine (Hashimoto, Fujita, Ishima, Chaki, & Iyo, 2008) and by perospirone, a $5-HT_{1A}$ receptor agonist (Hagiwara et al., 2008).

The social recognition test can be considered a "social version" of the object recognition test (Lemaire, Bohme, Piot, Roques, & Blanchard, 1994). Like the object recognition test, the social recognition test is a two-session procedure involving a resident rat and a juvenile intruder rat, where recognition at the second session is indicated by a decrease in investigation of an intruder previously introduced as compared with the introduction of a new animal. Using the social recognition test, it has been shown that increasing activity of NMDA receptors via blockade of the glycine transporter with the potential antipsychotic, SSR 504734, attenuates the long-term deficits induced by neonatal PCP (Depoortere et al., 2005). Similarly, social memory in normal adult rats is improved and the age-related deficits in social memory in aged rats reversed by acute treatment with ABT-239, an histamine H_3 receptor antagonist/inverse agonist (Fox et al., 2005). In an analogous fashion, scopolamine-induced social recognition deficits can be reversed by RO 4368554, a 5-HT_6 receptor antagonist (Schreiber et al., 2007).

3. Morris Water Maze

The procedure most commonly used for evaluating test substances on learning and memory is the MWM (Morris, 1981). In this procedure, rats or mice are placed in a circular water tank and left to find the escape platform just beneath the surface of the water and therefore not visible to the animal. On repeated exposure to the test situation, animals learn to find the escape platform more rapidly, usually in the presence of extra-maze visual cues. The procedure therefore represents a model of spatial learning. Acute PCP treatment in the rat impairs spatial memory in the MWM and this effect can be reversed by clozapine and other atypical antipsychotics (sertindole, risperidone) but not by haloperidol (Didriksen, Skarsfeldt, & Arnt, 2007; Okuyama et al., 1997). Likewise, acute MK-801-induced impairment of spatial learning in the MWM is attenuated by the α7 receptor agonist SSR 180711 (Pichat et al., 2007). As in the rat, repeated PCP treatment impairs spatial learning in the mouse and this effect has been reported to be reversed by co-treatment with clozapine but not haloperidol (Beraki, Kuzmin, Tai, & Ogren, 2008).

4. Operant-Delayed Alternation

Another procedure useful for evaluating drug effects on cognition, in particular short-term memory, is the delayed operant alternation procedure using a standard Skinner box (Roux, Hubert, Lenegre, Milinkevitch, & Porsolt, 1994). Previously trained rats are presented with a lever, either on the right or on the left side of the food dispenser. The rat presses on the lever and the lever is withdrawn. After a certain delay, two levers are presented and the rat has to press on the lever opposite to that presented previously to obtain a food reward (delayed alternation, delayed non-matching to sample). The left side of Fig. 6, taken from experiments in our laboratory, shows that vehicle-treated rats display delay-dependent forgetting as the delay is increased from 2.5 to 10 s. Acute administration of PCP (2 mg/kg s.c.), without disrupting operant behavior, induces a clear decrease in response accuracy suggesting a PCP-induced deficit in short-term memory. Data on the right side of Fig. 6 show that clozapine partially corrected the PCP-induced deficit up to 16 mg/kg p.o., a dose which started to disrupt

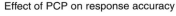

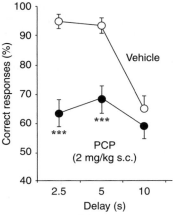

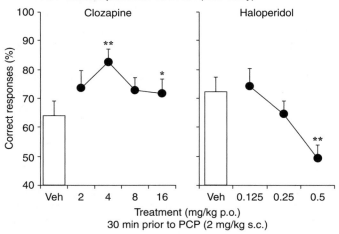

FIGURE 6   The effects of haloperidol and clozapine on the deficits in response accuracy induced by PCP (2 mg/kg i.p.) in a delayed alternation task in the male Rj:Wistar rat. In-house data generated using the method described by Roux et al. (1994).

operant behavior with fewer animals completing the task. In contrast, haloperidol failed to reverse the PCP-induced memory deficit and even exacerbated it at higher doses that disrupted operant behavior.

5. More Complex Procedures for Evaluating Cognition

The tests described in the preceding sections are commonly used in behavioral screening for activity against cognitive deficits. In case of positive effects, the most promising substances can be further evaluated in follow-up tests before initiating clinical trials. These tests will not be treated in detail here but could include tests of cognitive flexibility using attentional set-shifting tasks (Goetghebeur & Dias, 2009) or reversal learning (Idris, Repeto, Neill, & Large, 2005), whereas sustained attention can be evaluated using the 5-choice serial reaction time test (Chudasama & Robbins, 2006) in the rodent, or even the primate (Weed et al., 1999). These more complex procedures possess clear translational validity because of their similarities with neuropsychological tests performed in humans, such as the Wisconsin card sorting or the continuous performance tests. As a consequence, their predictive validity is likely to be relatively high (Day et al., 2008; Powell & Miyakawa, 2006).

C. Conditioned Avoidance Behavior

Selective blockade of the conditioned avoidance response (CAR) has long been considered as a selective and sensitive indicator of antipsychotic activity (Cook & Weidley, 1957; Wadenberg & Hicks, 1999). Animals can be trained to prevent the occurrence of an aversive stimulation, usually electric shock, by making a specific behavioral response. The CAR can be distinguished from passive avoidance (see above) in that the animal must engage in an active behavior to avoid the aversive stimulation.

Different behavioral paradigms come under the heading of CAR:

- one-way avoidance: the animal has to go to a specific place (jumping up onto a suspended pole, crossing to the other side of a two-compartment box) to avoid shock. Trials are repeated usually by manually replacing the animal in the starting position.
- two-way avoidance: the animal in a two-compartment box has to repeatedly "shuttle" from one side of the apparatus to the other to avoid shock.
- operant avoidance: the animal has to press on a lever to avoid shock.

A further distinction is between discriminated and non-discriminated avoidance. In discriminated avoidance the animal is repeatedly presented with an initially neutral stimulus (conditioned stimulus, CS) and has to perform the CAR within a short period of time, usually 5 s, otherwise it will receive the aversive stimulation (unconditioned stimulus, UCS). In non-discriminated avoidance, there is no CS apart from the environment itself, and the animal has to initiate the CAR without a warning signal.

In antipsychotic testing, three paradigms have traditionally been used, the one-way discriminated pole jump procedure (Cook & Weidley, 1957), the two-way discriminated shuttle box procedure (Bolles & Grossen, 1970), and the non-discriminated operant continuous avoidance procedure (Sidman,

1962). The procedures most used currently in antipsychotic development are the shuttle box and the Sidman procedures as they are readily automated.

The results obtained, however, have been very different. In one of the earliest publications on the effects of antipsychotics on the CAR (Cook & Weidley, 1957), using the discriminated pole jump procedure, the authors reported a specific blockade of avoidance responding at doses which were without effect on escape responding. These early findings have led to the persistent belief that selective blockade of avoidance behavior is an identifier of antipsychotic activity (Wadenberg & Hicks, 1999). Unfortunately, this principle appears to be procedure specific. In another early publication (Heise & Boff, 1962), using a non-discriminated Sidman procedure, neuroleptics blocked escape behavior at doses very close to those blocking the CAR, whereas with benzodiazepines the dose–ratio between escape and avoidance responding was considerably larger, that is, just the opposite of what was described by Cook and Weidley. Using the Sidman procedure in our laboratory, we have made similar observations to Heise and Boff with the typical antipsychotics (chlorpromazine, thioridazine, haloperidol), newer agents (sultopride, α-flupenthixol), and the atypical antipsychotic, clozapine (Fig. 7). All substances inhibited the CAR at doses which impaired escape behavior. Thus, although drug potency in CAR procedures appears to be highly correlated both with anti-DA activity and with clinical potency (Arnt, 1982; Olsen, Brennum, & Kreilgaard, 2008), the notion of selective blockade of the CAR as a specific predictor of antipsychotic efficacy is not generally true, or at best is dependent on the procedures employed.

V. Procedures for Evaluating EPS

EPS have been viewed as inextricably linked to the therapeutic efficacy of antipsychotics (Haase, 1978). Classical antipsychotics before clozapine induced a variety of symptoms generally grouped under the heading of EPS that occur at different times during antipsychotic treatment. Acute EPS symptoms (parkinsonism, dystonia, akathisia) develop early in the course of treatment, whereas tardive dyskinesias occur only after prolonged antipsychotic therapy. The acute phenomena represent a pharmacological consequence of drug administration, decrease when drug treatment is stopped, re-occur when drug treatment is reinstated, and in general can be attenuated by anticholinergics. Conversely, tardive dyskinesia occurs on discontinuation or reduction of drug treatment, is suppressed when drug treatment is reinstated, and tends to be exacerbated by treatment with anticholinergics (Casey, 1993). Acute EPS are considered as a manageable nuisance, whereas tardive dyskinesia is viewed as a debilitating and perhaps irreversible side effect of long-term treatment. Although generally considered to represent different forms of the same underlying drug-induced pathophysiology, EPS syndromes are clinically

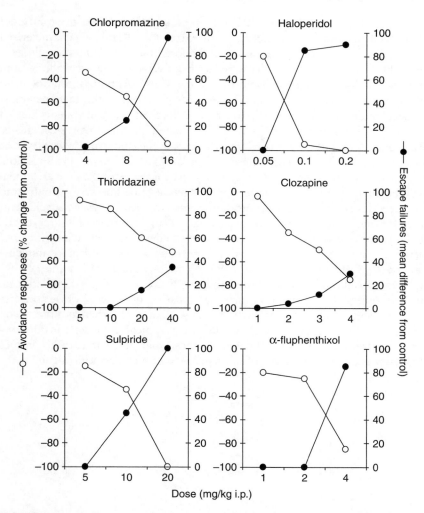

FIGURE 7 The effects of classical and atypical antipsychotics on Sidman avoidance responding in the male OLAC Lister Hooded rat. In-house data generated using the method described by Sidman (1962).

distinct from one another and may therefore require different animal procedures to assess the liability of novel substances to induce them.

A. Parkinsonism

Antipsychotic-induced parkinsonism is difficult to distinguish from idiopathic parkinsonism. Both are characterized by a triad of symptoms: tremor, rigidity, and akinesia (Weiden, 2007). Tremor, usually greatest at rest, includes rhythmic back and forth trembling of the extremities. Rigidity is characterized by cogwheel resistance during passively imposed motion. Akinesia includes a mask-like facial expression, decreased arm movements during walking, and reduced ability to initiate movement (Casey, 1993). Although none of these phenomena can be clearly identified in rodent behavior, the fact that most classical antipsychotics, but not clozapine, induce catalepsy in rodents has led to the catalepsy test being used for predicting parkinsonian side effects. Although many different procedures are used to measure catalepsy (Geyer & Ellenbroek, 2003; Sanberg, Bunsey, Giordano, & Norman, 1988; Simon, Langwinski, & Boissier, 1969), they all involve measures of the time an animal will remain in an unusual position imposed by the experimenter. In contrast to the early days of antipsychotic screening (Janssen, Niemegeers, & Schellekens, 1965), where catalepsy in rats was used as an identifier of antipsychotic activity, modern antipsychotic research seeks to demonstrate a wide difference between the doses showing potential therapeutic activity and those inducing catalepsy (Hoffman & Donovan, 1995; Natesan et al., 2008).

Data from our laboratory are shown in Fig. 8 using typical and atypical antipsychotics. Haloperidol induces catalepsy at doses very close to those inducing signs of therapeutic activity (Figs. 1 and 2), whereas little or no catalepsy is induced by clozapine or the other atypicals at doses considerably higher. Overall, the available data suggest that the capacity to induce catalepsy is a good predictor of antipsychotic-induced parkinsonism.

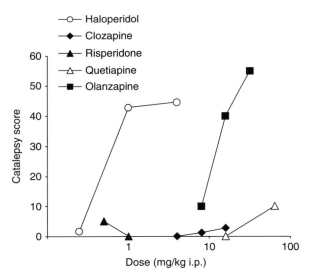

FIGURE 8   Cataleptic effects of typical and atypical antipsychotics in the male Rj:Wistar rat. In-house data generated using the method described by Simon et al. (1969).

B. Acute Dystonia

Antipsychotic-induced acute dystonia is characterized by involuntary muscle spasms, accompanied by briefly sustained or fixed abnormal postures including bizarre positions of the limbs and trunk, oculogyric crises, tongue protrusion, and torticollis (Casey, 1993).

Nothing resembling the above has been reported in rodents. On the other hand, purposeless chewing movements have been reported in rats that are increased by administration of certain antipsychotics, for example, haloperidol, *cis*-flupenthixol, trifluoperazine, fluphenazine, and sulpiride (Stewart, Rupniak, Jenner, & Marsden, 1988), all of which induce acute dystonia in humans (Deniker, Ginestet, & Loo, 1980). Clozapine, which is devoid of such effects in clinical use, does not alter chewing behavior even after chronic administration (Stewart et al., 1988). Furthermore the antipsychotic-induced chewing movements can be attenuated by centrally acting anticholinergic agents such as scopolamine or atropine, but not by the peripherally acting anticholinergic, methylscopolamine, suggesting the central origins of the effect. Although purposeless chewing in rats bears no clear resemblance to the spasmic nature of acute dystonia described in patients, pharmacologically the model would appear to possess a certain validity.

Clear acute dystonic phenomena have, however, been reported in different primate species, including old world macaques (Porsolt & Jalfre, 1981), baboons (Meldrum, Anlezark, & Marsden, 1977), new world cebus monkeys (Peacock & Gerlach, 1993), squirrel monkeys (Liebman & Neale, 1980), and marmosets (Fukuoka, Nakano, Kohda, Okuno, & Matsuo, 1997).

Figure 9 contains data we obtained in our laboratory with rhesus monkeys previously exposed to intermittent treatment with diverse antipsychotics over a 1–2 year period (Porsolt & Jalfre, 1981). These show that no dystonia was observed with typical antipsychotics like chlorpromazine and thioridazine or the atypical agent, clozapine at doses which were clearly behaviorally active, whereas marked dystonia was observed with two other typical neuroleptics, haloperidol and fluphenazine, known for their ability to induce acute dystonia in human (Deniker et al., 1980). Furthermore, the dystonia induced by haloperidol was clearly antagonized by scopolamine without attenuating the sedative effects of the compound (Fig. 10).

Overall, these data suggest that the primate, in contrast to the rat, constitutes a model of acute dystonia that is directly homologous to clinical observations in man and can thus be considered to possess clear translational validity.

C. Akathisia

Another EPS syndrome associated with antipsychotics is akathisia, a syndrome of subjective feelings of unrest accompanied by objective signs of

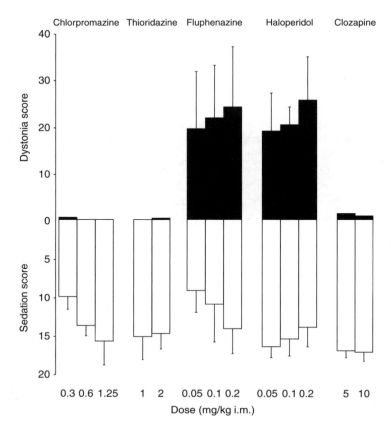

FIGURE 9 The acute dystonic and sedative effects of classical and atypical antipsychotics in the female rhesus monkey. Figure adapted from Porsolt and Jalfre (1981).

restlessness: pacing, rocking, marching on the spot, crossing and uncrossing the legs, and other repetitive non-purposeful actions (Casey, 1993).

The motor aspect of restlessness would appear difficult to model in the sense that most antipsychotics reduce spontaneous activity. There are, however, reports of hyperkinesias (stereotyped scratching, licking, and self-grooming) induced in dogs working on a complex operant schedule by haloperidol but not by clozapine (Bruhwyler, Chleide, Houbeau, Waegeneer, & Mercier, 1993), and of "flinging" behavior in monkeys repeatedly treated with haloperidol (Stewart et al., 1988) which may be related to motor akathisia.

Sachdev and Brune (2000) have suggested that antipsychotic-induced increases in defecation in rats habituated to the test environment may represent a model of the subjective component of akathisia. Indeed haloperidol and risperidone induced more fecal boli in habituated rats than those treated with clozapine, thioridazine, or chlorpromazine, which would appear to

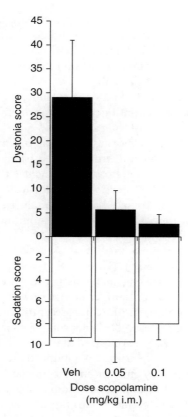

FIGURE 10 Antagonism by scopolamine of the acute dystonic effects induced by haloperidol (0.2 mg/kg i.m.) in the female rhesus monkey. Figure adapted from Porsolt and Jalfre (1981).

correspond to their clinical profiles (Sachdev & Saharov, 1998). On the other hand, drug-induced anxiety or more local drug effects on gastrointestinal transit could also explain such findings. Indeed, antipsychotic-induced defecation in habituated rats can be attenuated by treatment with anxiolytics that have limited efficacy in treating the subjective restlessness of akathisia (Russell, Hagenmeyer-Houser, & Sanberg, 1987).

Overall, the available data would appear too fragmentary to allow any firm conclusions about the usefulness of animal models of antipsychotic-induced akathisia.

D. Tardive Dyskinesia

Tardive dyskinesia is a syndrome of involuntary abnormal movements that occurs on reduction or cessation of long-term antipsychotic therapy.

The movements include chewing, tongue protrusion, lip smacking, puckering, paroxysms of rapid eye blinking, and choreoathetoid movements of the limbs and trunk (Casey, 1993). Some of the features, for example, orofacial movements, may resemble or even occur simultaneously with acute dystonia making differential diagnosis difficult.

Animal tests for tardive dyskinesia are hindered by the fact that antipsychotic treatment must be continued over considerable periods to model the slowly developing nature of the syndrome.

Thus in the rodent, periods of up to 1 year of antipsychotic treatment have been required to demonstrate an increased behavioral response to DA agonists thought to result from chronic treatment-induced hypersensitivity of central DA receptors (Clow, Jenner, Theodorou, & Marsden, 1979). In contrast to the clinical syndrome which is thought to be irreversible, these behavioral changes in the rodent disappear spontaneously within a brief period.

More convincing signs of tardive dyskinesia have been induced in monkeys. An early publication (Gunne & Barany, 1976) reported the occurrence of dyskinetic movements persisting for 1–6 years in cebus monkeys after cessation of years of haloperidol treatment. Acute treatment with two putative antipsychotics, the DA autoreceptor receptor agonist 3-PPP (Haggstrom, Gunne, Carlsson, & Wikstrom, 1983) and the benzamide sulpiride (Haggstrom, 1984) suppressed these signs. In the second study, treatment with sulpiride at the same time induced attacks of acute dystonia which could be reversed by anticholinergic medication. Similar findings have been reported for 3-PPP in cebus monkeys where tardive dyskinesia was induced by long-term treatment with fluphenazine enanthate (Kovacic, Le, & Clark, 1988). Other findings have suggested the effectiveness of the GABA agonist THIP (Andersson & Haggstrom, 1988).

Although these findings are encouraging, such models do not lend themselves readily for drug development programs because they are extremely time consuming.

VI. Conclusion

The present review on the behavioral procedures in animals useful for the evaluation of the potential antipsychotic activity of novel substances has covered the three major symptom domains of schizophrenia: positive symptoms, negative symptoms, and cognitive deficits with a review of methods for evaluating the principal side effects of antipsychotics, namely EPS.

Although a variety neurotransmitters have been hypothesized to play a role in schizophrenia (Marino et al., 2008), the systems most frequently implicated have been those related to central DA, 5-HT, and NMDA transmission. Manipulations of all three constitute the basis for tests aimed at evaluating positive symptoms. Agonists of central DA and 5-HT receptors and antagonists of central NMDA receptors induce recognizable behavioral effects in animals, including hyperactivity, stereotypies, and other bizarre behaviors, which have been suggested to model the excitation and bizarre behaviors typical of the florid manifestations of schizophrenia. Moreover, certain selective 5-HT$_2$ receptor agonists (mescaline, psilocybin, LSD) and NMDA antagonists (PCP, MK-801, ketamine) are known to induce hallucinations in man, reinforcing their heuristic utility as animal test procedures for evaluating treatments for positive symptoms.

The data reviewed suggested that the behavioral effects of DA agonists were particularly sensitive for detecting the antipsychotic activity of numerous clinically active substances, whether specific DA antagonists or atypical substances with a wider range of neurochemical targets. This was even true for substances with no marked affinity for central DA receptors such as the 5-HT$_{2A}$ antagonist M100907. Furthermore, the finding that the atypical agent clozapine appears to have more marked effects on DA agonist-induced hyperactivity than on stereotypies might reflect a more marked action of this substance on DA receptors in mesolimbic and cortical regions than in the striatum, thereby explaining its lower propensity to induce EPS. In contrast, although most of the antipsychotics reviewed potently antagonize the possibly hallucinatory effects of substances like mescaline, this action appears to reflect more the 5-HT antagonist properties of these substances, shared by other 5-HT antagonists that lack antipsychotic properties in man. Finally, although the hyperactivity and stereotypies induced by NMDA antagonists (PCP, MK-801) have heuristic value as models of florid schizophrenic symptoms, the behaviors induced in rodents appear insensitive to a wide range of antipsychotics including typical and atypical agents.

The negative symptoms of schizophrenia (emotional blunting, anhedonia, affective flattening, impoverished speech and thought, social withdrawal) possess the disadvantage that they are less specific to schizophrenia, and several are not amenable to modeling in animals. Anhedonia can be modeled in animals, but few data are available evaluating the effects of antipsychotics, although there are studies which suggest that the atypical agents olanzapine and quetiapine can reverse stress-induced anhedonia. A more interesting finding was that the immobility occurring during the forced swim test could be enhanced during and after repeated treatment with the NMDA antagonists and that this effect was attenuated by several atypical agents (clozapine, risperidone, olanzapine, quetiapine) but not by typical antipsychotics (haloperidol, pimozide, or chlorpromazine). This variant of the forced swim test might thus represent a model of affective flattening. Finally, social investigation in the social interaction test, usually a model for anxiety, is inhibited before and after repeated treatment with NMDA antagonists, and atypical antipsychotics (ziprasidone, aripiprazole, risperidone, and sometimes clozapine) but not the classical agent haloperidol can reverse this deficit.

Cognitive deficits in schizophrenia include impairments in attention, learning, and memory, all of which are also impaired in other psychiatric illnesses. PPI and LI represent models of attention. Considerable animal research has been performed with PPI, because PPI is clearly impaired in schizophrenics and can be measured by similar means in man and animals, providing translational validity to the model. Some data, including experiments from our laboratory, suggest that NMDA antagonist-induced deficits in PPI can be reversed by atypical, but not typical, antipsychotics. Conflicting findings have also been reported. LI would not appear to differentiate atypical from typical antipsychotics, although NMDA antagonist-induced deficits in LI may prove a useful new model of the cognitive deficit related to schizophrenia.

As concerns learning and memory, numerous models have shown deficits induced by NMDA antagonists, including object and social recognition tasks, the MWM, and an operant-delayed alternation task. The object recognition task is of particular interest from a translational point of view because object recognition is impaired in schizophrenic patients. Again some, but not all, studies have shown reversal of NMDA antagonist-induced deficits in this task by atypical but not typical antipsychotics, with similar findings for clozapine from our laboratory in an operant delayed alternation task. Overall, these data provide suggestive but nonconclusive evidence that atypical antipsychotics may alleviate glutamatergic antagonist-induced cognitive deficits in these animal models of learning and memory deficit.

The CAR in no way models the symptoms of schizophrenia and is therefore difficult to classify in terms of positive symptoms, negative symptoms, or cognitive deficit. The procedure has nonetheless been used for many years to characterize antipsychotic drug action. The data reviewed suggest that the CAR is clearly sensitive to antipsychotic drugs and that a high correlation exists between drug potency as measured in animals and that observed in man. On the other hand, it is less clear whether potential antipsychotics can be selectively identified on the basis of their effects on the CAR.

The procedures used to identify the propensity of novel substances to induce EPS are challenging since EPS refers to several apparently discrete disturbances: acutely occurring parkinsonism, dystonia and akathisia, and tardive dyskinesia after prolonged treatment. Catalepsy would appear to represent a useful model for antipsychotic-induced parkinsonism, while the dystonic reaction in primed monkeys appears to represent a homologous model of acute dystonia in man with clear translational validity. There is not as yet a convincing animal model of akathisia or an economically viable model of tardive dyskinesia. There is also no clear clinical evidence that the different manifestations of EPS are correlated. Indeed, phenomenologically they would appear to be distinct. If so, they should be evaluated separately during drug development. Acute dystonia, by its orofacial symptomatology, may resemble tardive dyskinesia, but the two disturbances are distinct in terms of their occurrence and their pharmacological response. The clear dystonic response to classical antipsychotics both in monkeys and in man and its absence with clozapine, together with the occurrence of tardive dyskinesia after chronic treatment with classical antipsychotics but not after clozapine, could, however, suggest that the acute dystonic reaction in monkeys might represent a predictor of the propensity of a novel substance to induce tardive dyskinesia after prolonged therapy.

The need for new animal models to evaluate novel compounds for the treatment of schizophrenia is currently a major area of concern, as highlighted in a number of recent reviews (Day et al., 2008; Markou et al., 2009) and by initiatives such as MATRICS and NEWMEDS (Geyer, 2008; Hughes, 2009). Such initiatives, together with the reconciliation of the multiple results reported for typical and atypical antipsychotics in the behavioral tests covered in the present review, are critical to improving the translational research necessary to generate novel and effective treatments for schizophrenia (Millan, 2008).

Acknowledgments

We thank Nathalie de Cerchio-Dorczynski for secretarial assistance.

Disclosure/Conflict of Interest: The authors are all employees of Porsolt & Partners, a contract research organization that specializes in preclinical animal pharmacology.

References

Adage, T., Trillat, A. C., Quattropani, A., Perrin, D., Cavarec, L., Shaw, J., et al. (2008). In vitro and in vivo pharmacological profile of AS057278, a selective d-amino acid oxidase inhibitor with potential anti-psychotic properties. *European Neuropsychopharmacology, 18,* 200–214.

Andersson, U., & Haggstrom, J. E. (1988). GABA agonists in cebus monkeys with neuroleptic-induced persistent dyskinesias. *Psychopharmacology (Berlin), 94,* 298–301.

Anisman, H., & Matheson, K. (2005). Stress, depression, and anhedonia: Caveats concerning animal models. *Neuroscience and Biobehavioral Reviews, 29,* 525–546.

Arnt, J. (1982). Pharmacological specificity of conditioned avoidance response inhibition in rats: Inhibition by neuroleptics and correlation to dopamine receptor blockade. *Acta Pharmacologica et Toxicologica, 51,* 321–329.

Auclair, A. L., Kleven, M. S., Besnard, J., Depoortere, R., & Newman-Tancredi, A. (2006). Actions of novel antipsychotic agents on apomorphine-induced PPI disruption: Influence of combined serotonin 5-HT1A receptor activation and dopamine D2 receptor blockade. *Neuropsychopharmacology, 31,* 1900–1909.

Bartholini, G. (1976). Differential effect of neuroleptic drugs on dopamine turnover in the extrapyramidal and limbic system. *Journal of Pharmacy and Pharmacology, 28,* 429–433.

Baruch, I., Hemsley, D. R., & Gray, J. A. (1988). Differential performance of acute and chronic schizophrenics in a latent inhibition task. *Journal of Nervous and Mental Disease, 176,* 598–606.

Bast, T., Zhang, W., Feldon, J., & White, I. M. (2000). Effects of MK801 and neuroleptics on prepulse inhibition: Re-examination in two strains of rats. *Pharmacology, Biochemistry, and Behavior, 67,* 647–658.

Becker, A., & Grecksch, G. (2004). Ketamine-induced changes in rat behaviour: A possible animal model of schizophrenia. Test of predictive validity. *Progress in Neuro-Psychopharmacology & Biological Psychiatry, 28,* 1267–1277.

Beraki, S., Kuzmin, A., Tai, F., & Ogren, S. O. (2008). Repeated low dose of phencyclidine administration impairs spatial learning in mice: Blockade by clozapine but not by haloperidol. *European Neuropsychopharmacology, 18,* 486–497.

Black, M. D., Varty, G. B., Arad, M., Barak, S., De, L. A., Boulay, D., et al. (2009). Procognitive and antipsychotic efficacy of glycine transport 1 inhibitors (GlyT1) in acute and neurodevelopmental models of schizophrenia: Latent inhibition studies in the rat. *Psychopharmacology (Berlin), 202,* 385–396.

Boissier, J. R., & Simon, P. (1965). Action de la caféine sur la motilité spontanée de la souris. *Archives Internationales de Pharmacodynamie et de Thérapie, 158,* 212–221.

Bolles, R. C., & Grossen, N. E. (1970). Function of the CS in shuttle-box avoidance learning by rats. *Journal of Comparative and Physiological Psychology, 70,* 165–169.

Boulay, D., Depoortere, R., Louis, C., Perrault, G., Griebel, G., & Soubrie, P. (2004). SSR181507, a putative atypical antipsychotic with dopamine D2 antagonist and 5-HT1A agonist activities: Improvement of social interaction deficits induced by phencyclidine in rats. *Neuropharmacology, 46,* 1121–1129.

Browman, K. E., Komater, V. A., Curzon, P., Rueter, L. E., Hancock, A. A., Decker, M. W., et al. (2004). Enhancement of prepulse inhibition of startle in mice by the H3 receptor antagonists thioperamide and ciproxifan. *Behavioural Brain Research, 153,* 69–76.

Bruhwyler, J., Chleide, E., Houbeau, G., Waegeneer, N., & Mercier, M. (1993). Differentiation of haloperidol and clozapine using a complex operant schedule in the dog. *Pharmacology, Biochemistry, and Behavior, 44,* 181–189.

Bunney, B. G., Bunney, W. E., & Carlsson, A., 1995. Schizophrenia and glutamate. In F. E. Bloom & D. J. Kupfer (Eds.), *Psychopharmacology: The fourth generation of progress* (pp. 1205–1214). New York: Raven Press.

Carlsson, A. (1988). The current status of the dopamine hypothesis of schizophrenia. *Neuropsychopharmacology, 1,* 179–186.

Carlsson, M., & Carlsson, A. (1989). The NMDA antagonist MK-801 causes marked locomotor stimulation in monoamine-depleted mice. *Journal of Neural Transmission, 75,* 221–226.

Casey, D. E. (1993). Neuroleptic-induced acute extrapyramidal syndromes and tardive dyskinesia. *Psychiatric Clinics of North America, 16,* 589–610.

Castagné, V., Cuénod, M., & Do, K. Q. (2004). An animal model with relevance to schizophrenia: Sex-dependent cognitive deficits in osteogenic disorder-Shionogi rats induced by glutathione synthesis and dopamine uptake inhibition during development. *Neuroscience, 123,* 821–834.

Castagné, V., Rougemont, M., Cuénod, M., & Do, K. Q. (2004). Low brain glutathione and ascorbic acid associated with dopamine uptake inhibition during rat's development induce long-term cognitive deficit: Relevance to schizophrenia. *Neurobiology of Disease, 15,* 93–105.

Castner, S. A., Goldman-Rakic, P. S., & Williams, G. V. (2004). Animal models of working memory: Insights for targeting cognitive dysfunction in schizophrenia. *Psychopharmacology (Berlin), 174,* 111–125.

Chudasama, Y., & Robbins, T. W. (2006). Functions of frontostriatal systems in cognition: Comparative neuropsychopharmacological studies in rats, monkeys and humans. *Biological Psychology, 73*, 19–38.

Cilia, J., Gartlon, J., Shilliam, C., Dawson, L., Moore, S., & Jones, D. (2009). Further neurochemical and behavioural investigation of Brattleboro rats as a putative model of schizophrenia. *Journal of Psychopharmacology*, in press.

Clow, A., Jenner, P., Theodorou, A., & Marsden, C. D. (1979). Striatal dopamine receptors become supersensitive while rats are given trifluoperazine for six months. *Nature, 278*, 59–61.

Cook, L., Tam, S. W., & Rohrbach, K. W. (1992). DuP 734 [1-(cyclopropylmethyl)-4-(2′(4″-fluorophenyl)-2′-oxoethyl)piperidine HBr], a potential antipsychotic agent: Preclinical behavioral effects. *Journal of Pharmacology and Experimental Therapeutics, 263*, 1159–1166.

Cook, L., & Weidley, E. (1957). Behavioral effects of some psychopharmacological agents. *Annals of the New York Academy of Sciences, 66*, 740–752.

Corbett, R., Zhou, L., Sorensen, S. M., & Mondadori, C. (1999). Animal models of negative symptoms: M100907 antagonizes PCP-induced immobility in a forced swim test in mice. *Neuropsychopharmacology, 21*, S211–S218.

Costall, B., Domeney, A. M., & Naylor, R. J. (1982). Behavioural and biochemical consequences of persistent overstimulation of mesolimbic dopamine systems in the rat. *Neuropharmacology, 21*, 327–335.

Costall, B., Marsden, C. D., Naylor, R. J., & Pycock, C. J. (1977). Stereotyped behaviour patterns and hyperactivity induced by amphetamine and apomorphine after discrete 6-hydroxydopamine lesions of extrapyramidal and mesolimbic nuclei. *Brain Research, 123*, 89–111.

Coyle, J. T. (2006). Glutamate and schizophrenia: Beyond the dopamine hypothesis. *Cellular and Molecular Neurobiology, 26*, 365–384.

Creese, I., Burt, D. R., & Snyder, S. R. (1976). Dopamine receptors and average clinical doses. *Science, 194*, 546.

Crow, T. J. (2007). How and why genetic linkage has not solved the problem of psychosis: Review and hypothesis. *American Journal of Psychiatry, 164*, 13–21.

Deegan, J. F., & Cook, L. (1958). A study of the anti-mescaline property of a series of CNS active agents in mice. *Journal of Pharmacology and Experimental Therapeutics, 122*, 17A.

den Boer, J. A., Vahlne, J. O., Post, P., Heck, A. H., Daubenton, F., & Olbrich, R. (2000). Ritanserin as add-on medication to neuroleptic therapy for patients with chronic or subchronic schizophrenia. *Human Psychopharmacology, 15*, 179–189.

Deniker, P., Ginestet, D., & Loo, H. (1980). *Maniement des médicaments psychotropes*. Paris: Doin.

Depoortere, R., Dargazanli, G., Estenne-Bouhtou, G., Coste, A., Lanneau, C., Desvignes, C., et al. (2005). Neurochemical, electrophysiological and pharmacological profiles of the selective inhibitor of the glycine transporter-1 SSR504734, a potential new type of antipsychotic. *Neuropsychopharmacology, 30*, 1963–1985.

Didriksen, M., Skarsfeldt, T., & Arnt, J. (2007). Reversal of PCP-induced learning and memory deficits in the Morris' water maze by sertindole and other antipsychotics. *Psychopharmacology (Berlin), 193*, 225–233.

Ellenbroek, B. A. (2004). Pre-attentive processing and schizophrenia: Animal studies. *Psychopharmacology (Berlin), 174*, 65–74.

Enna, S. J., & Williams, M. (2009). Challenges in the search for drugs to treat central nervous system disorders. *Journal of Pharmacology and Experimental Therapeutics, 329*, 404–411.

Ennaceur, A., & Delacour, J. (1988). A new one-trial test for neurobiological studies of memory in rats. 1: Behavioral data. *Behavioral and Brain Research, 31*, 47–59.

File, S. E., Ouagazzal, A. M., Gonzalez, L. E., & Overstreet, D. H. (1999). Chronic fluoxetine in tests of anxiety in rat lines selectively bred for differential 5-HT1A receptor function. *Pharmacology, Biochemistry, and Behavior, 62,* 695–701.

Floresco, S. B., Geyer, M. A., Gold, L. H., & Grace, A. A. (2005). Developing predictive animal models and establishing a preclinical trials network for assessing treatment effects on cognition in schizophrenia. *Schizophrenia Bulletin, 31,* 888–894.

Fox, G. B., Esbenshade, T. A., Pan, J. B., Radek, R. J., Krueger, K. M., Yao, B. B., et al. (2005). Pharmacological properties of ABT-239 [4-(2-{2-[(2R)-2-methylpyrrolidinyl] ethyl}-benzofuran-5-yl)benzonitrile]: II. Neurophysiological characterization and broad preclinical efficacy in cognition and schizophrenia of a potent and selective histamine H3 receptor antagonist. *Journal of Pharmacology and Experimental Therapeutics, 313,* 176–190.

Fukuoka, T., Nakano, M., Kohda, A., Okuno, Y., & Matsuo, M. (1997). The common marmoset (Callithrix jacchus) as a model for neuroleptic-induced acute dystonia. *Pharmacology, Biochemistry, and Behavior, 58,* 947–953.

Gabrovska, V. S., Laws, K. R., Sinclair, J., & McKenna, P. J. (2003). Visual object processing in schizophrenia: Evidence for an associative agnostic deficit. *Schizophrenia Research, 59,* 277–286.

Gaisler-Salomon, I., Diamant, L., Rubin, C., & Weiner, I. (2008). Abnormally persistent latent inhibition induced by MK801 is reversed by risperidone and by positive modulators of NMDA receptor function: Differential efficacy depending on the stage of the task at which they are administered. *Psychopharmacology (Berlin), 196,* 255–267

Galletly, C. (2009). Recent advances in treating cognitive impairment in schizophrenia. *Psychopharmacology (Berlin), 202,* 259–273.

Gardell, L. R., Vanover, K. E., Pounds, L., Johnson, R. W., Barido, R., Anderson, G. T., et al. (2007). ACP-103, a 5-hydroxytryptamine 2A receptor inverse agonist, improves the antipsychotic efficacy and side-effect profile of haloperidol and risperidone in experimental models. *Journal of Pharmacology and Experimental Therapeutics, 322,* 862–870.

Gardner, D. M., Baldessarini, R. J., & Waraich, P. (2005). Modern antipsychotic drugs: A critical overview. *CMAJ, 172,* 1703–1711.

Geyer, M. A. (2008). Developing translational animal models for symptoms of schizophrenia or bipolar mania. *Neurotoxicity Research, 14,* 71–78.

Geyer, M. A., & Ellenbroek, B. (2003). Animal behavior models of the mechanisms underlying antipsychotic atypicality. *Progress in Neuro-Psychopharmacology & Biological Psychiatry, 27,* 1071–1079.

Glick, S. D., & Zimmerberg, B. (1972). Amnesic effects of scopolamine. *Behavioral Biology, 7,* 245–254.

Goetghebeur, P., & Dias, R. (2009). Comparison of haloperidol, risperidone, sertindole, and modafinil to reverse an attentional set-shifting impairment following subchronic PCP administration in the rat—A back translational study. *Psychopharmacology (Berlin), 202,* 287–293.

Gogos, J. A., & Gerber, D. J. (2006). Schizophrenia susceptibility genes: Emergence of positional candidates and future directions. *Trends in Pharmacological Sciences, 27,* 226–233.

Grayson, B., Idris, N. F., & Neill, J. C. (2007). Atypical antipsychotics attenuate a sub-chronic PCP-induced cognitive deficit in the novel object recognition task in the rat. *Behavioural Brain Research, 184,* 31–38.

Gunne, L. M., & Barany, S. (1976). Haloperidol-induced tardive dyskinesia in monkeys. *Psychopharmacology (Berlin), 50,* 237–240.

Haase, H. J. (1978). Neuroleptics and the extrapyramidal system. *Arzneimittelforschung, 28,* 1536–1537.

Haggstrom, J. E. (1984). Effects of sulpiride on persistent neuroleptic-induced dyskinesia in monkeys. *Acta Psychiatrica Scandinavica. Supplementum, 311,* 103–108.

Haggstrom, J. E., Gunne, L. M., Carlsson, A., & Wikstrom, H. (1983). Antidyskinetic action of 3-PPP, a selective dopaminergic autoreceptor agonist, in Cebus monkeys with persistent neuroleptic-induced dyskinesias. *Journal of Neural Transmission, 58*, 135–142.

Hagiwara, H., Fujita, Y., Ishima, T., Kunitachi, S., Shirayama, Y., Iyo, M., et al. (2008). Phencyclidine-induced cognitive deficits in mice are improved by subsequent subchronic administration of the antipsychotic drug perospirone: Role of serotonin 5-HT1A receptors. *European Neuropsychopharmacology, 18*, 448–454.

Hargreaves, E. L., & Cain, D. P. (1995). MK801-induced hyperactivity: Duration of effects in rats. *Pharmacology, Biochemistry, and Behavior, 51*, 13–19.

Hashimoto, K., Fujita, Y., Ishima, T., Chaki, S., & Iyo, M. (2008). Phencyclidine-induced cognitive deficits in mice are improved by subsequent subchronic administration of the glycine transporter-1 inhibitor NFPS and D-serine. *European Neuropsychopharmacology, 18*, 414–421.

Hashimoto, K., Ishima, T., Fujita, Y., Matsuo, M., Kobashi, T., Takahagi, M., et al. (2008). Phencyclidine-induced cognitive deficits in mice are improved by subsequent subchronic administration of the novel selective alpha7 nicotinic receptor agonist SSR180711. *Biological Psychiatry, 63*, 92–97.

Heise, G. A., & Boff, E. (1962). Continuous avoidance as a base-line for measuring behavioral effects of drugs. *Psychopharmacologia, 3*, 264–282.

Hippius, H. (1989). The history of clozapine. *Psychopharmacology (Berlin), 99*(Suppl.), S3–S5.

Hoffman, D. C., & Donovan, H. (1995). Catalepsy as a rodent model for detecting antipsychotic drugs with extrapyramidal side effect liability. *Psychopharmacology (Berlin), 120*, 128–133.

Hughes, B. (2009). Novel consortium to address shortfall in innovative medicines for psychiatric disorders. *Nature Reviews. Drug Discovery, 8*, 523–524.

Idris, N. F., Repeto, P., Neill, J. C., & Large, C. H. (2005). Investigation of the effects of lamotrigine and clozapine in improving reversal-learning impairments induced by acute phencyclidine and D-amphetamine in the rat. *Psychopharmacology (Berlin), 179*, 336–348.

Ishiyama, T., Tokuda, K., Ishibashi, T., Ito, A., Toma, S., & Ohno, Y. (2007). Lurasidone (SM-13496), a novel atypical antipsychotic drug, reverses MK-801-induced impairment of learning and memory in the rat passive-avoidance test. *European Journal of Pharmacology, 572*, 160–170.

Ito, C. (2004). The role of the central histaminergic system on schizophrenia. *Drug News Perspectives, 17*, 383–387.

Janssen, P. A., Niemegeers, C. J., & Schellekens, K. H. (1965). Is it possible to predict the clinical effects of neuroleptic drugs (major tranquilizers) from animal data? I. "Neuroleptic activity spectra" for rats. *Arzneimittelforschung, 15*, 104–117.

Jones, B. J., Gallagher, B. J., III, Pisa, A. M., & McFalls, J. A., Jr. (2008). Social class, family history and type of schizophrenia. *Psychiatry Research, 159*, 127–132.

Karasawa, J., Hashimoto, K., & Chaki, S. (2008). D-Serine and a glycine transporter inhibitor improve MK-801-induced cognitive deficits in a novel object recognition test in rats. *Behavioural Brain Research, 186*, 78–83.

Kelly, C., & McCreadie, R. (2000). Cigarette smoking and schizophrenia. *Advances in Psychiatric Treatment, 6*, 327–331.

Keshavan, M. S., Tandon, R., Boutros, N. N., & Nasrallah, H. A. (2008). Schizophrenia, "just the facts": What we know in 2008 Part 3: Neurobiology. *Schizophrenia Research, 106*, 89–107.

Kovacic, B., Le, W. P., & Clark, D. (1988). Suppression of neuroleptic-induced persistent abnormal movements in Cebus apella monkeys by enantiomers of 3-PPP. *Journal of Neural Transmission, 74*, 97–107.

Lahti, A. C., Koffel, B., LaPorte, D., & Tamminga, C. A. (1995). Subanesthetic doses of ketamine stimulate psychosis in schizophrenia. *Neuropsychopharmacology, 13*, 9–19.

Large, C. H. (2007). Do NMDA receptor antagonist models of schizophrenia predict the clinical efficacy of antipsychotic drugs? *Journal of Psychopharmacology, 21*, 283–301.

Leite, J. V., Guimaraes, F. S., & Moreira, F. A. (2008). Aripiprazole, an atypical antipsychotic, prevents the motor hyperactivity induced by psychotomimetics and psychostimulants in mice. *European Journal of Pharmacology, 578*, 222–227.

Lemaire, M., Bohme, G. A., Piot, O., Roques, B. P., & Blanchard, J. C. (1994). CCK-A and CCK-B selective receptor agonists and antagonists modulate olfactory recognition in male rats. *Psychopharmacology (Berlin), 115*, 435–440.

Liebman, J., & Neale, R. (1980). Neuroleptic-induced acute dyskinesias in squirrel monkeys: Correlation with propensity to cause extrapyramidal side effects. *Psychopharmacology (Berlin), 68*, 25–29.

Liu, F., Grauer, S., Kelley, C., Navarra, R., Graf, R., Zhang, G., et al. (2008). ADX47273 [S-(4-fluoro-phenyl)-{3-[3-(4-fluoro-phenyl)-[1,2,4]-oxadiazol-5-yl]-piper   idin-1-yl}-metha-none]: A novel metabotropic glutamate receptor 5-selective positive allosteric modulator with preclinical antipsychotic-like and procognitive activities. *Journal of Pharmacology and Experimental Therapeutics, 327*, 827–839.

Lubow, R. E., & Moore, A. U. (1959). Latent inhibition: The effect of nonreinforced pre-exposure to the conditional stimulus. *Journal of Comparative and Physiological Psychology, 52*, 415–419.

Marino, M. J., Knutsen, L. J., & Williams, M. (2008). Emerging opportunities for antipsychotic drug discovery in the postgenomic era. *Journal of Medicinal Chemistry, 51*, 1077–1107.

Markou, A., Chiamulera, C., Geyer, M. A., Tricklebank, M., & Steckler, T. (2009). Removing obstacles in neuroscience drug discovery: The future path for animal models. *Neuropsychopharmacology, 34*, 74–89.

Marquis, K. L., Sabb, A. L., Logue, S. F., Brennan, J. A., Piesla, M. J., Comery, T. A., et al. (2007). WAY-163909 [(7bR,10aR)-1,2,3,4,8,9,10,10a-octahydro-7bH-cyclopenta-[b][1,4]diazepino[6,7,1hi]indole]: A novel 5-hydroxytryptamine 2C receptor-selective agonist with preclinical antipsychotic-like activity. *Journal of Pharmacology and Experimental Therapeutics, 320*, 486–496.

Martin, R. S., Secchi, R. L., Sung, E., Lemaire, M., Bonhaus, D. W., Hedley, L. R., et al. (2003). Effects of cannabinoid receptor ligands on psychosis-relevant behavior models in the rat. *Psychopharmacology (Berlin), 165*, 128–135.

Martinez, Z. A., Halim, N. D., Oostwegel, J. L., Geyer, M. A., & Swerdlow, N. R. (2000). Ontogeny of phencyclidine and apomorphine-induced startle gating deficits in rats. *Pharmacology, Biochemistry, and Behavior, 65*, 449–457.

McArthur, R. A., & Borsini, F. (2008). Animal and translational models for CNS drug discovery. Burlington MA: Academic Press.

McGrath, J., Saha, S., Chant, D., & Welham, J. (2008). Schizophrenia: A concise overview of incidence, prevalence, and mortality. *Epidemiologic Reviews, 30*, 67–76.

Meldrum, B. S., Anlezark, G. M., & Marsden, C. D. (1977). Acute dystonia as an idiosyncratic response to neuroleptics in baboons. *Brain, 100*, 313–326.

Meltzer, H. Y., Sturgeon, R. D., Simonovic, M., & Fessler, R. G. (1981). Phencyclidine as an indirect dopamine agonist. In E. F. Domino (Ed.), *PCP (Phencyclidine): Historical and current perspectives* (pp. 207–242). Ann Arbor, MI: NPP Books.

Meltzer, H. Y. (1989). Clinical studies on the mechanism of action of clozapine: the dopamine-serotonin hypothesis of schizophrenia. *Psychopharmacology (Berl), Suppl, 99*, S18–S27.

Millan, M. J. (2008). The discovery and development of pharmacotherapy for psychiatric disorders: A critical survey of animal and translational models and perspectives for their improvement. In R. A. McArthur & F. Borsini (Eds.), *Animal and translational models for CNS drug discovery (Vol. 1*, pp. 1–57). Burlington, MA: Academic Press.

Moran, P. M., Fischer, T. R., Hitchcock, J. M., & Moser, P. C. (1996). Effects of clozapine on latent inhibition in the rat. *Behavioural Pharmacology, 7*, 42–48.

Morris, B. J., Cochran, S. M., & Pratt, J. A. (2005). PCP: From pharmacology to modelling schizophrenia. *Current Opinion in Pharmacology*, *5*, 101–106.

Morris, R. G. (1981). Spatial localization does not require the presence of local cues. *Learning and Motivation*, *12*, 239–260.

Moser, P. C., Hitchcock, J. M., Lister, S., & Moran, P. M. (2000). The pharmacology of latent inhibition as an animal model of schizophrenia. *Brain Research. Brain Research Reviews*, *33*, 275–307.

Moser, P. C., Moran, P. M., Frank, R. A., & Kehne, J. H. (1996). Reversal of amphetamine-induced behaviours by MDL 100,907, a selective 5-HT2A antagonist. *Behavioural Brain Research*, *73*, 163–167.

Mouri, A., Noda, Y., Enomoto, T., & Nabeshima, T. (2007). Phencyclidine animal models of schizophrenia: Approaches from abnormality of glutamatergic neurotransmission and neurodevelopment. *Neurochemistry International*, *51*, 173–184.

Muscat, R., & Willner, P. (1989). Effects of dopamine receptor antagonists on sucrose consumption and preference. *Psychopharmacology (Berlin)*, *99*, 98–102.

Nabeshima, T., Mouri, A., Murai, R., & Noda, Y. (2006). Animal model of schizophrenia: Dysfunction of NMDA receptor-signaling in mice following withdrawal from repeated administration of phencyclidine. *Annals of the New York Academy of Sciences*, *1086*, 160–168.

Nagai, T., Noda, Y., Une, T., Furukawa, K., Furukawa, H., Kan, Q. M., et al. (2003). Effect of AD-5423 on animal models of schizophrenia: Phencyclidine-induced behavioral changes in mice. *Neuroreport*, *14*, 269–272.

Natesan, S., Reckless, G. E., Barlow, K. B., Nobrega, J. N., & Kapur, S. (2008). Amisulpride the "atypical" atypical antipsychotic–comparison to haloperidol, risperidone and clozapine. *Schizophrenia Research*, *105*, 224–235.

Nielsen, C. K., Arnt, J., & Sanchez, C. (2000). Intracranial self-stimulation and sucrose intake differ as hedonic measures following chronic mild stress: Interstrain and interindividual differences. *Behavioural Brain Research*, *107*, 21–33.

Ninan, I., & Kulkarni, S. K. (1999). Preferential inhibition of dizocilpine-induced hyperlocomotion by olanzapine. *European Journal of Pharmacology*, *368*, 1–7.

Noda, Y., Kamei, H., Mamiya, T., Furukawa, H., & Nabeshima, T. (2000). Repeated phencyclidine treatment induces negative symptom-like behavior in forced swimming test in mice: Imbalance of prefrontal serotonergic and dopaminergic functions. *Neuropsychopharmacology*, *23*, 375–387.

O'Neill, M. F., & Shaw, G. (1999). Comparison of dopamine receptor antagonists on hyperlocomotion induced by cocaine, amphetamine, MK-801 and the dopamine D1 agonist C-APB in mice. *Psychopharmacology (Berlin)*, *145*, 237–250.

Okuyama, S., Chaki, S., Kawashima, N., Suzuki, Y., Ogawa, S., Kumagai, T., et al. (1997). The atypical antipsychotic profile of NRA0045, a novel dopamine D4 and 5-hydroxytryptamine2A receptor antagonist, in rats. *British Journal of Pharmacology*, *121*, 515–525.

Olsen, C. K., Brennum, L. T., & Kreilgaard, M. (2008). Using pharmacokinetic-pharmacodynamic modelling as a tool for prediction of therapeutic effective plasma levels of antipsychotics. *European Journal of Pharmacology*, *584*, 318–327.

Olszewski, R. T., Wegorzewska, M. M., Monteiro, A. C., Krolikowski, K. A., Zhou, J., Kozikowski, A. P., et al. (2008). Phencyclidine and dizocilpine induced behaviors reduced by N-acetylaspartylglutamate peptidase inhibition via metabotropic glutamate receptors. *Biological Psychiatry*, *63*, 86–91.

Orsetti, M., Canonico, P. L., Dellarole, A., Colella, L., Di, B. F., & Ghi, P. (2007). Quetiapine prevents anhedonia induced by acute or chronic stress. *Neuropsychopharmacology*, *32*, 1783–1790.

Orsetti, M., Colella, L., Dellarole, A., Canonico, P. L., Ferri, S., & Ghi, P. (2006). Effects of chronic administration of olanzapine, amitriptyline, haloperidol or sodium valproate in naive and anhedonic rats. *The International Journal of Neuropsychopharmacology, 9,* 427–436.

Owen, M. J., Williams, H. J., & O'Donovan, M. C. (2009). Schizophrenia genetics: Advancing on two fronts. *Current Opinion in Genetics & Development, 19,* 266–270.

Palucha-Poniewiera, A., Klodzinska, A., Stachowicz, K., Tokarski, K., Hess, G., Schann, S., et al. (2008). Peripheral administration of group III mGlu receptor agonist ACPT-I exerts potential antipsychotic effects in rodents. *Neuropharmacology, 55,* 517–524.

Peacock, L., & Gerlach, J. (1993). Effects of several partial dopamine D2 receptor agonists in Cebus apella monkeys previously treated with haloperidol. *European Journal of Pharmacology, 237,* 329–340.

Petersen, R. C., & Stillman, R. C. (1978). Phencyclidine: An overview. In R. C. Petersen & R. C. Stillman (Eds.), *Phencyclidine (PCP) abuse: An appraisal* (pp 1–17). Rockville, MD: National Institute on Drug Abuse.

Phillips, A. G., Blaha, C. D., & Fibiger, H. C. (1989). Neurochemical correlates of brain-stimulation reward measured by ex vivo and in vivo analyses. *Neuroscience and Biobehavioral Reviews, 13,* 99–104.

Pichat, P., Bergis, O. E., Terranova, J. P., Urani, A., Duarte, C., Santucci, V., et al. (2007). SSR180711, a novel selective alpha7 nicotinic receptor partial agonist: (II) efficacy in experimental models predictive of activity against cognitive symptoms of schizophrenia. *Neuropsychopharmacology, 32,* 17–34.

Porsolt, R. D., Bertin, A., & Jalfre, M. (1977). Behavioral despair in mice: A primary screening test for antidepressants. *Archives Internationales de Pharmacodynamie et de Thérapie, 229,* 327–336.

Porsolt, R. D., Bertin, A., & Jalfre, M. (1978). "Behavioural despair" in rats and mice: Strain differences and the effects of imipramine. *European Journal of Pharmacology, 51,* 291–294.

Porsolt, R. D., & Jalfre, M. (1981). Neuroleptic-induced acute dyskinesias in rhesus monkeys. *Psychopharmacology (Berlin), 75,* 16–21.

Pouzet, B., Didriksen, M., & Arnt, J. (2002). Effects of the 5-HT(6) receptor antagonist, SB-271046, in animal models for schizophrenia. *Pharmacology, Biochemistry, and Behavior, 71,* 635–643.

Powell, C. M., & Miyakawa, T. (2006). Schizophrenia-relevant behavioral testing in rodent models: A uniquely human disorder? *Biological Psychiatry, 59,* 1198–1207.

Qiao, H., Noda, Y., Kamei, H., Nagai, T., Furukawa, H., Miura, H., et al. (2001). Clozapine, but not haloperidol, reverses social behavior deficit in mice during withdrawal from chronic phencyclidine treatment. *Neuroreport, 12,* 11–15.

Ross, C. A., Margolis, R. L., Reading, S. A., Pletnikov, M., & Coyle, J. T. (2006). Neurobiology of schizophrenia. *Neuron, 52,* 139–153.

Roux, S., Hubert, I., Lenegre, A., Milinkevitch, D., & Porsolt, R. D. (1994). Effects of piracetam on indices of cognitive function in a delayed alternation task in young and aged rats. *Pharmacology, Biochemistry, and Behavior, 49,* 683–688.

Rung, J. P., Carlsson, A., Markinhuhta, K. R., & Carlsson, M. L. (2005). The dopaminergic stabilizers (–)-OSU6162 and ACR16 reverse (+)-MK-801-induced social withdrawal in rats. *Progress in Neuro-Psychopharmacology and Biological Psychiatry, 29,* 833–839.

Rung, J. P., Carlsson, A., Ryden, M. K., & Carlsson, M. L. (2005). (+)-MK-801 induced social withdrawal in rats; a model for negative symptoms of schizophrenia. *Progress in Neuro-Psychopharmacology and Biological Psychiatry, 29,* 827–832.

Russell, K. H., Hagenmeyer-Houser, S. H., & Sanberg, P. R. (1987). Haloperidol-induced emotional defecation: A possible model for neuroleptic anxiety syndrome. *Psychopharmacology (Berlin), 91,* 45–49.

Sachdev, P. S., & Brune, M. (2000). Animal models of acute drug-induced akathisia—A review. *Neuroscience and Biobehavioral Reviews, 24,* 269–277.

Sachdev, P. S., & Saharov, T. (1998). Effects of specific dopamine D1 and D2 receptor antagonists and agonists and neuroleptic drugs on emotional defecation in a rat model of akathisia. *Psychiatry Research*, *81*, 323–332.

Sams-Dodd, F. (1999). Phencyclidine in the social interaction test: An animal model of schizophrenia with face and predictive validity. *Reviews in the Neurosciences*, *10*, 59–90.

Sanberg, P. R., Bunsey, M. D., Giordano, M., & Norman, A. B. (1988). The catalepsy test: Its ups and downs. *Behavioral Neuroscience*, *102*, 748–759.

Sarter, M. (2004). Animal cognition: Defining the issues. *Neuroscience and Biobehavioral Reviews*, *28*, 645–650.

Schreiber, R., Vivian, J., Hedley, L., Szczepanski, K., Secchi, R. L., Zuzow, M., et al. (2007). Effects of the novel 5-HT(6) receptor antagonist RO4368554 in rat models for cognition and sensorimotor gating. *European Neuropsychopharmacology*, *17*, 277–288.

Serretti, A., De Ronchi, D., Lorenzi, C., & Berardi, D. (2004). New antipsychotics and schizophrenia: A review on efficacy and side effects. *Current Medicinal Chemistry*, *11*, 343–358.

Shadach, E., Gaisler, I., Schiller, D., & Weiner, I. (2000). The latent inhibition model dissociates between clozapine, haloperidol, and ritanserin. *Neuropsychopharmacology*, *23*, 151–161.

Sidman, M. (1962). An adjusting avoidance schedule. *Journal of Experimental Analysis of Behavior*, *5*, 271–277.

Simon, P., & Chermat, R. (1972). Recherche d'une interaction avec les stéréotypiesprovoquées par l'amphétamine chez le rat. *Journal de Pharmacologie*, *3*, 235–238.

Simon, P., Langwinski, R., & Boissier, J. R. (1969). Comparaison de différents tests d'évaluation de la catalepsie chez le rat. *Therapie*, *24*, 985–995.

Snigdha, S., & Neill, J. C. (2008a). Efficacy of antipsychotics to reverse phencyclidine-induced social interaction deficits in female rats—A preliminary investigation. *Behavioural Brain Research*, *187*, 489–494.

Snigdha, S., & Neill, J. C. (2008b). Improvement of phencyclidine-induced social behaviour deficits in rats: Involvement of 5-HT1A receptors. *Behavioural Brain Research*, *191*, 26–31.

Southam, E., Cilia, J., Gartlon, J. E., Woolley, M. L., Lacroix, L. P., Jennings, C. A., et al. (2009). Preclinical investigations into the antipsychotic potential of the novel histamine H3 receptor antagonist GSK207040. *Psychopharmacology (Berlin)*, *201*, 483–494.

Spedding, M., Jay, T., Costa e Silva, J., & Perret, L. (2005). A pathophysiological paradigm for the therapy of psychiatric disease. *Nature Reviews. Drug Discovery*, *4*, 467–476.

Spielewoy, C., & Markou, A. (2003). Withdrawal from chronic phencyclidine treatment induces long-lasting depression in brain reward function. *Neuropsychopharmacology*, *28*, 1106–1116.

Stewart, B. R., Rupniak, N. M., Jenner, P., & Marsden, C. D. (1988). Animal models of neuroleptic-induced acute dystonia. *Advances in Neurology*, *50*, 343–359.

Stone, J. M., Morrison, P. D., & Pilowsky, L. S. (2007). Glutamate and dopamine dysregulation in schizophrenia—A synthesis and selective review. *Journal of Psychopharmacology*, *21*, 440–452.

Suemaru, K., Yasuda, K., Umeda, K., Araki, H., Shibata, K., Choshi, T., et al. (2004). Nicotine blocks apomorphine-induced disruption of prepulse inhibition of the acoustic startle in rats: Possible involvement of central nicotinic alpha7 receptors. *British Journal of Pharmacology*, *142*, 843–850.

Sun, T., Hu, G., & Li, M. (2009). Repeated antipsychotic treatment progressively potentiates inhibition on phencyclidine-induced hyperlocomotion, but attenuates inhibition on amphetamine-induced hyperlocomotion: Relevance to animal models of antipsychotic drugs. *European Journal of Pharmacology*, *602*, 334–342.

Swerdlow, N. R., Weber, M., Qu, Y., Light, G. A., & Braff, D. L. (2008). Realistic expectations of prepulse inhibition in translational models for schizophrenia research. *Psychopharmacology (Berlin)*, *199*, 331–388.

Tanaka, K., Suzuki, M., Sumiyoshi, T., Murata, M., Tsunoda, M., & Kurachi, M. (2003). Subchronic phencyclidine administration alters central vasopressin receptor binding and social interaction in the rat. *Brain Research*, *992*, 239–245.

Thiebot, M. H., Kloczko, J., Chermat, R., Soubrie, P., Puech, A. J., & Simon, P. (1982). A simple model for studying benzodiazepines: Potentiation of hyperactivity induced by cocaine in mice. *Drug Development Research*, *1*, 135–143.

Toda, M., & Abi-Dargham, A. (2007). Dopamine hypothesis of schizophrenia: Making sense of it all. *Current Psychiatry Report*, *9*, 329–336.

Turgeon, S. M., & Hoge, S. G. (2003). Prior exposure to phencyclidine decreases voluntary sucrose consumption and operant performance for food reward. *Pharmacology, Biochemistry, and Behavior*, *76*, 393–400.

Vanover, K. E., Weiner, D. M., Makhay, M., Veinbergs, I., Gardell, L. R., Lameh, J., et al. (2006). Pharmacological and behavioral profile of N-(4-fluorophenylmethyl)-N-(1-methylpiperidin-4-yl)-N′-(4-(2-methylpropylo xy)phenylmethyl) carbamide (2R,3R)-dihydroxybutanedioate (2:1) (ACP-103), a novel 5-hydroxytryptamine(2A) receptor inverse agonist. *Journal of Pharmacology and Experimental Therapeutics*, *317*, 910–918.

Wadenberg, M. L., & Hicks, P. B. (1999). The conditioned avoidance response test re-evaluated: Is it a sensitive test for the detection of potentially atypical antipsychotics? *Neuroscience and Biobehavioral Reviews*, *23*, 851–862.

Wang, D., Noda, Y., Zhou, Y., Nitta, A., Furukawa, H., & Nabeshima, T. (2007). Synergistic effect of galantamine with risperidone on impairment of social interaction in phencyclidine-treated mice as a schizophrenic animal model. *Neuropharmacology*, *52*, 1179–1187.

Wassef, A., Baker, J., & Kochan, L. D. (2003). GABA and schizophrenia: A review of basic science and clinical studies. *Journal of Clinical Psychopharmacology*, *23*, 601–640.

Webber, M. A., & Marder, S. R. (2008). Better pharmacotherapy for schizophrenia: What does the future hold? *Current Psychiatry Reports*, *10*, 352–358.

Weed, M. R., Taffe, M. A., Polis, I., Roberts, A. C., Robbins, T. W., Koob, G. F., et al. (1999). Performance norms for a rhesus monkey neuropsychological testing battery: Acquisition and long-term performance. *Brain Research. Cognitive Brain Research*, *8*, 185–201.

Weiden, P. J. (2007). EPS profiles: The atypical antipsychotics are not all the same. *Journal of Psychiatric Practice*, *13*, 13–24.

Weiner, D. M., Burstein, E. S., Nash, N., Croston, G. E., Currier, E. A., Vanover, K. E., et al. (2001). 5-hydroxytryptamine2A receptor inverse agonists as antipsychotics. *Journal of Pharmacology and Experimental Therapeutics*, *299*, 268–276.

Weiner, I., Gaisler, I., Schiller, D., Green, A., Zuckerman, L., & Joel, D. (2000). Screening of antipsychotic drugs in animal models. *Drug Development Research*, *50*, 235–249.

Williams, H. J., Owen, M. J., & O'Donovan, M. C. (2009). New findings from genetic association studies of schizophrenia. *Journal of Human Genetics*, *54*, 9–14.

Williams, M. (2009). Commentary: Genome-based CNS drug discovery—D-Amino acid oxidase (DAAO) as a novel target for antipsychotic medications: Progress and challenges. *Biochemical Pharmacology*, *78*, 1360–1365.

Willner, P. (1991). Methods for assessing the validity of animal models of human psychopathology. In A. Boulton, G. Baker, & M. Martin-Iverson (Eds.), *Animal models in psychiatry* (pp. 1–23). Clifton, MJ: The Humana Press.

Willner, P., Papp, M., Phillips, G., Maleeh, M., & Muscat, R. (1990). Pimozide does not impair sweetness discrimination. *Psychopharmacology (Berlin)*, *102*, 278–282.

Zou, H., Zhang, C., Xie, Q., Zhang, M., Shi, J., Jin, M., et al. (2008). Low dose MK-801 reduces social investigation in mice. *Pharmacology, Biochemistry, and Behavior*, *90*, 753–757.

Alexander Scriabine[*] and Daniel U. Rabin[†]

[*]Guilford, Connecticut, 06437
[†]The France Foundation, Old Lyme, Connecticut 06371

New Developments in the Therapy of Pulmonary Fibrosis

Abstract

Fibrosis is a normal response to injury. When it becomes excessive, however, it can interfere with the normal function of various organs. In the lungs fibrosis can lead to interstitial pneumonias. Idiopathic pulmonary fibrosis (IPF) is a chronic interstitial pneumonia of unknown cause and poor prognosis. It is characterized by clinical, radiologic, and histologic criteria. The frequently used therapy of steroids (e.g. prednisolone) and immunosuppressants (e.g. azathioprine) has not been shown to be effective. No drugs for the therapy of IPF are approved in the United States. Bosentan, pirfenidone, and N-acetyl cysteine are currently in clinical trials with preliminary results suggesting they may prolong the life expectancy of patients with IPF. New

Advances in Pharmacology, Volume 57
1054-3589/08 $35.00
10.1016/S1054-3589(08)57011-6

approaches to the treatment of IPF have been proposed. They include endothelial and cytokine antagonists, and antioxidants. Preclinical and clinical studies with these drugs in IPF are reviewed in this chapter. Their antifibrotic activity has been demonstrated in cell culture as well as *in vivo* in bleomycin-induced fibrosis in mice or rats. Better translation of preclinical findings to clinical medicine will help in the discovery and development of new drugs for the treatment of IPF.

I. Introduction

In spite of substantial progress in drug development during the last century, there are still many conditions that cannot be cured or even controlled. The need to find better therapeutics to treat cancer or Alzheimer's disease is widely recognized, with current research efforts producing many new leads. While there are other lethal disorders without adequate therapy, in many cases, the search for drugs to treat them is low on the priority lists of government laboratories and pharmaceutical companies. Some of these neglected conditions are rare, others common. However, if the incidence is low in developed countries, the financial returns for new drugs to treat them are very limited. In some cases the medical need, the potential market, and the opportunity for drug discovery have not yet been recognized by either the scientific community in general or the pharmaceutical industry in particular. Among these are antifibrotic agents. Currently, there are no antifibrotic drugs approved for this use in the United States, although there is a substantial medical need and potential market for such compounds. While the field of antifibrotic drugs is still in its infancy, it is now taking its first steps. During the last few years new targets were identified that are likely to be exploited during the next decade. Described in this chapter are proposed pharmacological approaches for the treatment of a particular fibrotic disorder, idiopathic pulmonary fibrosis (IPF). Drugs effective in IPF are likely to be useful in the therapy of some of the other fibrotic conditions as well.

II. Fibrosis and Fibrogenesis

Fibrosis, deposition of fibrous material at a site of injury, is a normal repair process. The initial response to injury is formation of a clot. This is followed by an inflammatory response involving local vasodilation, an increase in vascular permeability, and an accumulation of leukocytes and monocytes. Cytokines, secreted initially by blood or endothelial cells, transform monocytes into M_1 or M_2 macrophages. M_1 macrophages form tissue necrosis factor alpha (TNF_α), while M_2 macrophages generate transforming growth factor beta (TGF$_\beta$), the major profibrotic cytokine. TGF$_\beta$ stimulates endothelial cells to undergo endothelial-to-mesenchymal transitions (EMTs) and form myofibroblasts that control many other factors responsible for fibrogenesis (Acharaya et al., 2008; Koli, Myllarniemi, Keski-Oja, & Kinnula, 2008; Prud'homme, 2007; Trojanowska, 2008). In fibroblasts the fibrogenic response is mediated by TGF$_\beta$, connective tissue growth factor (CTGF, CCN2) and endothelin-1 (ET-1) (Leask, 2008). Many other cytokines, chemokines, and enzymes, formed by myofibroblasts, also contribute to fibrogenesis (Table I).

TABLE I   Targets for Antifibrotic Drugs—Profibrotic Growth Factors, Cytokines, and Enzymes

Factor	Function	References
TGF$_\beta$	Regulation of fibrogenesis, gene expression, induction of ROS, CTGF, ECM, ET-1	Koli et al. (2008), Lönn, Morén, Raja, Dahl, & Moustakas (2009)
ROS	Activation of latent TGF$_\beta$	Koli et al. (2008), Sullivan, Ferris, Pociask, and Brody (2008)
PDGF	Chemoattraction, mitosis, maintenance of connective tissue	Trojanowska (2008)
TNF$_\alpha$	Regulation of TGF$_\beta$ expression	Sullivan et al. (2008)
ET-1	Mediation of profibrotic effects of TGF$_\beta$	Leask (2008)
CTGF	Enhancement of ET-1 and TGF$_\beta$	Leask (2008)
IL-1	Enhancement of inflammation and fibrosis	Gasse et al. (2007)
IL-13	Upregulation of TGF$_\beta$ receptors,	Murray et al. (2008)
IGF II	Increase in ECM production	Hsu & Feghali-Bostwick (2008)
NOX enzymes	Increase of ROS formation	Lambeth, Krause, & Clark (2008)
MCP-3/ CCL7	Activation of TGF$_\beta$ and type I collagen	Ong et al. (2009)
TLR9	Enhancement of myofibroblasts differentiation	Meneghin et al. (2008)
FRA-2	Increase of fibrogenesis, vascular remodeling	Efert et al. (2008)
Smad3	Mediation of profibrogenic effects of TGF$_\beta$	Gauldie et al. (2006)
Arginase-1	Activation of macrophages	Mora et al. (2006)
Dril-l	Activation of TGF$_\beta$ target genes	Lin et al. (2008)

TGF-β, transforming growth factor-β; ROS, reactive oxygen species; PDGF, platelet-derived growth factor; TNF$_\alpha$, tumor necrosis factor α; ET-1, endothelin-1; CTGF, connective tissue gowth factor; IL-1, interleukin-1; IL-13, interleukin-13; IGF II, insulin growth factor II; NOX enzymes, nicotinamide adenine dinucleotide phosphate oxidases; MCP-3/CCL7, monocyte chemoattractant protein-3/chemokineCCL7 (chemokine (C–C motif) ligand-7); TLR9, toll-like receptor 9; FRA-2, Fos-related protein-2; Smad3, signal transducing transcriptional protein 3; Dril-1, dead ringer-like-1; ECM, extracellular matrix.

TABLE II Targets for Antifibrotic Drugs—Antifibrotic Factors, Cytokines, and Enzymes

Factor	Function	Reference
uPA	Activation of plasminogen	Gharaee-Kermani, Hu, Phan, & Gyetko (2008)
IP-10	Reduction of fibroblast migration	Tager et al. (2004)
ECSOD	Scavenging of ROS	Gao, Kinnula, Myllärniem, & Oury (2008)
FRNK	Reduction of myofibroblast differentiation	Ding, Gladson, Wu, Hayasaka, & Olman (2008)
Calveolin-1	Decrease in TGFβ signaling	Del Galdo et al. (2008)
LPA	Antioxidant activity	Ley and Zarbock (2008)
ld-1	Inhibition of Dril-1	Lin et al. (2008)
CRP	Inhibition of fibroblasts migration and p38 activated MAPK	Kikuchi et al. (2009), Nagase, Rennard, & Takazawa (2009)

uPA, urokinase plasminogen activator; IP-10, interferon-gamma inducible protein of 10 kDa; ECSOD, extracellular superoxide dismutase; FRNK, focal adhesion kinase-related nonkinase; LPA, lipophospatidic acid; ld-1, transcriptional regulator inhibitor of differentiation-1; CRP, C-reactive protein; ROS, reactive oxygen species; Dril-1, dead ringer-like-1; MAPK, mitogen-activated protein kinase.

Activated myofibroblasts produce matrix proteins including type I and III collagens (Ong et al., 2009). Synthesis and deposition of matrix proteins constitutes a remodeling phase that leads to formation of a scar. The process of fibrogenesis is complicated not only by the multiplicity of endogenous profibrotic factors, but also by the presence of antifibrotic chemokines and enzymes (Table II).

The final phase of the wound repair process is scar resolution. This involves a decrease in collagen synthesis and/or an increase in collagen degradation. This phase is controlled largely by matrix metalloproteinases (MMPs) and their endogenous inhibitors (TIMPs, tissue inhibitors of metalloproteinases). In all phases of fibrogenesis, the pro- and antifibrotic factors are in a state of delicate balance. Disruption of this balance can lead to disease. Interested readers can find a more detailed review of the factors involved in recent articles on this topic (Lupher & Gallatin, 2006; Wilson & Wynn, 2009; Wynn, 2008).

III. Fibrotic Diseases

As a repair process, fibrosis is initially beneficial. It becomes pathological, however, if it is not properly controlled and/or the initial cause of injury persists. Excessive fibrosis can interfere with the normal function of vital organs, such as the heart, lungs, kidney, or liver, and can lead to death. While fibrosis is tissue specific, many aspects of its development are common in different organs, so that the same therapeutic approaches may be

TABLE III   Fibrotic Diseases

Autoimmune myocarditis	Pleural fibrosis
Renal fibrosis	Pulmonary fibrosis
Cystic fibrosis	Retroperitoneal fibrosis
Endomyocardial fibrosis	Sarcoidosis
Eosophageal fibrosis	Scleroderma
Liver cirrhosis	Systemic sclerosis
Macular degeneration	Uterine fibrosis
Mixed connective tissue disease	

applicable to many, if not all, fibrotic diseases. For example, enhanced upregulation or activation of $TGF_{\beta 1}$ is reported to contribute to the development of pulmonary fibrosis (Sullivan et al., 2008; Willis & Borok, 2007), renal fibrosis (Liu, 2004; Qi, Chen, Poronnik, & Pollock, 2008), and even scleroderma (Trojanowska, 2008). Moreover, EMT is implicated in pulmonary fibrotic diseases (Borok, 2009; Willis & Borok, 2007) and renal fibrosis (Liu, 2004). The involvement of these same factors in other fibrotic diseases is likely, although not yet established. Table III lists the major fibrotic disorders. Fibrosis also plays a contributory role in other conditions, such as rheumatoid arthritis and lupus erythematosus.

A. Pulmonary Fibrosis

Pulmonary fibrosis is not a single disease, but multiple diffuse parenchymal disorders of the lungs. These conditions are usually classified according to their cause or origin. Deposition of particulate matter in the lungs can lead to occupational diseases, such as silicosis (Akgun et al., 2008; Cohen, Patel, & Green, 2008), beryllium-induced lung disease (Fontenot & Amicosante, 2008) or asbestosis (Kamp, 2009), while hypersensitivity to molds can cause aspergillosis (Vlahakis & Aksamit, 2001), or farmer's lung disease (Reboux et al., 2007). Certain drugs and other chemicals are known or are suspected to cause pulmonary fibrosis (Table IV). It should be noted that some of the drugs, such as azathioprine and methotrexate, that are currently used to treat pulmonary fibrosis are also suspected of causing it in some patients.

B. Interstitial Lung Disease and Idiopathic Pulmonary Fibrosis

The precise etiology of pulmonary fibrosis cannot always be established and patients are often diagnosed as having idiopathic interstitial lung disease (ILD). This is not a single condition, but rather is a group of interstitial pneumonias that are differentiated primarily by lung histology. The classification and treatment of ILDs has been the subject of international

TABLE IV   Drugs Known or Suspected to Cause Pulmonary Fibrosis

Adalimubab	Melphalan
Azathioprine	Methotrexate
Amiodarone	Methamphetamine
Amphotericin B	Methylphenidate
Bortezomib	Minocycline
Busulfan	Mitomycin
Bleomycin	Nitrofurantoin
Bromocriptine	Peplomycin
Carmustine (BCNU)	Practolol
Cefotaxime	Procainamide
Chlorambucil	Rifampicin
Cyclophosphamide	Sirolimus
Clindamycin	Sulfsalazine
Cocaine	Tamoxifen
Gold salts	Timolol
Heroin	Imipenem–cilastatin
	Vinblastine

controversy that has led to establishment of guidelines (American Thoracic Society/European Respiratory Society (ATS/ERS), 2002; Brash, 2006; Rogliani et al., 2008; Wells & Hirani, 2008). There are at least nine idiopathic interstitial pneumonias, the most common of which is IPF (Table V)

The incidence of IPF in the United States is more than 30,000 cases per year, and the prevalence is currently more than 80,000 patients (ATS/ERS, 2002; Raghu, Weycker, Edelsberg, Bradford, & Oster, 2006, www.pilotfor-ipf.org). Most cases are diagnosed between the ages of 40 and 70, with two thirds being older than 60 years at presentation. IPF is slightly more prevalent in males, especially in the elderly.

Although the cause of IPF is not known, the condition has been characterized by radiologic, histologic and clinical findings (ATS/ERS, 2002; Maher, Wells & Laurent, 2007). Typical high-resolution computed tomography (HRCT) findings in IPF include irregular reticular opacities, subpleural, posterior, lower-lobe predominance, traction bronchiectasis,

TABLE V   Idiopathic Interstitial Pneumonias

Usual interstitial pneumonia	UIP
Idiopathic pulmonary fibrosis	IPF
Desquamative interstitial pneumonia	DIP
Respiratory bronchiolitis	RB
Lymphoid interstitial pneumonia	LIP
Cryptogenic organizing pneumonia	COP
Diffuse alveolar damage	DAD
Acute interstitial pneumonia	AIP
Nonspecific interstitial pneumonia	NSIP

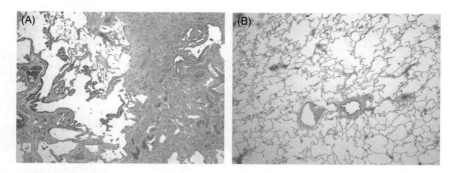

FIGURE I   Fibrotic and normal human lung. Photographs were taken with 5× objective. (A) Lung from a patient with IPF. Note massive remodeling with extensive scarring, destruction of normal alveoli, "honeycombs," and residual small airways. Fibroblastic foci can only be seen with higher magnification. (B) Normal human lung architecture with a small bronchiole and an artery. (Courtesy of Robert Homer, MD, Ph.D., Professor of Pathology and Internal Medicine, Yale University School of Medicine, New Haven, CT.)

honeycombing, minimal ground-glass opacities, and lymph node enlargement. Features not typical of IPF that should trigger consideration of an alternative diagnosis include pleural effusion, pleural thickening, moderate ground glass opacities, nodules, and scattered cysts (ATS/ERS, 2002). The typical histological findings in usual interstitial pneumonia (UIP) are destruction of alveoli, extensive scaring, scattered foci of proliferating fibroblasts, "honeycomb" changes in subpleural parenchyma, as well as hyperplasia of type II pneumocytes. There appears to be an increased apoptosis of type II alveolar cells, while myofibroblasts are relatively resistant to apoptosis. Some of these pathological changes can be seen on Fig. 1. Infiltrates with lymphocytes and plasma cells can be occasionally seen at the earlier stages of the disease but are usually absent in advanced cases. Proliferating fibroblasts can only be seen at higher power. Clinical symptoms include dry cough, dyspnea on exertion, end-inspiratory rales, and impaired gas exchange.

IPF has a poor prognosis, with the life expectancy being 3–5 years after diagnosis. Prognosis is determined primarily by cardiopulmonary exercise testing, though emerging biomarkers such as surfactant proteins (Kinder et al., 2009), KL-6 (mucinous high-molecular-weight glycoprotein expressed on type II pneumocytes) (Yokoyama et al., 2006), and fibrocytes (Moeller et al., 2009) promise to improve prognostic accuracy. The clinical course is characterized by a decline of pulmonary function over time. Maximal oxygen uptake (VO_2 max) below 8.3 ml/kg/min has been correlated with high mortality (Fell et al., 2009). The cause of death is usually multiple organ failure after acute exacerbation (AE) of the disease. While exacerbations can occur at any time after diagnosis, they usually happen a few years after the initial diagnosis. A case of AE in the early stage of the disease has been recently described (Sakamoto et al., 2009).

Alveolar epithelial cell injury is believed to be the initiating event in IPF. The cause of epithelial injury is unknown, although viral infection is thought to be a culprit. Indeed, herpes virus deoxyribonucleic acid (DNA) has been consistently detected in the lungs of patients with IPF (Tang et al., 2003). Chronic pulmonary infection with γ-herpes virus 68 (MHV68) produces pulmonary fibrosis in mice lacking interferon-γ receptor (IFNγR$^{-/-}$) (Mora et al., 2005) and Epstein–Barr virus (EBV)-induced alveolar epithelial cell injury leads to the increased expression of TGF$_{β1}$ in human cell lines (Malizia et al., 2008). According to one case report (Ankermann, Claviez, Wagner, Krams, & Riedel, 2003), an acute EBV virus infection in a child led to pulmonary fibrosis that was successfully resolved by steroids. Tsukamoto et al. (2000) detected EBV virus DNA in 24 out of 25 patients with IPF, while in nine out of 29 lung specimens from IPF patients cuboidal epithelial cells stained positively for EBV latent protein-1 (LMP-1). Lawson et al. (2008) found expression of herpes simplex virus protein in type II alveolar epithelial cells from 15 out of 23 IPF patients. These and other findings suggest that in some cases herpes simplex or other viruses may have caused IPF or played a role in its progression.

Another observation that tends to support the viral hypothesis relates to the origin of dry cough. According to Wells & Hirani (2008), the pathogenesis of cough in IPF is poorly understood and may be related to an increase in the sensitivity of sensory receptors rather than to pulmonary pathology. It is usually associated with sneezing and nasopharyngeal irritation and may conceivably represent another manifestation of a chronic systemic viral infection.

Another possible cause of epithelial injury in IPF is gastroesophageal reflux disease (GERD) which can result in chronic aspiration of gastric acid. The association of GERD with IPF was first proposed by Mays, Dubois, & Hamilton (1976) and further supported by Tobin, Pope & Pellegrini (1988). The evidence for the role of GERD in the pathogenesis of IPF was recently reviewed by Pashinsky, Jaffin & Lile (2009).

Genetic factors appear to predispose some to fibrotic diseases (Verleden et al., 2001). Occasional familial occurrence of IPF is linked to chromosomes 4, 5, and 11, and surfactant protein 1 and telomerase genes are viewed as susceptibility genes for this condition (Steele & Brown, 2007). The familial form of IPF, which is characterized by autosomal-dominant inheritance, affects less than 10% of IPF patients. In some of these individuals, genes encoding the protein or RNA components of telomerase have been identified (Armanios et al., 2007). Genetic defects in surfactant protein A2 have been associated with IPF as shown by Wang et al. (2009), while Alder et al. (2008) found that telomeres in alveolar epithelium and leukocytes of patients with IPF are shortened and that this shortening is not likely to be due to telomerase mutation. These findings suggest a deficiency in the regenerative capacity of epithelial cells in patients with IPF (Blasco, 2007;

Behr & Thannickal, 2009). Serial analysis of gene expression was used by Boon et al. (2009) to generate profiles from lung biopsies of six patients with slow and of six with rapidly progressing IPF. They found that transcripts distinguished the stable from rapidly progressing form of IPF and identified a gene (Plunc) that was previously not associated with this disorder.

The existence of various "forms" of IPF, familial versus sporadic, or slow versus rapidly progressing, suggests it may not be a single disease. The exclusion of all possible causes and identification of contributing factors at the time of initial diagnosis is highly important for prognostic and therapeutic purposes.

C. Animal Models of Pulmonary Fibrosis

Reliable animal disease models greatly facilitate drug development, even when the precise trigger of a disease is unknown. Since this is the case with IPF, the availability of an animal model is particularly important for successful development of antifibrotic drugs. The standard models of pulmonary fibrosis are bleomycin-treated rodents. Experimental pulmonary fibrosis was first produced with bleomycin in dogs (Fleischman et al., 1971) and subsequently reproduced in mice by Adamson & Bowden (1974). Extensive reviews of the bleomycin model and of its use in pulmonary research were recently published (Gauldie & Kolb, 2008; Moeller, Ask, Warburton, Gauldie, & Kolb, 2008; Moore & Hogaboam, 2008). A single intratracheal administration of bleomycin produces pulmonary fibrosis in rodents, with a maximal effect at between 20 and 28 days after exposure to the drug. Thereafter fibrosis slowly resolves. The cause and the spontaneous resolution of fibrosis differentiate this model from IPF in humans, although it is similar with respect to the production of cytokines and free radicals. Moeller et al. (2008) listed published studies on the prevention or treatment of bleomycin-induced fibrosis in laboratory animals. They point out that to mimic clinical situations, the potential antifibrotic drugs should be administered after, and not prior to, the development of bleomycin-induced fibrosis. Antioxidants, angiotensin-converting enzyme inhibitors, angiotensin antagonists, immunosuppressants, macrolide antibiotics, and many other agents are reported to reduce fibrosis in bleomycin-treated animals. Most of the drugs were never tested for antifibrotic activity in humans whereas others were ineffective in clinical trials. However, the fact that pirfenidone is effective in this model, and has yielded promising clinical results in a phase III trial, suggests the potential utility of this model in drug discovery (Iyer, Gurujeyalakshmi, & Giri, 1999a, 1999b).

Other drugs or chemicals known to produce pulmonary fibrosis in humans are also used in the search for potential antifibrotic drugs. For example, Cantor et al. (1984) produced amiodarone-induced fibrosis in hamsters, while Kennedy et al. (1988) used amiodarone to induce injury in perfused rabbit lungs. Further, Leeder, Brien, and Massey (1994) demonstrated a reduction of amiodarone-induced pulmonary toxicity by N-acetyl cysteine (NAC), and antioxidants reduce silica -induced pulmonary fibrosis in mice (Lombard-Gillooly & Hubbard, 1993). Pulmonary fibrosis is also produced in rats by paraquat (Satomi, Sakaguchi, Kasahara, & Akahori, 2007). The angiotensin-converting enzyme inhibitors captopril and enalapril reduce paraquat-induced pulmonary fibrosis in rats (Ghazi-Khansari et al., 2007), and hexavalent chromium-induced fibrosis is reduced in rats by vitamins C and E (Hemmati, Nazari, Ranjbari, & Torfi, 2008). Parra et al. (2008) induced pulmonary fibrosis in mice by butyl-hydroxytoluene and found it to be histologically identical to fibrosis in humans with IPF. Ask et al. (2008) have induced pulmonary fibrosis in rats by adenoviral gene transfer of TGF$_\beta$ and thereafter assessed progression of the disease by noninvasive techniques.

Attempts have also been made to develop *in vitro* models of pulmonary fibrosis. As an example, cadmium chloride in combination with TGF$_\beta$ produces fibrosis in rat lung slice cultures (Lin et al., 1998) and Nakayama et al. (2008) report that pirfenidone inhibits the effects of TGF$_{\beta 1}$ on protein expression in cultured human fibroblasts.

It appears that adequate technology for the preclinical evaluation of potential antifibrotic drugs is available, although it is obvious that neither animal models nor *in vitro* techniques mimic the human condition in all respects.

IV. Search for Antifibrotic Drugs

A. Endothelin Antagonists

ET-1 is one of the three isoforms of endothelin, a peptide secreted by endothelial cells (Hickey, Rubani, Paul, & Highsmtith, 1985). All three isoforms bind to two types of endothelin receptors, ET$_A$ (endothelin receptor, type A) and ET$_B$ (endothelin receptor, type B). ET-1 is a 21 amino acid protein that was isolated, sequenced, and cloned by Yanagisawa et al. (1988). A highly potent vaso- and bronchoconstrictor, endothelin has been implicated in many pulmonary diseases, including fibrosis (Abraham, 2008; Fagan, McMurtry, & Rodman, 2001; Jain, Shaul, Borok, Wills, & Brigham, 2007; Kim & Chapman, 2007). ET-1 is mitogenic in endothelial and vascular smooth muscle cells, and is upregulated in lungs of patients with IPF. Through ET$_A$ and ET$_B$ receptors, ET-1 promotes EMT, conversion of epithelial to fibroblasts-like cells, and the synthesis of collagen types I and III. Through ET$_A$ receptors it inhibits MMP-1 and activates TGF$_{\beta 1}$ signaling (Jain et al., 2007; Kim & Chapman, 2007; Kim et al., 2006). These and other findings strongly suggest that ET-1 is a profibrotic mediator and therefore likely to play a role in the development of IPF.

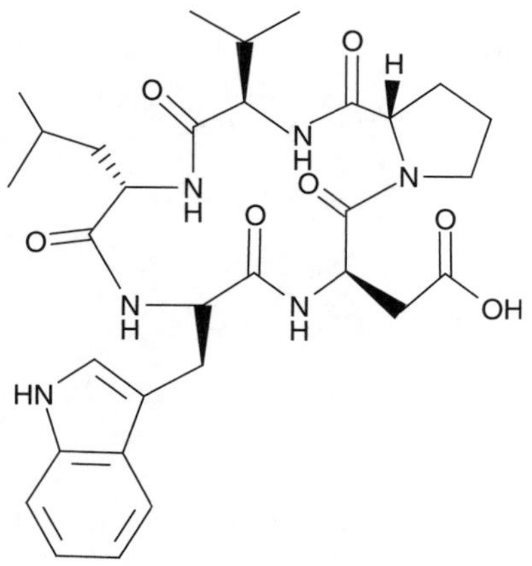

BQ-123

FIGURE 2   Chemical structure of BQ-123, the first-generation endothelin antagonist.

Since the discovery of endothelin, many ET-1 receptor antagonists have been synthesized and studied. The first antagonists were developed at Banyu Pharmaceutical Company in Japan (Kojiri et al., 1991). These agents are peptides produced by *Streptomyces misakiensis*, a strain isolated from a soil sample. Based on these leads, Ishikawa et al. (1992) prepared numerous other cyclic peptides with selective ET_A receptor antagonist activity. Among them is the most widely studied ET_A receptor antagonist, cyclic pentapeptide, BQ-123 (cyclo(–D-Asp–L-Pro–D-Val–L-Leu–D-Trp–)) (Fig. 2) (Moreland, 1994). The pharmacology of BQ-123 has been studied in many *in vitro* and *in vivo* systems. In the lungs, BQ-123 antagonizes ET-1-induced contractions of isolated animal or human pulmonary arteries and attenuates monocrotaline- or hypoxia-induced elevation of pulmonary arterial pressure in rats. The proliferative effect of ET-1 in cultured human pulmonary arterial smooth muscle cells is reduced by BQ-123 (Zamora, Dempsey, Walchak, & Stelzner, 1993).

The pharmacology of another peptide, a selective ET_B receptor antagonist, N-*cis*-2,6-dimethylpiperidinocarbonyl-L-γ-methylleucyl-D-1-methoxy-carbonyltryptophanyl-D-norleucine (BQ-788), is reviewed by Okada and Nishikibe (2002). In most of the experimental studies, BQ-123 and BQ-788 are used as tools to investigate differential physiological roles of ET receptors. The studies suggest the possible utility of ET_A-selective or nonspecific ET-1 antagonists as a treatment for systemic or pulmonary hypertension, as well as in heart failure. Neither BQ-123 nor BQ-788 is effective orally.

Attempts to develop nonpeptide, small molecule ET-1 inhibitors at Hoffmann-La-Roche led to the discovery of bosentan (Clozel & Salloukh, 2005; Clozel et al., 1994) (Fig. 3). Bosentan antagonizes the binding of ET-1

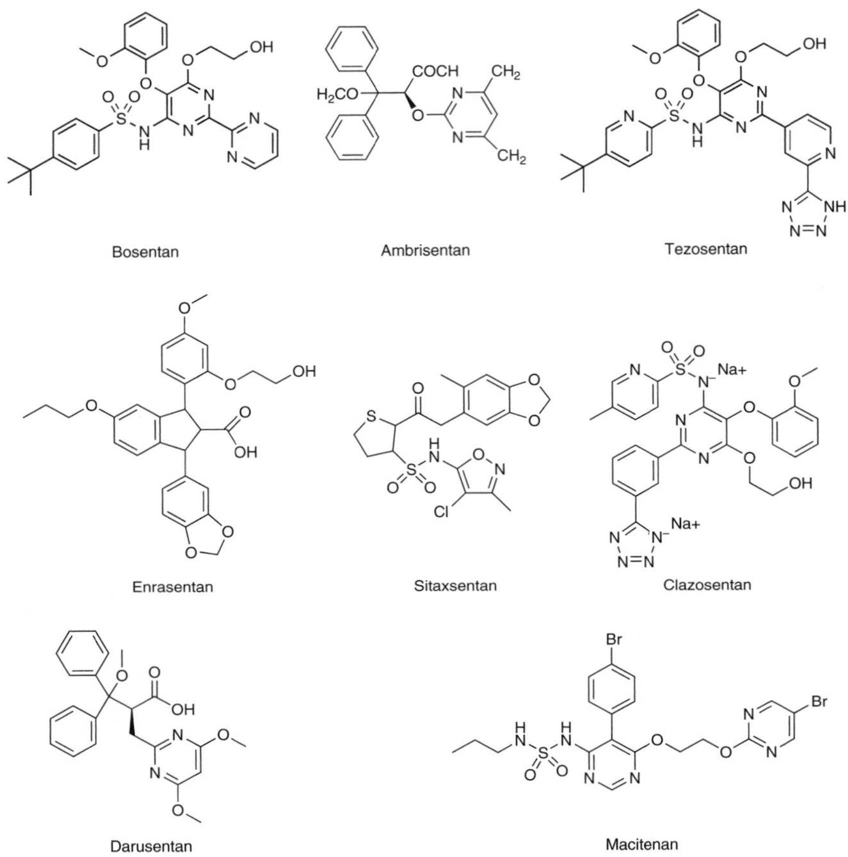

FIGURE 3   Chemical structures of second-generation endothelin antagonists.

to ET_A receptors ($K_i = 4.7$ nM) in human smooth muscle cell cultures and blocks ET_B receptors in rat trachea ($pA_2 = 6$). At 1 mg/kg p.o. and higher doses, bosentan blocks the pressor effects of ET-1 in rats. These and other results indicate that bosentan was the first nonpeptide orally active and highly potent ET_A and ET_B receptor antagonist.

The initial clinical studies with bosentan were conducted in patients with systemic hypertension (Krum, Viscoper, Lacourciere, Budde, & Charlon, 1998). At daily doses ranging from 100 to 2,000 mg, bosentan displayed antihypertensive activity. At 500 mg daily its effect was similar to 20 mg of enalapril. Its antihypertensive effect was not associated with the reflex activation of the sympathetic nervous system. During short-term oral therapy, bosentan displays beneficial hemodynamic effects in patients with chronic heart failure (Kiowski, Sutch, Oechslin, & Bertel, 2001). However, a larger trial using 500 mg b.i.d. (twice per day) was terminated early because of a high incidence of abnormal liver function tests. In subsequent studies bosentan was administered at 125 mg b.i.d. In a large trial (1,613 patients with severe heart failure) bosentan failed to produce significant improvements in mortality, hospitalization rate, or clinical status (Rubin & Roux, 2002). Fluid retention appeared to be one of the possible causes for its failure. These data notwithstanding, some advocated another heart failure trial with bosentan at a lower dose and/or in combination with a strong diuretic (Kaira, Moon, & Coats, 2002). The sponsor of bosentan, Hoffmann-La-Roche, did not pursue the heart failure indication and development of the drug was taken over by Actelion. Actelion placed emphasis on a new indication, pulmonary arterial hypertension. The rationale for this selection was based on the reports that ET-1 is overexpressed in the lungs of patients with pulmonary hypertension (Giaid et al., 1993), and that bosentan prevents or reverses hypoxia-induced pulmonary hypertension in rats (Chen et al., 1995). In the first randomized, placebo-controlled study in patients with pulmonary hypertension, bosentan (125 mg b.i.d., for 12 weeks) improved exercise capacity and cardiopulmonary hemodynamics (Channick et al., 2001). These findings were confirmed and extended in a study by Rubin et al. (2002). Bosentan, 62.5 mg per day for 4 weeks followed by 125 or 250 mg for 12 weeks, improved 6-min walking distance (6-MWD), Borg dyspnea index, and time to clinical deterioration. In subsequent clinical studies in various patient populations, bosentan consistently improved the dyspnea score, but had variable effects on 6-MWD (Opitz, Ewert, Kirch, & Pittrow, 2008). Bosentan (Tracleer®) is approved in the United States for the treatment of pulmonary hypertension with a warning of potential liver injury and a contraindication in pregnancy. The warning is based on increases in aminotransferases levels (over $3\times$ the upper limit of normal) in 11% of patients. The contraindication is based on the finding of teratogenic effects of bosentan in rats at 60 and 300 mg/kg/day (Physicians' Desk Reference, 2009).

Since ET-1 is profibrotic (Shi-Wen et al., 2007) and bosentan reduces collagen deposition in rats with bleomycin-induced pulmonary fibrosis (Park, Saleh, Giaid, & Michel, 1997), the possibility was considered that bosentan may have beneficial effect in patients with IPF. One of the initial clinical trials (Bosentan Use in Interstitial Lung Disease, BUILD-1, King et al., 2008) involved 159 patients at 29 centers in five European countries, the United States and Israel. Bosentan, at 62.5 and 125 mg b.i.d., had no effect on 6-MWD after 12 months of therapy. However, it appeared to reduce the combined end point of disease progression or death and had beneficial effects in seven out of eight domains of the quality of life. The authors concluded that the results were sufficiently encouraging to continue clinical trials with bosentan in patients with IPF.

Ambrisentan (Letairis®) is the second endothelin antagonist approved for the treatment of pulmonary hypertension in the United States. It is more selective than bosentan for ET_A receptors, its bioavailability is higher and its elimination half-life longer (Cheng, 2008; Croxtall & Keam, 2008; MacIntyre, Dhaun, Goddard, & Webb, 2008, Vatter & Seifert, 2006). In three double-blind randomized clinical trials ambrisentan, at 2.5–10 mg/day, improved 6-MWD, dyspnea score, and functional data. Thirty out of 31 patients with pulmonary hypertension, who discontinued either bosentan or sitaxsentan because of transaminase elevation, tolerated ambrisentan (McGoon et al., 2008). Two clinical trials are underway to assess the safety and efficacy of ambrisentan in patients with IPF (NCT00768300 and NCT00879229).

Other ET-1 antagonists (Fig. 3) were synthesized and developed as treatments for pulmonary or systemic hypertension, or heart failure. Nonselective ET-1 antagonists, tezosentan (Torre-Amione et al., 2001) and enrasentan (Cosenzi, 2003), as well as ET_A-selective antagonists, sitaxsentan (Barst et al., 2004, 2006; Zaca et al., 2009), clazosentan (Roux et al., 1997), and darusentan (Epstein, 2008; Prie, Leung, Cernacek, Ryan, & Dupuis, 1997), were studied in animals and humans. More recently, Iglarz et al. (2008) developed macitentan, a nonselective ET-1 antagonist with improved physicochemical properties and higher lipophilicity than other members of this class. There is, however, no published information on the antifibrotic activity of any of these ET-1 antagonists, except bosentan. Thus, the possibility remains that some of them could be useful in the management of fibrotic diseases.

B. Antioxidants

The disturbance of pulmonary antioxidant/oxidant balance leading to oxidative stress is thought to be one of the major factors contributing to the pathogenesis of IPF (Kinnula, 2008; Kinnula, Fattman, Tan, & Oury, 2005; Kinnula & Myllärniemi, 2008; Rahman, Biswas, Saibal, & Kode, 2006; Rahman, Yang, & Biswas, 2008; Rahman et al., 1999; Walters, Cho, & Kleeberger, 2008). Reactive oxygen species (ROS) production by alveolar macrophages is increased in patients with IPF (Cantin, North, Felis, Hubbard, & Crystal, 1987; Strausz, Muller-Querheim, Steppling, & Ferlinz, 1990). While superoxide anion (O_2^-), hydrogen peroxide (H_2O_2), peroxynitrite, and hydroxyl radicals (OH^-) act as signaling molecules, they also damage proteins, lipids, and other cellular macromolecules, activate TGF_β and other profibrotic cytokines, and consequently enhance fibrogenesis. Antioxidant defenses consist of endogenous as well as exogenous scavengers and catalytic antioxidants. In patients with IPF this defense system appears to be overwhelmed by ROS even though the alveolar levels of nonenzymatic antioxidants may be elevated (Markart et al., 2009). Production of ROS in lung macrophages is also increased in animals with bleomycin-induced fibrosis (Inghilleri, Morbini, Oggionni, Barni, & Fenoglio, 2006), and fibrosis is prevented or reduced in these animals by the administration of antioxidants (Kilinç et al., 1993). ROS are required for the development of bleomycin-induced fibrosis in mice (Manoury et al., 2005). Taken together, these data support the notion that antioxidant therapy may have a beneficial effect in the treatment of IPF.

On the basis of their mechanism of action, antioxidants are subdivided in two major categories: (1) scavengers that react with ROS forming less toxic species and (2) catalytic antioxidants that are not consumed when reacting with ROS (Day, 2008).

I. Antioxidant Scavengers

Many antioxidant scavengers either occur naturally in the body and/or are regularly present in the human diet. Glutathione (GT), vitamins E and C, polyphenols, and uric acid belong to this group. Numerous antioxidant polyphenols are present in plants, vegetables, and fruits. Indeed, curcumin (Biswas, McClure, Jimenez, Megson, & Rahman, 2005; Rahman, Biswas, & Kirkham, 2006) and resveratrol (Sener, Topaloglu, Sehirtli, Ercan, & Gedik, 2007) (Fig. 4) ameliorate bleomycin-induced pulmonary fibrosis in rats. Attenuation of amiodarone-induced pulmonary fibrosis in rats by vitamin E is associated with suppression of TGFβ gene expression (Card, Racz, Brien, & Massey, 2003).

GT is a major antioxidant in lung. In addition to its antioxidant activity, GT suppresses the proliferation of human lung fibroblasts (Cantin, Larivee, & Begin, 1990) and regulates the fibrogenic effects of TGFβ (Ono et al.,

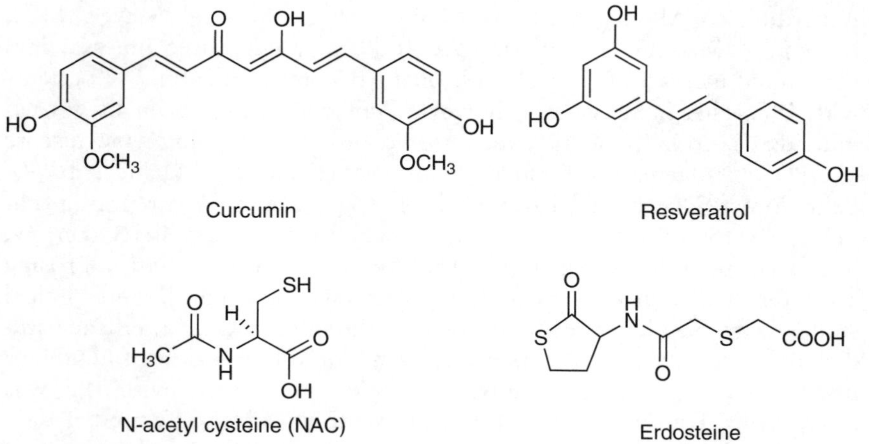

FIGURE 4 Chemical structures of antioxidants with putative antifibrotic activity.

2009). Moreover, GT levels in the epithelial lining fluid are decreased in patients with IPF (Beeh et al., 2002). Since GT does not readily penetrate the cell membrane, and has bronchoconstrictor activity, most experimental and clinical studies were performed with its thiol precursor, NAC. Other thiols or prodrugs known to be metabolized to thiols, such as erdosteine, have also been shown to prevent bleomycin-induced fibrosis in laboratory animals (Day, 2008; Sogut et al., 2004; Yildirim et al., 2005).

2. N-Acetyl Cysteine (NAC)

NAC was synthesized in 1961 and patented by Mead Johnson in 1965. Its use as a mucolytic in the treatment of respiratory diseases was reviewed by Ziment (1986) and in the treatment of acetaminophen overdose by Smilkstein, Knapp, Kulig, & Rumack (1988). Subsequently, NAC was found to restore GT levels and consequently antioxidant defense mechanisms in pulmonary diseases (Ruffman & Wendel, 1991). At 400 mg/kg in drinking water, NAC reduces lung collagen content in mice with bleomycin-induced pulmonary fibrosis (Shahzeidi, Sarnstrand, Jeffery, McAnulty, & Laurent, 1991). The effectiveness of NAC in bleomycin-induced fibrosis was confirmed by Hagiwara, Ishii, and Kitamura (2000) in mice and by Mata et al. (2003), Cortijo et al. (2001), Serrano-Mollar et al. (2003), and Yildirim et al. (2005) in rats. In endothelial cells from bovine pulmonary artery, NAC at 10 mM in combination with 10 mM GT and 5 mM cysteine inhibited $TGF_{\beta 1}$ activity (White, Maloney, Lee, Lanzillo, & Fanburg, 1999). Meurer, Lahme, Tihaa, Weiskirchen, and Gressner (2005) reported that in rat hepatic stellate cells NAC downregulates TGF_β signaling. These observations could explain the mechanism of the antifibrotic action of NAC.

During the last 15 years, numerous clinical reports described antioxidant and antifibrotic effects of NAC in patients with pulmonary diseases. According to Meyer, Buhl, & Magnussen (1994) and Meyer, Buhl, Kampf, & Magnussen (1995), NAC, 600 mg t.i.d. (three times a day) for 5 days, increases GT levels in bronchoalveolar lavage fluid of patients with IPF. This increase was, however, not consistently seen in normal individuals or in patients with chronic obstructive pulmonary disease (COPD) (Bridgeman, Marsden, Selby, Morrison, & MacNee, 1994). Behr, Maier, Degenkolb, Krombach, & Vogelmeier (1997) reported that NAC, 600 mg t.i.d. for 12 weeks along with immunosuppressive therapy, improved pulmonary function tests (PFTs) in patients with fibrosing alveolitis. Gillissen & Novak (1998) reviewed preclinical and clinical studies with NAC and recommended that long-term clinical efficacy studies be undertaken with it as a treatment for IPF and other pulmonary diseases. A pilot clinical study with NAC in patients with IPF was reported by Tomioka et al. (2005). In this trial, NAC (352 mg per day) was administered by inhalation for 12 months to 10 patients with IPF, while 12 other patients received bromhexine HCl as a control. NAC had no effect on pulmonary function, 6-MWD, or quality of life, but slightly reduced exercise desaturation, improved ground-glass score in HRCT, and decreased mucin-like glycoprotein (KL-6) serum levels. The authors concluded that NAC may delay disease progression. The interest in NAC was revived by the report by Demedts et al. (2005) who treated IPF patients with NAC, 600 mg t.i.d., p.o. for 1 year along with prednisone and azathioprine ("standard therapy"). The results indicated that vital capacity (VC) and diffusing capacity for carbon monoxide were better preserved in patients receiving NAC than in those receiving "standard therapy" alone. Hunninghake (2005) suggested that beneficial effects of NAC in patients with IPF may be due to prevention of the toxic effects of prednisone and azathioprine and pointed out the need for a long-term clinical trial with NAC alone. The planned PANTHER (Prednisone, Azathioprine, and N-acetyl cysteine: a study THat Evaluates Response in IPF) will test NAC alone and in combination with prednisone and azathioprine.

3. Catalytic Antioxidants

The endogenous catalytic antioxidant defense system in human lung consists of many enzymes and proteins (Day, 2008; Kinnula & Myllär-niemi, 2008). These are expressed primarily in bronchial and alveolar epithelium, but also in macrophages and inflammatory cells. Of particular importance are three superoxide dismutases (SODs): MnSOD, CuZnSOD, and ECSOD (extracellular SOD) as well as heme oxygenase-1 (Lakari, Paako, Pietarinen-Runtti, & Kinnula, 2000; Lakari et al., 2001), glu-tathione-S-transferases, and peroxidases (Hayes, Flanagan, & Jowsay, 2005). The protective effect of ECSOD was extensively studied in experimental fibrosis models (Gao et al., 2008; Oury et al., 2002). Mice lacking ECSOD are more sensitive to asbestos-induced fibrosis than normal animals (Fattman, Tan, Toblewski, & Oury, 2006) and bleomycin-induced pulmonary damage is enhanced in animals lacking this enzyme (Fattman et al., 2003). It was also found that ECSOD is only barely detectable in the fibrotic lesions of a diseased human lung (Kinnula et al., 2006) and TGFβ inhibits expression of ECSOD in alveolar epithelial and other cells (Stralin & Marklund, 2001).

Inhibition of fragmentation of collagen (types I and IV) as well as of heparan sulfate proteoglycans by ECSOD is likely to play a role in its antifibrotic activity (Gao et al., 2008). It is thought that ECSOD polymorphisms may determine genetic variability in the susceptibility of some individuals to pulmonary fibrosis (Kinnula et al., 2006).

4. SOD Mimetics

Although SOD and similar enzymes can theoretically be useful in the therapy of fibrotic diseases, smaller molecules mimicking the effects of SOD, but with higher cell permeability, were thought to be more desirable candidates for this use. Such compounds were synthesized and developed as treatments for cardiovascular diseases such as atherosclerosis, septic shock, hypertension, and ischemia/reperfusion injury. The pharmacological properties and potential therapeutic use of SOD mimetics were reviewed by Cuzzocrea, Riley, Caputi, & Salvemini (2001), Kinnula & Crapo (2003), Day (2008), Rabkin & Klassen (2008), and Wozniak & Czyz (2008). There are three classes of Mn-containing SOD mimetics: macrolytics, salens, and porphyrins.

The macrolytic M40403 (S–S dimethyl substituted biscyclohexylpyridine) has been shown to protect rats from carrageenan-induced pleurisy and to improve survival of rats subjected to splanchnic artery occlusion and reperfusion (Cuzzocrea et al., 2001b; Salvemini et al., 2001). M40403 also prevents myocardial injury caused by hyperglycemia in perfused rat hearts (Di Filippo et al., 2004) and reduces antigen-induced respiratory abnormalities and airway inflammation in sensitized guinea pigs (Masini et al., 2005). Reversal of endothelial dysfunction in apoE^0 mice by M40403 was explained by inhibition of NAD(P)H (reduced β-nicotinamide dinucleotide phosphate) oxidase (Jiang, Guo, Salvemini, & Dusting, 2003).

Salens protect rats from ischemic brain injury (Baker et al., 1998) and one of them (EUK-8, manganese N,N^1-bis(salicylidene) ethylenediamine chloride), ameliorates acute lung injury in endotoxemic swine (Gonzalez et al., 1995). Two other compounds, EUK-134 [manganese 3-methoxy-N, N^1 bis(saliclidene) ethylenediamine chloride] and tempol (4-hydroxy-2,2,6,6-tetramethylpiperidine-N-oxyl), are reported to reduce the renal toxicity of paraquat by dismutation or scavenging of superoxide anions and reduction of hydroxyl ion generation (Samai, Sharpe, Gard, & Chatterjee, 2007). The SOD mimetic and superoxide scavenging activities of Mn(II)- and Cu(II)-complexes of monensin were described by Fisher, Lau, and Naughton (2005).

Damaging cellular effects of peroxynitrite can be blocked by metalloporphyrins (Rabkin & Klassen, 2008), and bleomycin-induced pulmonary fibrosis in mice is attenuated by MnTBAP [(manganese (III) tetrakis(4-benzoic acid porphyrin)] (Oury et al., 2001). An orally active catalytic metalloporphyrin, AEOL 11207 [5,15-bis(methoxycarbonyl)-10,20-bis-trifluoromethyl-porphyrinato manganese(III) chloride], displays neuroprotective activity and antagonizes methylphenyltetrahydropyridine toxicity in mice suggesting possible utility in the treatment of Parkinson's disease (Liang, Huang, Fulton, Day, & Patel, 2007). Although the potential of superoxide dismutase mimetics in the treatment of COPD was recognized by Bowler, Barnes, & Crapo (2004), only a few laboratory, and no clinical, studies have been published on the effects of these compounds in the treatment of these conditions.

C. Other Leads

I. Animal Studies

Cortijo et al. (2009) reported beneficial effects of roflumilast, a phosphodiesterase-4 (PDE4) inhibitor (Fig. 5) in bleomycin-induced fibrosis in mice and rats. Of particular interest was their finding that roflumilast, 1 or 5 mg/kg/day p.o., alleviates fibrosis not only in preventive (roflumilast on days 1–14 after bleomycin) but also in therapeutic protocols (roflumilast on days 7–12 after bleomycin), while methhylprednisolone, 10 mg/kg/day p.o., was effective only in the preventive protocol. Intratracheal administration of roflumilast to rats has also been shown to reverse antigen-induced reduction in forced vital capacity (FVC) (Chapman et al., 2007). The therapeutic use of PDE4 inhibitors in IPF may be, however, limited by their emetic effects.

A selective cyclooxygenase-2 (COX-2) inhibitor, meloxicam, reduced bleomycin-induced pulmonary fibrosis in mice (Arafa, Abdel-Wahab, El-Shaafeey, Badary, & Hamada, 2007). Since meloxicam also has antioxidant activity, its effect may not be due solely to COX-2 inhibition.

Fabre et al. (2008) studied the role of 5-HT (5-hydroxytryptamine, serotonin) in fibrogenesis and found that both, 5-HT_{2A} (5-hydroxytryptamine receptor, subtype 2A) or 5-HT_{2B} (5-hydroxytryptamine receptor, subtype 2B) receptor antagonists, reduced bleomycin-induced fibrosis in mice. These agents reduced lung messenger ribonucleic acid (mRNA) levels of transforming growth factor $TGF_{\beta 1}$, CTGF, and plasminogen activator inhibitor-1. It had been previously reported that 5-HT induces TGF_β mRNA in rat mesangial cells through the 5-HT_{2A} receptor subtype (Grewal, Mukhin, Garnovskaya, Raymond, & Greene, 1999).

According to Yildirim et al. (2006), melatonin at 4 mg/kg/day for 16 days reduces the fibrosis score and prevents an increase in lung hydroxyproline content of rats with bleomycin-induced pulmonary fibrosis. This effect is associated with the reduction in lung catalase activity, but not superoxide dismutase or GT peroxidase activities. These findings suggest that melatonin may prevent pulmonary fibrosis by reducing protein and lipid peroxidation.

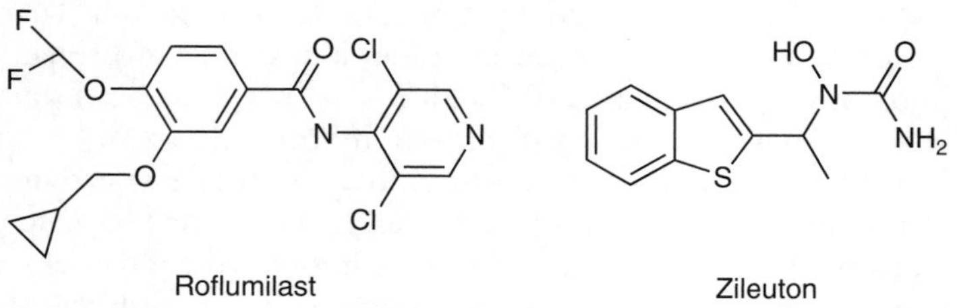

Roflumilast   Zileuton

FIGURE 5 Chemical structures of putative antifibrotics, PDE4 inhibitor roflumilast, and 5-lipoxygenase inhibitor, zileuton.

Borie et al. (2008) studied the antifibrotic effects of pasireotide (SOM230), a new somatostatin analog. Pasireotide reduces lung collagen content, as well as TGF_β and CTGF mRNA in mice with bleomycin-induced fibrosis and reduces α-1 collagen-1 mRNA expression in TGF_β-stimulated human fibroblasts.

The renin–angiotesin system has been implicated in fibrogenesis (Border & Noble, 2001) and the antifibrotic effects of angiotensin II receptor antagonists and of angiotensin-converting enzyme inhibitors in animals have been described (Molteni et al., 2000; Wang, Ibarra-Sunga, Verlinski, Pick, & Uhal, 2000). Intratracheally administered antisense oligonucleotides against angiotensinogen mRNA alleviates bleomycin-induced pulmonary fibrosis in mice (Li et al., 2007). Retrospective analysis of survival of IPF patients treated with angiotensin converting inhibitors revealed, however, no difference in survival between them and those IPF subjects not receiving these inhibitors (Nadrous, Ryu, Douglas, Decker, & Olson, 2004).

Pharmacological inhibition of leukotrienes with either the 5-lipoxygenase inhibitor zileuton {N-(1-benzo[b]thien-2-ylethyl)-N-hydroxyurea} (Fig. 5) or the $cysLT_1$ (leukotriene receptor-1) receptor antagonist MK-571 (3-(3-(2-(7-quinolyl) phenyl(3-dimethyl amino-3 oxopropyl) thio) methyl)thio) propanoic acid reduces bleomycin-induced pulmonary fibrosis in mice (Failla et al., 2006). These findings support the role of leukotrienes in fibrogenesis and provide another target for antifibrotic drugs. A phase II clinical trial with zileuton in IPF patients has been initiated at the University of Michigan.

Since many cytokines require copper for their activity, tetrathiomolybdate, a copper-binding molecule, has been evaluated and found to reduce bleomycin-induced fibrosis in mice (Brewer, Dick, Ullenbruch, Jin, & Phan, 2004).

A TGF_β-neutralizing antibody, GC-1008 (human anti-TGF_β monoclonal antibody), was designed to interact with all three TGF_β isoforms and is currently being tested in patients with either cancer or IPF (Grutter et al., 2008).

The potential role for protein kinase inhibitors in the therapy of fibrotic disorders was recently reviewed by Garneau-Tsodikova and Thannickal (2008). Because inhibitors of focal adhesion kinase and of protein kinase B/phosphoinositide 3-kinase (PKB/AKT) reduce the resistance of myofibroblasts to apoptosis they display antifibrotic activity.

Antiproliferative kinase inhibitors with appropriate selectivity could have utility in the therapy of fibrotic diseases. A systematic pharmacological study of prototype kinase inhibitors might be informative and could provide a specific mechanistic approach to the development of antifibrotic drugs. If the selective inhibition of an isoform of p38 mitogen-activated protein kinase (MAPK) by pirfenidone is confirmed, inhibitors of the p38 MAPK pathway (Xing et al., 2009; Zhang, Shen, & Lin, 2007) can be tested as candidates for new antifibrotic agents.

D. Clinical Studies

Anticoagulants, such as warfarin or heparin added to prednisolone, were reported to increase the 1-year survival rate of patients with IPF (Kubo et al., 2005). However, this finding was questioned by Nagai, Handa, and Kim (2008).

In laboratory studies IFNγ-1b has been shown to inhibit collagen synthesis, reduce the expression of profibrotic cytokines, and inhibit fibroblast proliferation (Eickelberg et al., 2001; Narayanan, Whitney, Souza, & Raghu, 1992). During the last decade, clinical studies with IFNγ-1b in patients with IPF produced some favorable, but largely negative, results (Antoniou et al., 2005, 2006, 2008; Nagai et al., 2008; Raghu, 2006; Raghu et al., 2004; Ziesche, Hofbauer, Wittmann, Petkov, & Block, 1999).

The results of a large multicenter, randomized, placebo-controlled trial of IFNγ-1b in patients with IPF (INternational study of Survival outcomes in idiopathic Pulmonary fibrosis with InterRfErone gamma-1b, INSPIRE) were recently published (King et al., 2009). The trial included 826 patients in 81 centers in North America and seven European countries. The majority of patients (551) received IFNγ-1b for the first 2 weeks at 100 μg b.i.d. twice a week and subsequently at 200 μg, t.i.d., s.c. Other patients received placebo. The primary end point was survival. The trial was discontinued after the second interim analysis (median duration of treatment = 64 weeks) as it did not demonstrate efficacy. The mortality rate was 15% in drug-treated and 13% in placebo-treated patients. Development of this drug for IPF has been suspended.

Colchicine was reported to inhibit fibroblast proliferation and collagen synthesis in a human fibroblast cell line (Entzian et al., 1997) and to decrease expression of TGFβ in the lung tissue of patients with IPF (Tzortzaki et al., 2007). In a group of 10 IPF patients, colchicine (0.6 mg/day for 12 weeks) decreased the dyspnea index and produced selective improvements in CT scans (Addrizzio-Harris et al., 2002). However, it was ineffective in a trial with 167 patients (Douglas, Ryu, & Schroeder, 2000) and in 30 patients with mild to moderate IPF (Fiorucci et al., 2008).

Imatinib (Gleevec®) is an inhibitor of *bcr-abl* tyrosine kinase with antineoplastic activity. It also inhibits platelet-derived growth factor (PDGF), vascular endothelial growth factor, and basic fibroblast growth factor (bFGF). It is approved for the treatment of chronic myeloid leukemia, gastrointestinal (GI) stromal tumors, and is under clinical evaluation as a treatment for many other cancers (Buchdunger, O'Reilly, & Wood, 2002). Since PDGF signaling is reported to be involved in fibrogenesis (Abdollahi et al., 2005), and imatinib prevents bleomycin-induced pulmonary fibrosis in mice

(Aono et al., 2005), it was tested and found to be effective in a few patients with scleroderma-associated pulmonary fibrosis (Distler & Distler, 2009). Dasatinib and nilotinib are two other tyrosine kinase inhibitors with PDGF inhibitory properties that have been shown to display antifibrotic effects *in vitro* and *in vivo* (Akhmetshina et al., 2008). However, reports of imatinib-induced pneumonitis (Yamasawa, Sugiyama, Y., Bando, M., & Ohnol, S., 2008) may limit its usefulness in IPF.

Etanercept (Enbrel®) is a soluble TNF_α receptor that acts as a TNF_α carrier, blocking its action. It is widely used clinically in the treatment of rheumatoid arthritis, polyarthritis, and psoriasis. Etanercept prevents bleomycin-induced pulmonary fibrosis in mice and reduces lung collagen content after bleomycin treatment (Piguet & Vesin, 1994). It was tested in 88 patients with clinically progressive IPF (Jackson & Fell, 2008; Raghu et al., 2008). At 25 mg, s.c., twice a week for 48 weeks, etanercept produced no significant effects on efficacy end points (PFTs), but appeared to slow disease progression. Another trial based on mortality as an end point was recommended and one is now in progress (www.ClinicalTrials.gov). Reports on etanercept causing fatal fibrosing alveolitis or pulmonary fibrosis are, however, likely to complicate its further evaluation in patients with pulmonary diseases (Diez Pina et al., 2008; Tengstrand, Ernestam, Engvall, Rydvald, & Hafstrom, 2005).

V. Pirfenidone

Pirfenidone (Fig 6), a synthetic small molecule with antifibrotic properties, is approved in Japan for the treatment of IPF. Pirfenidone has been investigated in various models of fibrosis as well as in human fibrotic diseases.

A. Pharmacology

Multiple mechanisms of action have been investigated for pirfenidone, including inhibition of TGF_β-stimulated collagen synthesis (Card, Racz,

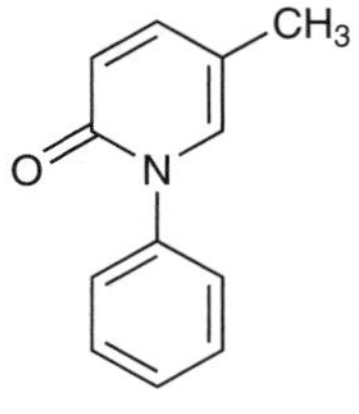

FIGURE 6   Chemical structure of pirfenidone.

Brien, Margolin, & Massey, 2003), suppression of proinflammatory cyto-kines, and inhibition of fibroblast proliferation (Cain et al., 1998, Guru-jeyalakshmi, Hollinger, & Giri, 1999). Recent experiments raise the possibility that pirfenidone acts as a superoxide scavenger in complex with iron (Mitani et al., 2008). As a primary molecular target for pirfenidone has not been identified, chemical optimization with increased potency and selectivity has yet to be described.

The antifibrotic effects of pirfenidone have been examined in animal models such as rat hepatic cirrhosis (Salazar-Montes, Ruiz-Corro, López-Reyes, Castrejón-Gómez, & Armendáriz-Borunda, 2008), rodent models of renal disease (Cho, Smith, Branton, Penzak, & Kopp, 2007), mouse cyclophosphamide-induced lung fibrosis (Kehrer & Margolin, 1997), and hamster bleomycin-induced lung fibrosis (Iyer, Margolin, Hyde, & Giri, 1998; Iyer et al., 1995). The rodent lung disease systems are probably better models for environmentally induced pulmonary fibrosis than IPF, but positive results lend support to proceeding with human clinical trials.

Increased collagen synthesis in the bleomycin hamster model of lung fibrosis involves overexpression of gene products for procollagen, TGF_{β}, and fibronectin (Raghow, Lurie, Seyer, & Kang, 1985). Iyer and colleagues examined the effects of pirfenidone on gene expression in this model (Iyer et al., 1999a, 1999b) and found that pirfenidone (at 0.5% in food) decreased bleomycin-induced inflammation, overexpression of procollagen I and III genes, and an increase in TGF_{β} gene transcription. These results suggest that pirfenidone has multiple effects, including anti-inflammatory activity, free radical scavenging, and modulation of gene expression.

The *in vivo* anti-inflammatory actions of pirfenidone were also demon-strated in the endotoxic shock model (Cain et al., 1998), where it displays both prophylactic and therapeutic effects (Oku, Nakazato, Horikawa, Tsuruta, & Suzuki, 2002). Liver TGF_{β} is elevated by i.p. injection of lipopolysaccharide and D-galactosamine, but p.o. administration of 500 mg/kg pirfenidone 5 min before or 4 h after challenge significantly blunted the action of these substances. Pirfenidone significantly suppresses serum TNF_{α}, interleukin (IL)-12, and $IFN\gamma$, but markedly enhances IL-10 levels when administered 5 min prior to endotoxin challenge. Murine macrophages (line RAW264.7) express TNF_{α} when exposed to lipopolysac-charide *in vitro*. This effect is suppressed at the translational level by 1.6 mM pirfenidone (Nakazato, Oku, Yamane, Tsuruta, & Suzuki, 2002).

The expression of heat shock protein (HSP) 47, a collagen-specific chaperone, is upregulated in mice by bleomycin. Kakugawa et al. (2004) showed that pirfenidone treatment of such animals reduced the increase in histologic lung fibrosis score, normalized the increase in lung hydro-xyproline content, and reduced F4/80 macrophage numbers in the lung, the overexpression of α-smooth muscle actin, and the overexpression of HSP47.

To examine the relevance of these molecular changes to human IPF, Kakugawa et al. (2005) examined surgical lung biopsy material from patients with idiopathic UIP, cardiovascular disease (CVD)-associated UIP, and idiopathic nonspecific interstitial pneumonia (NSIP). The expression level of HSP47 in type II pneumocytes from patients with idiopathic UIP was significantly higher than that found with CVD-associated UIP and idiopathic NSIP. The expression of HSP47 in fibroblasts was significantly higher in idiopathic UIP and idiopathic NSIP than in CVD-associated UIP. The expression of type I procollagen in type II pneumocytes was significantly higher in idiopathic UIP than in idiopathic NSIP, and the expression of alpha-SMA in fibroblasts was significantly higher in idiopathic UIP than in idiopathic NSIP. These data from human ILD tissue suggest that the cell and animal models may have relevance to human IPF, and that the changes induced by pirfenidone may have positive effects in the management of pulmonary disease.

When cultured normal human lung fibroblasts (NHLF) are stimulated with $TGF_{\beta 1}$ there is an increase in mRNA and protein levels of HSP47 and collagen type I (Nakayama et al., 2008). These effects are reduced in a dose-dependent manner by pirfenidone, with an IC_{50} for the transcriptional changes of approximately 0.5 mg/ml (3 mM). Though the free drug concentration in culture is certainly less, the high concentration required for $TGF_{\beta 1}$ functional antagonism raises a question about the specificity of pirfenidone action.

Similar effects have been observed in a rat model of chemically induced liver fibrosis (Di Sario et al., 2004). Induction of fibrosis with dimethylnitrosamine (DMN) results in increased mRNA levels of $TGF_{\beta 1}$, procollagen I and several other products, with pirfenidone reducing these increases and lowering collagen deposition.

According to a press release placed online (http://www.redorbit.com/news/496688) on May 8, 2006, InterMune scientists identified the principal mechanisms of action of pirfenidone as selective inhibition of an isoform of p38 gamma kinase and attenuation of TGF_{β}—induced collagen synthesis.

Oku et al. (2008) compared the antifibrotic action of pirfenidone (30 or 100 mg/kg/day p.o., t.i.d.) with that of prednisolone (3 or 15 mg/kg/day p.o., q.d. (every day)) in mice with bleomycin-induced fibrosis. Both drugs were administered daily for approximately 30 days. Only pirfenidone inhibited fibrosis and suppressed the increases in pulmonary levels of bFGF, $TGF_{\beta 1}$, stromal cell-derived factor 1α (SDF-1$_\alpha$), IL-18 and IFNγ, while both drugs attenuated increases in IL$_{1\beta}$, IL-6, monocyte chemotactic protein (MCP)-1, and IL-12p40 (subunit of interleukin-12). These findings suggest that in bleomycin-treated mice, pirfenidone at this dose has broad spectrum anti-inflammatory and antifibrotic actions.

B. Clinical Studies

The cellular and *in vivo* effects of pirfenidone in laboratory animals set the stage for trials to test its antifibrotic actions in human IPF. The pharmacokinetic (PK) properties of pirfenidone were studied in older healthy adults (Rubino, Bhavnani, Ambrose, Forrest, & Loutit, 2009). A dose of 801 mg t.i.d. was the maximum used in recent phase III efficacy/safety trials. Rubino et al. (2009) examined single dose PK at this dose, as well as the effect of food and antacid on drug exposure. In fasted subjects the maximal plasma concentration of pirfenidone was attained within 0.5 h, while in fed individuals this occurred in 3.0–3.5 h. Approximately 80% of the drug (or metabolite) was accounted for in urine. The estimates for the terminal elimination half-life of pirfenidone ranged between 2.4 and 2.9 h, and the median maximum concentration of the drug in the fasted state was approximately twice that in the fed state. Food resulted in a slight but significant decrease in the AUC (area under the concentration–time curve). Since GI side effects correlated with C_{max} (maximal drug concentration), the authors suggest that administration of pirfenidone with food could minimize the adverse effects with minor loss of total drug exposure.

Several pilot clinical trials tested pirfenidone in human fibrotic diseases, including advanced liver fibrosis (Armendariz-Borunda et al., 2006), secondary progressive multiple sclerosis (Walker, Giri, & Margolin, 2005), and focal segmental glomerulosclerosis (Cho et al., 2007). The largest trials, however, were performed in patients with IPF.

Based on encouraging results from open label trials (Nagai et al., 2002; Nicod, 1999; Raghu, Johnson, Lockhart, & Mageto, 1999), a placebo-controlled prospective random control trial of pirfenidone was performed in patients with IPF (Azuma et al., 2005). A probable or definite HRCT diagnosis with typical clinical features was required for entry. These features included bibasilar inspiratory crackles, abnormal PFTs, and increased serum levels of KL-6, and the surfactant proteins A (SP-A) and D (SP-D). Additionally, patients had adequate oxygenation at rest and an SpO_2 (oxygen saturation, measured by oximeter) of 90% or less during exertion while breathing air within 1 month before enrollment. The primary end point was the change in the lowest SpO_2 during a 6-min walk test (6-MWT). Patients were randomized at a ratio of 2:1, pirfenidone: placebo. A total of 107 patients were evaluated for efficacy. The pirfenidone dose was gradually increased to 600 mg t.i.d.

The trial was terminated by the safety monitoring board after 9 months because of an imbalanced occurrence of AEs, with 5 AEs in the 35 patients in the placebo arm and no AEs in the 75 patients in the pirfenidone arm. Since the study was terminated prior to the planned 1 year, the primary efficacy end point was not evaluable. When the 80 patients in both groups who completed the 6-MWT were compared to each other instead of baseline, there was a significant difference at both 6 and 9 months ($p = 0.0069$ and 0.0305, respectively).

At 9 months, more patients in the pirfenidone group experienced increases in SpO_2 and FVC, while fewer in that group experienced declines in these two parameters. While the positive trends in these secondary end points are encouraging, they can serve only as hypothesis generating because of the unusual circumstances of the trial. Despite these changes, neither dyspnea nor the quality of life was affected by the study medication, and there were no significant changes in serum SP-D or KL-6 measurements between groups.

A follow-up, phase III, double-blind, placebo-controlled clinical study of pirfenidone by Shionogi was reported on the company web site (www. shionogi.co.jp). The study was comprised of pirfenidone groups and a placebo arm (1,800 mg pirfenidone, 108 patients; 1,200 mg pirfenidone, 55 patients; placebo, 104 patients). The primary end point was change in FVC, and there were several secondary end points: progression-free survival (disease progression defined as death or more than 10% decrease in VC) and change of lowest SpO_2 from baseline to 1 year. Although both treatment groups had less loss of FVC than the placebo group (each $p = 0.04$), the SpO_2 changes were not significant. The high-dose group had better progression-free survival than the placebo group ($p = 0.03$), but the low-dose group did not differ significantly from the placebo group ($p = 0.065$).

It is possible that with a different dosing scheme and with more patients the significance of the findings would be increased.

CAPACITY 1 and CAPACITY 2 were two phase III international randomized placebo-controlled clinical trials of pirfenidone in IPF patients. Although the data have not been published, partial results have been released on the sponsor's web site (www.intermune.com) and have been presented at the 2009 American Thoracic Society meeting (Noble et al., 2009). A total of 779 patients participated. In CAPACITY 1, 344 patients were randomized at 1:1 to receive either 2,403 mg pirfenidone per day or placebo. In CAPACITY 2, 435 patients were randomized at 2:1:2 to receive either 2403 mg/day or 1197 mg/day of pirfenidone, or placebo. The study completion rate was similar in all groups, ranging from 92 to 95%. The treatment completion rates were 82–85% in the pirfenidone groups, and 90% in both placebo groups. The primary end point of both CAPACITY studies was change in percent predicted FVC after 72 weeks of treatment, evaluated with a nonparametric rank ANCOVA. In the CAPACITY 2 study, the primary end point was met ($p = 0.001$), whereas it was not in CAPACITY 1 ($p = 0.501$). An exploratory analysis of pooled primary end point data from both studies resulted in a p-value of 0.005. The change in percent predicted FVC for the placebo and 2,403 mg groups is shown in Table VI. The change in the pirfenidone arms is the same in CAPACITY 1 and

TABLE VI Change in Percent Predicted Forced Vital Capacity at Study (CAPACITY 1 or 2) Conclusion (72 Weeks) and at the Half-Way Point

| | CAPACITY 1 | | | CAPACITY 2 | | |
	Pirfenidone N = 171	Placebo N = 173	p-value	Pirfenidone N = 174	Placebo N = 174	p-value
Week 36	−1.91	−3.86	0.011	−2.25	−5.30	<0.001
Week 72	−6.49	−7.23	0.501	−6.49	−9.55	0.001

N, number of patients; dose of pirfenidone = 2,403 mg/day; adapted from InterMune web site.

CAPACITY 2 (–6.45%), while the change in the placebo arms are different (–7.23 and –9.55%, respectively).

The major adverse events (an incidence ≥1.5 times in the pirfenidone groups versus the placebo groups) were GI (nausea, dyspepsia, vomiting) and skin (photosensitivity, rash) reactions. The low pirfenidone dose group was reported to have fewer side effects than the high-dose group. Though there were discordant results in the CAPACITY studies, the results suggest that this agent may be effective in the treatment of IPF.

VI. Gene Therapy

During the last 20 years, many attempts were made to use gene therapy in experimental pulmonary fibrosis. For example, bleomycin does not cause fibrosis in transgenic mice deficient in murine plasminogen activator inhibitor-1 (PAI-1) (Eitzman et al., 1996). Sisson, Hattori, Xu, & Simon (1999) found that bleomycin-induced fibrosis can be successfully treated in mice by the adenovirus-mediated transfer of urokinase-type plasminogen activator (uPA) gene to the lungs. Intratracheal transfer of Smad7 (signal transducing transcriptional protein 7, antagonist of TGFβ signaling), but not of Smad6 gene, prevents bleomycin-induced pulmonary fibrosis in mice (Nakao et al., 1999). According to Kapoor (2008), the potential applications of Smad7 gene therapy are promising. Cyclin-dependent kinase inhibitor p21 is known to prevent apoptosis. Inoshima et al. (2004) used, therefore, adenoviral transfer of human p21 gene to reduce bleomycin-induced fibrosis in mice. The IL-10 gene has been found to suppress production and activation of TGFβ in the lungs of mice even if delivered after fibrosis is established (Nakagome et al., 2006). According to Kijiyama et al. (2006), intratracheal transfer of tissue factor pathway inhibitor gene inhibits bleomycin-induced fibrosis in rats. Attempts to regulate TGFβ1-induced collagen gene expression were reviewed by Cutroneo, White, Phan, and Ehrlich (2006).

The first candidate gene for IPF (ELMOD2) was identified by Hodgson et al. (2006). Decreased levels of ELMOD2 mRNA were found in six cases of sporadic IPF by the same investigators. Yang et al. (2007) profiled RNA from lungs of patients with sporadic and familial interstitial pneumonias and identified transcriptional differences. The evidence for genetic predisposition to infiltrative lung diseases was reviewed by Steele and Brown (2007).

Transfection of a soluble TGF type II receptor gene into the skeletal muscle either before or after bleomycin attenuates pulmonary fibrosis in mice (Yamada et al., 2007).

Silencing of connective tissue factor (CTGF) gene by a small interfering ribonucleic acid (siRNA)-expressing plasmid decreases differentiation of myofibroblasts and deposition of extracellular matrix proteins in human lung fibroblasts culture (Lin et al., 2008). According to Griesenbach and Alton (2009), gene transfer to the airway epithelial cells has many obstacles. For example, the viral gene transfer agents stimulate immunity and are, therefore, not suitable for the therapy of chronic diseases. Clinical trials with nonviral vectors are now in progress.

VII. Conclusion

During the last decade, extensive research has been conducted on IPF and therapeutic approaches to treat this condition. New targets for drug development, as well as new leads, were identified. However, there are still no Food and Drug Administration-approved drugs for treating this condition.

There have been several barriers to developing effective therapeutics for IPF. One is the fact that IPF is considered an orphan disease because of its prevalence, lessening the urgency for finding a cure. Because the population in developed countries is rapidly aging, IPF is becoming a more common disorder. It is anticipated that companies will begin to look more favorably on drug development in this area as it is becoming apparent that fibrotic diseases as a group may share the same therapeutic targets. In this case, drugs developed for the treatment of pulmonary fibrosis may be useful in the therapy of renal, myocardial, hepatic, and other fibrotic diseases as well, broadening the use of such agents.

The complexity of fibrogenesis and the multiplicity of profibrotic and antifibrotic factors are other reasons for the failure to develop effective drugs. With the advancement of basic research in fibrosis many new targets for drug development have been discovered. However, these discoveries have yet to be translated through to drug discovery and clinical testing. In addition, the consolidation of the pharmaceutical industry has resulted in more focused research programs and less enthusiasm for undertaking higher risk projects that lack "proof of concept."

There is also a justifiable skepticism about the relevance of the *in vitro* or animal research methodology that is currently used in drug discovery. The findings of cell culture experiments are not always applicable to the whole organism, and results obtained in mice or rats may not be relevant to humans. Although the bleomycin-induced fibrosis in rodents test tends to identify false positive leads, it might be relevant for early stage IPF. Animal models are often more sensitive than patients in clinical trials, as experimental animals are homogenous in genetic background, sex, age, weight, general health, and diet. Compounds which are safe and effective at reasonable doses in a "therapeutic" protocol of bleomycin-induced fibrosis should be considered for optimization and eventual clinical evaluation.

Lack of patentability, toxicity, ignorance of the molecular target, or questionable "drugability" of potential antifibrotic drugs are common barriers to their development. In today's highly competitive environment, few companies are willing to pay for the development of a generic agent like NAC for the treatment of IPF without proprietary protection. Also, some of the drugs identified as antifibrotics belong to chemical classes known for their toxicity, extensive metabolism, or poor bioavailability and, therefore, are not considered good candidates for development.

It is conceivable that a blockade of only one profibrotic factor cannot stop or reverse fibrogenesis. A drug combination product designed to affect multiple fibrogenic pathways may be required for the effective therapy of IPF. It is also recognized that TGFβ and other profibrotic cytokines have many critical biological functions, such that their complete blockade could have serious adverse effects. The fact that pirfenidone, one of the few promising drugs, attenuates, rather than completely inhibits, the activity of numerous profibrotic factors, supports the concept of a broad-spectrum approach to antifibrotic therapy.

Another strategy is to search for drugs to enhance resolution of fibrosis. It has been shown that experimental hepatic fibrosis in rodents can be resolved by drugs (Iredale et al., 1998; Mitchell et al., 2009; Tang, Yang, & Li, 2009; Tsai et al., 2008), and that myocardial fibrosis in a transgenic rabbit model of cardiomyopathy is completely reversed by NAC (Lombardi et al., 2009). The reversibility of pulmonary fibrosis is a controversial subject. It has been suggested that in pulmonary fibrosis the loss of basement membrane, and consequently of normal lung architecture, establishes the point of no return (Strieter, 2008). Perhaps at earlier stages of the disease pulmonary fibrosis is reversible. Unfortunately, the mechanism of resolution of fibrosis is poorly understood and only a few approaches for the development of fibrolytic targets have been identified. Expression of TIMPs is decreased, while apoptosis of activated hepatic stellate cells is increased during recovery from hepatic fibrosis (Iredale et al., 1998; Issa et al., 2001). Drugs could conceivably facilitate these events. Blockade of $\alpha_v\beta_3$ integrin, stimulation of apoptosis of myofibroblasts by M1 macrophages, or of conversion of M2 to M1 macrophages, may enhance resolution of fibrosis (Zhou et al., 2004; Lupher & Gallatin, 2006).

A better understanding of fibrogenesis and fibrolysis will greatly facilitate discovery and development of new antifibrotic drugs. Based on past experience, many more years are needed to advance the knowledge base of this field to a level adequate for successful design and development of drugs capable to selectively modifying fibrosis in humans. In the interim, available leads should be optimized on the basis of their activity in mice with bleomycin-induced fibrosis or a similar model. If the end point of a clinical trial is mortality, the same end point should be used in an animal model.

There is also an urgent need for better biomarkers for use in clinical trials. The duration of trials of drugs for treating IPF can be substantially reduced in time and cost if mortality is replaced by an end point based on a meaningful biomarker.

Preclinical and clinical studies with pirfenidone and NAC in pulmonary fibrosis reviewed in this article revealed major delays in the development of these drugs. The antifibrotic effectiveness of pirfenidone in animals has been known for 14 years (Iyer et al., 1995) and in humans for 10 years (Nicod, 1999), while the safety of NAC in patients with pulmonary fibrosis was reported 15 years ago (Meyer et al., 1994). As of today (September 2009) these drugs are not yet available for the therapy of IPF in the United States.

Acknowledgments

The authors are grateful to Robert Homer, MD, Ph.D., Professor of Pathology and Medicine, Yale University School of Medicine, New Haven, CT for providing Fig. 1 and to Mrs. Barbara Botti, Cheshire, CT for preparation of Figs. 2–5.

Conflict of Interest: Alexander Scriabine, MD has no conflict of interest. Daniel U. Rabin, Ph.D. is an employee of the France Foundation, sponsor of the PILOT™ Continuing Medical Education Initiative. InterMune® (a biopharmaceutical company focused on development of innovative therapy in pulmonology and hepatology) is the commercial supporter of PILOT™.

References

Abdollahi, A., Li, M., Ping, G., Plathow, C., Domhan, S., Kiessling, F., et al. (2005). Inhibition of platelet-derived growth factor attenuates pulmonary fibrosis. *Journal of Experimental Medicine, 201,* 925–935.

Abraham, D. (2008). Role of endothelin in lung fibrosis. *European Respiratory Review*, *17*, 145–150.

Acharaya, P. S., Majumdar, S., Jacob, M., Hayden, J., Mrass, P., Weninger, W., et al. (2008). Fibroblast migration is mediated by CD-44-dependent TGFβ activation. *Journal of Cell Science*, *121*, 1393–1402.

Adamson, I. Y., & Bowden, D. H. (1974). The pathogenesis of bleomycin-induced pulmonary fibrosis in mice. *American Journal of Pathology*, *77*, 185–197.

Addrizzio-Harris, D. J., Harkin, T. J., Tchou-Wong, K. M., McGuiness, G., Goldberg, G., Cheng, D., et al. (2002). Mechanism of colchicine's effect in the treatment of asbestosis and idiopathic pulmonary fibrosis. *Lung*, *180*, 61–72.

Akgun, M., Araz, O., Akkurt, I., Eroglu, A., Alper, F., Saglam, F., et al. (2008). An epidemic of silicosis among denim sandblasters. *European Respiratory Journal*, *32*, 1295–1303.

Akhmetshina, A., Dees, C., Pileckyte, M., Maurer, B., Axmann, R., Jungel, A., et al. (2008). Dual inhibition of c-abl and PDGF receptor signaling by disatinib and nilotinib for the treatment of dermal fibrosis. *The FASEB Journal*, *22*, 2214–2222.

Alder, J. K., Chen, J. J., Lancaster, L., Danoff, S., Su, S. C., Cogan, J. D., et al. (2008). Short telomeres are a risk factor for idiopathic pulmonary fibrosis. *Proceedings of the National Academy of Sciences, USA*, *105*, 13051–13056.

Ankermann, T., Claviez, A., Wagner, H. J., Krams, M., & Riedel, F. (2003). Chronic interstitial lung disease with lung fibrosis in a girl: Uncommon sequelae of Epstein-Barr virus infection. *Pediatric Pulmonology*, *35*, 234–238.

Antoniou, K. M., Nicholson, A. G., Dimadi, M., Malagari, K., Latsi, P., Rapti, A., et al. (2006), Long-term clinical effects of interferon-gamma-1b and colchicine in pulmonary fibrosis. *European Respiratory Journal*, *28*, 496–504.

Antoniou, K. M., Tzortzaki, E. G., Alexandrakis, M. G., Zervou, M., Tzanakis, N., Sfiridaki, K., et al. (2005). Investigations of IL-18 and IL-12 in induced sputum of patients with IPF before and after treatment with interferon gamma-1b. *Sarcoidosis Vasculitis & Diffuse Lung Diseases*, *22*, 204–209.

Antoniou, K. M., Tzanakis, N., Tzortzaki, E. G., Malagari, K., Koutsopoulos, A. V., Alexandrakis, M., et al. (2008). Different angiogenic CXC chemokine levels in bronchoalveolar lavage fluid after interferon gamma-1b therapy in idiopathic pulmonary fibrosis patients. *Pulmonary Pharmacology & Therapeutics*, *21*, 840–844.

Aono, Y., Nishioka, Y., Inayama, M., Ygai, M., Kishi, J., Uehara, H., et al. (2005). Imatinib as a novel antifibrotic agent in bleomycin-induced pulmonary fibrosis in mice. *American Journal of Respiratory and Critical Care Medicine*, *171*, 1279–1285.

Arafa, H. M. M., Abdel-Wahab, M. H., El-Shaafeey, M. F., Badary, O. A., & Hamada, F. M. (2007). Anti-fibrotic effect of meloxicam in a murine lung fibrosis model. *European Journal of Pharmacology*, *564*, 181–189.

Armanios, M. Y., Chen, J. J., Cogan, J. D., Alder, R. J., Ingersoll, R. G., Markin, C., et al. (2007). Telomerase mutations in families with idiopathic pulmonary fibrosis. *New England Journal of Medicine*, *356*, 1317–1326.

Armendariz-Borunda, J., Islas-Carbajal, M. C., Meza-Garcia, E., Rincon, A. R., Lucano, S., Sandoval, A. S., et al. (2006). A pilot study in patients with established advanced liver fibrosis using pirfenidone. *Gut*, *55*, 1663–1665.

Ask, K., Labiris, R., Farkas, L., Moeller, A., Froese, A., Farncombe, T., et al. (2008). Comparison between conventional and "clinical" assessment of lung fibrosis. *Journal of Translational Medicine*, *6*, 16.

ATS/ERS (2002). International multidisciplinary consensus classification of the idiopathic interstitial pneumonias. *American Journal of Respiratory and Critical Care Medicine*, *165*, 277–304.

Azuma, A., Nukiwa, T., Tsuboi, E., Suga, M., Abe, S., Nakata, K., et al. (2005). Double-blind, placebo-controlled trial of pirfenidone in patients with idiopathic pulmonary fibrosis. *American Journal of Respiratory and Critical Care Medicine*, *171*, 1040–1047.

Baker, K., Marcus, C. B., Huffman, K., Kruk, H., Malfroy, B., & Doctorow, S. R. (1998). Synthetic combined superoxide dismutase/catalase mimetics are protective as a delayed treatment in a rat stroke model: A key role for reactive oxygen species in ischemic brain injury. *Journal of Pharmacology and Experimental Therapeutics, 284,* 215–221.

Barst, R. J., Langleben, D., Badesh, D., Frost, A., Lawrence, E. C., Shapiro, S., et al. (2006). Treatment of pulmonary arterial hypertension with the selective endothelin-A receptor antagonist, sitaxsentan. *Journal of the American College of Cardiology, 47,* 2049–2056.

Barst, R. J., Langleben, D., Frost, A., Horn, E. M., Oudiz, R., Shapiro, S., et al. (2004). Sitaxsentan therapy for pulmonary arterial hypertension. *American Journal of Respiratory and Critical Care Medicine, 169,* 441–447.

Beeh, K. M., Beier, J., Haas, I. C., Kornmann, O., Micke, B., & Buhl, R. (2002). Glutathione deficiency of the lower respiratory tract in patients with idiopathic pulmonary fibrosis. *European Respiratory Journal, 19,* 1119–1123.

Behr, J., Maier, K., Degenkolb, B., Krombach, F., & Vogelmeier, C. (1997). Antioxidative and clinical effects of high-dose N-acetylcysteine in fibrosing alveolitis. Adjunctive therapy to maintenance immunosuppression. *American Journal of Respiratory and Critical Care Medicine, 156,* 1897–1901.

Behr, J., & Thannickal, V. J. (2009). Update in diffuse parenchymal lung disease 2008. *American Journal of Respiratory and Critical Care Medicine, 179,* 439–444.

Biswas, S. K., McClure, D., Jimenez, L. A., Megson, I. L., & Rahman, I. (2005). Curcumin induces glutathione biosynthesis and inhibits NF-kappaB activation and interleukin-8 release in alveolar epithelial cells: Mechanism of free radical scavenging activity. *Antioxidants & Redox Signaling, 7,* 32–41.

Blasco, M. A. (2007). Telomere length, stem cells and aging. *Nature Chemical Biology, 3,* 640–649.

Boon, K., Bailey, N. W., Yang, J., Steele, M. P., Groshong, S., Kervitsky, D., et al. (2009). Molecular phenotypes distinguish patients with relatively stable from progressive idiopathic pulmonary fibrosis (IPF). *PLoS one, 4,* e5134 [Electronic Resource].

Border, W. A., & Noble, P. W. (2001). Maximizing hemodynamic-independent effects of angiotensin II antagonists in fibrotic diseases. *Seminars in Nephrology, 21,* 563–572.

Borie, R., Fabre, A., Prost, F., Marchal-Somme, J., Lebtahi, R., Marchand-Adam, S., et al. (2008). Activation of somatostatin receptors attenuates pulmonary fibrosis. *Thorax, 63,* 251–258.

Borok, Z. (2009). Role of alpha-3-integrin in EMT and pulmonary fibrosis. *Journal of Clinical Investigation, 119,* 7–10.

Bowler, R. P., Barnes, P. J., & Crapo, J. D. (2004). The role of oxidative stress in chronic obstructive pulmonary disease. *Journal of Chronic Obstructive Pulmonary Disease, 1,* 255–277.

Brash, F. (2006). Interstitielle Lungenerkrankungen. *Pathologie, 27,* 116–132.

Brewer, G. J., Dick, R., Ullenbruch, M. R., Jin, H., & Phan, S. H. (2004). Inhibition of cytokines by tetrathiomolybdate in the bleomycin model of pulmonary fibrosis. *Journal of Inorganic Biochemistry, 98,* 2160–2167.

Bridgeman, M. M. E., Marsden, M., Selby, C., Morrison, D., & MacNee, W. (1994). Effect of N-acetyl cysteine on the concentrations of thiols in plasma, bronchoalveolar lavage fluid and lung tissues. *Thorax, 49,* 670–675.

Buchdunger, E., O'Reilly, T., & Wood, J. (2002). Pharmacology of imatinib. *European Journal of Cancer, 38*(Suppl. 5), 528–536.

Cain, W. C., Stuart, R. W., Lefkowitz, D. L., Starnes, J. D., Margolin, S., & Lefkowitz, S. S. (1998). Inhibition of tumor necrosis factor and subsequent endotoxin shock by pirfenidone. *International Journal of Immunopharmacology, 20,* 685–695.

Cantin, A. M., Larivee, B., & Begin, R. O. (1990). Extracellular glutathione suppresses human lung fibroblasts proliferation. *American Journal of Respiratory Cell and Molecular Biology, 3,* 79–85.

Cantin, A. M., North, S. L., Felis, G. A., Hubbard, R. C., & Crystal, R. G. (1987). Oxidant-mediated epithelial cell injury in idiopathic pulmonary fibrosis. *Journal of Clinical Investigation, 79*, 1665–1673.

Cantor, J. O., Osman, M., Cerreta, J. M., Suarez, R., Mandi, I., & Turino, G. M. (1984). Amiodarone-induced pulmonary fibrosis in hamsters. *Experimental Lung Research, 6*, 1–10.

Card, J. W., Racz, W. J., Brien, J. F., Margolin, S. B., & Massey, T. E. (2003). Differential effects of pirfenidone on acute pulmonary injury and ensuing fibrosis in the hamster model of amiodarone-induced pulmonary toxicity. *Toxicological Sciences, 75*, 169–180.

Card, J. W., Racz, W. J., Brien, J. F., & Massey, T. E. (2003). Attenuation of amiodarone-induced pulmonary fibrosis by vitamin E is associated with suppression of transforming growth factor β_1 gene expression but not prevention of mitochondrial dysfunction. *Journal of Pharmacology and Experimental Therapeutics, 304*, 277–283.

Chapman, R. W., House, A., Jones, H., Richard, J., Celly, C., Prelusky, D., et al. (2007). Effect of inhaled roflumilast on the prevention and resolution of allergen-induced late phase airflow obstruction in Brown Norway rats. *European Journal of Pharmacology, 571*, 215–221.

Channick, R. N., Simonneau, G., Sitbon, O., Robbins I. M., Frost, A., Tapson, V. F., et al. (2001). Effects of dual endothelin receptor antagonist bosentan in patients with pulmonary hypertension: A randomized placebo-controlled study. *Lancet, 358*, 1119–1123.

Chen, S. J., Chen, Y. F., Meng, Q. C., Durand, J., Dicarlo, V. S., & Oparil, S. (1995). Endothelin receptor antagonist bosentan prevents and reverses hypoxic pulmonary hypertension in rats. *Journal of Applied Physiology, 79*, 2122–2133.

Cheng, J. W. M. (2008). Ambrisentan for the management of pulmonary arterial hypertension. *Clinical Therapeutics, 30*, 825–833.

Cho, M. E., Smith, D. C., Branton, M. H., Penzak, S. R., & Kopp, J. B. (2007). Pirfenidone slows renal function decline in patients with focal segmental glomerulosclerosis. *Clinical Journal of the American Society of Nephrology, 2*(5), 906–913.

Clozel, M., Breu, V., Gray, G. A., Kalina, B., Löffler, B.-M., Burri, K., et al. (1994). Pharmacological characterization of bosentan, a new potent orally active nonpeptide endothelin receptor antagonist. *Journal of Pharmacology and Experimental Therapeutics, 270*, 228–235.

Clozel, M., & Salloukh, H. (2005). Role of endothelin in fibrosis and anti-fibrotic potential of bosentan. *Annals of Medicine, 37*, 2–12.

ClinicalTrials website (http://www.clinicaltrials.gov/ct2/results?term=etanercept). Assessed August 2009.

Cohen, R. A. C., Patel, A., & Green, F. H. Y. (2008). Lung disease caused by exposure to coal mine and silica dust. *Seminars in Respiratory and Critical Care Medicine, 29*, 651–661.

Cortijo, J., Cerda-Nicolas, M., Serrano, J., Bioque, G., Estrela, J. M., Santangelo, F., et al. (2001). Attenuation by oral N-acetylcysteine of bleomycin-induced lung injury in rats. *European Respiratory Journal, 17*, 1228–1235.

Cortijo, J., Iranzo, A., Milara, X., Mata, M., Cerdá-Nicolás, M., Ruiz-Sauri, A., et al. (2009). Roflumilast, a phosphodiesterase 4 inhibitor, alleviates bleomycin-induced lung injury. *British Journal of Pharmacology, 156*, 534–544.

Cosenzi, A. (2003). Enrasentan, an antagonist of endothelin receptors. *Cardiovascular Drug Reviews, 21*, 1–16.

Croxtall, J. D., & Keam, S. J. (2008). Ambrisentan. *Drugs, 68*, 2195–2204.

Cutroneo, K. R., White, S. L., Phan, S. H., & Ehrlich, H. P. (2006). Therapies for bleomycin-induced lung fibrosis through regulation of $TGF_{\beta1}$ induced collagen gene expression. *Journal of Cellular Physiology, 211*, 585–589.

Cuzzocrea, S., Riley, D. P., Caputi, A. P., & Salvemini, D. (2001a). Antioxidant therapy: A new pharmacological approach in shock, inflammation and ischemia/reperfusion injury. *Pharmacological Reviews, 53*, 135–159.

Cuzzocrea, S., Mazzoni, E., Dugo, L., Caputi, A. P., Aston, K., Riley, D. P., et al. (2001b). Protective effects of a new stable, highly active SOD mimetic, M40401 in splanchnic artery occlusion and reperfusion. *British Journal of Pharmacology, 132,* 19–29.

Day, B. J. (2008). Antioxidants as potential therapeutics for lung fibrosis. *Antioxidants & Redox Signaling, 10,* 355–371.

Del Galdo, F., Lisanti, M. P., & Jimenez, S. A. (2008). Caveolin-1, transforming growth factor-β receptor internalization, and the pathogenesis of systemic sclerosis. *Current Opinion in Rheumatology, 20,* 713–719.

Demedts, M., Behr, J., Buhl, R., Costabel, U., Dekhuijzen, R., Jansen, H. M., et al. (2005). High-dose acetylcysteine in idiopathic pulmonary fibrosis. *New England Journal of Medicine, 353,* 2229–2242.

Di Filippo, C., Cuzzocrea, S., Marfella, R., Fabbroni, V., Scollo, G., Berrino, L., et al. (2004). M40403 prevents myocardial injury by acute hyperglycemia. *European Journal of Pharmacology, 497,* 65–74.

Di Sario, A., Bendia, E., Macarri, G., Candelaresi, C., Taffetani, S., Marzioni, M., et al. (2004). The anti-fibrotic effect of pirfenidone in rat liver fibrosis is mediated by downregulation of procollagen alpha1(I), TIMP-1 and MMP-2. *Digestive and Liver Disease, 36,* 744–751.

Diez Pina, J. M., Vazquez Gomez, O., Mayoralas Alises, S., Garcia Jimenez, J. D., Alvaro Alvarez, D., & Rodriguez Bolado, M. P. (2008). Etanercept as a possible trigger of fatal pulmonary fibrosis [Spanish]. *Archivos de Broncopneumologia, 44,* 393–395.

Ding, Q., Gladson, C. L., Wu, H., Hayasaka, H., & Olman, M. A. (2008). Fokal adhesion kinase (FAK)-related non-kinase inhibits myofibroblast differentiation through different MAPK activation in a FAK-dependent manner. *Journal of Biological Chemistry, 283,* 26839–26849.

Distler, J. H. W., & Distler, O. (2009). Imatinib as a novel therapeutic approach for fibrotic disorders. *Rheumatology, 48,* 2–4.

Douglas, W. W., Ryu, J. H., & Schroeder, D. R. (2000). Idiopathic pulmonary fibrosis: Impact of oxygen and colchicine, prednisolone, or no therapy on survival. *American Journal of Respiratory and Critical Care Medicine, 161,* 1172–1178.

Efert, R., Hasselblatt, P., Rath, M., Popper, H., Zenz, R., Komnenovic, V., et al. (2008). Development of pulmonary fibrosis through a pathway involving the transcription factor Fra-2/AP-1. *Proceedings of the National Academy of Sciences, USA, 105,* 10525–10530.

Eickelberg, O., Pansky, A., Koehler, E., Bihl, M., Tamm, M., Hildebrand, P., et al. (2001). Molecular mechanisms of TGFβ antagonism by interferon γ and cyclosporine A in lung fibrosis. *FASEB Journal, 15,* 797–806.

Eitzman, D. T., McCoy, R. D., Zheng, X., Fax, W. P., Shen, T., Ginsburg, D., et al. (1996). Bleomycin-induced pulmonary fibrosis in transgenic mice that either lack or overexpress the murine plasminogen activator inhibitor-1 gene. *Journal of Clinical Investigation, 97,* 232–237.

Entzian, P., Schlaak, M., Seitzer, U., Bufe, A., Acil, Y., & Zabel, P. (1997). Antiiflammatory and antifibrotic properties of colchicines: Implications for idiopathic pulmonary fibrosis. *Lung, 175,* 41–51.

Epstein, B. J. (2008). Efficacy and safety of darusentan: A novel endothelin receptor antagonist. *The Annals of the Pharmacotherapy, 42,* 1060–1069.

Fabre, A., Marchal-Somme, J., Marchand-Adam, S., Quesnel, C., Borie, R., Dehoux, M., et al. (2008). Modulation of bleomycin-induced fibrosis by serotonin receptor antagonists in mice. *European Journal of Pharmacology, 32,* 426–436.

Fagan, K., McMurtry, I. F., & Rodman, D. M. (2001). Role of endothelin-1 in lung disease. *Respiratory Research, 2,* 90–101.

Failla, M., Genovese, T., Mazzon, E., Gili, E., Muià, C., Sortino, M., et al. (2006). Pharmacological inhibition of leukotrienes in an animal model of bleomycin-induced acute lung injury. *Respiratory Research, 7,* 137.

Fattman, C. L., Chang, L.-Y., Termin, T. A., Petersen, L., Enghild, J. J., & Oury, T. D. (2003). Enhanced bleomycin-induced pulmonary damage in mice lacking extracellular superoxide dismutase. *Free Radical Biology and Medicine, 35,* 763–771.

Fattman, C. L., Tan, R. J., Toblewski, J. M., & Oury, T. D. (2006). Increased sensitivity to asbestos lung injury in mice lacking extracellular superoxide dismutase. *Free Radical Biology and Medicine, 40,* 601–607.

Fell, C. D., Liu, L. X., Motika, C., Kazerooni, E. A., Gross, B. H., Travis, W. D., et al. (2009). The prognostic value of cardiopulmonary exercise testing in idiopathic pulmonary fibrosis. *American Journal of Respiratory and Critical Care Medicine, 179,* 402–407.

Fiorucci, E., Lucantoni, G., Paone, G., Zotti, M., Li, B. E., Serpilli, M., et al. (2008). Colchicine, cyclophosphamide and prednisone in the treatment of mild-moderate idiopathic pulmonary fibrosis: Comparison of three currently available therapeutic regimens. *European Review for Medical and Pharmacological Sciences, 12,* 105–111.

Fisher, A. E. O., Lau, G., & Naughton, D. P. (2005). Lipophilic ionophore complexes as superoxide dismutase mimetics. *Biochemical and Biophysical Research Communications, 329,* 930–933.

Fleischman, R. W., Baker, J. R., Thompson, G. R., Schaeppi, U. H., Illievski, V. R., Conney, D. A., et al. (1971). Bleomycin-induced interstitial pneumonia in dogs. *Thorax, 26,* 675–682.

Fontenot, A. P., & Amicosante, M. (2008). Metal-induced diffuse lung disease. *Seminars in Respiratory and Critical Care Medicine, 29,* 662–669.

Gao, F., Kinnula, V. L., Myllärniemi, M., & Oury, T. D. (2008). Extracellular superoxide dismutase in pulmonary fibrosis. *Antioxidants & Redox Signaling, 10,* 343–354.

Garneau-Tsodikova, S., & Thannickal, V. J. (2008). Protein kinase inhibitors in the treatment of pulmonary fibrosis. *Current Medicinal Chemistry, 15,* 2632–2640.

Gasse, P., Mary, C., Guenon, I., Noulin, N., Charron, S., Schnyder, B., et al. (2007). IL-1R1/MyD88 signaling and the inflammasome are essential in pulmonary inflammation and fibrosis in mice. *Journal of Clinical Investigation, 117,* 3786–3799.

Gauldie, J., & Kolb, M. A. (2008). Animal models of pulmonary fibrosis: How far from effective reality? *American Journal of Physiology. Lung Cellular and Molecular Physiology, 294,* L151.

Gauldie, J., Kolb, M., Ask, K., Martin, G., Bonniaud, P., & Warburton, D. (2006). Smad3 signaling involved in pulmonary fibrosis and emphysema. *Proceedings of the American Thoracic Society, 3,* 696–702.

Gharaee-Kermani, M., Hu, B., Phan, S. H., & Gyetko, M. R. (2008) The role of urokinase in idiopathic pulmonary fibrosis and implication for therapy. *Expert Opinion on Investigational Drugs, 17,* 905–916.

Ghazi-Khansari, M., Mohammadi-Karakani, A., Sotoudeh, M., Mokhtary, P., Pour-Esmaeil, E., & Maghsoud, S. (2007). Antifibrotic effect of captopril and enalapril on paraquat-induced fibrosis in rats. *Journal of Applied Toxicology, 27,* 342–349.

Giaid, A., Yanagisawa, M., Langleben, D., Michel, R. P., Levy, R., Shainhib, H., et al. (1993). Expression of endothelin-1 in the lungs of patients with pulmonary hypertension. *New England Journal of Medicine, 328,* 1732–1739.

Gillissen, A., & Nowak, D. (1998). Characterization of N-acetylcysteine and ambroxol in antioxidant therapy. *Respiratory Medicine, 92,* 609–623.

Gonzalez, P. K., Zhuang, J., Doctorow, S. R., Malfroy, B., Benson, P. F., Menconi, M. J., et al. (1995). EUK-8, a synthetic superoxide dismutase and catalase mimetic, ameliorates acute lung injury in endotoxemic swine. *Journal of Pharmacology and Experimental Therapeutics, 275,* 798–806.

Grewal, J. S., Mukhin, Y. V., Garnovskaya, M. N., Raymond, J. R., & Greene, E. L. (1999). Serotonin 5-HT$_{2A}$ receptor induces TGF$_{\beta 1}$ expression in mesangial cells via ERK: Proliferative and fibrotic signals. *American Journal of Physiology, 276*(6 Pt 2), F922–F930.

Griesenbach, U., Alton, E. W., & UK Cystic Fibrosis Gene Therapy Consortium. (2009). Gene transfer to the lung: Lessons learned from more than 2 decades of CF gene therapy. *Advanced Drug Delivery Reviews, 61*, 128–1390.

Grutter, C., Wilkinson, T., Turner, R., Podichetty, S., Finch, D., McCourt, M., et al. (2008). A cytokine-neutralizing antibody as a structural mimetic of 2 receptor interactions. *Proceedings of National Academy of Sciences, USA, 105*, 20251–20156.

Gurujeyalakshmi, G., Hollinger, M. A., & Giri, S. N. (1999). Pirfenidone inhibits PDGF isoforms in bleomycin hamster model of lung fibrosis at the translational level. *American Journal of Physiology, 276*(2 Pt 1), L311–L318.

Hagiwara, S. I., Ishii, Y., & Kitamura, S. (2000). Aerosolized administration of N-acetylcysteine attenuates lung fibrosis induced by bleomycin in mice. *American Journal of Respiratory and Critical Care Medicine, 162*, 225–231.

Hayes, J. D., Flanagan, J. U., & Jowsay, I. R. (2005). Glutathione transferases. *Annual Review of Pharmacology and Toxicology, 45*, 51–88.

Hemmati, A. A., Nazari, Z., Ranjbari, N., & Torfi, A. (2008). Comparison of preventive effects of vitamin C and E on hexavalent chromium induced pulmonary fibrosis in rat. *Inflammopharmacology, 16*, 195–197.

Hickey, K. A., Rubani, G. B., Paul, R. J., & Highsmtith, R. F. (1985). Characterization of a coronary vasoconstrictor produced by cultured endothelial cells. *American Journal of Physiology, 248*, C550–C556.

Hodgson, U., Pulkkinen, V., Dixon, M., Peyrard-Janvid, M. R., Lahermo, P., Ollikainen, V., et al. (2006). ELMOD2 is a candidate gene for familial idiopathic pulmonary fibrosis. *American Journal of Human Genetics, 79*, 149–154.

Hsu, E., & Feghali-Bostwick, C. A. (2008). Insulin-like growth factor-II is increased in systemic sclerosis-associated pulmonary fibrosis and contributes to the fibrotic process via Jun N-terminal kinase and phosphotidylinositol-3 kinase dependent pathways. *American Journal of Pathology, 172*, 1580–1590.

Hunninghake, G. W. (2005). Antioxidant therapy for idiopathic pulmonary fibrosis. *New England Journal of Medicine, 353*, 2285–2287.

Iglarz, M., Binkert, C., Morrison, K., Fischli, W., Gatfield, J., Treiber, A., et al. (2008). Pharmacology of macitentan, an orally active tissue-targeting dual endothelin receptor antagonist. *Journal of Pharmacology and Experimental Therapeutics, 327*, 736–745.

Inghilleri, S., Morbini, P., Oggionni, T., Barni, R., & Fenoglio, C. (2006). In situ assessment of oxidant and nitrogenic stress in bleomycin pulmonary fibrosis. *Histochemistry and Cell Biology, 125*, 661–669.

Inoshima, I., Kuwano, K., Hamada, N., Yoshimi, M., Maeyama, T., Hagimoto, N., et al. (2004). Induction of CDK inhibitor p21 gene as a new therapeutic strategy against pulmonary fibrosis. *American Journal of Physiology. Lung Cellular and Molecular Physiology, 286*, L727–733.

InterMune web site. http://www.intermune.com /wt/itmin/reach. pirfenidone-IPF. Accessed August 2009.

Iredale, J. P., Benyon, R. C., Pickering, J., McCullen, M., Northrop, M., Pawley, S., et al. (1998). Mechanisms of spontaneous resolution of rat liver fibrosis. *Journal of Clinical Investigation, 102*, 538–549.

Ishikawa, K., Fukami, T., Nagase, T., Fujita, K., Hayama, T., Niiyama, R., et al. (1992). Cyclic pentapeptide endothelin antagonists with high ET$_A$ selectivity. Potency and selectivity-enhancing modifications. *Journal of Medicinal Chemistry, 35*, 2139–2142.

Issa, R., Williams, E., Trim, N., Kendall, T., Arthur, M. J., Reichen, J., et al. (2001). Apoptosis of hepatic cells: Involvement in resolution of biliary fibrosis and regulation by soluble growth factors. *Gut, 48*, 548–557.

Iyer, S. N., Gurujeyalakshmi, G., & Giri, S. N. (1999a). Effects of pirfenidone on procollagen gene expression at the transcriptional level in bleomycin hamster model of lung fibrosis. *Journal of Pharmacology and Experimental Therapeutics, 289*, 211–218.

Iyer, S. N., Gurujeyalakshmi, G., & Giri, S. N. (1999b). Effects of pirfenidone on transforming growth factor-beta gene expression at the transcriptional level in bleomycin hamster model of lung fibrosis. *Journal of Pharmacology and Experimental Therapeutics, 291*, 367–373.

Iyer, S. N., Margolin, S. B., Hyde, D. M., & Giri, S. N. (1998). Lung fibrosis is ameliorated by pirfenidone fed in diet after the second dose in a three-dose bleomycin-hamster model. *Experimental Lung Research, 24*, 119–132.

Iyer, S. N., Wild, J. S., Schiedt, M. J., Hyde, D. M., Margolin, S. B., & Giri, S. N. (1995). Dietary intake of pirfenidone ameliorates bleomycin-induced lung fibrosis in hamsters. *Journal of Laboratory and Clinical Medicine, 125*, 779–785.

Jackson, R. M., & Fell, C. D. (2008). Etanercept for idiopathic pulmonary fibrosis. Lessons on clinical trial design. *American Journal of Respiratory and Critical Care Medicine, 178*, 889–891.

Jain, R., Shaul, P. W., Borok, Z., Wills, B., & Brigham, C. (2007). Endothelin-1 induces alveolar epithelial-mesenchimal transition through endothelin type A receptor-mediated production of TGF-beta1. *American Journal of Respiratory Cell and Molecular Biology, 37*, 38–47.

Jiang, F., Guo, Y., Salvemini, D., & Dusting, G. J. (2003). Superoxide dismutase mimetic M40403 improves endothelial function in apolipoprotein(E)-deficient mice. *British Journal of Pharmacology, 139*, 1127–1134.

Kaira, P. R., Moon, J. C. C., & Coats, J. (2002). Do results of the ENABLE (Endothelin Antagonist Bosentan for Lowering Cardiac Events in Heart Failure) study spell the end for non-selective endothelin antagonism in heart failure? *International Journal of Cardiology, 85*, 195–197.

Kakugawa, T., Mukae, H., Hayashi, T., Ishii, H., Abe, K., Fujii, T., et al. (2004). Pirfenidone attenuates expression of HSP47 in murine bleomycin-induced pulmonary fibrosis. *European Respiratory Journal, 24*, 57–65.

Kakugawa, T., Mukae, H., Hayashi, T., Ishii, H., Nakayama, S., Sakamoto, N., et al. (2005). Expression of HSP47 in usual interstitial pneumonia and nonspecific interstitial pneumonia. *Respiratory Research, 6*, 57.

Kamp, D. W. (2009). Asbestos-induced lung diseases: An update. *Translational Research: The Journal of Laboratory and Clinical Medicine, 153*, 143–152.

Kapoor, S. (2008). Smad7 gene transfer therapy: Therapeutic applications beyond colonic fibrosis. *European Journal of Clinical Investigation, 38*, 876–877.

Kehrer, J. P., & Margolin, S. B. (1997). Pirfenidone diminishes cyclophosphamide-induced lung fibrosis in mice. *Toxicology Letters, 90*, 125–132.

Kennedy, J. P., Gordon, G. B., Paky, A., McShane, A., Adkinson, N. F., Peters, S. P., et al. (1988). Amiodarone causes acute oxidant lung injury in ventilated and perfused rabbit lungs. *Journal of Cardiovascular Pharmacology, 12*, 23–1236.

Kijiyama, N., Ueno, H., Sugimoto, I., Sasaguri, Y., Yatera, K., Kido, M., et al. (2006). Intratracheal gene transfer of tissue factor pathway inhibitor attenuates pulmonary fibrosis. *Biochemical and Biophysical Research Communications, 339*, 1113–1119.

Kikuchi, K., Kohiyama, T., Yamauchi, Y., Kato, J., Takami, K., Okasaki, H., et al. (2009). C-reactive protein modulates human lung fibroblast migration. *Experimental Lung Research, 35*, 48–58.

Kilinç, C., Ozean, O., Karaoz, E., Sunguroglu, K., Kuluay, T., & Karaca, L. (1993). Viamin E reduces bleomycin-induced fibrosis in mice: Biochemical and morphological studies. *Journal of Basic and Clinical Physiology and Pharmacology, 4*, 249–269.

Kim, K. K., & Chapman, H. A. (2007). Endothelin-1 as initiator of epithelial-mesenchymal transition. Potential role for endothelin-1 during pulmonary fibrosis. *American Journal of Respiratory Cell and Molecular Biology, 37*, 1–2.

Kim, K. K., Kugler, M. C., Wolters, P. J., Robillard, L., Galvez, M. G., Bruwell, A. N., et al. (2006). Alveolar epithelial cell mesenchymal transition develops in vivo during pulmonary fibrosis and is regulated by the extracellular matrix. *Proceedings of the National Academy of Sciences, USA, 103,* 13180–13185.

Kinder, B. W., Brown, K. K., McCormack, F. X., Ix, J. H., Kervitsky, A., Schwarz, M. I., et al. (2009). Serum surfactant protein-A is a strong predictor of early mortality in idiopathic pulmonary fibrosis. *Chest, 135,* 1557–1563.

King, T. E., Albera, C., Bradford, V. Z., Costabel, U., Homel, P., Lancaster, L., et al. (2009). Effect of interferon-gamma-1b on survival in patients with idiopathic pulmonary fibrosis (INSPIRE): A multicentre, randomized, placebo-controlled trial. *Lancet, 374,* 222–228.

King, T. E., Behr, J., Brown, K. K., du Bois, R. M., Lancaster, L., deAndrade, J. A., et al. (2008). BUILD-1: A randomized placebo-controlled trial of bosentan in idiopathic pulmonary fibrosis. *American Journal of Respiratory and Critical Care Medicine, 177,* 75–81.

Kinnula, V. L. (2008). Redox imbalance and lung fibrosis. *Antioxidants & Redox Signaling, 10,* 249–252.

Kinnula, V. L., & Crapo, J. D. (2003). Superoxide dismutases in the lung and human lung diseases. *American Journal of Respiratory and Critical Care Medicine, 167,* 1600–1619.

Kinnula, V. L., Fattman, C. L., Tan, R. J., & Oury, T. D. (2005). Oxidative stress in pulmonary fibrosis: A possible role for redox modulatory therapy. *American Journal of Respiratory and Critical Care Medicine, 172,* 417–422.

Kinnula, V. L., Hodgson, U. A., Lakari, E. K., Tan, R. J., Sormunen, R. T., Soini, Y. M., et al. (2006). Extracellular superoxide dismutase has a highly specific localization in idiopathic pulmonary fibrosis/usual interstitial pneumonia. *Histopathology, 49,* 66–74.

Kinnula, V. L., & Myllärniemi, M. (2008). Oxidant-antioxidant imbalance as a potential contributor to the progression of human pulmonary fibrosis. *Antioxidants & Redox Signaling, 10,* 727–738.

Kiowski, W., Sutch, G., Oechslin, E., & Bertel, O. (2001). Hemodynamic effects of bosentan in patients with chronic heart failure. *Heart Failure Reviews, 6,* 325–334.

Kojiri, K., Ihara, M., Nakajima, S., Kawanura, K., Funashi, K., Yano, M., et al. (1991). Endothelin-binding inhibitors, BE-18257A and BE-18257B.1. Taxonomy, fermentation, isolation and characterization. *Journal of Antibiotics, 44,* 1342–1347.

Koli, K., Myllarniemi, M., Keski-Oja, J., & Kinnula, V. L. (2008). Transforming growth factor-beta activation in the lung: Focus on fibrosis and reactive oxygen species. *Antioxidants & Redox Signaling, 10,* 333–342.

Krum, H., Viscoper, R. J., Lacourciere, Y., Budde, M., & Charlon, V. (1998). The effect of an endothelin-receptor antagonist, bosentan, on blood pressure in patients with hypertension, *New England Journal of Medicine, 338,* 784–791.

Kubo, H., Nakayama, K., Yanai, M., Suzuki, T., Yamaya, M., Watanabe, M., et al. (2005). Anticoagulant therapy for idiopathic pulmonary fibrosis. *Chest, 128,* 1475–1482.

Lakari, E., Paako, P., Pietarinen-Runtti, P., & Kinnula, V. L. (2000). Manganese superoxide dismutase and catalase are coordinately expressed in the alveolar region in chronic interstitial pneumonias and granulomatous diseases of the lung. *American Journal of Respiratory and Critical Care Medicine, 161,* 615–621.

Lakari, E., Pylkas, P., Pietarinen-Runtti, P., Paako, P., Soini, Y., & Kinnula, V. L. (2001). Expression and regulation of hemeoxygenase 1 in healthy human lungs and interstitial lung disorders. *Human Pathology, 32,* 1257–1263.

Lambeth, J. D., Krause, K. H., & Clark, R. A. (2008). NOX enzymes as novel targets for drug development. *Seminars in Immunopathology, 30,* 339–363.

Lawson, W. E., Crossno, P. F., Polosukhin, V. V., Roldan, J., Cheng, D.-S., Lane, K. B., et al. (2008). Endoplasmic reticulum stress in alveolar epithelial cells is prominent in IPF: Association with altered surfactant protein processing and herpes virus infection. *American Journal of Physiology. Lung Cellular and Molecular Physiology, 294,* L1119–L1126.

Leask, A. (2008). Targeting the TGFβ, endothelin-1 and CCN2 axis to combat fibrosis in scleroderma, *Cellular Signalling, 20,* 1409–1414.

Leeder, R. G., Brien, J. F., & Massey, T. E. (1994). Investigation of the role of oxidative stress in amiodarone-induced pulmonary toxicity in the hamster. *Canadian Journal of Physiology and Pharmacology, 72*, 613–621

Ley, K., & Zarbock, A. (2008). From lung injury to fibrosis. *Nature Medicine, 14*, 20–21.

Li, X., Zhuang, J., Rayford, H., Zhang, H., Shu, R., & Uhal, B. D. (2007). Attenuation of bleomycin-induced pulmonary fibrosis by intratracheal administration of antisense oligonucleotides against angiotensinogen mRNA. *Current Pharmaceutical Design, 13*, 1257–1268.

Liang, L.-P., Huang, J., Fulton, R., Day, B. J., & Patel, M. (2007). An orally active metalloporphyrin protects against 1-methyl-4-phenyl-1,2,3,6-tetrahydropyridine neurotoxicity in vivo. *Journal of Neuroscience, 27*, 4326–4333.

Lin, C. J., Yang, P. C., Hsu, M. T., Yew, F. H., Liu, T. Y., Shun, C., et al. (1998). Induction of pulmonary fibrosis in organ-cultured rat lung by cadmium chloride and transforming factor—beta1. *Toxicology, 127*, 157–166.

Lin, L., Zhou, Z., Zheng, L., Alber, S., Watkins, S., Ray, P., et al. (2008). Cross talk between Id1 and its interactive protein Dril1 mediate fibroblasts responses to transforming growth factor-beta in pulmonary fibrosis. *American Journal of Pathology, 173*, 337–346.

Liu, Y. (2004). Epithelial to mesenchymal transition in renal fibrinogenesis: Pathological significance, molecular mechanism, and therapeutic intervention. *Journal of the American Society of Nephrology, 15*, 1–12.

Lombard-Gilloly, K., & Hubbard, A. K. (1993). Modulation of silica-induced lung injury by reducing lung non-protein sulfhydryls with buthionine sulfoximine. *Toxicology Letters, 66*, 305–315.

Lombardi, R., Rodriguez, G., Chen, S. N., Ripplinger, C. M., Li, W., Chen, J., et al. (2009). Resolution of established cardiac hypertrophy and fibrosis and prevention of systolic dysfunction in a transgenic rabbit model of human cardiomyopathy through thiol-sensitive mechanism. *Circulation, 119*, 1398–1407.

Lönn, P., Morén, A., Raja, E., Dahl, M., & Moustakas, A. (2009). Regulating the stability of TGFβ receptors and Smads. *Cell Research, 19*, 21–35.

Lupher, M. J., Jr., & Gallatin, W. M. (2006). Regulation of fibrosis by the immune system. *Advances in Immunology, 89*, 245–288.

MacIntyre, I. M., Dhaun, N., Goddard, J., & Webb, D. J. (2008). Ambrisentan and its role in the management of pulmonary arterial hypertension, *Drugs of Today, 44*, 875–885.

Maher, T. M., Wells, A. U., & Laurent, G. J. (2007). Idiopathic pulmonary fibrosis: Multiple causes and multiple mechanisms? *European Respiratory Journal, 30*, 835–839.

Malizia, A. P., Keating, D. T., Smith, S. M., Walls, D., Doran, P. P., & Egan, J. J. (2008). Alveolar epithelial injury with Epstein-Barr virus upregulates TGFβ1 expression. *American Journal of Physiology. Lung Cellular and Molecular Physiology, 295*, L451–L460.

Manouri, B., Nenan, S., Leclerc, O., Guenon, I., Boichot, E., Planquois, J.-M., et al. (2005). The absence of reactive oxygen species production protects mice against bleomycin-induced pulmonary fibrosis. *Respiratory Research, 6*, 11–23.

Markart, P., Luboeinski, T., Korfei, M., Schmidt, R., Wygrecka, M., Mahavadi, P., et al. (2009). Alveolar oxidative stress is associated with elevated levels of nonenzymatic low-molecular-weight antioxidants in patients with different forms of chronic fibrosing interstitial lung diseases. *Antioxidants & Redox Signaling, 11*, 227–240.

Masini, E., Bani, D., Vannacci, A., Pierpaoli, S., Mannaioni, P. F., Comhair, S. A. A., et al. (2005). Reduction of antigen-induced respiratory abnormalities and airway inflammation in sensitized guinea pigs by a superoxide mimetic. *Free Radical Biology & Medicine, 39*, 520–531.

Mata, M., Ruiz, A., Cerda, M., Martinez-Losa, M., Cortijo, J., Santangelo, F., et al. (2003). Oral N-acetylcysteine reduces bleomycin-induced lung damage and mucin Muc5ac expression in rats. *European Respiratory Journal, 22*, 900–905.

Mays, E. E., Dubois, J. J., & Hamilton, G. B. (1976). Pulmonary fibrosis associated with trachiobronchial aspiration: A study of the frequency of hiatal hernia and gastroesophageal reflux in interstitial fibrosis of obscure etiology. *Chest*, *69*, 512–515.

McGoon, M. D., Frost, A. E., Oudiz, R. J., Badesh, D. B., Galle, N., Olschewski, H., et al. (2008) Ambrisentan therapy in patients with pulmonary arterial hypertension who discontinued bosentan or sitaxsentan due to liver function test abnormalities. *Chest*, *135*, 122–129.

Meneghin, A., Choi, E. S., Evanoff, H. L., Kunkel, S. L., Martinez, F. J., Flaherty, K. R., et al. (2008). TLR-9 is expressed in idiopathic interstitial pneumonia and its activation promotes in vitro myofibroblast differentiation. *Histochemistry and Cell Biology*, *130*, 979–992.

Meurer, S. K., Lahme, B., Tihaa, L., Weiskirchen, R., & Gressner, A. M. (2005). N-acetyl-L-cysteine suppresses TGFβ signaling at distinct molecular steps: The biochemical and biological efficacy of a multifunctional, antifibrotic drug. *Biochemical Pharmacology*, *70*, 1026–1034.

Meyer, A. B., Buhl, R., Kampf, S., & Magnussen, H. (1995). Intravenous N-acetylcysteine and lung glutathione in patients with pulmonary fibrosis and normals. *American Journal of Respiratory and Critical Care Medicine*, *152*, 1055–1060.

Meyer, A. B., Buhl, R., & Magnussen, H., (1994). The effect of oral N-acetylcysteine on lung glutathione levels in idiopathic pulmonary fibrosis. *European Respiratory Journal*, *7*, 431–436

Mitani, Y., Sato, K., Muramoto, Y., Karakawa, T., Kitamado, M., Iwanaga, T., et al. (2008). Superoxide scavenging activity of pirfenidone-iron complex. *Biochemical and Biophysical Research Communications*, *372*, 19–23.

Mitchell, C., Couton, D., Couty, J. P., Anson, M., Crain, A. M., Bizet, V., et al. (2009). Dual role of CCR2 in the constitution and the resolution of liver fibrosis in mice. *American Journal of Pathology*, *174*, 1766–1775.

Moeller, A., Ask, K., Warburton, D., Gauldie, J., & Kolb, M. (2008). The bleomycin animal model: A useful tool to investigate treatment options for idiopathic pulmonary fibrosis? *International Journal of Biochemistry & Cell Biology*, *40*, 362–382.

Moeller, A., Gilpin, S. E., Ask, K., Cox, G., Cook, D., Gauldie, J., et al. (2009) Circulatimg fibrocytes are an indicator of poor prognosis in idiopathic pulmonary fibrosis. *American Journal of Respiratory and Critical Care Medicine*, *179*, 588–594.

Molteni, A., Moulder, J. F., Cohen, E. F., Ward, W. F., Fish, B. L., Taylor, J. M., et al. (2000). Control of radiation-induced pneumopathy and lung fibrosis by angiotensin-converting enzyme inhibitors and an angiotensin, II receptor blocker. *International Journal of Radiation Biology*, *76*, 523–532.

Moore, B. B., & Hogaboam, C. M. (2008). Animal models of human lung disease. *American Journal of Physiology. Lung Cellular and Molecular Physiology*, *294*, L152–L160.

Mora, A. L., Torres-Gonzales, E., Rojas, M., Ritzenthaler, J., Xu, J., Roman, J., et al. (2006). Activation of alveolar macrophages via the alternative pathway in herpes virus-induced lung fibrosis. *American Journal of Respiratory Cell and Molecular Biology*, *35*, 466–473.

Mora, A. L., Woods, C. R., Garcia, A., Xu, J., Rojas, M., Speck, S. H., et al. (2005). Lung infection with γ-herpesvirus induces progressive pulmonary fibrosis in Th2-biased mice. *American Journal of Physiology. Lung Cellular and Molecular Physiology*, *289*, L711–L721.

Moreland, S. (1994). BQ-123, a selective ET$_A$ receptor antagonist. *Cardiovascular Drug Reviews*, *12*, 48–69.

Murray, L. A., Argentieri, R. L., Farrell, F. X., Bracht, M., Sheng, H., Whitaker, B., et al. (2008). Hyper-responsiveness of IPF/UIP fibroblasts: Interplay between TGFbeta1, IL-13 and CCL2. *International Journal of Biochemistry & Cell Biology*, *40*(10), 2174–2182.

Nadrous, H. F., Ryu, J. H., Douglas, W. W., Decker, P. A., & Olson, E. J. (2004). Impact of angiotensin-converting enzyme inhibitors and statins on survival in idiopathic pulmonary fibrosis. *Chest, 126*, 438–446.

Nagai, S., Handa, T., & Kim, D. S. (2008). Pharmacotherapy in patients with idiopathic pulmonary fibrosis. *Expert Opinion on Pharmacotherapy, 9*, 1909–1925.

Nagai, S., Hamada, K., Shigematsu, M., Taniyama, M., Yamauchi, S., & Izumi, T. (2002). Open-label compassionate use one year-treatment with pirfenidone to patients with chronic pulmonary fibrosis. *Internal Medicine, 41*(12), 1118–1123.

Nagase, T., Rennard, S. I., & Takazawa, H. (2009). C-reactive protein modulates human fibroblasts migration. *Experimental Lung Research, 35*, 48–58.

Nakagome, K., Dohl, M., Okunishi, K., Tanaka, R., Miyazaki, J., & Yamamoto, K. (2006). In vivo IL-10 gene delivery attenuates bleomycin-induced pulmonary fibrosis by inhibiting the production and activation of TGF_β in the lung. *Thorax, 61*, 886–894.

Nakao, A., Fujii, M., Matsumura, R., Kumano, K., Saoto, Y., Miyazono, K., et al. (1999). Transient gene transfer and expression of Smad7 prevents bleomycin-induced lung fibrosis in mice. *Journal of Clinical Investigation, 104*, 5–11.

Nakayama, S., Mukae, H., Sakamoto, N., Kakugawa, T., Yoshioka, S., Soda, H., et al., (2008). Pirfenidone inhibits the expression of HSP47 in TGF_β-stimulated human lung fibroblasts. *Life Sciences, 82*, 210–217.

Nakazato, H., Oku, H., Yamane, S., Tsuruta, Y., & Suzuki, R. (2002). A novel anti-fibrotic agent pirfenidone suppresses tumor necrosis factor-alpha at the translational level. *European Journal of Pharmacology, 446*(1–3), 177–185.

Narayanan, A. S., Whitney, J., Souza, A., & Raghu, G. (1992). Effect of gamma-interferon on collagen synthesis by normal and fibrotic human lung fibroblasts. *Chest, 101*, 1326–1331.

Nicod, L. P. (1999). Pirfenidone in idiopathic pulmonary fibrosis. *Lancet, 354*, 268–269.

Noble, P. W., Albera, C., Bradford, W., Costabel, U., Kardatzke, D., King, T., Jr., et al. (2009). The CAPACITY (CAP) trials: Randomized, double-blind, placebo-controlled, phase III trials of pirfenidone (PFD) in patients with idiopathic pulmonary fibrosis (IPF). *American Journal of Respiratory and Critical Care Medicine, 179*, A1129.

Okada, M., & Nishikibe, M. (2002). BQ-788, a selective endothelin ET_B receptor antagonist. *Cardiovascular Drug Reviews, 20*, 53–66.

Oku, H., Nakazato, H., Horikawa, T., Tsuruta, Y., & Suzuki, R. (2002). Pirfenidone suppresses tumor necrosis factor-alpha, enhances interleukin-10 and protects mice from endotoxic shock. *European Journal of Pharmacology, 446*(1–3), 167–176.

Oku, H., Shimizu, T., Kawabata, T., Nagira, M., Hikita, I., Ueyama, A., et al. (2008). Anti-fibrotic action of pirfenidone and prednisolone: Different effects on pulmonary cytokines and growth factors in bleomycin-induced murine pulmonary fibrosis. *European Journal of Pharmacology, 590*, 400–408.

Ong, V. H., Carulli, M. T., Xu, S., Khan, K., Lindahl, G., Abraham, D. J., et al. (2009) Cross-talk between MCP-3 and TGF_β promotes fibroblasts collagen biosynthesis. *Experimental Cell Research, 315*, 151–161.

Ono, A., Utsugi, M., Masubuchi, K., Ishizuka, T., Kawata, T., Shimizu, Y., et al. (2009). Glutathione redox regulates TGF_β–induced fibrogenic effects through Smad3 activation. *FEBS Letters, 583*, 357–362.

Opitz, C. F., Ewert, R., Kirch, W., & Pittrow, D. (2008). Inhibition of endothelin receptors in the treatment of pulmonary arterial hypertension: Does selectivity matter? *European Heart Journal, 29*, 1936–1948.

Oury, T. D., Schaefer, L. M., Fattman, C. L., Choi, A., Weck, K. E., & Watkins, S. C. (2002). Depletion of pulmonary EC-SOD after exposure to hypoxia. *American Journal of Physiology. Lung Cellular and Molecular Physiology, 283*, L777–L784.

Oury, T. D., Thakker, K., Menache, M., Chang, L. Y., Crapo, J. D., & Day, B. J. (2001). Attenuation of bleomycin-induced pulmonary fibrosis by a catalytic antioxidant metalloporphyrin. *American Journal of Respiratory Cell and Molecular Biology, 25,* 164–169.

Park, S. H., Saleh, D., Giaid, A., & Michel, R. P. (1997). Increased endothelin-1 in bleomycin-induced pulmonary fibrosis and the effect of an endothelin receptor antagonist. *American Journal of Respiratory and Critical Care Medicine, 156,* 600–608.

Parra, E. R., Boufelli, G., Berthanha, F., Samorano, Lde, P., Aguiar, A. C., Jr., et al. (2008). Temporal evolution of epithelial, vascular and interstitial lung injury in an experimental model of idiopathic pulmonary fibrosis induced by butyl-hydroxytoluene. *International Journal of Experimental Pathology, 89,* 350–357.

Pashinsky, Y. Y., Jaffin, B. W., & Lile, V. R. (2009). Gastroesophageal reflux disease and idiopathic pulmonary fibrosis. *The Mount Sinai Journal of Medicine, New York, 76,* 24–29.

Physicians' Desk Reference, 63rd Edition (2009). *Tracleer®.* 3289–3292. Montvale, NJ, USA, also available on www.PDR.net

Piguet, P. F., & Vesin, C. (1994). Treatment by human recombinant soluble TNF receptor of pulmonary fibrosis induced by bleomycin or silica in mice. *European Respiratory Journal, 7,* 515–518.

Prie, S., Leung, T. K., Cernacek, P., Ryan, J. W., & Dupuis, J. (1997). The orally active ET_A receptor antagonist (+)-(S)-2-(4,6-dimethoxy-pyrimidin-2-yloxy)-3-methoxy-3,3-diphe-nyl-propionic acid (LU 135252) prevents the development of pulmonary hypertension and endothelial metabolic dysfunction in monocrotaline-treated rats. *Journal of Pharmacology and Experimental Therapeutics, 282,* 1312–1318.

Prud'homme, G. J. (2007). Pathobiology of transforming growth factor beta in cancer, fibrosis and immunologic disease. *Laboratory Investigation, 87,* 1077–1091.

Qi, W., Chen, X., Poronnik, P., & Pollock, C. A. (2008). Transforming growth factor-β/connective tissue growth factor axis in the kidney. *International Journal of Biochemistry & Cell Biology, 40,* 9–13.

Rabkin, S. W., & Klassen, S. S. (2008). Metalloporphyrins as a therapeutic drug class against peroxynitrite in cardiovascular diseases involving ischemic reperfusion injury. *European Journal of Pharmacology, 586,* 1–8.

Raghow, R., Lurie, S., Seyer, J. M., & Kang, A. H. (1985). Profiles of steady state levels of messenger RNAs coding for type I procollagen, elastin, and fibronectin in hamster lungs undergoing bleomycin-induced interstitial pulmonary fibrosis. *Journal of Clinical Investigation, 76(5),* 1733–1739.

Raghu, G. (2006). Idiopathic pulmonary fibrosis: Treatment options in pursuit of evidence-based approach. *European Respiratory Journal, 28,* 463–465.

Raghu, G., Johnson, W. C., Lockhart, D., & Mageto, Y. (1999). Treatment of idiopathic pulmonary fibrosis with a new antifibrotic agent, pirfenidone: Results of a prospective, open-label Phase II study. *American Journal of Respiratory and Critical Care Medicine, 159(4 Pt 1),* 1061–1069.

Raghu, G., Brown, K. K., Bradford, W. Z., Starko, K., Noble, P. W., Schwartz, D. A., et al. (2004). A placebo-controlled trial of interferon gamma-1b in patients with pulmonary fibrosis. *New England Journal of Medicine, 350,* 125–133.

Raghu, G., Brown, K. K., Costabel, U., Cottin, V., du Bois, R. M., Lasky, J. A., et al. (2008). Treatment of idiopathic pulmonary fibrosis with etanercept: An exploratory, placebo-controlled trial. *American Journal of Respiratory and Critical Care Medicine, 178,* 948–955.

Raghu, G., Weycker, D., Edelsberg, J., Bradford, W. Z., & Oster, G. (2006) Incidence and prevalence of idiopathic pulmonary fibrosis. *American Journal of Respiratory and Critical Care Medicine, 174(7),* 810–816.

Rahman, I., Biswas, S. K., & Kirkham, P. A. (2006). Regulation of inflammation and redox signaling by dietary phenols. *Biochemical Pharmacology, 72,* 1439–1452.

Rahman, I., Biswas, S. K., Saibal, K., & Kode, A. (2006). Oxidant and antioxidant balance in the airways and airway diseases. *European Journal of Pharmacology, 533,* 222–239.

Rahman, I., Skwarska, E., Henry, M., Davis, M., O'Connor, C. M., FitsGerald, M. X., et al. (1999). Systemic and pulmonary oxidative stress in idiopathic pulmonary fibrosis. *Free Radical Biology & Medicine, 27*(1–2), 60–68.

Rahman, I., Yang, S.-R., & Biswas, S. K. (2008). Current concepts of redox signaling in the lungs. *Antioxidants & Redox Signaling, 8*, 681–689.

Reboux, G., Plarroux, R., Roussel, S., Millon, L., Bardonnet, K., & Daphin, J.-C. (2007). Assessment of four serological techniques in the immunological diagnosis of farmer's lung disease. *Journal of Medical Microbiology, 56*, 1317–1321.

RedOrbit website. http://www.redorbit.com/news/496688, accessed August 2009.

Rogliani, P., Mura, M., Porrtta, M. A., & Sattini, C. (2008) New Perspectives in the treatment of idiopathic pulmonary fibrosis. *Therapeutic Advances in Respiratory Disease, 2*, 75–93.

Roux, S., Breu, V., Giller, T., Neidhort, W., Ramuz, H., Coassolo, P., et al. (1997). Ro 61–1790, a new hydrosoluble endothelin antagonist: General pharmacology and effects on experimental cerebral vasospasm. *Journal of Pharmacology and Experimental Therapeutics, 283*, 1110–1118.

Rubin, L. J., Badesh, D. B., Barst, R. J., Galie, N., Black, C. M., Keogh, A., et al. (2002). Bosentan therapy for pulmonary arterial hypertension. *New England Journal of Medicine, 346*, 896–903.

Rubino, C. M., Bhavnani, S. M., Ambrose, P. G., Forrest, A., & Loutit, J. S. (2009). Effect of food and antacids on the pharmacokinetics of pirfenidone in older healthy adults. *Pulmonary Pharmacology & Therapeutics, 22*(4), 279–285.

Rubin, L. J., & Roux, S. (2002). Bosentan: A dual endothelin receptor antagonist. *Expert Opinion on Investigational Drugs, 11*, 991–1002.

Ruffman, R., & Wendel, A. (1991). GSH rescue by N-acetylcysteine. *Klinische Wochenschrift, 69*, 857–862.

Sakamoto, K., Taniguchi, H., Kondoh, Y., Ono, K., Hasegawa, Y., & Kitaichi, M. (2009). Acute exacerbation of idiopathic pulmonary fibrosis as the initial presentation of the disease. *European Respiratory Review, 18*, 120–132.

Salazar-Montes, A., Ruiz-Corro, L., López-Reyes, A., Castrejón-Gómez, E., & Armendáriz-Borunda, J. (2008). Potent antioxidant role of pirfenidone in experimental cirrhosis. *European Journal of Pharmacology, 595*(1–3), 69–77.

Salvemini, D., Mazzon, E., Dugo, L., Riley, D. P., Serraino, I., Caputi, A. P., et al. (2001). Pharmacological manipulation of the inflammatory cascade by the superoxide dismutase mimetic, M40403. *British Journal of Pharmacology, 132*, 815–827.

Samai, M., Sharpe, M. A., Gard, P. R., & Chatterjee, P. K. (2007). Comparison of the effects of the superoxide dismutase mimetics EUK-134 and tempol on paraquat-induced neurotoxicity. *Free Radical Biology & Medicine, 43*, 528–534.

Satomi, Y., Sakaguchi, K., Kasahara, Y., & Akahori, F. (2007). Novel and extensive aspects of paraquat-induced pulmonary fibrogenesis: Comparative and time-course microarray analyses to fibrogenic and non-fibrogenic rats. *Journal of Toxicological Sciences, 32*, 529–553.

Sener, G., Topaloglu, N., Sehirtli, A. O., Ercan, F., & Gedik, N. (2007). Resveratrol alleviates bleomycin-induced lung injury in rats. *Pulmonary Pharmacology & Therapeutics, 20*, 642–649.

Serrano-Mollar, A., Closa, D., Prats, N., Blesa, S., Martinez-Losa, M., Cortijo, J., et al. (2003). In vivo antioxidant treatment protects against bleomycin-induced lung damage in rats. *British Journal of Pharmacology, 138*, 1037–1048.

Shahzeidi, S., Sarnstrand, B., Jeffery, P. K., McAnulty, R. I., & Laurent, G. J. (1991). Oral N-acetylcysteine reduces bleomycin-induced collagen deposition in the lungs of mice. *European Respiratory Journal, 4*, 845–852.

Shionogi website: www.shionogi.co.jp/index-e/pirfenidone. English. Accessed August 2009.

Shi-wen, X., Kennedy, L., Renzoni, E. A., Bou-Gharios, G., du Bois, R. M., Black, C. M., et al. (2007). Endothelin is a downstream mediator of profibrotic responses to transforming growth factor beta in human lung fibroblasts. *Arthritis & Rheumatism, 56*, 4189–4194.

Sisson, T. H., Hattori, N., Xu, Y., & Simon, R. H. (1999). Treatment of bleomycin-induced pulmonary fibrosis by transfer of urokinase-type plasminogen activator genes. *Human Gene Therapy, 10*, 2315–2323.

Smilkstein, M. J., Knapp, G. L., Kulig, K. W., & Rumack, B. H. (1988). Efficacy of oral N-acetylcysteine in the treatment of acetoaminophen overdose. *New England Journal of Medicine, 319*, 1557–1562.

Sogut, S., Ozyurt, H., Armutcu, F., Kart, L., Iraz, M., Akyol, O., et al. (2004). Erdosteine prevents bleomycin-induced pulmonary fibrosis in rats. *European Journal of Pharmacology, 494*, 213–220.

Steele, M. P., & Brown, K. K. (2007). Genetic predisposition to respiratory diseases: Infiltrative lung diseases (2007). *Respiration, 74*, 601–608.

Stralin, P., & Marklund, S. L. (2001). Vasoactive factors and growth factors alter vascular smooth muscle cell EC-SOD expression. *American Journal of Physiology. Heart and Circulatory Physiology, 281*, H1621–H1629.

Strausz, J., Muller-Querheim, J., Steppling, H., & Ferlinz, R. (1990) Oxygen radical production by alveolar inflammatory cells in idiopathic pulmonary fibrosis. *The American Review of Respiratory Disease, 141*, 129–133.

Strieter, R. M., (2008). What differentiates normal lung repair and fibrosis? *Proceedings of the American Thoracic Society, 5*, 305–310.

Sullivan, D. E., Ferris, M., Pociask, D., & Brody, A. R. (2008). The latent form of $TGF_{\beta 1}$ is induced by TNF_α through an ERK specific pathway and is activated by asbestos-derived reactive oxygen species in vitro and in vivo *Journal of Immunotoxicology, 5*, 145–149.

Tager, A. M., Kradin, R. L., LaCamera, P., Bercury, S. D., Campanella, G. S. V., Leary, C. P., et al. (2004). Inhibition of pulmonary fibrosis by the chemokine IP-10/CXCL10. *American Journal of Respiratory Cell and Molecular Biology, 31*, 395–404.

Tang, X., Yang, J., & Li, J. (2009). Accelerative effect of leflunomide on recovery from hepatic fibrosis involves TRAIL-mediated hepatic stellate cell apoptosis. *Life Sciences, 84*, 552–557.

Tang, Y.-W., Johnson, J. E., Browning, P. J., Cruz-Gervis, R. A., Davis, A., Graham, B. S., et al. (2003). Herpesvirus DNA is consistently detected in lungs of patients with idiopathic pulmonary fibrosis. *Journal of Clinical Microbiology, 41*, 2633–2640.

Tengstrand, B., Ernestam, S., Engvall, I.-L., Rydvald, Y., & Hafstrom, I. (2005) TNF blockade in rheumatoid arthritis can cause severe fibrosing alveolitis. Six case reports [Swedish]. *Lekartidningen, 102*, 3788–3790.

Tobin, R. W., Pope, C. E., & Pellegrini, C. A. (1988). Increased prevalence of gastroesophageal reflux in patients with idiopathic pulmonary fibrosis. *American Journal of Respiratory and Critical Care Medicine, 158*, 1804–1808.

Tomioka, H., Kuwata, Y., Imanaka, K., Hashimoto, K., Ohnishi, H., Tada, K., et al. (2005). A pilot study of aerosolized N-acetylcysteine for idiopathic pulmonary fibrosis. *Respirology, 10*, 449–455.

Torre-Amione, G., Durand, J. B., Nagueh, S., Vooletich, M. T., Kobrin, I., & Pratt, C. (2001). A pilot safety trial of prolonged (48 h) infusion of the dual endothelin receptor antagonist tezosentan in patients with advanced heart failure. *Chest, 120*, 460–466.

Trojanowska, M. (2008). Role of PDGF in fibrotic diseases and systemic sclerosis. *Rheumatology, 47*, 2–4.

Tsai, J. H., Liu, J. Y., Wu, T. T., Ho, P. C., Shyu, J. C., Hsieh, Y. S., et al. (2008). Effects of silymarin on the resolution of liver fibrosis induced by carbon tetrachloride in rats. *Journal of Viral Hepatitis, 15*, 508–514.

Tsukamoto, K., Hayakawa, H., Sato Chida, K., Nakamura, H., & Miura, K. (2000). Involvement of Epstein-Barr virus latent membrane protein1 in disease progression in patients with idiopathic pulmonary fibrosis. *Thorax*, *55*, 958–961.

Tzortzaki, E. G., Antoniou, K. M., Zervou, M. I., Koutsopoulos, A., Tzanakis, N., Plataki, M., et al. (2007). Effects of antifibrotic agents on TGF-beta1, CTGF and IFN-gamma expression in patients with idiopathic pulmonary fibrosis. *Respiratory Medicine*, *101*, 1821–1829.

Vatter, H., & Seifert, V. (2006). Ambrisentan, a non-peptide endothelin receptor antagonist. *Cardiovascular Drug Reviews*, *24*, 63–76.

Verleden, G. M., duBois, R. M., Bouros, R. M., Drent, D., Millar, M., Muller-Quernheim, A., et al. (2001). Genetic predisposition and pathogenetic mechanisms of interstitial lung diseases of unknown origin. *European Respiratory Journal*, *32* (Suppl.), 17s–29s.

Vlahakis, N. E., & Aksamit, T. R. (2001) Diagnosis and treatment of allergic bronchopulmonary aspergillosis. *Mayo Clinic Proceedings. Mayo Clinic*, *76*, 930–938.

Walker, J. E., Giri, S. N., & Margolin, S. B. (2005). A double-blind, randomized, controlled study of oral pirfenidone for treatment of secondary progressive multiple sclerosis. *Multiple Sclerosis*, *11*, 149–158.

Walters, D. M., Cho, H.-Y., & Kleeberger, S. R. (2008). Oxidative stress and antioxidants in the pathogenesis of pulmonary fibrosis: A potential role for Nrf2. *Antioxidants & Redox Signaling*, *10*, 321–332.

Wang, R., Ibarra-Sunga, O., Verlinski, L., Pick, R., & Uhal, B. D. (2000). Abrogation of bleomycin-induced epithelial apoptosis and lung fibrosis by captopril or by a caspase inhibitor. *American Journal of Physiology. Lung Cellular and Molecular Physiology*, *279*, L143–L151.

Wang, Y., Kuan, P. J., Xing, C., Conkhite, J. T., Torres, F., Rosenblatt, R. L., et al. (2009). Genetic defects in surfactant protein A2 are associated with pulmonary fibrosis and lung cancer. *American Journal of Human Genetics*, *84*, 52–59

Wells, A. U., & Hirani, N. (2008). Interstitial lung disease guideline. *Thorax*, *63*(Suppl. 5), 1–58.

White, A. C., Maloney, E. K., Lee, S.-L., Lanzillo, J. J., & Fanburg, B. L. (1999). Reduction of endothelial cell related TGFβ activity by thiols. *Endothelium*, *6*, 231–234.

Willis, B. C., & Borok, Z. (2007). TGFβ-induced EMT: Mechanisms and implications for fibrotic lung diseases. *American Journal of Physiology. Lung Cellular and Molecular Physiology*, *293*, L525–L534.

Wilson, M. S., & Wynn, T. A. (2009). Pulmonary fibrosis: Pathogenesis, etiology and regulation. *Mucosal Immunology*, *2*, 103–121.

Wozniak, M., & Czyz, M. (2008). Superoxide dismutase mimetics: Possible clinical applications [Polish]. *Postepy Higieny I Medycyny do Swiadczalne*, *62*, 613–624.

Wynn, T. A. (2008). Cellular and molecular mechanisms of fibrosis. *Journal of Pathology*, *214*, 199–210

Xing, L., Sheh, H. S., Selness, S. R., Devraj, R. V., Walker, J. K., Devadas, B., et al. (2009). Structural bioinformatics-based prediction of exceptional selectivity of p38MAP kinase inhibitor PH-797804. *Biochemistry*, *48*, 6402–6411.

Yamada, M., Kuwano, K., Maeyama, T., Yoshimi, M., Hamada, N., Fukumoto, J., et al. (2007). Gene transfer of soluble transforming factor type II receptor by in vivo electroporation attenuates lung injury and fibrosis. *Journal Clinical Pathology*, *60*, 916–920.

Yamasawa, H., Sugiyama, Y., Bando, M., & Ohno, S. (2008). Drug-induced pneumonitis associated with imatinib mesylate in a patient with idiopathic pulmonary fibrosis. *Respiration*, *75*, 350–354.

Yanagisawa, M., Kurihara, H., Kimura, S., Tomobe, Y., Kobayashi, M., Mitsui, Y., et al. (1988). A novel potent vasoconstrictor peptide produced by vascular endothelial cells. *Nature*, *332*, 411–415.

Yang, I. V., Burch, L. H., Steele, M. P., Savov, J. D., Hollingsworth, E., McElvania-Tekippe, K. G., et al. (2007). Gene expression profiling of familial and sporadic interstitial pneumonia. *American Journal of Respiratory and Critical Care Medicine, 175*, 45–54.

Yildirim, Z., Kotuk, M., Erdogan, H., Iraz, M., Yagmurca, M., Kuku, I., et al. (2006). Preventive effect of melatonin on bleomycin-induced lung fibrosis in rats. *Journal of Pineal Research, 40*, 27–33.

Yildirim, Z., Kotuk, M., Traz, M., Kuku, I., Ulu, R., Armutcu, F., et al. (2005). Attenuation of bleomycin-induced lung fibrosis by oral sulfhydryl containing antioxidants in rats: Erdosteine and acetylcysteine. *Pulmonary Pharmacology & Therapeutics, 18*, 367–373.

Yokoyama, A., Kondo, K., Nakajima, M., Matsushima, T., Takahashi, T., Nishimura, M., et al. (2006). Prognostic value of circulating KL-6 in idiopathic pulmonary fibrosis. *Respirology, 11*(2), 164–168.

Zaca, V., Metra, M., Danesi, R., Lombardi, C., Verzura, G., & Dei Cas, L. (2009). Successful switch to sitaxsentan in a patient with HIV-related pulmonary arterial hypertension and late intolerance to nonselective endothelin receptor blockade. *Therapeutic Advances in Respiratory Disease, 3*, 11–14.

Zamora, M. A., Dempsey, E. C., Walchak, S. J., & Stelzner, T. J. (1993). BQ123, an ET_A receptor antagonist, inhibits endothelin-1-mediated proliferation of human pulmonary artery smooth muscle cells. *Am J Respir Cell Med Biol, 9*, 429–433.

Zhang, J., Shen, B., & Lin, A. (2007). Novel strategies for inhibition of the p38 MAPK pathway. *Trends in Pharmacological Sciences, 28*, 286–295.

Zhou, X., Murphy, F. R., Gehdu, N., Zhang, J., Iredale, J. P., & Benyon, R. C. (2004). Engagement of $\alpha_v\beta_3$ integrin regulates proliferation and apoptosis of hepatic stellate cells. *Journal of Biological Chemistry, 279*, 23996–24006.

Ziesche, R., Hofbauer, E., Wittmann, K., Petkov, V., & Block, L. H. (1999). A preliminary study of long-term treatment with interferon gamma 1-b and low dose prednisolone in patients with idiopathic pulmonary fibrosis. *New England Journal of Medicine, 341*, 1264–1269.

Ziment, I. (1986). Acetylcysteine: A drug with an interesting past and a fascinating future. *Respiration, 60*, 26–30.

Index

Contents of Previous Volumes